ESSENTIALS
OF
FAMILY
PRACTICE

ESSENTIALS OF FAMILY PRACTICE

ROBERT E. RAKEL, M.D.

Professor and Chairman, Department of Family Medicine;
Associate Dean for Academic and Clinical Affairs
Baylor College of Medicine, Houston, Texas

W.B. SAUNDERS COMPANY
A Division of Harcourt Brace & Company
Philadelphia/London/Toronto/Montreal/Sydney/Tokyo

W.B. SAUNDERS COMPANY
A Division of
Harcourt Brace & Company

The Curtis Center
Independence Square West
Philadelphia, Pennsylvania 19106

Library of Congress Cataloging-in-Publication Data

Rakel, Robert E.
    Essentials of family practice / Robert E. Rakel.
       p. cm.
    ISBN 0-7216-4227-6
      1. Family medicine.   I. Title.
    RC46.R33 1993
    610—dc20   92-1219

Essentials of Family Practice   ISBN 0-7216-4227-6

Printed in the United States of America.

Last digit is the print number: 9   8   7   6   5   4   3   2

CONTRIBUTORS

LOIS A. ADDISON, M.A., M.L.T.
Primary Care Laboratory Medicine Consultant, Dunrobin, Ontario, Canada
Interpreting Laboratory Tests

ANDREW M. BARCLAY, M.D.
Professor and Chairman, Department of Family and Community Medicine, University of Kansas School of Medicine—Wichita; Attending Staff, HCA Wesley Medical Center; Attending Staff, St. Francis Regional Medical Center; Attending Staff, St. Joseph Medical Center, Wichita, Kansas
Clinical Case Studies (Genetic Counseling)

ALEXANDER BERGER, M.D.
Professor, Department of Family and Community Medicine, Eastern Virginia Medical School, Norfolk, Virginia; Director, Portsmouth Family Medicine Residency; Maryview Hospital; Portsmouth General Hospital, Portsmouth, Virginia
Clinical Case Studies (Blurred Vision)

WENDY S. BIGGS, M.D.
Chief Resident, Department of Family Medicine, Baylor College of Medicine, Houston, Texas
Problem Solving in Family Medicine

F. MARIAN BISHOP, Ph.D., M.S.P.H.
Professor and Chairman, Department of Family and Preventive Medicine, University of Utah School of Medicine, Salt Lake City, Utah
Interviewing Techniques

ALAN BLUM, M.D.
Assistant Professor, Department of Family Medicine, Baylor College of Medicine; Attending Physician, St. Luke's Episcopal Hospital; Active Staff, The Methodist Hospital, Houston, Texas
Clinical Case Studies (Approaches to Patients Who Smoke)

JAMES H. BRAY, Ph.D.
Associate Professor, Department of Family Medicine, Baylor College of Medicine; Medical Staff, St. Luke's Episcopal Hospital; Medical Scientist, The Methodist Hospital, Houston, Texas
The Family's Influence on Health

BARUCH A. BRODY, Ph.D.
Leon Jaworski Professor of Biomedical Ethics, Baylor College of Medicine; Professor of Philosophy, Rice University, Houston, Texas
Ethics in Family Medicine

H. JAMES BROWNLEE, M.D.
Interim Chairman and Associate Professor, Department of Family Medicine, University of South Florida School of Medicine; Director, Family Practice Residency, Bayfront Medical Center; Bayfront Medical Center; All Children's Hospital, St. Petersburg, Florida
Clinical Case Studies (Stiff Joints)

ERICH E. BRUESCHKE, M.D.

Vice Dean, Rush Medical College; Professor and Chairman, Department of Family Medicine, Rush-Presbyterian-St. Luke's Medical Center; Senior Attending Physician, Rush-Presbyterian-St. Luke's Medical Center; Attending Physician, Christ Hospital and Medical Center, Chicago, Illinois

Clinical Case Studies (Upset Stomach and Headache)

WALTER L. CALMBACH, M.D.

Assistant Professor, Department of Family Practice, University of Texas Health Science Center; Staff Physician, Member, Emergency Center Committee, Medical Center Hospital, San Antonio, Texas

Clinical Case Studies (Knee Injury; Low Back Pain)

DAVID C. CAMPBELL, M.D., M.Ed.

Clinical Associate Professor, Department of Family Medicine, St. Louis University; Program Director, Family Medicine Residency, Deaconess Hospital, St. Louis, Missouri

Clinical Case Studies (Leg Pain)

THOMAS L. CAMPBELL, M.D.

Associate Professor of Family Medicine, Associate Professor of Psychiatry, University of Rochester School of Medicine and Dentistry; Attending Physician, Highland Hospital, Rochester, New York

The Family's Influence on Health

RICHARD D. CLOVER, M.D.

Associate Professor, Department of Family Medicine, University of Texas Medical Branch—Galveston; John Sealy Hospital; St. Mary's Hospital of Galveston, Galveston, Texas

Clinical Case Studies (Fever and Runny Nose; Sinus Congestion)

JANE E. CORBOY, M.D.

Assistant Professor, Department of Family Medicine, Baylor College of Medicine; Medical Director, Baylor Family Practice Center; Staff Physician, St. Luke's Episcopal Hospital; Staff Physician, Texas Children's Hospital; Staff Physician, The Methodist Hospital, Houston, Texas

Clinical Case Studies (Nosebleed; Chest Pain)

JAMES C. COYNE, Ph.D.

Professor, Department of Family Practice, University of Michigan Medical School; University of Michigan Medical Center, Ann Arbor, Michigan

Clinical Case Studies (Excessive Sleepiness and Fatigue)

EARL R. CROUCH, Jr., M.D.

Professor and Chairman, Department of Ophthalmology, Associate Professor, Department of Pediatrics, Eastern Virginia Medical School; Chairman, Professional Information Committee, American Association of Pediatric Ophthalmology and Strabismus; Sentara Norfolk General Hospital; Sentara Leigh Hospital; Children's Hospital of the Kings Daughters; Director of Pediatric Ophthalmology and Strabismus, Eastern Virginia Medical School, Norfolk, Virginia

Clinical Case Studies (Blurred Vision)

MICHAEL A. CROUCH, M.D., M.S.P.H.

Associate Professor, Department of Clinical Family Medicine, Baylor College of Medicine; Staff Physician, St. Luke's Episcopal Hospital; Staff Physician, The Methodist Hospital; Courtesy Staff, Texas Children's Hospital, Houston, Texas

Family Dynamics; Clinical Case Studies (Preschool Physical Exam)

LARRY CULPEPPER, M.D., M.P.H.

Associate Professor, Department of Family Medicine, Brown University, Providence, Rhode Island; Memorial Hospital, Pawtucket, Rhode Island; Women and Infant's Hospital, Rochester, New York

How to Read Medical Journals

DANIEL J. DERKSEN, M.D.

Assistant Professor, Department of Family and Community Medicine, University of New Mexico School of Medicine; University of New Mexico Medical Center, Albuquerque, New Mexico
Clinical Case Studies (Vomiting and Low Back Pain)

CHARLES E. DRISCOLL, M.D.

Professor and Head, Department of Family Practice, University of Iowa College of Medicine; Active Staff, Mercy Hospital of Iowa City; Active Staff, University of Iowa Hospitals and Clinics, Iowa City, Iowa
Clinical Case Studies (Sexual Dysfunction)

C. EDWARD EVANS, M.B., M.R.C.S.

Professor, Department of Family Medicine, McMaster University; Active Staff, McMaster University Medical Center, Hamilton, Ontario, Canada
Patient Compliance

PATRICK J. FAHEY, M.D.

Associate Professor, Department of Family Medicine, The Ohio State University College of Medicine; Attending Physician, Family Medicine, The Ohio State University Hospitals; Attending Physician in Family Medicine, Children's Hospital; Courtesy Staff, Family Medicine, Park Medical Center, Columbus, Ohio
Clinical Case Studies (Nutritional Problems in the Elderly)

RICHARD E. FINLAYSON, M.D.

Consultant, Department of Psychiatry and Psychology, Consultant, Department of Family Medicine, Mayo Clinic and Mayo Foundation; Associate Professor, Department of Psychiatry, Mayo Medical School; Rochester, Minnesota
Clinical Case Studies (Memory Loss)

PAUL M. FISCHER, M.D.

Professor, Department of Family Medicine, Medical College of Georgia, Augusta, Georgia
Interpreting Laboratory Tests

WILLIAM L. FRANZEN, Jr., P.T.

Private Practice, Orthopedic and Sports Physical Therapy of St. Louis, St. Louis, Missouri
Clinical Case Studies (Leg Pain)

ROBERT E. FROELICH, M.D.

Inpatient Psychiatric Services, Veterans Affairs Medical Center, Salt Lake City, Utah
Interviewing Techniques

CHARLETTE GALLAGHER-ALLRED, Ph.D., R.D.

Clinical Assistant Professor, Department of Family Medicine, The Ohio State University; Nutrition Consultant, Department of Nutrition and Public Affairs, Ross Laboratories, Columbus, Ohio
Clinical Case Studies (Nutritional Problems in the Elderly)

JOHN P. GEYMAN, M.D.

Professor of Family Medicine, School of Medicine, University of Washington; University of Washington Medical Center, Seattle, Washington
Clinical Case Studies (Palpitations and Sweating)

ROLAND A. GOERTZ, M.D.

Assistant Clinical Professor of Family Medicine, The University of Texas Health Science Center at San Antonio, San Antonio, Texas; Medical Director, PCA Health Plans of Texas, Austin, Texas
Clinical Case Studies (Shortness of Breath)

DAVID GONZALEZ, M.D.
Director, Sports Medicine Clinic, University of Delaware, Newark, Delaware
Clinical Case Studies (Leg Pain)

R. BRIAN HAYNES, M.D., Ph.D.
Professor of Clinical Epidemiology, Professor of Medicine, McMaster University Faculty of Health Sciences; Active Staff, Chedoke-McMaster Hospital; Affiliate Staff, Hamilton Civic Hospitals, Hamilton, Ontario, Canada
Patient Compliance

WARREN A. HEFFRON, M.D.
Professor and Chairman, Department of Family, Community, and Emergency Medicine, University of New Mexico School of Medicine; University of New Mexico Hospital, Albuquerque, New Mexico
Disease Prevention

JOSEPH HOBBS, M.D.
Associate Professor, Medical College of Georgia; Staff, Georgia War Veterans Nursing Home; Director, Family Medicine Inpatient Service, Augusta, Georgia
Clinical Case Studies (Chronic Fatigue)

MARSHA C. HOLLEMAN, M.D., M.P.H.
Assistant Professor, Department of Family Medicine, Baylor College of Medicine; Active Staff, St. Luke's Episcopal Hospital; Active Staff, The Methodist Hospital; Courtesy Staff, Texas Children's Hospital, Houston, Texas
Clinical Case Studies (Normal Pregnancy; Abdominal Pain)

WARREN L. HOLLEMAN, Ph.D.
Assistant Professor, Department of Family Medicine, Baylor College of Medicine, Houston, Texas
Ethics in Family Medicine; Home Care

RICHARD. L. HOLLOWAY, Ph.D.
Professor, Vice Chairman, and Chief, Division of Family Medicine Academic Programs, Department of Family and Community Medicine, Medical College of Wisconsin, Milwaukee, Wisconsin
Research in Family Medicine

JERRY E. JONES, M.D., M.S.
Associate Professor, University of Alabama, School of Medicine, Tuscaloosa Program; Active Staff, Druid City Hospital, Tuscaloosa, Alabama
Clinical Case Studies (Diarrhea)

WAYNE J. KATON, M.D.
Professor, Department of Psychiatry, Adjunct Professor, Department of Family Medicine, Chief, Division of Consultation Liaison Psychiatry, University of Washington Medical School, Seattle, Washington
Clinical Case Studies (Palpitations and Sweating)

LOUIS A. KAZAL, Jr., M.D.
Assistant Professor, Department of Family Medicine, Baylor College of Medicine; Attending Physician, St. Luke's Episcopal Hospital; Attending Physician, The Methodist Hospital; Courtesy Staff, Texas Children's Hospital, Houston, Texas; Courtesy Staff, Star Valley Hospital, Afton, Wyoming
Clinical Case Studies (Laceration)

SANFORD R. KIMMEL, M.D.
Associate Professor of Clinical Family Medicine, Medical College of Ohio; Medical College Hospitals; St. Vincent Medical Center; The Toledo Hospital, Toledo, Ohio
Clinical Case Studies (Short Child)

PAMELA M. KIRCHER, M.D.

Clinical Instructor, Department of Family Medicine, Baylor College of Medicine; Staff Physician, The Hospice at the Texas Medical Center; Courtesy Staff, Southwest Memorial Hospital, Houston, Texas

Home Care (Case Study)

GREG L. LEDGERWOOD, M.D.

Associate Clinical Professor, University of Washington School of Medicine; Active Staff, Mid Valley Hospital, Omak, Washington; Courtesy Staff, Central Washington Hospital, Wenatchee, Washington; Active Staff, Valley Care Center, Okanogan, Washington

Clinical Case Studies (Recurrent Ear Infections; Multiple Allergies)

RICHARD E. LUTZ, M.D.

Assistant Professor of Pediatrics, University of Kansas School of Medicine; Attending Physician, Pediatric Section, HCA Wesley Medical Center; Attending Physician, Pediatric Section, St. Francis Regional Medical Center; Attending Physician, Pediatric Section, St. Joseph Hospital, Wichita, Kansas

Clinical Case Studies (Genetic Counseling)

CHRISTINE C. MATSON, M.D.

Vice Chair and Associate Professor, Department of Family Medicine, Baylor College of Medicine; Associate Chief, Family Medicine Section, St. Luke's Episcopal Hospital; Deputy Chief, Family Medicine Section, The Methodist Hospital, Houston, Texas

Clinical Case Studies (Breast Discomfort)

HARRY E. MAYHEW, M.D.

Professor and Chairman, Department of Family Medicine, Medical College of Ohio; Chairman, Division of Family Medicine, Medical College Hospital, Toledo, Ohio

Clinical Case Studies (Vomiting and Low Back Pain)

JOHN W. McCALL, III, Ph.D.

Assistant Professor, Department of Family Medicine, University of Tennessee, Memphis, Tennessee

How to Read Medical Journals

KAY F. McFARLAND, M.D.

Professor of Medicine, Department of Medicine, University of South Carolina, Columbia, South Carolina

Clinical Case Studies (Diabetes Mellitus; Intermittent Tachycardia)

SUSAN M. MILLER, M.D., M.P.H.

Assistant Professor, Departments of Family Medicine and Internal Medicine, Baylor College of Medicine; Attending Physician, St. Luke's Episcopal Hospital; Attending Physician, The Methodist Hospital; Courtesy Staff, Texas Children's Hospital; Medical Director, Thomas Street Clinic, Harris County Hospital District, Houston, Texas

Clinical Case Studies (Weight Loss and Diarrhea)

ALAN G. MOORE, M.D.

Department of Obstetrics and Gynecology, Houston Northwest Medical Center, Houston, Texas

Clinical Case Studies (Amenorrhea; Vaginal Bleeding)

R. MICHAEL MORSE, M.D.

Associate Professor of Family Medicine, University of Virginia School of Medicine; Medical Director, Foundation Institute for Quality Health, University of Virginia Health Services; University of Virginia Medical Center, Charlottesville, Virginia

Disease Prevention

STEVEN D. MORSE, M.D.

Attending Physician and Associate Director, Department of Emergency Medicine, Montgomery Hospital, Norristown, Pennsylvania

Clinical Case Studies (Severe Lethargy; Confusion with Lethargy)

CHARLES M. PLOTZ, M.D., Med.Sc.D.

Chairman, Department of Family Practice, State University of New York, Brooklyn, New York

Stiffness in Fingers

JOHN G. PRICHARD, M.D., M.HS.

Clinical Associate Professor, UCLA School of Medicine; Director of Clinical Affairs and Chief, Medical Services, Ventura County Medical Center, Ventura, California

Clinical Case Studies (Cough; Fever and Chest Pain)

ROBERT E. RAKEL, M.D.

Richard M. Kleberg, Sr. Professor and Chairman, Department of Family Medicine, Baylor College of Medicine; Associate Dean for Academic and Clinical Affairs, Baylor College of Medicine; Attending Physician, St. Luke's Episcopal Hospital; Attending Physician, The Methodist Hospital, Houston, Texas

The Family Physician; Care of the Dying Patient; The Scope of Family Practice; Developing Communication Skills; Using Consultants; The Problem-Oriented Medical Record

JANET P. REALINI, M.D.

Associate Professor, Department of Family Practice, University of Texas Health Science Center; Attending Physician, Medical Center Hospital, San Antonio, Texas

Clinical Case Studies (Contraception)

SHELLEY P. ROATEN, Jr., M.D.

Associate Professor, Department of Family Practice and Community Medicine, University of Texas Southwestern Medical Center, Dallas, Texas; Active Staff, Hillcrest Baptist Medical Center; Active Staff, Providence Health Center, Waco, Texas

Clinical Case Studies (Skin Irritation; Recurring Rash)

Wm. MacMILLAN RODNEY, M.D.

Professor and Chair, Department of Family Medicine, The University of Tennessee, Memphis; Family Practice Residency, St. Francis Hospital; Family Practice Residency, Baptist Hospital, Memphis, Tennessee

Clinical Case Studies (Fatigue; Heartburn)

JOHN C. ROGERS, M.D., M.P.H.

Associate Professor and Director of Predoctoral Section and Fellowship Program, Department of Family Medicine, Baylor College of Medicine; Active Staff, St. Luke's Episcopal Hospital; Active Staff, The Methodist Hospital; Courtesy Staff, Texas Children's Hospital, Houston, Texas

Research in Family Medicine; Problem Solving in Family Medicine

JOHN S. ROLLAND, M.D.

Associate Clinical Professor of Psychiatry and Co-Director, Center for Family Health, The University of Chicago; Lecturer, Department of Psychiatry, Yale University School of Medicine, New Haven, Connecticut; Attending Physician, University of Chicago Hospitals, Chicago, Illinois

The Family Impact of Illness and Disability

SUSAN SCHOOLEY, M.D.

Chairman, Department of Family Practice, Henry Ford Health System, Detroit, Michigan

The Family's Influence on Health

THOMAS L. SCHWENK, M.D.

Associate Professor and Chairman, Department of Family Practice, University of Michigan; Attending Physician, University of Michigan Hospitals, Ann Arbor, Michigan

Clinical Case Studies (Excessive Sleepiness and Fatigue)

ROBERT SMITH, M.D.

Professor and Director Emeritus, Department of Family Medicine, Director, Headache Center, University of Cincinnati; Attending Member of Faculty, University Hospital, Cincinnati, Ohio

Clinical Case Studies (Headache)

STEPHEN J. SPANN, M.D.

Evalyn Matheson Phillips and Claurice M. Phillips, M.D. Professor in Family Medicine and Chairman, Department of Family Medicine, The University of Texas Medical Branch at Galveston; John Sealy Hospital (UTMB); St. Mary's Hospital of Galveston, Galveston, Texas

Clinical Case Studies (Sinus Congestion; Fever and Runny Nose)

ROBERT H. SPRINKLE, M.D., Ph.D.

Assistant Professor and Assistant Director for Education in the Center for Health Policy Research and Education, Duke University; Assistant Professor of Pediatrics, Duke University Medical Center; Assistant Professor of Public Policy Studies, Institute of Policy Sciences and Public Affairs, Duke University; Co-Director, Division of Policy and Ethics, Duke-UNC Comprehensive Sickle Cell Center, Durham, North Carolina

Clinical Case Studies (Newborn Care)

NANCY GRAY STEVENS, M.D., M.P.H.

Assistant Professor, Family Medicine, University of Washington Medical School; Active Staff, University of Washington Medical Center, Seattle, Washington

Clinical Case Studies (Palpitations and Sweating)

PORTER STOREY, M.D.

Clinical Assistant Professor of Medicine and Family Medicine, Baylor College of Medicine; Consultant in Neuro-Oncology, University of Texas, M.D. Anderson Cancer Center; Medical Director, The Hospice at the Texas Medical Center, Houston, Texas

Care of the Dying Patient

JOHN E. SUTHERLAND, M.D.

Professor, Department of Family Practice, Southern Illinois University School of Medicine; St. John's Hospital; Memorial Medical Center, Springfield, Illinois

Clinical Case Studies (Vaginitis)

E. LEE TAYLOR, Jr., M.D.

Associate Dean and Assistant to the Executive Vice President, Amarillo Regional Academic Health Center; Professor, Department of Family Medicine, Texas Tech University Health Sciences Center; Northwest Texas Hospital; High Plains Baptist Hospital, Amarillo, Texas

Economics of Medical Practice

JAN C. UPDIKE, M.D.

Associate Professor of Family Medicine, University of South Carolina; Richland Memorial Hospital, Columbia, South Carolina

Clinical Case Studies (Diabetes Mellitus; Intermittent Tachycardia)

SUSAN VANDERBERG-DENT, M.D.

Assistant Chairman for Educational Programs, Associate Professor of Department of Family Medicine, Director of Predoctoral Education, Department of Family Medicine, Rush Medical College; Associate Attending Physician, Department of Family Medicine, Rush-Presbyterian-St. Luke's Medical Center; Active Attending Physician, Christ Hospital and Medical Center, Chicago, Illinois)

Clinical Case Studies (Upset Stomach and Headache)

DONALD S. WILLIAMSON, Ph.D.

Professor of Clinical Family Medicine, Department of Family Medicine, Baylor College of Medicine; Staff, Psychiatry Section, Internal Medicine Service, St. Luke's Episcopal Hospital, Houston, Texas

Family Dynamics

PREFACE

This book is designed to be a companion to the fourth edition of *The Textbook of Family Practice* and to serve as a resource for medical students enrolled in courses teaching the essentials of our discipline. Although it was originally envisioned as a condensed version of *The Textbook,* it quickly became apparent that this objective would be better served by selecting the most appropriate chapters and developing new material as needed to address most closely the needs of medical students. As a result, most of the material in this book is new and not found in the fourth edition.

Clinical information is presented in an entirely different manner from that found in *The Textbook.* Patients are discussed in more than forty separate case studies just as they would present to their family physician with complaints such as fatigue, back pain, headache, or cough. Using the SOAP format, problem-solving methods typical of those used in family practice are used to develop a differential diagnosis. The potential diagnoses are discussed and the patient followed in a manner characteristic of actual practice. Test questions follow each chapter and case study.

Numerous tables, decision trees, and line drawings enhance the chapters and case studies. Of particular merit are the drawings in the case on laceration in Chapter 20 and the tables in Chapter 19, Interpreting Laboratory Tests.

We hope this text will heighten medical students' awareness of the basics of family practice and the thought processes required in primary care. The concept of continuing comprehensive care is essential knowledge for all students regardless of intended specialty, but it is absolutely vital to those entering primary care.

As with any publishing project, this book did not happen by itself. I am indebted to the family practice faculty and family physicians in private practice who provided most of the material for this book. They drew on their practice experience and generously shared it with our medical students. The tasks of coordinating deadlines, communicating with authors, and generally moving the book forward fell to Roxy Cuddy, my editorial assistant. This text would not have been possible without her.

My most special thanks and appreciation is reserved for my wife, Peggy, who has long abided my passion for the written word and supported with great understanding my need to edit and write. She has endured publication of this volume and four editions of *The Textbook* with much good humor and grace.

ROBERT E. RAKEL, M.D.

CONTENTS

THE FAMILY PHYSICIAN

ROBERT E. RAKEL

The family physician provides continuing, comprehensive care in a personalized manner to patients of all ages and to their families, regardless of the presence of disease or the nature of the presenting complaint. Family physicians accept responsibility for managing an individual's total health needs while maintaining an intimate, confidential relationship with the patient. The family physician personally takes care of most of the patient's health needs; for the remainder of the patient's problems, the physician selects appropriate consulting physicians or other health professionals to assist in care. The efforts of all health professionals are coordinated by the family physician, who has ongoing responsibility for the patient's care.

Family medicine is the body of knowledge and the skills that constitute the medical discipline; when applied to the care of patients and their families, this discipline becomes the specialty of family practice. Family medicine emphasizes responsibility for total health care—from the first contact and initial assessment through the ongoing care of chronic problems (from prevention through rehabilitation). Coordination and integration of all necessary health services with the least amount of fragmentation are important features of the discipline.

THE JOY OF FAMILY PRACTICE

The rewards in family practice come largely from knowing patients intimately over time, sharing their trust, respect, and friendship. The thrill of family practice is the close bond (actually friendship) that develops with patients. This bond is strengthened with each physical or emotional crisis in a person's life when he or she turns to the family physician for help.

It is especially rewarding when the family physician cares for a newly married couple, delivers their first baby, sees them frequently for well-child care, and provides ongoing care for the parents, the growing child, and subsequent children. No other medical specialty is so privileged. To participate in a family's life in such a close and intimate manner is uniquely rewarding.

The practice of family medicine involves the joy of greeting old friends in every examining room, and the variety of problems encountered keeps one professionally stimulated and perpetually challenged. In contrast, physicians practicing in narrow specialties often lose their enthusiasm for medicine after seeing the same problem hundreds of times. The variety of family medicine sustains the excitement and precludes boredom.

Devotion to continuing, comprehensive, personalized care; to early detection and management of illness; to the prevention of disease and maintenance of health; and to the ongoing management of patients in a community setting uniquely qualify the family physician to deliver primary care.

DEVELOPMENT OF THE SPECIALTY

About 1923, Francis Peabody commented that the swing of the pendulum toward specialization had reached its apex and that modern medicine had fragmented the health care delivery system to too great a degree. He called for a rapid return of the generalist physician who would give comprehensive, personalized care.

Dr. Peabody's declaration proved premature; society and the medical establishment were not ready for such a proclamation. The trend toward specialization gained momentum through the 1950s, and fewer physicians entered general practice. In the early 1960s, leaders in the field of general practice began advocating a seemingly paradoxical solution to reverse the trend and correct the scarcity of general practitioners—the creation of still another specialty. However, the physicians envisioned a specialty that embodied the knowledge, skills, and ideals they knew as primary care. In 1966, the concept of a new specialty in primary care received official recognition in two separate reports published 1 month apart. The first of these was the *Report of the Citizens' Commission on Graduate Medical Education of the American Medical Association,* also known as the Millis Commission Report. The second report came from the Ad Hoc Committee on Education for Family Practice of the Council of Medical Education of the American Medical Association, also called the Willard Committee. Three years later, the American Board of Family Practice (ABFP) came into being as the 20th medical specialty board, thus giving birth to the specialty of family practice.

Much of the impetus for the Millis and Willard reports came from the American Academy of General Practice, which was renamed the American Academy of Family Physicians (AAFP) in 1971. The name change reflected a desire to increase emphasis on family-oriented health care and to gain academic acceptance for the new specialty of family practice.

The ABFP has distinguished itself by being the first specialty board to require recertification (every 6 years) to ensure the ongoing competence of its members. Among basic requirements for certification and recertification, the ABFP had included continuing education—the foundation on which the American Academy of General Practice had been built when organized in 1947. A member of the ABFP must participate in 50 hours of acceptable continuing education activity each year to be eligible for recertification. Once eligible, a candidate's competence is examined by cognitive testing and performance evaluation. The ABFP's emphasis on quality of education, knowledge, and performance has facilitated the rapid increase in prestige for the family physician in our health care system. The obvious logic of the ABFP's emphasis on continuing education to maintain required knowledge and skills has been adopted by other specialties and state medical societies.

DEFINITIONS

FAMILY PRACTICE. The AAFP and ABFP have defined family practice as

> ... the medical specialty that provides continuing and comprehensive health care for the individual and the family. It is the specialty in breadth that integrates the biological, clinical and behavioral sciences. The scope of family practice encompasses all ages, both sexes, each organ system and disease entity.

Any definition of family practice must be built on a base of data that is appropriate to the activities of physicians practicing the specialty. For this reason, the curriculum for training family physicians is designed to represent realistically the skills and body of knowledge they will require in practice. This curriculum definition relies heavily on an accurate analysis of the problems seen and the skills used by family physicians in their practices. The almost randomly educated primary physician of previous years is being replaced by one specifically prepared to address the kinds of problems likely to be encountered in practice. For this reason, the "model office" is an essential component of all family practice residency programs.

PRIMARY CARE. The specialty of family practice is designed specifically to deliver primary care, which was reaffirmed in 1990 by the AAFP Congress of Delegates to mean

> ... a form of medical care delivery that emphasizes first-contact care and assumes ongoing responsibility for the patient in both health maintenance and therapy of illness. It is personal care involving a unique interaction and communication between the patient and the physician. It is comprehensive in scope and includes the overall coordination of the care of the patient's health problems, be they biological, behavioral or social. The appropriate use of consultants and community resources is an important part of effective primary care.

AAFP REPORTER

Because many physicians deliver primary care in different ways and with varying degrees of preparation, the staff of the ABFP further clarified the definition:

> Primary care is a form of delivery of medical care that encompasses the following functions:
>
> 1. It is "first-contact" care, serving as a point-of-entry for the patient into the health care system;
> 2. It includes continuity by virtue of caring for patients over a period of time, both in sickness and in health;
> 3. It is comprehensive care, drawing from all the traditional major disciplines for its functional content;
> 4. It serves a coordinative function for all the health-care needs of the patient;
> 5. It assumes continuing responsibility for individual patient follow-up and community health problems; and
> 6. It is a highly personalized type of care.

PERSONALIZED CARE

> It is much more important to know what sort of patient has a disease than what sort of disease a patient has.

SIR WILLIAM OSLER

Family physicians do not just treat patients; they care for people. This caring function of family medicine emphasizes the personalized approach to understanding the patient as a person, respecting the person as an individual, and showing compassion for his or her discomfort. Compassion means co-suffering and reflects the physician's willingness somehow to share the patient's anguish and understand what the sickness means to that person. Compassion is an attempt to "feel" along with the patient. Pellegrino states that "we can never *feel* with another person when we pass judgment as a superior, only when we see our own frailties as well as his." Pellegrino goes on to comment that a compassionate authority figure is effective only when others can receive the "orders" without being humiliated. The physician must not "put down" the patients but must be ever ready, in Galileo's words,

> ...to pronounce that wise, ingenuous, and modest statement—"I don't know."

Compassion, practiced in these terms in each patient encounter, is the irreducible base for mitigating the inherent dehumanizing tendencies of today's highly institutionalized and technologically oriented patient care.

Physicians engaged primarily in hospital-based medicine must make a stronger effort to maintain personalized care because of the added exposure to and the necessary use of devices and techniques directed toward specific diseases. The physician should guard against thinking in terms of diseases and instead think in terms of patients who have problems needing attention. The whole-person approach to patient care is hampered by focusing primarily on the disease; specific diseases require specific treatments and tend to direct the physician's attention away from other needs of the patient.

Peabody noted that "The treatment of a disease may be entirely impersonal; the care of a patient must be completely personal." If an intimate relationship with patients remains our primary concern as physicians, high-quality medical care will persist, regardless of the way it is organized and financed. For this reason, family practice emphasizes consideration of the individual patient in the full context of his or her life rather than the episodic care of a presenting complaint. The Millis Commission Report stresses that the family physician

> . . . focuses not upon individual organs and systems but upon the whole man who lives in a complex social setting; and knows that diagnosis or treatment of a part often overlooks major causative factors and therapeutic opportunities.

It is generally recognized that medicine has become depersonalized owing to the rapid rise of superspecialization and technology. Theodore F. Fox, as editor of *The Lancet* wrote:

> I know, too, that we must get used to a world in which ices no longer taste of cream, nor new potatoes of new potatoes; and . . . ghastly plastic flowers seem to be commoner than real ones. But nobody is going to persuade me that a nice receptionist, some good notes, and an internist keeping office hours adds up to a personal doctor who knows me and my home. Even if you throw in a psychiatric social worker, I still feel that I am being put off with a plastic substitute for the real thing. And I am supported in this belief by the knowledge that when personal medical care is abolished, it is sooner or later re-invented.

Family physicians assess the illnesses and complaints presented to them, dealing personally with the majority and arranging special assistance for a few. The family physician serves as the patients' advocate, explaining the causes and implications of illness to patients and their families, and serves as an advisor and confidant to the family—both individually and collectively. The family physician receives many intellectual satisfactions from this practice, but the greatest reward arises from the depth of human understanding and personal satisfaction inherent in family practice.

Patients have adjusted somewhat to a more impersonal form of health care delivery and frequently look to institutions rather than to individuals for their health care—yet their need for personalized concern and compassion remains. Tumulty found that patients consider a good physician one who (1) shows genuine interest in them, (2) thoroughly evaluates their problems, (3) demonstrates compassion, understanding, and warmth, and (4) provides clear insight into what is wrong and what must be done to correct it.

The family physician's relationship with each patient should reflect compassion, understanding, and patience, combined with a high degree of intellectual honesty. The physician must be thorough in approaching problems but also possess a keen sense of humor. He or she must be capable of encouraging in each patient optimism, courage, insight, and the self-discipline necessary for recovery.

CHARACTERISTICS AND FUNCTIONS OF THE FAMILY PHYSICIAN

Attributes of the Family Physician

The following characteristics are certainly desirable for all physicians, but they are of greatest importance for the physician in family practice.

1. A strong sense of responsibility for the total, ongoing care of the individual and the family during health, illness, and rehabilitation.
2. Compassion and empathy, with a sincere interest in the patient and the family.
3. A curious and constantly inquisitive attitude.
4. Enthusiasm for the undifferentiated medical problem and its resolution.
5. An interest in the broad spectrum of clinical medicine.
6. The ability to deal comfortably with multiple problems occurring simultaneously in one patient.
7. A desire for frequent and varied intellectual and technical challenges.
8. The ability to support children during growth and development and during their adjustment to family and society.
9. The ability to assist patients in coping with everyday problems and in maintaining stability in the family and community.
10. The capacity to act as coordinator of all health resources needed in the care of a patient.
11. A continuing enthusiasm for learning and for the satisfaction that comes from maintaining current medical knowledge through continuing medical education.
12. The ability to maintain composure in times of stress and to respond quickly with logic, effectiveness, and compassion.
13. A desire to identify problems at the earliest possible stage (or to prevent disease entirely).
14. A strong wish to maintain maximum patient satisfaction, recognizing the need for continuing patient rapport.
15. The skills necessary to manage chronic illness and to ensure maximal rehabilitation following acute illness.
16. An appreciation for the complex mix of physical, emotional, and social elements in holistic and personalized patient care.
17. A feeling of personal satisfaction derived from intimate relationships with patients that naturally develop over long periods of continuous care, as opposed to the short-term pleasures gained from treating episodic illnesses.
18. A skill for and commitment to educating patients and families about disease processes and the principles of good health.

The ideal family physician is an explorer, driven by a persistent curiosity and the desire to know more. He or she is part theologian, as was Paracelsus; part politician, as was Benjamin Rush; and part humorist, as was Oliver Wendell Holmes. At all times, however, he or she holds the care of the patient—the whole patient—as a primary goal.

Continuing Responsibility

One of the essential functions of the family physician is the willingness to accept ongoing responsibility for managing a patient's medical care. Once a patient or a family has been accepted into the physician's practice, responsibility for care is both total and continuing. The Millis Commission chose the phrase "primary physician" to emphasize the concept of primary responsibility for the patient's welfare; however, the term "primary care physician" is more popular and refers to any physician who provides first-contact care.

The family physician's commitment to patients does not cease at the end of illness but is a continuing responsibility, regardless of the patient's state of health or the disease process. There is no need to identify the beginning or endpoint of treatment, since care of a problem can be reopened at any time—even though a later visit may be primarily for another problem. This prevents the family physician from focusing too narrowly on one problem and helps maintain a perspective on the total patient in his or her environment. Peabody felt that much patient dissatisfaction results from the physician's neglecting to assume personal responsibility for supervision of the patient's care:

> For some reason or other, no one physician has seen the case through from beginning to end, and the patient may be suffering from the very multitude of his counselors.

Accurate Diagnosis

The physician who is well acquainted with the patient not only provides more personal and humane medical care but does so more economically than the physician involved only in episodic care. The physician who knows his or her patients well can assess the nature of their problems more rapidly and accurately. Because of the intimate, ongoing relationship, the family physician is under less pressure to exclude diagnostic possibilities by use of expensive laboratory and radiologic procedures than is the physician who is unfamiliar with the patient.

The greater the degree of continuing involvement with a patient, the more capable the physician is in detecting early signs and symptoms of organic disease and functional problems. Patients with problems arising from emotional and social conflicts can be managed most effectively by a physician who has intimate knowledge of the individual and of his or her family and community background. This knowledge comes only from insight gained by observing the patient's long-term patterns of behavior and responses to changing stressful situations. This longitudinal view is particularly useful in the care of children and allows the physician to be more effective in assisting children to reach their full potential. The closeness that develops between physicians and young patients increases a physician's ability to aid the patient with problems that occur during later periods in life—such as adjustment to puberty, problems with marriage or employment, and changing social pressures. As the family physician maintains this continuing involvement with successive generations within a family, the ability to manage intercurrent problems increases with knowledge of the total family background.

Improved Insight

By virtue of this ongoing involvement and intimate association with the family, the family physician develops a perceptive awareness of a family's nature and style of operation. This ability to observe families over time allows valuable insight that improves the quality of medical care provided to an individual patient. One of the greatest challenges in family medicine is the need to be alert to the changing stresses, transitions, and expectations of family members over time and to the effect that these and other family interactions have on the health of individuals.

Although the family is the family physician's primary concern, his or her skills are equally applicable to the individual living alone or to people in other varieties of family living. Individuals with alternative forms of family living interact with others who have significant effects on their lives. The principles of group dynamics and interpersonal relationships that affect health are equally applicable to everyone.

The family physician needs to assess an individual's personality so that presenting symptoms can be appropriately evaluated and given the proper degree of attention and emphasis. A complaint of abdominal pain may be treated lightly in one patient who frequently presents with minor problems, but the same complaint would be investigated immediately and in depth in another individual who has a more stoic personality. The decision regarding which studies to perform and when is influenced by knowledge of the patient's lifestyle, personality, and previous response pattern. The greater the degree of knowledge and insight into the patient's background, which is gained through years of previous contact, the more capable the physician is in making an appropriate early and rapid assessment of the presenting complaint. The less background information the physician has to rely on, the greater is the need to depend on costly laboratory studies and the more likely is overreaction to the presenting symptom. Families receiving continuing comprehensive care have fewer incidences of hospitalization, fewer operations, and fewer physician visits for illnesses compared with those who have no regular physician. This is due, at least in part, to the physician's knowledge of the patients, seeing them earlier for acute problems and thus preventing complications that would require hospitalization, being available by telephone, and seeing them more frequently in the office for health supervision. Care is also less expensive, since there is less need to rely on x-ray and laboratory procedures and visits to emergency rooms.

Proper Training

The quality of our health care system is being eroded by physicians' being trained extensively at great expense to practice in one area and instead practicing in another, such as anesthesiologists practicing in emergency rooms and surgeons practicing as generalists.

Primary care, to be done well, requires extensive training specifically tailored to the problems frequently seen in primary care. These include the early detection, diagnosis, and treatment of depression; the early diagnosis of cancer (especially of the breast and the colon); the management of gynecologic problems; and the care of those with chronic and terminal illnesses.

The United States has the most expensive health care system in the world, with 12% of the gross national product devoted to health care. Schroeder believes that this situation will continue as long as the system accepts a high concentration of specialists, fee-for-service payment, patient self-referral directly to specialists, practice of specialties by physicians who have not gone through the specialty certification process, and a high dependency on specialists for primary care.

Patient Self-Referral

Clearly, the increasing complexity of our health care system multiplies expense and wastefulness when a patient self-diagnoses problems or selects a specialist rather than developing a firm and ongoing relationship with a family physician. The most efficient and cost-effective system involves a single personal physician who ensures the most logical and economical management of a problem. Medical care should be available to patients in the precise degree needed—neither too extensive nor too limited. This ensures that simple problems will not be magnified out of proportion. The more complex and involved a diagnostic process is, the more costly it becomes, and the greater is the potential for error.

The need for a primary physician who accepts continuing responsibility for patient care is emphasized by Michael Balint in his concept of "collusion of anonymity" (also see Chap. 13). In this situation, the patient is seen by a variety of physicians, not one of whom is willing to accept total management of the problem. Important decisions are made—some good, some bad—but without anyone's feeling fully responsible for them.

Francis Peabody examined the futility of a patient's making the rounds from one specialist to another without finding relief because he

> . . . lacked the guidance of a sound general practitioner who understood his physical condition, his nervous temperament and knew the details of his daily life. Many a patient who on his own initiative had sought out specialists has had minor defects extenuated so that they assume a needless importance and has even undergone operations that might well have been avoided. These are often pathetically tragic figures as they veer from one course of treatment to another—like ships that lack a guiding hand upon the helm, they swing from tack to tack with each new gust of wind but get no nearer to Port of Health because there is no pilot to set the general direction of their course.

The family physician also must be committed to managing the common chronic illnesses that have no known cure but for which continuing management by a personal physician is all the more necessary to maintain an optimal state of health for the patient.

Comprehensive Care

The term "comprehensive medical care" spans the entire spectrum of medicine. The effectiveness with which a physician delivers primary care depends on the degree of expertise attained during training and practice. The family physician must be comprehensively trained to acquire all the medical skills necessary to care for the majority of patient problems. The greater the number of disciplines omitted from the family physician's training and practice, the more frequent is the need to refer minor problems to another physician. A truly comprehensive primary physician adequately manages acute infections, biopsies skin and other lesions, repairs lacerations, treats musculoskeletal sprains and minor fractures, removes foreign bodies, treats vaginitis, provides obstetric care and care for the newborn infant, gives supportive psychotherapy, and supervises diagnostic procedures. The needs of a family physician's patient will range from a routine physical examination, when the patient feels well and wishes to identify potential risk factors, to a problem that calls for referral to one or more narrowly specialized physicians with highly developed technical skills. The family physician must be aware of the variety and complexity of skills and facilities available to help manage patients and must match these to the individual's specific needs, giving full consideration to the patient's personality and expectations.

Management of an illness involves much more than a diagnosis and an outline for treatment. It also requires an awareness of all the factors that may aid or hinder an individual's recovery from illness. This requires consideration of religious beliefs; social, economic, or cultural problems; personal expectations; and heredity. The outstanding clinician recognizes the effects that spiritual, intellectual, emotional, social, and economic factors have on a patient's illness.

The family physician's ability to confront relatively large numbers of unselected patients with undifferentiated conditions and carry on a therapeutic relationship over time is a unique primary care skill. The skilled family physician will have a higher level of tolerance for the uncertain than will his or her consultant colleague.

The World Health Organization, the United Nations, and other organizations sponsored the World Conference on Medical Education in Edinburgh, Scotland, in 1988, which addressed the need for reform in medical education. The meeting made a number of recommendations to medical schools in its "Edinburgh Declaration":

1. Enlarge the range of settings in which educational programs are conducted to include all health resources of the community, not hospitals alone.

2. Ensure that curriculum content reflects national health priorities and the availability of affordable resources.

3. Ensure continuity of learning throughout life, shifting emphasis from the passive methods so widespread now to more active learning, including self-directed and independent study as well as tutorial methods.

4. Build both curriculum and examination systems

to ensure the achievement of professional competence and social values, not merely the retention and recall of information.

5. Train teachers as educators, not solely as experts in content, and reward education excellence as fully as excellence in biomedical research or clinical practice.

6. Complement instruction about the management of patients with increased emphasis on promotion of health and prevention of diseases.

7. Pursue integration of education in science and education in practice, also using problem solving in clinical and community settings as a base for learning.

8. Employ selection methods for medical students that go beyond intellectual ability and academic achievement to include evaluation of personal qualities.

9. Encourage and facilitate cooperation between the ministries of health, ministries of education, community health services, and other relevant bodies in joint policy development, program planning, implementation, and review.

10. Ensure admission policies that match the numbers of students trained with national needs for doctors.

11. Increase the opportunity for joint learning, research, and service with other health and health-related professions as part of the training for teamwork.

12. Clarify responsibility and allocate resources for continuing medical education.

Interpersonal Skills

One of the foremost skills of the family physician is the ability to utilize effectively the knowledge of interpersonal relations in the management of patients. This powerful element of clinical medicine is perhaps the specialty's most useful tool. Modern society considers the medical care system inadequate in those situations in which understanding and compassion are important to the patient's comfort and recovery from illness. Physicians are too often seen as lacking this personal concern and as being unskilled in understanding personal anxiety and feelings. There is an obvious need to nourish the seed of compassion and concern for sick people with which students enter medical school.

Family practice emphasizes the integration of compassion, empathy, and personalized concern to a greater degree than does a more technical or task-oriented specialty. Some of the earnest solicitude of the old country doctor and his untiring compassion for people must be incorporated as the effective, yet impersonal modern medical procedures are applied. The patient should be viewed compassionately as a person in distress who needs to be treated with concern, dignity, and personal consideration. He or she has a right to be given some insight into his or her problems, a reasonable appraisal of the potential outcome, and a realistic picture of the emotional, financial, and occupational expenses involved in his or her care. To relate well to patients, a physician must develop compassion and courtesy, the ability to establish rapport and to communicate effectively, the ability to gather information rapidly and to

organize it logically, the skills required to identify all significant patient problems and to manage these problems appropriately, the ability to listen, the skills necessary to motivate people, and the ability to observe and detect nonverbal clues (see Chap. 9).

Accessibility

Just as good rapport is therapeutic, so too is the mere *availability* of the physician. The feeling of security that the patient gains just by knowing he or she can "touch" the physician, either in person or by phone, is in itself therapeutic and has a comforting and calming influence. Accessibility is an essential feature of primary care. Services must be available when needed and should be within geographic proximity. When primary care is not available, many individuals turn to hospital emergency departments. Emergency room care is, of course, fine for emergencies, but it is no substitute for the personalized, long-term, comprehensive care a family physician can provide.

Diagnostic Skills: Undifferentiated Problems

The family physician, above all, must be an outstanding diagnostician. Skills in this area must be honed to perfection, since problems are usually seen in their early, undifferentiated state and without the degree of resolution that usually is present by the time patients are referred to consulting specialists. This is a unique feature of family practice, because symptoms seen at this stage are often vague and nondescript, with signs being either minimal or absent. Unlike the consulting specialist, the family physician does not evaluate the case after it has been preselected by another physician, and the diagnostic procedures used by the family physician must be selected from the entire spectrum of medicine.

EARLY CLUES. At this stage of disease, there are often only subtle differences between the early symptoms of serious disease and those of self-limiting, minor ailments. To the inexperienced person, the clinical pictures may appear identical, but to the astute and experienced family physician, one symptom will be more suspicious than another because of the greater probability that it signals a potentially serious illness. Diagnoses are frequently made on the basis of probability, and the likelihood that a specific disease is present frequently depends on the incidence of the disease relative to the symptom seen in the physician's community during a given time of year.

The Russian exile and author Alexander Solzhenitsyn points out the value of the family physician's ability to recognize and respond to the subtle, early symptoms of illness:

The family doctor is a figure without whom the family cannot exist in a developed society. He knows the needs of each member of the family, just as the mother knows their tastes. There's no shame in taking to him some trivial complaint you'd never take to the outpatient clinic, which entails getting an appointment card and waiting your turn, and where there's a quota of nine patients an hour. And yet all neglected illnesses arise out of these trifling complaints. *How many adult human beings are there, now, at this minute, rushing about in mute panic wishing they could find a doctor, the kind of person to whom they can pour out the fears they have deeply concealed or even found shameful?* [Emphasis added]

CANCER WARD, ALEXANDER SOLZHENITSYN

Approximately one-fourth of all patients seen will never be assigned a final, definitive diagnosis, since the resolution of a presenting symptom or a complaint will come before a specific diagnosis can be made. Pragmatically, this is an efficient method that is less costly and achieves high patient satisfaction—even though it may be disquieting to the purist physician who feels that a thorough workup and specific diagnosis should always be obtained.

The family physician is an expert in the rapid assessment of a problem presented for the first time. He or she evaluates its potential significance, often making a diagnosis by exclusion rather than by inclusion, after making certain the symptoms are not those of a serious problem. Once assured, he or she allows some time to elapse, using time as one of his or her most efficient diagnostic aids. Follow-up visits are scheduled at appropriate intervals to watch for subtle changes in the presenting symptoms. The physician usually identifies the symptom that has the greatest discriminatory value and watches it more closely than other symptoms. The most significant clue of the true nature of the illness may depend on subtle changes in this key symptom. The family physician's effectiveness is often determined by his or her knack for perceiving the hidden or subtle dimensions of illness and following them closely.

VALUE OF THE HISTORY.   The maxim that an accurate history is the most important factor in arriving at an accurate diagnosis is especially appropriate in family medicine, since symptoms may be the only obvious feature of an illness at the time it is presented to the family physician. Further inquiry into the nature of the symptoms, time of onset, extenuating factors, and other unique subjective features may provide the only diagnostic clues available at such an early stage. Above all, the family physician must be a skilled clinician with the ability to evaluate symptoms, verbal and nonverbal communication, and early signs of illness in order to choose those diagnostic tests that are of greatest value in diagnosing a problem early.

The family physician attempts to minimize the degree of morbidity resulting from illness. For example, he or she pays close attention to the complete eradication of a urinary tract infection in an effort to prevent permanent damage that could result in renal failure, requiring expensive and incapacitating renal dialysis or a kidney transplant. Similar examples include the early identification of carcinoma in situ of the cervix to prevent the lethal spread of uterine carcinoma, as well as the early identification of a dysplastic hip, which, if undetected, could result in a permanent deformity.

REASON FOR VISIT.   The family physician must be a perceptive humanist, alert to early identification of new problems. Arriving at an early diagnosis may, in fact, be of less importance than determining the real reason the patient came to the physician. The symptoms may be due to a self-limiting or acute problem, but anxiety or fear may be the true precipitating factor. Although the symptom may be hoarseness that has resulted from postnasal drainage accompanying an upper respiratory tract infection, the patient may fear it is caused by a laryngeal carcinoma similar to that recently found in a friend or celebrity. Clinical evaluation must rule out the possibility of laryngeal carcinoma, but the patient's fears and apprehension regarding this possibility also must be allayed. Similarly, a 42-year-old man with influenza and pleuritic chest pain may be anxious and apprehensive because his father died at age 45 of an acute myocardial infarction. (In fact, a frequent reason for a patient's requesting a complete checkup and electrocardiogram is the recent heart attack of an acquaintance at work.) Mild thrombophlebitis in a 35-year-old woman could bring her to the physician in a more anxious state than is warranted because her mother died from a pulmonary embolus, or a housewife's anxiety about breast cancer may well stem from a friend's recent mastectomy.

HAND ON THE DOORKNOB SYNDROME.   This phenomenon is familiar to every experienced physician. It occurs at the end of a patient visit. When the patient is ready to leave, he or she says, "You don't think this pain could be cancer do you?" It is not until the patient feels "safe"—that escape is guaranteed if the patient receives an unwanted or unwelcome answer—that he or she feels confident enough to reveal the true reason for the visit. It may have been (and often is) that a friend of the patient's recently was found to have cancer or a celebrity recently died from cancer. It is important to be alert and receptive to these last-minute messages and take the time to address them adequately so the patient's anxiety is allayed.

Every physical problem has an emotional component, and although this factor is usually minimal, it can be extremely significant. A patient's personality, fears, and anxieties all play a role in every illness and are important factors to consider in all primary care.

The Family Physician as Coordinator

Francis Peabody, professor of medicine at Harvard Medical School from 1921 to 1927, was a man ahead of his time; his comments remain appropriate today:

Never was the public in need of wise, broadly trained advisors so much as it needs them today to guide them through the complicated maze of modern medicine. The extraordinary development of medical science with its consequent diversity of medical specialists and the increasing limitations in the extent of special fields, the very factors indeed which are creating specialists, in themselves create a new demand. Not for men who are experts along narrow lines but for men who are in touch with many lines.

The family physician, by virtue of his or her breadth of training in a wide variety of medical disciplines, has unique insights into the skills possessed by physicians in the more limited specialties. The family physician is best prepared to select specialists whose skills can be applied most appropriately to a given case as well as to coordinate the activities of each so that they are not counterproductive. The AAFP has described this role of the family physician:

As long as there is a need for health care services, there will be a need for a physician who assumes continuing responsibility for the health care of the patient as an individual, and for the family as the basic social unit of society. Such a physician must possess a basic core of knowledge current through constant use. This physician must be proficient in basic techniques and must know when patients require more sophisticated skills.

As medicine becomes more specialized and complex, the family physician's role as the integrator of health services becomes increasingly important. The family physician not only facilitates the patient's access to the whole health care system but also interprets the activities of this system to the patient, explaining the nature of the illness, the implication of the treatment, and the effect of both on the patient's way of life. The following statement from the Millis Commission Report concerning expectations of the patient is especially appropriate:

The patient wants someone of high competence and good judgment to take charge of the total situation, someone who can serve as coordinator of all the medical resources that can help solve his problem. He wants a company president who will make proper use of his skills and knowledge of more specialized members of the firm. He wants a quarterback who will diagnose the constantly changing situation, coordinate the whole team, and call on each member for the particular contributions that he is best able to make to the team effort.

Such breadth of vision is important for a coordinating physician. He or she must have a realistic overview of the problem and an awareness of the many alternative routes in order to select the most appropriate one. As Pellegrino has stated:

It should be clear, too, that no simple addition of specialties can equal the generalist function. To build a wall one needs more than the aimless piling up of bricks, one needs an architect. Every operation which analyzes some part of the human mechanism requires to be balanced by another which synthesizes and coordinates.

The complexity of modern medicine frequently involves a variety of health professionals, each with highly developed skills in a particular area. In planning a patient's care, the family physician, having established rapport with the patient and family and having knowledge of the patient's background, personality, fears, and expectations, is best able to select and coordinate the activities of appropriate individuals from the large variety of medical disciplines. He or she can maintain effective communication among those involved, as well as function as the patient's advocate and interpret to the patient and family the many unfamiliar and complicated procedures being used. This prevents any one consulting physician, unfamiliar with the concepts or actions of all others involved, from ordering a test or medication that would conflict with other treatment. J. E. Dunphy has described the value of the surgeon and the family physician working closely as a team:

It is impossible to provide high quality surgical care without that knowledge of the whole patient which only a family physician can supply. When their mutual decisions . . . bring hope, comfort and ultimately, health to a gravely ill human being, the total experience is the essence and the joy of medicine.

The ability to orchestrate the knowledge and skills of diverse professionals is a skill to be learned during training and cultivated in practice. It is not an automatic attribute of all physicians or merely the result of exposure to a large number of professionals. These coordinator skills extend beyond the traditional medical disciplines into the many community agencies and allied health professions as well. For the family physician to be an effective coordinator, it is essential that all pertinent health information be channeled through him or her—regardless of what institution, agency, or individual renders the service. The family physician helps remove barriers to health care, whether they be economic, emotional, social, or occupational. Because of his or her close involvement with the community, the family physician is ideally suited to being the integrator of the patient's care, coordinating the skills of consultants when appropriate, and involving community nurses, social agencies, the clergy, or other family members when needed. A knowledge of community health resources and a personal involvement with the community can be used to maximum benefit not only for diagnostic and therapeutic purposes but also to achieve the best possible level of rehabilitation.

REFERENCES

Ad Hoc Committee on Education for Family Practice of the Council on Medical Education of the American Medical Association (Willard Committee). Meeting the Challenge of Family Practice. Chicago, American Medical Association, September 1966.

American Academy of Family Physicians. Official Definition of Family Practice and Family Physician (AAFP Publication No. 303). Kansas City, Mo., AAFP, 1986.

American Academy of Family Physicians. Official AAFP definition of primary care. AAFP Reporter 1975; 2(6):1.

Balint M. The Doctor, His Patient and the Illness. New York, Pitman, 1965.

Citizens' Commission on Graduate Medical Education of the American Medical Association (Millis Commission). The Graduate Education of Physicians. Chicago, American Medical Association, August 1966.

Dunphy JE. Responsibility and authority in American surgery. Bull Am Coll Surg 1964; 49:9.

Fox TF. The personal doctor and his relation to the hospital. Lancet 1960; 1:743.

Geyman JP. Family Practice: Foundation of Changing Health Care. New York, Appleton-Century-Crofts, 1980.

McWhinney IR. An Introduction to Family Medicine. New York, Oxford University Press, 1981.

Osler W. Aequanimitas, with Other Addresses, 3d ed. Philadelphia, Blakiston, 1932.

Peabody FW. Doctor and Patient. New York, Macmillan, 1930.

Pellegrino ED. The generalist function in medicine. JAMA 1966; 198:541.

Pellegrino ED. Humanism and the Physician. Knoxville, Tenn., University of Tennessee Press, 1979.

Schroeder SA. Western European responses to physician oversupply. JAMA 1984; 252(3):373–384.

Tumulty PA. What is a clinician and what does he do? N Engl J Med 1970; 283(1):20–24.

Tumulty PA. The Effective Clinician: His Methods and Approach to Diagnosis and Care. Philadelphia, W.B. Saunders, 1973.

QUESTIONS

1. Which of the following are attributes of family medicine?
   a. Continuing comprehensive care
   b. Boredom
   c. Variety
   d. Personal care
   e. Primarily inpatient care

2. The American Medical Association's Report of the Citizens' Commission on Graduate Medical Education
   a. Was published in 1975.
   b. Is known as the Willard report.
   c. Was instrumental in establishing the American Board of Family Practice.
   d. Is known as the Millis report.
   e. Resulted in the name change of the American Academy of General Practice to the American Academy of Family Physicians.

3. Match the following.
   a. AAFP
   b. AAGP
   c. ABFP
   d. Organized in 1947
   e. Established in 1969
   f. Named in 1971
   g. Medicine's 20th primary specialty board
      (1) American Academy of General Practice
      (2) American Academy of Family Practice
      (3) American Board of Family Physicians
      (4) American Board of Family Practice
      (5) American Academy of Family Physicians

4. The American Board of Family Practice
   a. Was the first specialty board to require recertification.
   b. Requires 50 hours of CME annually.
   c. Requires a written examination every 6 years.
   d. Establishment was promoted by the Millis and Willard reports.

5. Which of the following are important components of residency training in family practice?
   a. Exposure to and experience in managing problems frequently seen in practice
   b. Abdominal surgery
   c. Prenatal care
   d. A model office
   e. Management of psychosocial and economic problems

Answers appear on page 445.

2

THE SCOPE OF FAMILY PRACTICE

ROBERT E. RAKEL

The specialty of family practice emphasizes training in ambulatory care skills in an appropriately realistic environment using patients representing a cross section of a community and incorporating those problems most frequently encountered by physicians practicing primary care. It is more realistic to train a primary care physician in a community atmosphere, providing exposure to the diseases and problems most closely approximating those he or she will encounter during practice. The ambulatory care skills and knowledge that most medical graduates need cannot be taught totally within the tertiary medical center.

The lack of relevance in the referral medical center also applies to the hospitalized patient. Figure 2–1, which is derived from data accumulated in the United States and Great Britain, places the health problems of an average community in perspective. In an adult population of 1000 people aged 16 years or older, 750 will experience at least one illness or injury during an average month. Most of these people will be managed by self-treatment, but 250 patients will consult a physician. Of these, 5 patients will be referred for consultation to another physician, and 9 will be hospitalized—8 of them in a community hospital and one in a university medical center. It is obvious that patients seen in the medical center (frequently the majority of cases used for teaching) represent atypical samples of illness occurring within the community. Students exposed only in this manner develop an unrealistic concept of the kinds of medical problems prevalent in society. It focuses their training on knowledge and skills of limited usefulness in later practice.

PRACTICE CONTENT

The first major system for classifying disease was the International Classification of Disease, which was modified for use in the United States and became the International Classification of Diseases Adapted for Use in the United States. This was further modified by hospitals into the Hospital International Classification of Diseases Adapted for Use in the United States, which in-

cluded perinatal mortality and psychiatric problems and contained more than 4000 items. This classification system had major deficiencies when applied to the problems most frequently encountered by practicing family physicians, so the Royal College of General Practitioners developed a classification system pertinent to its members' needs in the administration of ambulatory care. That system served as a nucleus for an international classification of problems seen by practicing family physicians throughout the world. The sponsoring organization is the World Organization of National Colleges, Academies, and Academic Associations of General Practitioners/Family Physicians (WONCA). The classification was developed by an international working party, which gave it the name International Classification of Health Problems in Primary Care, also called Ich-Pic and Pri-Care. The working party conducted a large-scale international trial that isolated the 371 items most commonly encountered by family physicians. In this manner, a large number of problems included in the International Classification of Disease but infrequently encountered in family practice have been eliminated. The International Classification of Health Problems in Primary Care is compatible with the larger International Classification of Disease, however, and can be used interchangeably or expanded at will.

The National Ambulatory Medical Care Survey conducted by the National Center for Health Statistics of the United States Department of Health and Human Services has, since 1975, annually reported the problems seen by office-based physicians (in all specialties) in the United States. A symptom classification was developed to document the complaints presented by patients to physicians in their offices. The National Ambulatory Medical Care Survey reverses the previous trend of evaluating the prevalence of disease after the fact (measuring causes of death or diagnosis upon discharge from a hospital) by evaluating the presenting complaints or symptoms at the onset of the illness. This change in approach is a formidable and difficult task but one that is yielding a large amount of new and valuable information. The 20 most common symptoms or reasons prompting office visits in 1989 are shown in Table 2–1

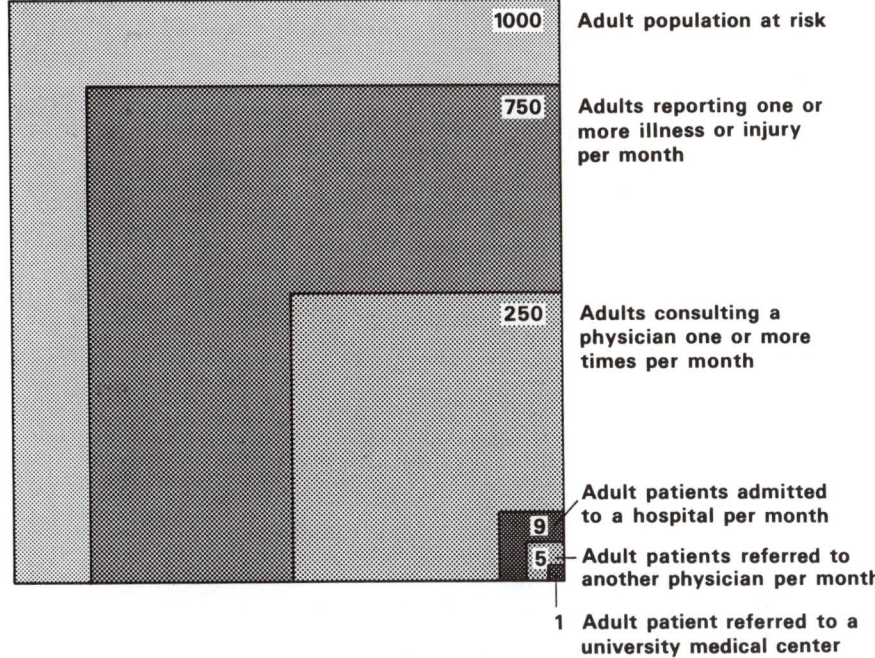

Figure 2–1. Number of persons experiencing illness or injury during an average month, per 1000 adult population. (From White KL, Williams F, and Greenberg B. Ecology of medical care. N Engl J Med 1961; 265:885, with permisssion.)

1000 Adult population at risk

750 Adults reporting one or more illness or injury per month

250 Adults consulting a physician one or more times per month

9 Adult patients admitted to a hospital per month

5 Adult patients referred to another physician per month

1 Adult patient referred to a university medical center per month

and the diagnoses arrived at during those visits are shown in Table 2–2. Much of the excitement of family practice comes from the variety of problems encountered in practice and the freedom to enjoy the challenges of hospital care as well as those of the outpatient setting.

"Clustering" is a system of classifying problems encountered in practice by grouping diagnoses according to similar pathophysiologic conditions. This permits a more comprehensive yet concise description of problems seen. Table 2–3 lists the most common diagnostic clusters seen by family physicians in the outpatient setting, and Table 2–4 lists the most common diagnoses for hospitalized patients. Greater than 50% of all hospital diagnoses can be identified in the top 14 clusters.

The broad range of disorders seen by family physicians is evident by comparing the outpatient and inpatient diagnoses. Most of the problems cared for in the hospital, such as congestive heart failure, do not even appear on the list of problems commonly seen in the office. In the Rosenblatt study, 23% of all patient encounters took place in the hospital, and the family physicians surveyed felt that hospital care was an important and rewarding part of their practice.

As interest in primary care continues to grow and data continue to be collected, increasing information will be available as to what problems are being seen in practices throughout the country. Data from studies such as these, combined with ABFP surveys and audits of office records, will enable family practice training programs to revise their curricula according to the realities of everyday practice.

TABLE 2–1. PRINCIPAL REASONS FOR OFFICE VISITS IN THE UNITED STATES (ALL SPECIALTIES)

RANK	PRINCIPAL REASON FOR VISIT	NUMBER OF VISITS (000)	PERCENT
1	General medical examination	27,909	4.0
2	Cough	24,997	3.6
3	Prenatal examination	24,056	3.5
4	Symptoms referable to the throat	16,972	2.5
5	Postoperative visit	16,660	2.4
6	Well-baby examination	14,831	2.1
7	Earache or ear infection	14,468	2.1
8	Back symptoms	13,744	2.0
9	Skin rash	12,325	1.8
10	Stomach pain, cramps, and spasms	12,313	1.8
11	Fever	11,634	1.7
12	Vision dysfunctions	10,253	1.5
13	Hypertension	10,055	1.5
14	Knee symptoms	9,816	1.4
15	Blood pressure test	9,792	1.4
16	Headache, pain in head	9,609	1.4
17	Headcold, upper respiratory infection	8,669	1.3
18	Nasal congestion	8,647	1.2
19	Chest pain and related symptoms	8,399	1.2
20	Neck symptoms	8,112	1.2
All other reasons		419,439	60.6

Source: From DeLozier JE, Gagnon RO. 1989 Summary: National Ambulatory Medical Care Survey (Advance Data from Vital and Health Statistics No. 203). Hyattsville, Md., National Center for Health Statistics, 1991. (*Reprinted with permission.*)

Office Visits

Available data concerning primary care indicate that more people use this type of medical service than any other kind and that, contrary to popular opinion, sophisticated medical technology is not normally either required or overused in basic primary care encounters

TABLE 2–2. RANKING OF OFFICE VISITS BY DIAGNOSIS (ALL SPECIALTIES)

RANK	DIAGNOSIS	PERCENT	CUMULATIVE PERCENT
1	Essential hypertension	4.0	4.0
2	Normal pregnancy	3.4	7.4
3	General medical examination	2.9	10.3
4	Otitis media, suppurative and unspecified	2.9	13.2
5	Acute upper respiratory infection	2.3	15.5
6	Health supervision of infant or child	2.3	17.8
7	Diabetes mellitus	1.9	19.7
8	Allergic rhinitis	1.7	21.4
9	Bronchitis, not specified	1.6	23.0
10	Acute pharyngitis	1.6	24.6
11	Chronic sinusitis	1.3	25.9
12	Neurotic disorders	1.2	27.1
13	Diseases of sebaceous glands	1.2	28.3
14	Disorders of refraction and accommodation	1.1	29.4
15	Sprains and strains of back, except sacroiliac	1.1	30.5
16	Asthma	1.0	31.5
17	Contact dermatitis, other eczema	0.9	32.4
18	Cataract	0.9	33.3
19	Osteoarthrosis, allied disorders	0.9	34.2
20	Chronic ischemic heart disease, except angina pectoris	0.8	35.0

Source: Constructed from information from DeLozier JE, Gagnon RO. 1989 Summary: National Ambulatory Medical Care Survey (Advance Data from Vital and Health Statistics No. 203). Hyattsville, Md., National Center for Health Statistics, 1991. *(Used with permission.)*

TABLE 2–3. FREQUENCY OF MOST COMMON DIAGNOSIS CLUSTERS FOR OUTPATIENT FAMILY PRACTICE

RANK	DIAGNOSIS CLUSTER	PERCENT	CUMULATIVE PERCENT
1	General medical examination	14.5	14.5
2	Acute upper respiratory tract infection	7.9	22.4
3	Hypertension	7.0	29.4
4	Soft-tissue injuries	3.9	33.3
5	Acute sprains, strains	3.1	36.4
6	Prenatal and postnatal care	3.0	39.4
7	Depression/anxiety	2.9	42.3
8	Ischemic heart disease	2.6	44.9
9	Diabetes	2.4	47.3
10	Dermatitis/eczema	2.1	49.4
11	Degenerative joint disease	2.0	51.4
12	Urinary tract infection	2.0	53.4
13	Obesity	1.7	55.1
14	Acute lower respiratory tract infection	1.7	56.8
15	Nonfungal skin infection	1.6	58.4
16	Infectious diarrhea/gastroenteritis	1.5	59.9
17	Vaginitis, vulvitis, cervicitis	1.3	61.2
18	Fractures/dislocations	1.2	62.4
19	Otitis media	1.2	63.6
20	Emphysema, chronic bronchitis, chronic obstructive pulmonary disease	1.2	64.8
21	Medical/surgical aftercare	1.1	65.9
22	Peptic ulcer diseases	1.0	66.9
23	Headache	0.9	67.8
24	Bursitis, synovitis, tenosynovitis	0.8	68.6
25	Low back pain	0.8	69.4
26	Sinusitis	0.8	70.2
27	Chronic rhinitis	0.7	70.9
28	Fibrositis, myalgia, arthralgia	0.7	71.6
29	Menstrual disorders	0.6	72.2
30	Asthma	0.5	72.7

Source: Constructed from Rosenblatt RA, Cherkin DC, Schneeweiss R, et al. The structure and content of family practice: current status and future trends. J Fam Pract 1982; 15(4):681–722, Tables 8 and 12. *(Used with permission.)*

TABLE 2–4. TOP 30 CLUSTERS OF HOSPITAL DIAGNOSES BY OFFICE-BASED GENERAL AND FAMILY PHYSICIANS

RANK	DIAGNOSIS	PERCENT	CUMULATIVE PERCENT
1	Ischemic heart disease (including myocardial infarction)	7.9	7.9
2	Pregnancy, normal and complicated	6.2	14.1
3	Malignant neoplasm	6.2	20.3
4	Back pain, radiculopathy	4.3	24.6
5	Cerebrovascular disease	4.0	28.6
6	Pneumonia	3.1	31.7
7	Diabetes mellitus	3.1	34.8
8	Congestive heart failure	2.7	37.5
9	Chronic obstructive pulmonary disease	2.7	40.2
10	Appendicitis/appendectomy	2.3	42.5
11	Fractures and dislocations (except femur)	2.3	44.8
12	Surgical aftercare	2.0	46.8
13	Cholecystitis	1.9	48.7
14	Peptic ulcer disease	1.8	50.5
15	Benign diseases of uterus	1.7	52.2
16	Fracture of femur	1.6	53.8
17	Diarrheal disease	1.6	55.4
18	Hernias of abdominal wall without obstruction	1.4	56.8
19	Kidney stone	1.4	58.2
20	Diseases of urinary tract	1.4	59.6
21	Diseases of intestine and peritoneum (NEC)*	1.3	60.9
22	Upper respiratory tract infection and influenza	1.2	62.1
23	Essential benign hypertension	1.1	63.2
24	Abnormal menstrual bleeding	1.0	64.2
25	Pyogenic infections of skin and subcutaneous tissue	0.9	65.1
26	Diverticulitis of colon	0.9	66.0
27	Pelvic inflammatory disease	0.8	66.8
28	Gastrointestinal obstruction	0.8	67.6
29	Arthritis	0.8	68.4
30	Anemia	0.7	69.1

*NEC = not elsewhere classified.
Source: Modified from Rosenblatt RA, Cherkin DC, Schneeweiss R, et al. The structure and content of family practice: Current status and future trends. J Fam Pract 1982; 15(4):681–722. *(Used with permission.)*

(Gold and Azevedo). Indeed, most primary care visits arise from patients requesting care for relatively uncomplicated problems, many of which are self-limiting but which cause them concern or discomfort. Treatment is often symptomatic, consisting of pain relief or anxiety reduction rather than a ''cure.'' The greatest level of cost efficiency results when these patients' needs are satisfied while the self-limiting course of the disease is recognized without incurring unnecessary costs for additional tests.

Only 1.0% of all physician visits made during 1989 ended in hospital admissions, and only 2.9% were referred to other physicians (DeLozier and Gagnon).

Each year 77% of people in the United States make at least one visit to a physician (Adams and Benson). In 1989, the average was 2.8 office visits per person (DeLozier and Gagnon). Females averaged 3.3 visits per person per year, and males had 2.3 visits per person per year. The annual visit rate ranged from 1.9 visits per person per year for young adults 15 to 24 years of age to more than twice that (5.9 visits per person per year) for those 75 years of age and older. Approximately 30% of all visits were made to physicians in general and family practice.

House Calls

At one time, house calls were a routine feature of medical practice in the United States. As general practice declined, so did the number and frequency of house calls. However, the house call continues to be a valuable tool used by family physicians to develop a thorough understanding of patients and their environment, and family practice residencies are encouraged to include house calls in their training programs.

The cost-containment pressures that arose in the 1980s with the advent of diagnostic related groups and professional review organizations have led to a resurgence in home care. More patients with acute as well as chronic illnesses are being managed at home, and the home-care industry has grown at a rate of 20% a year, whereas the availability of nursing home beds has increased only 2% annually (Kavesh).

Elderly patients, especially the frail elderly, often have

considerable difficulty getting to and from the physician's office. The patient is more comfortable and under less stress at home and more problems can be identified, leading to improved care. Ramsdell and coworkers have shown that home-visit assessments reveal two new problems and up to eight new treatment recommendations when home visits follow physician office-based assessments. Home visits may be the only way to identify some environmental hazards and to accurately evaluate the patient's functional status.

PHYSICIAN SUPPLY

The 1988 report of the American Medical Association's Council on Long Range Planning and Development notes that although the number of family physicians will increase by 9% by the year 2000, the U.S. population will increase by 12.3%. Also, managed-care systems will place increased demands on the need for family physicians, thus decreasing even further the number available in some rural areas.

The Graduate Medical Education National Advisory Committee in 1980 projected a surplus of 150,000 physicians in the United States by the year 2020, with the greatest need in primary care. Mulhausen and McGee project an even greater demand for primary care physicians than was estimated by the Graduate Medical Education National Advisory Committee.

Another federally convened group, the Council on Graduate Medical Education and the American Medical Association Center for Health Policy Research have issued reports indicating more conservative estimates of physician surplus but emphasizing that whatever the numbers, there will be a significant shortage of family physicians and psychiatrists and a significant excess of pediatricians, internal medicine subspecialists, and obstetricians and gynecologists.

If the growth in physician supply continues, American Medical Association analysts warn that "soon some physicians might not have enough work to stay proficient, and the status of the profession might decline." Similarly, the quality of primary care will decline as physicians trained in a surplus subspecialty practice primary care without retraining. Rhee and associates showed that when physicians practice outside their specialty areas, the relative quality of their performance declines.

Table 2–5 presents the percentage of physicians practicing in each specialty in the United States and Canada. It is clear that Canada has a much larger percentage of primary care physicians than does the United States, es-

TABLE 2–5. PERCENTAGE OF ACTIVE PHYSICIANS BY SPECIALTY IN THE UNITED STATES AND CANADA, 1989

	USA	CANADA
Allergy	0.31	0.10
Anesthesiology	4.22	3.98
Cardiovascular disease	2.73	1.16
Dermatology	1.22	0.80
Emergency medicine	2.29	0.38
Family practice	7.71	11.89
Gastroenterology	1.20	0.49
General practice	4.01	41.05
General surgery	6.51	4.31
Internal medicine	16.23	6.89
Neurology	1.50	0.98
Neurologic surgery	0.72	0.38
Obstetrics/gynecology	5.51	3.03
Ophthalmology	2.66	1.90
Orthopedic surgery	3.12	1.85
Otolaryngology	1.33	1.11
Pathology	2.73	2.02
Pediatrics	6.57	3.56
Plastic surgery	0.75	0.69
Psychiatry	6.46	6.00
Pulmonary diseases	1.00	0.59
Radiology	4.59	3.96
Thoracic surgery	0.35	0.10
Urologic surgery	1.54	1.00
Other	14.75	1.78
TOTAL	100.00	100.00

Sources: From Roback G, Randolph L, Seldman B. Physician Characteristics and Distribution in the United States. Chicago, American Medical Association, 1990, and Health and Welfare Canada. Health Personnel in Canada, Ottawa, Canada, 1990. *(Used with permission.)*

pecially when 60% of U.S. internists are in subspecialties. Family practice is clearly the largest primary care discipline and the only one whose goal is to produce primary care physicians.

As much-needed changes in the American medical system are implemented, it is essential that more attention is paid to the problem of physician and specialty maldistribution. Paul Beeson has commented:

> I have no doubt at all that a good family doctor can deal with the great majority of medical episodes quickly and competently. A specialist, on the other hand, feels that he must be thorough, not only because of his training but also because he has a reputation to protect. He, therefore, spends more time with each patient and orders more laboratory work. The result is a waste of doctors' time and patients' money. This not only inflates the national health bill, but also creates an illusion of doctor shortage when the only real need is to have the existing doctors doing the right things.

REFERENCES

Adams PF, Benson V. Current Estimates from the National Health Interview Survey, 1989: National Cancer for Health Statistics. Vital Health Stat [10] 1990; 176.

American Medical Association Council on Long Range Planning and Development. The Future of Family Practice. Chicago, American Medical Association, 1988.

Beeson PB. Some good features of the British National Health Service. J Med Ed 1974; 49:43.

DeLozier JE, Gagnon RO. 1989 Summary: National Ambulatory Medical Care Survey (Advance Data from Vital and Health Statistics No. 203). Hyattsville, Md., National Center for Health Statistics, 1991.

Gold M, Azevedo D. The content of adult primary care episodes. Public Health Rep 1982; 97:48.

Graduate Medical Education National Advisory Committee (GMENAC). Final Report, vol. 1 [DHHS Pub. No. (HRA) 81-651]. Hyattsville, Md., Health Resources Administration, September 1980.

Kavesh WN. Home care: process, outcome, cost. Annu Rev Gerontol Geriatr 1986; 6:135–195.

Mulhausen R, McGee J. Physician need: An alternative projection from a study of large, prepaid group practices. JAMA 1989; 261(13):1930–1934.

Ramsdell JW, Swart JA, Jackson JE, Renvall M. The yield of a home visit in the assessment of geriatric patients. J Am Geriatr Soc 1989; 37(1):17–24.

Rhee S, Luke R, Lyons T, Payne B. Domain of practice and the quality of physician performance. Med Care, 1981; 19(1):14–23.

Roback G, Randolph L, Seldman B. Physician Characteristics and Distribution in the United States. Chicago, American Medical Association, 1990.

Rosenblatt RA, Cherkin DC, Schneeweiss R, et al. The structure and content of family practice: Current status and future trends. J Fam Pract 1982; 15(4):681–722.

White KL, Williams F, Greenberg B. Ecology of medical care. N Engl J Med 1961; 265:885.

QUESTIONS

1. In an average community of 1000 people, each month
    a. 750 people will be ill or injured.
    b. 500 people will see a physician.
    c. 9 people will be hospitalized.
    d. 5 people will be hospitalized in a university medical center.
    e. Only 2% of those visiting a physician will be referred to another physician.

2. The National Ambulatory Medical Care Survey (NAMCS) conducted by the U.S. Department of Health and Human Services since 1975
    a. Documents problems seen by all physicians in their office practices.
    b. Documents presenting symptoms and diagnoses made in both outpatient and inpatient care.
    c. Is an accurate assessment of the kinds of problems comprising primary care.
    d. Notes that hypertension is the most common diagnosis among patients seen in physicians' offices.

3. In the United States,
    a. Over 75% of people visit a physician's office at least once a year.
    b. The average patient will visit a physician about three times a year.
    c. The elderly (those over 75 years of age) will visit a physician twice as often as the average person.
    d. 30% of all physician visits are to general or family physicians.
    e. 5% of all physician visits require hospital admission.

4. One reason why Canada and Britain have more cost-effective health care systems than the United States is
    a. That they have fewer psychiatrists.
    b. That they have more primary care physicians than consultants.
    c. That they have fewer plastic surgeons.
    d. That they have a lower cost of living.
    e. That they have no health maintenance organizations (HMOs).

Answers appear on page 445.

3

ETHICS IN FAMILY MEDICINE

WARREN L. HOLLEMAN and BARUCH A. BRODY

Economic, social, legal, and political factors have combined, in recent years, to effect major changes in medical practice and health care policy. Concern for patient rights and patient autonomy, as well as the demands of third-party payers, has transformed the practice of medicine. The ethical issues discussed in this chapter have taken on new dimensions as a result of this transformation.

MEDICINE AS A RELATIONSHIP AND AS A PROFESSION

At its most fundamental level, the practice of medicine should not be regarded as a science, an art, or a business, even though each of these elements is essential. The practice of medicine—particularly primary care medicine—is rooted, instead, in a relationship between the patient as person and the physician as professional (Jonsen, Siegler, and Winslade; Smith and Churchill; Siegler). Two problems currently threaten the quality of that relationship: a misunderstanding of patient autonomy and inappropriate third-party intervention.

When physicians respect the autonomy of their patients so that patients take control of their own health care, the physician is in danger of becoming a hired hand of the patient and the physician–patient relationship is in danger of degenerating into a purely commercial relationship. Patients "own" their bodies, but they should not "own" their physicians. Physicians have an obligation to practice within professional standards of care as well as a right to refrain from doing anything that would violate their own moral and religious conventions (Christie and Hoffmaster). Physicians must respect the autonomy of their patients, but they also must avoid the temptation to shirk their own professional and moral responsibilities and must nurture a cooperative relationship with the patient. This is no easy task, but it is through cooperation that the physician and the patient can best work together toward a common goal—to maintain the health of the patient.

The physician–patient relationship also suffers when outside parties interfere inappropriately. When third-party payers set the standard of care, the physician is in danger of becoming a hired hand of the third party. The physician must balance competing loyalties between patients and third parties as well as between professional standards and personal beliefs. In this era of third-party payers, the physician–patient relationship can no longer be exclusive, but it must remain primary. In the remainder of this section we examine two areas in which these problems are particularly prominent: work-related visits and benefits-related visits.

Work- and School-Related Evaluations

Preemployment examinations, work-release evaluations, school-absence excuses, and athletic physicals comprise a major component of many primary care practices. Inappropriate third-party interventions in this area challenge the primacy of the physician–patient relationship and the integrity of the medical profession. The following guidelines have been suggested (Holleman and Matson; Holleman and Holleman; Rosenstock and Hagopian; Kelman) and should help alleviate some of the problems most commonly associated with these evaluations.

The purpose of the preemployment examination is to determine a person's fitness for work, to protect workers from illnesses and injuries, to protect employers from the costs of preventable job-related illnesses and injuries, and to collect baseline data for the future treatment of such illnesses and injuries. To enable the physician to make such an evaluation, the employer must provide the physician with a detailed job description, including physical requirements, psychologic strains, and exposure to toxins. The physician should then tell the employer whether the prospective employee can perform the job without posing a risk to self or others. As discussed below, the physician should not release any medical records to the employer but should keep them on file as baseline data. At the beginning of the evaluation, the physician should advise the patient of the investigative nature of the visit. The physician must warn the prospective employee regarding health risks of the particular occupation (e.g., toxins affecting pregnancies, stresses affecting hypertensive patients) and must tell him or her of any problems detected in the course of the evaluation, regardless of their effect on job performance.

Work-release evaluations, school-release evaluations, and athletic physicals should be performed in accordance with the same guidelines as preemployment physicals, but they do present some additional problems of their own. Most work- and school-release evaluations involve short-term absences for minor problems for which there are few, if any, objective findings. Often workers and students present after their illness or injury has resolved. These absences often reflect personal, family, or job-related problems that are not strictly medical in nature. Investigating such problems for employers and school administrators damages the physician–patient relationship and discredits medicine as a healing profession. Patients will have difficulty trusting a physician who investigates on one occasion but offers therapy on another. We recommend that physicians encourage employers and school administrators to develop nonmedical strategies for policing casual absenteeism. Physicians who do perform these evaluations should minimize the harm to the physician–patient relationship and to the integrity of the profession by evaluating only in the context of treatment and by refusing to release confidential medical information to employers and school administrators.

Benefits-Related Evaluations

Many patients present to primary care physicians seeking to be certified as eligible for workers' compensation, long-term disability, group or individual medical insurance, Medicare, Medicaid, and veterans' benefits. Many others have already been certified and are seeking proper care under the terms of these programs. Physicians must be familiar with the details of the various programs so as to enable their patients to benefit appropriately from them. Physicians also must be aware of the potential abuses of such programs so as to help protect those who legitimately qualify from being harmed by those who do not. For example, if a patient presents with an on-the-job injury but also requests treatment for some other problem, the physician should file separate bills so that the workers' compensation fund only pays for job-related illnesses and injuries. Physicians who detect intentional abuse should attempt to identify the reasons for the abuse, particularly in the case of habitual, long-term abusers (Alexander; Whiting). Long-term abuse of benefits programs can be prevented only if primary care physicians insist that patients receive continuing comprehensive care from one physician or from a small team of physicians who know the patient well.

SPECIAL PROBLEMS IN PRIMARY CARE SETTINGS

Having introduced the concept of medicine as a relationship and as a profession and having seen what this concept means in many primary care contexts, we turn in the next sections to problem areas that challenge our understanding of the physician–patient relation and of the professional character of medicine.

Confidentiality

The principle of confidentiality is one of the most widely accepted and historically influential principles governing the patient–physician relationship in Western cultures. The Hippocratic oath mandates that the physician not divulge "whatsoever I shall see or hear in the course of my profession as well as outside my profession in my intercourse with men, if it be what should not be published abroad." The 1980 Principles of Medical Ethics of the American Medical Association mandate that the physician "shall safeguard patient confidences within the constraints of the law."

Confidentiality is important as a way of encouraging patients to be frank in their communications with physicians, as a way of physicians keeping an implicit promise to patients that their confidence will be respected, and as a way of emphasizing the patient's right to privacy. In all these ways, preserving confidentiality strengthens the relationship between an autonomous patient and a professional physician.

As the delivery of health care has changed from the model of a single physician caring for individual patients to the model of a team of health care workers in an institutional setting providing care to a wide variety of patients, the mandate of confidentiality has changed. The emphasis has switched from physicians keeping secrets to information about patients being divulged only to those members of the health care team and those institutional employees who have a need for the information, either to provide appropriate care or to meet appropriate institutional needs (e.g., monitoring of quality of care or organizing reimbursement). The underlying theme remains that information should not be provided to anyone else without the patient's consent.

This last point deserves special emphasis because it structures the decision as to when it is appropriate to provide information about the patient to insurance companies and to employers. Providing such information is perfectly appropriate if the patient consents; otherwise, it is not. For this reason, patients are commonly asked to authorize the release of information to particular individuals; the principle of confidentiality is not breached if information is provided pursuant to such a release (Bruce). However, the scope of information supplied and the persons to whom it is supplied are determined by the patient's instructions. Thus, if a patient requests a statement certifying that he or she is fit to return to work, it is not appropriate for the physician to provide to the employer a full account of the patient's illness and treatment; all that should be provided is the requested statement about the patient's fitness to return to work.

There are circumstances in which our society has judged that the need for information outweighs the principle of confidentiality; these are the circumstances in which the physician is required by law to disclose otherwise confidential information regardless of the wishes of the patient. The exact circumstances vary from jurisdiction to jurisdiction and are determined by state statutes and court decisions. Common circumstances include certain types of judicial proceedings, suspected abuse of dependent individuals such as children and the frail elderly, venereal and communicable diseases, and gunshot wounds (Bruce). In recent years, following the *Tarasoff* decision in California (Tarasoff), the concept has emerged that physicians are obligated to warn and/or to take measures to protect third parties threatened by the behavior of their patients, even if doing so involves a breach of confidentiality. The scope of that principle is far from clear (Mills et al.); one obvious controversial example is whether physicians should warn the spouses or regular sexual partners of patients who test positively for the AIDS virus about the threat this illness poses to them (Dickens).

The principle of confidentiality extends to not providing information to family members of competent adult patients unless the patients want the information to be shared. Often, it will be clear that the patient has no concern about the sharing of information with his or her family. In cases of doubt, the patient should be consulted, especially if the information is of a sensitive nature or if there is evidence of family discord. An appropriate practice upon admitting a patient to a hospital is to ask the patient to identify a particular family member, if any, to whom information should be provided for distribution to the family if the patient is not capable of fulfilling that role (e.g., in the immediate postoperative period).

Certain cases are particularly troublesome. Among the most troublesome are those involving teenage patients. Information about pediatric patients is, of course, provided directly to the parents of the patients and not to the patients themselves; information about adult patients is, of course, provided directly to the patient and not the patient's parents. What about teenage patients seeking abortions, contraceptive advice, or treatment for venereal diseases, substance abuse, or psychiatric problems? Unless confidentiality can be guaranteed, such patients may not seek out the care they need. If confidentiality is protected, such patients may not get the parental counseling and support from which they could also benefit. Considerable confusion exists about the morally appropriate and legally mandated approach to confidentiality of information involving adolescent patients (Holder; Morrissey et al.). Equally troubling are cases involving elderly patients who are less than fully competent but far from totally demented. Families of such patients often ask physicians to provide them with information about the patient's condition, information that they may not want to share with the patient. Such a request may be perfectly appropriate for the clearly incompetent demented patient, whereas it is obviously inappropriate for normal geriatric patients. How to handle cases that fall between these two extremes is unclear.

Informed Consent

The principle of informed consent is a much more recently articulated principle than the principle of confidentiality; the actual phrase "informed consent" first appeared in 1957 in the court case *Salgo* v. *Leland Stanford Jr. University Board of Trustees*. It has come, however, to be accepted as a fundamental principle governing the relation between patients and physicians.

The principle's basic mandate is that a physician must obtain the free and informed consent of a patient, if the patient is competent to give that consent, or of the patient's surrogate, if the patient is not competent, before medical treatment is provided. Two exceptions are normally recognized. The first (the *emergency exception*) is invoked when emergency treatment is necessary to protect the patient's life or health and consent cannot be obtained in a timely fashion. The second (the *therapeutic privilege*) is invoked when there is strong reason to believe that the very attempt to obtain consent will be harmful to the patient because of the psychologic impact of the information conveyed (Rozovsky).

Several complementary accounts of the significance of the principle of informed consent are available. One stresses the clinical benefits (in terms of building trust and obtaining compliance) from a therapeutic regimen begun as a result of a joint patient–physician decision rather than as a result of a unilateral physician decision. The other stresses the patient's right to control what happens to his or her body; the resulting obligation of the physician to obtain informed consent is the way in which the physician respects this right.

The standard practice in many institutions is to obtain written documentation of informed consent primarily (if not exclusively) in cases of invasive procedures. This practice should not be understood to mean that the principle of informed consent does not apply to other medical interventions; it applies to all of them. Signed consent forms are merely written evidence of the informed consent already obtained, and the practice reflects the prudent desire to obtain written documentation in cases in which potential liability is highest. Informed consent, as opposed to the written documentation of that consent, should be obtained in all cases, both as a way of obtaining clinical benefits and as a way of respecting patient's rights.

There has been considerable disagreement about the amount and type of information that must be supplied to the patient. Obviously, only a portion of the relevant information known by the physician can be conveyed to the patient. Moreover, any attempt to provide too much information may result in the physician overwhelming and confusing the patient. Some selection of information is required, and the disagreement centers around which principle of selection to adopt.

Two different proposals have been adopted by America's courts (Rozovsky). The first is the *professional practice standard*, which maintains that a consent is informed if the patient has been provided the information that reasonable medical practitioners would normally provide under similar circumstances. The second is the *rea-*

TABLE 3-1. ELEMENTS OF INFORMED CONSENT UNDER REASONABLE PERSON STANDARD

Nature of the patient's condition (e.g., hypertension)

Description of the treatment proposed (e.g., particular medication)

Benefits of proposed treatment (e.g., control of hypertension and resulting lowering of risk of disease)

Risks of proposed treatment (e.g., side effects for that medication)

Alternatives (e.g., other medications, diet and exercise, no intervention)

Costs of proposed treatment

Source: From Rakel RE. Textbook of Family Practice, 4th ed. Philadelphia, W.B. Saunders, 1990. *(Reprinted with permission.)*

sonable person standard, which maintains that a consent is informed if the patient has been provided the information that a reasonable person would need to have in order to make a decision about whether to undergo the therapy in question. The information to be provided would presumably fall under the categories shown in Table 3–1.

Most commentators have argued for the second standard, since it better corresponds to the goals of informed consent, but a majority of courts have adopted the usually less demanding professional practice standard (Rozovsky). Clinicians are, we believe, best advised to adopt the usually more stringent reasonable person standard, since it provides all the clinical and moral benefits of obtaining informed consent while firmly ensuring that the legal requirement of informed consent is satisfied. Clinicians also must be careful to provide that information using terminology that patients are likely to understand.

A very difficult problem arises when one is dealing with patients whose competency is impaired. Informed consent is obtained from the patient when the patient is clearly competent and from the patient's surrogate (a legally appointed guardian, if available, or the closest family member) if the patient is clearly incompetent. What, however, should one do when the patient's mental capacities are clearly impaired but present to some degree? This problem is partially alleviated when one remembers that the assessment of the patient's competency is not an assessment of the patient's total ability to manage all his or her affairs; it is just the assessment of whether at this movement the patient can (1) receive the information relevant to giving or refusing informed consent for this particular treatment, (2) remember that information, (3) appropriately assess and use that information to make a decision, and (4) make a decision (Brody). Although no formal test exists to ensure that the patient has the capacity to perform items 1 to 4 in the list, a careful discussion with the patient will usually enable the physician to ascertain whether these criteria are satisfied. If doubt remains, one should obtain consent from both the patient and the surrogate.

A second difficulty involves teenage patients. Informed consent is obtained from parents before one treats children, but from patients once they become adults. How should physicians treat teenage patients? Most states have passed special laws allowing physicians to treat them after obtaining only their consent when (1) the treatment is for venereal disease, pregnancy or contraception, or drug-related problems, (2) they are living away from their parents and are responsible for their own affairs, or (3) they are married. Other cases (particularly abortion) are more problematic (Holder; Morrissey et al.).

The Noncompliant Patient

Implicit in the principle of informed consent, the principle that medical treatment can only be provided after the patient has freely and knowingly consented to it, is the concept that a patient may choose not to comply with the physician's recommendations and that the choice not to comply must be respected. This concept can easily be misunderstood, however, leading to a quick and facile acceptance of a patient's noncompliance before its meaning is properly understood.

Several studies of noncompliance (Applebaum and Roth; Connelly and Campbell) have indicated that the majority of cases of noncompliance involve failures of communication, lack of trust due to previous bad experiences with the physician in question or others, and psychologic and psychopathologic factors. Only a minority of cases involve a true value difference between the physician and the patient. This finding has profound implications for the clinical management of noncompliance. Physicians confronting noncompliant patients need to assess the noncompliance, evaluate its cause, and react appropriately. Table 3–2 indicates how such a noncompliance assessment would proceed. In short, morality does not call on the physician to accept at face value every episode of noncompliance on the part of the patient. Doing so may in fact constitute a form of disrespect for the patient. What morality does call for is a full evaluation of the cause of the noncompliance, appropriate responses, where possible, to eliminate the cause, and respect for the patient's noncompliance only when it is an informed and competent refusal that is based on a difference between the patient's and the physician's values.

Even in those cases in which noncompliance represents an informed and competent refusal of the physician's recommendations because the patient's values differ, there may well exist alternative, second-best forms

TABLE 3-2. EVALUATION OF NONCOMPLIANCE

CAUSE	CLINICAL RESPONSE
Problem in communication	Patient should be reinformed about the need for treatment
Failure of trust	Address question of mistrust Involve other physicians who may be trusted
Psychologic factors	Treat anxiety, depression, and so on
Value conflict	Respect patient wishes

Source: From Rakel RE. Textbook of Family Practice, 4th ed. Philadelphia, W.B. Saunders, 1990. *(Reprinted with permission.)*

of treatment that could be mutually acceptable. Consider a patient who refuses to stay in a hospital for a full evaluation because the patient is concerned about the need to be home to handle personal problems. Such a patient should be scheduled for an outpatient evaluation, even if it is not as satisfactory as a full evaluation in the hospital. (More examples of such compromises are provided later.) Respecting patient values in cases of noncompliance is not a matter of letting the patient win a power struggle; it is, more often, finding a mutually acceptable (even though not necessarily optimal) course of action. A failure to seek out such alternatives may often represent a lack of respect for the patient.

A form of noncompliance that deserves special attention is the patient who does not fill the prescription the physician writes. This is sometimes due to the patient's financial condition. The optimal medication, from the physician's perspective, may cost too much from the patient's perspective. Particularly when dealing with patients who have high medication bills because they need so many drugs or with patients who have very limited means, physicians should raise the question of cost frankly and explore less expensive but satisfactory (even if not optimal) medications.

A similar problem often arises when one considers the question of side effects of various drugs. Different patients with different values and different tolerances may find certain side effects unacceptable. The physician should certainly not assume that a pattern of side effects that is acceptable to the physician will be acceptable to the patient. An important recent study (Croog et al.) has stressed the significance of these matters in connection with the choice of antihypertensive agents, considering the implications of different agents for sexual dysfunction. Taking the patient's values into account in deciding which antihypertensive medication to order is a far clearer example of respecting the patient's values than simply accepting a patient's noncompliance with a prescription for a particular antihypertensive medication. This point can, of course, be generalized to other cases.

SPECIAL PROBLEMS IN TERTIARY CARE SETTINGS

Quality of care can be improved by careful attention to the components examined thus far: the physician–patient relation, medicine as a profession, confidentiality, informed consent, and the promotion of patient compliance. When the focus shifts from primary care provided by the family physician to care provided by subspecialists in tertiary care settings, new problems arise and old problems become even more complicated. The next two sections examine ways of resolving some of these problems.

Referrals

Decisions regarding referrals and consultations (see Chapter 15 of Rakel, *Textbook of Family Practice,* for the distinction between referrals and consultations) are often accompanied by great confusion. Referrals to subspecialists practicing in tertiary care institutions can provoke anxiety on the part of patients. The referring physician risks losing a patient and a substantial amount of money and is subject to embarrassment if a mistake is discovered. Referrals sometimes degenerate into power struggles between subspecialists and generalists. Because primary care is a community-based discipline, there is much debate and little consensus as to the primary care physician's role in the tertiary care setting (Christie and Hoffmaster). The following guidelines about appropriate referrals and about continuity through referrals are intended to help clarify these responsibilities and thus ease the tension and improve the quality of care.

Decisions to use consultants should be based on a realistic assessment of the potentialities and limitations of family medicine as a discipline, of onself as a physician, and of the facilities available in one's geographic region. Unfortunately, a number of other factors (financial and institutional as well as medical) often cloud the decision-making process and disrupt relations between primary and tertiary care physicians (Weiss).

Many subspecialists in oversubscribed areas have taken it upon themselves to practice primary care as a means of bolstering their incomes, despite their inadequate training in this area (Sigel and Sigel; Aiken et al.; Gillette). Conversely, primary care physicians sometimes feel pressured to go beyond their areas of expertise for financial and professional reasons: They fear losing the patient and the income and fear that their seeking consultation might reinforce the misconception that primary care physicians are inferior (Perkoff; Weary; Sussman et al.).

Knowing when to use consultants requires courage and humility. Courage is the ability to act competently and wisely without being swayed by irrational fears. Some primary care physicians, motivated by unrealistic fears of mistakes and exposure, refer too early. Humility, on the other hand, is the willingness to recognize one's *actual* limitations and to act accordingly. Some primary care physicians, unaware of their limitations, refer too late. A proper combination of courage and humility, along with good working relationships with subspecialists, can prevent most of the problems involved in referring or seeking consultation too early or too late.

Even if the primary care physician does decide to refer the patient, he or she remains the patient's primary physician (Christie and Hoffmaster). Equipped with a strong knowledge of general medicine, of the patient's medical history, and of the patient's personal traits, and committed to treating the disease in the context of the person and the person in the context of the family, the primary care physician is ideally suited to manage the patient throughout the referral.

When initiating a referral, the primary care physician's responsibilities are to educate the patient as to the reasons for referral, to recommend a subspecialist or treatment center best suited to the patient's medical and personal needs, to prepare the patient for what lies ahead, and to provide the specialist with data relevant to the patient's illness. Even after the referral, the primary care physician remains responsible for the quality of the patient's care. This may require translating medical jargon to patients or patient preferences to subspecialists and hospital staff, coordinating the activities of the various consultants, mediating disputes between consultants, ensuring that confidentiality is maintained by the health care team, and counseling patients and their families. The referral process is not complete until the subspecialist and the primary physician have discussed all findings, treatments, results, and recommendations and the patient has discussed these with the primary care physician (Christie and Hoffmaster; McPhee et al.; Rakel and Williamson).

Sometimes subspecialists disagree as to how to manage a particular disorder. Consider the different way that surgeons and cardiologists may treat carotid artery disease. Or consider the range of approaches, within particular subspecialties, in treating certain disorders: differences among gynecologists regarding indications for a hysterectomy and differences among neonatologists in managing severely handicapped infants. This makes the referring physician's task a difficult and delicate one. The referring physician must be aware of the differences between subspecialties and between particular physicians within a subspecialty. The referring physician must know the patient and the patient's family well enough to recommend the appropriate subspecialist. In many cases, the principle of informed consent will mandate that the referring physician educate the patient and the family to the strengths and weaknesses of the available options. Primary care physicians should help their patients find a subspecialist who will be appropriate to both their medical needs and their personal preferences (Froom et al.).

Financial Gatekeeping

The soaring costs of health care have led corporations and government agencies to develop prospective payment systems and capitation plans, with primary care physicians often serving as gatekeepers of the health care network. It is hoped that this will save money and streamline the referral process. On the other hand, this might drive a bureaucratic wedge into the physician–patient relationship, allow money to compete with quality in determining the standard of care, and inhibit the physician's freedom to practice an individualized style of medicine.

Prospective reimbursement systems (such as the Medicare diagnosis-related group system) save money by limiting the reimbursement available to physicians, thereby encouraging them to do less. Designers of such systems have the legitimate right to require physicians to avoid wasteful procedures and referrals; this prevents unnecessary expenditures and ensures a more just distribution of health care expenditures. Such limitations do not, however, preclude the physician's responsibility to offer the patient the best possible care within the limitations set by those policies. When particular patients require care in excess of the normal level of reimburse-

ment, the primary care physician confronts a major ethical dilemma.

Considerable controversy exists as to whether physicians should do everything that they believe may benefit each patient without regard to costs or other societal considerations (Levinsky) or whether physicians must not be allowed to ignore the bottom line (Aaron and Schwartz). Traditionalists tend to ignore the fact that financial considerations have always limited the quality of care available to the poor. The question we are now confronting is whether these considerations may legitimately limit the quality of care available to everyone.

In caring for individual patients, physicians should distinguish between providing what the patient wants and what the patient needs. The controversy concerns whether all procedures and services likely to benefit the patient—as evidenced by outcome data—should be made available to the patient. When patients request unnecessary or marginally beneficial procedures and services, however, physicians must refuse.

It is often recommended (Fried) that if societal costs necessitate that care be withdrawn from or limited for certain patients, these decisions must be made not at the bedside but at the policy level, prior to and apart from particular situations and applications. Such difficult policy decisions should not be made by physicians alone but should be negotiated at the policy level by the three major competing parties in the health care delivery system: institutional representatives, whose concern it is that the bills be paid; physicians, whose interest is professional integrity and personal income; and patients, who want the best care and the maximum choice at the lowest price (Pellegrino and Thomasma). It is an open question whether these recommendations are reasonable, realistic, and appropriate (Brody).

THE PHYSICIAN AS HUMAN BEING

The medical profession has, in the past few decades, achieved truly impressive gains in the battle against sickness, suffering, and death. Diseases that killed their victims just a generation ago are now manageable, curable, or even preventable. Yet physicians seem remarkably inept at maintaining their own health and well-being; they suffer high rates of alcoholism, substance abuse, divorce, burnout, and suicide (Hilfiker; Jonsen). Why can't the healers heal themselves, and what can they do to get on the road to recovery? To deal with these problems, we recommend that physicians learn to distinguish between competence and perfectionism, dedication and "workaholism," and compassion and sentimentalism.

In medical school and residency, young doctors often learn to put their careers ahead of self and family (Gerber). This dedication is, in some ways, good. Young physicians want to do everything they can to help their patients. But this is often coupled with an unrealistic perception of their capabilities and those of their profession. They allow their egos to become too closely identified with their successes and failures. They become obsessed with insecurity (they are not good enough) and guilt (they do not work hard enough). They worry that they might have missed a diagnosis and fear that their patients will die or suffer unnecessarily. Physicians are not supposed to make mistakes, but they do. Their profession requires staying on top of an ever-expanding field of knowledge, adeptness at a wide range of techniques and skills, making the right decision when fatigued or hassled or angry, picking up on subtle clues or poorly articulated symptoms, and juggling a plethora of human needs at once. Mistakes are inevitable, but talking about them is taboo. The only place mistakes are openly discussed, it seems, is the courtroom (Hilfiker). To be more effective clinicians, physicians must learn to acknowledge their capacity to err and must learn to discuss errors in a constructive manner. Physicians who do not admit their mistakes are doomed to repeat them. Physicians who discuss their mistakes can learn from them and experience healing in the process.

The physician who takes the time to care for personal and family needs is a more effective clinician because he or she is better able to cope with the stresses and strains of a demanding profession. And, in the case of primary care physicians whose patients know them well, the physician will become a role model for personal health and fitness.

Another area in which physicians must learn to accept their humanity, and the humanity of their patients, is in the area of emotions. Clinicians must help patients recognize, express, and interpret their emotions. Clinicians must become aware of their own emotions, recognize their clinical value, and learn how to express and interpret them. The physician who ignores the emotions dehumanizes the physician–patient relationship. The primary care physician who improperly expresses, utilizes, or interprets emotional factors deprofessionalizes that relationship (Zinn; Frankel; Katz). Traditionally, physicians have been trained to maintain objectivity, affective neutrality, and clinical detachment. To be scientific, however, does not preclude recognizing the legitimacy of emotions or the necessity of empathy as a legitimate clinical and moral response to suffering. Sometimes a patient's feelings offer a clue to his or her symptoms. Sometimes a physician's feelings in response to a patient offer a clue to the patient's problem (Zinn). Suffering patients need a physician who will suffer alongside them and who will help them to express and interpret their feelings (Reich). When their patients suffer, physicians suffer too. The physician who suffers alongside a suffering patient or family allows the opportunity for healing of self as well as of the patient or family. Many of the physician's feelings, however, cannot be expressed appropriately in the clinical encounter. To maintain personal well-being, therefore, the physician must find appropriate outlets for expression and interpretation. Balint groups, support groups, and case conferences can serve this function, along with informal conversations with colleagues, staff, spouses, and friends. Many physicians find outlets for expression and interpretation through the arts. Some keep journals, some write stories or poems, and some fulfill this need through painting, photography, or drama.

The ethical questions faced by physicians have been transformed, in ways we have indicated, by changing economic, social, legal, and political factors. In the end, however, the ethics of medicine remains committed to a view of the patient–physician relationship as a relationship between two autonomous human beings—a patient who is suffering and seeks help and a physician who maintains his or her humanity as well as his or her professionalism.

REFERENCES

Aaron H, Schwartz W. The Painful Prescription: Rationing Hospital Care. Washington, Brookings Institute, 1984.

Aiken, LH, Lewis CE, Craig J, et al. The contributions of specialists to the delivery of primary care: A new perspective. N Engl J Med 1979; 300:1363–1370.

Alexander E Jr. A "truth in mending" act (commentary). JAMA 1980; 243:1239–1240.

Applebaum P, Roth L. Patients who refuse treatment in medical hospitals. JAMA 1983; 250:1296–1301.

Brody BA. Life and Death Decision Making. New York, Oxford University Press, 1988.

Bruce JA. Privacy and Confidentiality of Health Care Information. Chicago, American Hospital Association, 1984.

Christie RJ, Hoffmaster CB. Ethical Issues in Family Medicine. New York, Oxford University Press, 1986.

Connelly J, Campbell C. Patients who refuse treatment in medical offices. Arch Intern Med 1987; 147:1829–1833.

Croog S, et al. Sexual symptoms in hypertensive patients. Arch Intern Med 1988; 148:788–794.

Dickens BM. Legal limits of AIDS confidentiality. JAMA 1988; 259:3449–3451.

Frankel BL. Affective neutrality (a piece of my mind). JAMA 1986; 256:515.

Fried C. Rights and health care—Beyond equity and efficiency. N Engl J Med 1975; 293:241–245.

Froom J, Feinbloom RI, Rosen MG. Risks of referral. J Fam Pract 1984; 18:623–626.

Gerber LA. Married to Their Careers: Career and Family Dilemmas in Doctors' Lives. New York, Tavistock Publications, 1983.

Gillette RD. The delivery of "primary care" by specialists. N Engl J Med 1979; 301:893–894.

Hilfiker D. A Physician Looks at His Work. New York, Pantheon Books, 1985.

Holder A. Legal Issues in Pediatrics and Adolescent Medicine. New Haven, Conn., Yale University Press, 1985.

Holleman WL, Holleman MC. School and work release evaluations. JAMA 1988; 260:3629–3634.

Holleman WL, Matson CC. Preemployment evaluations: Dilemmas for the family physician. J Am Board Fam Pract 1991; 4:95–101.

Jonsen AR, Siegler M, Winslade WJ. Clinical Ethics: A Practical Approach to Ethical Decisions in Clinical Medicine, 2d ed. New York, Macmillan, 1986.

Jonsen AR. Watching the doctor. N Engl J Med 1983; 308:1531–1535.

Katz RL. Empathy: Its Nature and Uses. London, The Free Press of Glencoe, Collier-Macmillan, 1963.

Kelman GR. The preemployment medical examination. Lancet 1985; 2:1231–1233.

Levinsky NG. The doctor's master. N Engl J Med 1984; 311:1573–1575.

McPhee SJ, Lo B, Saika GY, Meltzer R. How good is communication between primary care physicians and subspecialty consultants? (special report). Arch Intern Med 1984; 144:1265–1268.

Mills M, Sullivan G, Eth S. Protecting third parties: A decade after Tarasoff. Am J Psychiatry 1987; 144:68–74.

Morrissey J, Hofmann A, Thrope J. Consent and Confidentiality in the Health Care of Children and Adolescents. New York, The Free Press, 1986.

Pellegrino EG, Thomasma DC. A Philosophical Basis of Medical Practice: Toward a Philosophy and Ethic of the Healing Professions. New York, Oxford University Press, 1981.

Perkoff GT. Ethical aspects of the physician surplus: Implications for family practice. J Fam Pract 1986; 22:455–460.

Rakel RE. Use of consultants. In Rakel RE (ed.): Textbook of Family Practice, 4th ed. Philadelphia, W.B. Saunders, 1990, pp. 247–258.

Reich WT. Speaking of suffering: A moral account of compassion. Soundings 1989; 72:83–108.

Rosenstock L, Hagopian A. Ethical dilemmas in providing health care to workers. Ann Intern Med 1987; 107:575–580.

Rozovsky F. Consent to Treatment: A Practical Guide. Boston, Little, Brown, 1984.

Siegler M. The progression of medicine: From physician paternalism to patient autonomy to bureaucratic parsimony. Arch Intern Med 1985; 145:713.

Sigel L, Sigel B. The role of subspecialists in primary medical care. Perspect Biol Med 1980; 24:122–128.

Smith HL, Churchill LR. Professional Ethics and Primary Care Medicine: Beyond Dilemmas and Decorum. Durham, N.C., Duke University Press, 1986.

Sussman EJ, Tsiaras WG, Soper KA. Diagnosis of diabetic eye disease. JAMA 1982; 247:3231–3234.

Tarasoff v. Regents of California 118 Cal. Rptr. 129 (1974).

Weary PE. Behold, the gatekeeper cometh (commentary). Int J Dermatol 1984; 23:33–35.

Weiss BD. Family practice in hospitals (commentary). JAMA 1985; 253:549–550.

Weiss BD. The effect of malpractice insurance costs on family physicians' hospital practices. J Fam Pract 1986; 23:55–58.

Whiting RK. The anxious manipulator and disability (letter). J Occup Med 1977; 19:655.

Zinn WM. Doctors have feelings too. JAMA 1988; 259:3296–3298.

QUESTIONS

1. What does it mean to say that medicine is a "relationship" and a "profession"?

2. Why is respect for patient autonomy important, and how far should a physician go in respecting patient autonomy?

3. In what ways can third parties interfere with the physician–patient relationship, and what can the physician do to balance properly the relation with the patient and competing third parties?

4. Why is it important to maintain confidentiality in the physician–patient relationship? Under what circumstances should the protection of confidentiality take a back seat to other concerns?

5. What are the two major exceptions to standard informed consent practices? Which two standards are usually invoked in determining how much information to tell the patient?

6. What are some of the major causes of noncompliance? What strategies should be used in caring for such patients?

7. What are the referring physician's responsibilities toward the patient after referral?

8. What are the advantages and disadvantages of prospective reimbursement systems, and what can the family physician do to mitigate the disadvantages?

9. What factors contribute to perfectionism, "workaholism," and alcoholism among physicians, and what can medical students, residents, and physicians do to maintain good physical, emotional, and spiritual health?

Answers are in the text.

4

FAMILY DYNAMICS

MICHAEL A. CROUCH and DONALD S. WILLIAMSON

Understanding what goes on in families can help physicians take better care of patients. Family dynamics reflect and influence the physical, mental, and spiritual health of the individuals in a family. Physicians who understand these interactions within families and between families and society can take better care of their patients.

All happy families are alike; every unhappy family is unhappy in its own way.

TOLSTOY

All happy families are more or less dissimilar; all unhappy families are more or less alike.

NABOKOV

Physicians who follow the same patients over long periods of time come to understand what led Tolstoy and Nabokov to make their paradoxical observations. At one extreme, happy families radiate a sense of integrity and caring. Adult members espouse and live by clear human values, express feelings appropriately, communicate effectively, and share power while negotiating decisions. All family members—children, adolescents, and adults—are encouraged to develop their own life goals and emotional independence while staying connected with the family as a whole. Happy families cope relatively well with adversity, often coming out of a crisis stronger for the experience. Thus happy families tend to have a similar atmosphere and ability to function well, even under increased levels of stress. Individual happy families differ widely, however, in how they organize and conduct family life, and their members tend toward a healthy diversity in many ways.

Instead of integrity, unhappy families radiate a sense of chaos or rigidity, reflecting a high level of chronic underlying anxiety. Despite this, unhappy families can be caring when life circumstances are calm. When such families are stressed, however, their members tend to shift quickly into counterproductive modes of clinging, assaulting, or escaping. When the levels of individual and family anxiety rise, emotional reactions tend to override rational responses. Family members may adopt personal values from authority figures, such as parents or clergy, or from friends and other peers without considering their logical and emotional consistency. Alternatively, family members may form values by reacting in opposition to the espoused or actual values of influential people, again without critical analysis of their merits and drawbacks. At one extreme of emotionality, members of unhappy families may experience and express intense feelings, many of which are negative. This style creates a heated family atmosphere. At the opposite extreme, family members may shut off, blunt, or hide their feelings, creating a cold atmosphere. Communication tends to be chaotic, rigid, or sparse, paralyzing decision-making processes and creating coercive power differentials between spouses and among family members.

Unhappy families tend to view individual differences and independence as disloyalty that threatens their precarious survival. Because of their marginal emotional reserve, such families have great difficulty dealing with stressors, expected or unexpected. Despite their numerous liabilities, many unhappy families have an admirable spirit of dogged persistence in the face of generations of trials and sorrow. Physicians who appreciate this fortitude can be very helpful to such families and can derive great satisfaction from serving as a needed advocate and ally.

The preceding discussion assumes that families can be validly sorted into two dichotomous categories. Various labels have been used for this purpose: good versus bad, and functional versus dysfunctional, and so on. Reality, however, is more complicated. Most families exhibit fluctuating mixtures of happy and unhappy features. For this reason, the majority of families have been referred to by researchers and family therapists as "midrange families." Each midrange family has its own strengths and vulnerabilities. Physicians can be most effective by helping families capitalize on their strengths and deal with their vulnerabilities in healthier ways.

It has become fashionable to regard virtually all families as dysfunctional, particularly with respect to co-dependency. Such pejorative labeling unnecessarily stigmatizes the average human experience. A more objective, systemic view would be that families do the best they can with their genetic endowment, social learning, and life circumstances. Physicians can sometimes be most helpful by encouraging patients to think and feel less judgmental about their own families while learning to handle family problems more responsibly.

Preconceptions about the general nature of the family have limited usefulness and are fraught with hazards. Assuming that unverified generalizations, especially negative stereotypes, apply to the unique family dynamics of a particular patient may interfere with attempts to understand and help that individual. Some common generalizations involve the nature and purposes of the family.

DEFINITION OF FAMILY

Many definitions of family are based on normative values of heterosexuality, marriage, and reproduction. Such definitions overlook numerous nonnormative family forms that have existed in most cultures for thousands of years. More varied family forms have become much more common in the last half of the 20th century. In fact, the stereotypical nuclear family, consisting of a breadwinner father, homemaker mother, and one or more nonadult biologic offspring, is present in only 7% of all households in the United States. One simple, broad definition of family is as "a significant group of intimates with a history and a future [together]" (Ransom and Vandervoort). This embraces virtually any group that might think of itself as "family." A more complicated definition (Ramsey and Lewis) refers to the multigenerational emotional system:

The family is a small social system made up of individuals related to each other, biologically or by reason of strong affections and loyalty, that comprises a permanent household (or cluster of households) and persists over decades. . . . The operative emotional field of the family at any given moment may include three generations.

Although this definition assumes more permanence than is seen in many families, people usually form new families with the intention of maintaining them long term. Even after two people are divorced, the emotional field of a newly constituted family includes the former partners, particularly if children are involved. For individuals who know little or nothing about their parents or grandparents, mysterious attitudes about the family's past often perpetuate current problems.

PURPOSES OF THE FAMILY

The family has been viewed idealistically as the "key link in the chain of being" (Nisbet). In contrast, it has been portrayed cynically as an "institution for the systematic production of physical and mental illness in its members" (Montagu). One major purpose of the family is to help its members satisfy their needs for physical and emotional survival. Some families have difficulty providing for basic physical needs—food, clothing, and shelter. Obtaining health care for illness is problematic for many more families. If basic physical needs are not well met, emotional needs are very unlikely to be met adequately.

THE FAMILY EMOTIONAL SYSTEM

In general, the more intense and precarious a family's struggle to meet basic needs, the less likely it is that fam-

ily members will trust others and feel loved. Material and financial security, however, does not guarantee fulfillment of emotional needs. Emotional development is strongly influenced by general human tendencies and the particular circumstances in one's family of origin. Family members are connected by emotion, so the family is essentially an emotional system. All family members participate in and are influenced by what has been called "family emotionality" (Bowen).

Multigenerational Family Anxiety

Family members seek to meet their needs mainly through interactions heavily influenced by two opposite emotional urges. The desire to be emotionally close to one's spouse or lover, parents, and children probably derives from the reproductive urge and biologic bonding, as well as from the material survival advantages of the small group. On the other hand, the urge to be a separate and somewhat autonomous individual is a logical extension of the self-preservation instinct, seen in other animal species as territoriality and aggression. Exaggeration of either preference can unbalance the behavior of a given individual or family. In American society, women have been socialized toward togetherness with their children and with other women, whereas men have been encouraged to seek separateness through work and competitive sports. The extreme outcome for a woman is the "supermom," who is overinvested in her children and who lacks societally valued job skills. The extreme outcome for a man is the "workaholic," who is distant from his wife and children because of work and who meets some of his togetherness needs by watching or playing sports or drinking with other men during what leisure time he allows himself.

Human beings tend to have considerable trouble integrating their rational thoughts with their feelings. This is especially true in difficult situations that evoke strong emotions. Some families appear better able to foster the necessary maturity to temper emotion with reason, even under stress. Likewise, such families can allow feelings to guide reason when this is appropriate. Members of these families have relatively little chronic anxiety, and they tend to cope well with acute anxiety. Members of families that have lived with high levels of anxiety for generations become acutely more anxious with less provocation and do not cope well with stress.

Although acute anxiety commands more attention, chronic anxiety probably influences health more adversely in the long run. In this discussion, the term "chronic anxiety" denotes a vague mental dissonance and uneasiness, of which the individual is often not fully aware. This definition (Bowen) differs from the conventional definition of anxiety. The physiologic alterations and pathophysiologic changes accompanying chronic anxiety are more subtle unless they are compounded by overlapping acute anxiety or the development of a more tangible manifestation, such as peptic ulcer disease.

Family therapists (Bowen, Kerr) have described numerous ways in which individuals and families experience and express chronic anxiety. Physicians see many people who develop physical and mental symptoms as manifestations of their chronic anxiety about their home life and work situations. Depression, headaches, irritable bowel syndrome, sleep disorders, and chronic fatigue are among the most common stress-related health problems.

Difficulties with intimate relationships are another predictable mode for experiencing anxiety. Individuals tend to select partners whose levels of chronic anxiety and intellectual–emotional maturity are similar to their own. Much of the time emotional reactions preempt the formulation of more thoughtful responses to the actions and perceived slights of others. Individuals with higher levels of chronic anxiety tend to become overinvolved with each other emotionally. Their sense of self relies too much on the approval and co-dependency of their partner.

Especially early in the history of a relationship, overinvolvement may look and feel quite positive ("being in love"). Each individual may overfunction in certain ways that benefit the partnership (work outside the home, domestic work, parenting) while underfunctioning in other respects (drinking too much, mismanaging finances). Eventually, one or both partners suffer from a lack of emotional breathing space. They may get into nonproductive conflict more quickly, more often, and more intensely. At the other extreme, some anxious persons go to great lengths to avoid conflict, perhaps because of a fear of being abandoned if they openly express their negative feelings. In either event, important issues remain unresolved.

Distancing from others emotionally is another way of handling one's anxiety. Historically, men have been more likely than women to distance themselves from other family members, both while they live in the household and after leaving the household through separation or divorce. Completely cutting off communication with one's parent, child, or sibling signals severe chronic anxiety, usually about particularly "toxic" family issues that have been passed along for several generations.

Events and situations from a family's past continue to influence succeeding generations. Someone whose grandmother had diabetes mellitus with severe complications such as blindness, amputations, and kidney failure may be genetically predisposed to developing diabetes. Knowing about this risk often generates considerable fear about one's own vulnerability to disability and early death. Patients who openly acknowledge their fear may make more conscientious efforts to avoid becoming overweight. Successfully maintaining a healthy weight status can, in turn, keep their level of anxiety down. In contrast, many patients who deny their vulnerability to diabetes become increasingly obese and develop a variety of somatic symptoms (back pain, headaches) that mask underlying depression. Physicians who focus on the somatic symptoms without exploring their meaning miss both the depression and the fear of developing diabetes. Astute physicians who explore patients' attitudes about personal health can help decrease the likelihood that emotional factors will trigger the emergence of diabetes or other serious illnesses to which such patients are predisposed. Probing patients'

beliefs about such chronic problems as hypertension also can pave the way for improved health care outcomes (e.g., better control of blood pressure and prevention of stroke).

Psychosocial events in a family's past also may affect the health of family members. If a woman and her mother both became pregnant as unmarried teenagers, the woman may show ambivalence about her teenage daughter's emerging sexuality. Hypervigilance by the mother may actually increase the daughter's likelihood of repeating the family pattern of teenage pregnancy, as well as her risk of acquiring sexually transmitted diseases or of developing sexual dysfunction. Sexual and physical abuse often occur in successive generations of families as expressions of anxiety and troubled relationships. Women in unhappy marriages often visit physicians for minor somatic symptoms. Women abused first by their fathers or mothers and then by their husbands have difficulty admitting the abuse to physicians and find it even harder to terminate abusive relationships. The prospect of divorce may be a difficult issue for families with strong religious values and no previous experience with marital dissolution or for families with many failed marriages.

Triangulation in Families

Anxiety tends to escalate when two-person relationships are stressed by life circumstances. Sometimes anxiety is diminished or redistributed by involving a third person in the dyadic relationship ("triangling"). A child may become a referee or peacemaker for his or her parents' conflictual marriage. In some families, a child develops worsening symptoms of a physical illness such as asthma when conflict occurs, distracting attention from the conflict. In more dysfunctional families, a child may be blamed for the family's problems and treated harshly as a scapegoat. Another common form of triangling is the extramarital affair, which can restabilize a precarious family system or precipitate marital separation and divorce, depending on what the participants learn about themselves from the experience. Substance abuse may be a form of triagulation. The workaholic may use work as the third point of a triangle with his or her spouse. (This tendency is common among physicians.)

ASSESSING FAMILY DYNAMICS

Family composition and structure can be elicited quickly with pertinent questions on a health history questionnaire or by doing a genogram (Crouch). A genogram is a biopsychosocial family tree. It records considerable information about family illnesses and also shows the clinician where the family is in its life cycle. Vulnerable life-cycle phases include middle-aged parents with teenage children, adolescents leaving the home, and aging and dying grandparents.

A genogram can be drawn in skeletal form during one of the first few visits—ideally the first visit—and then it can be elaborated as indicated during subsequent visits (see Chap. 14). The genogram often reveals important family patterns of illness, disease, and psychosocial problems (Fig. 4–1). The longevity of male and female members of previous and current generations provides clues to the genetic vulnerability of family members to life-threatening illness. Information about the occurrences of heart disease, cancer, depression and anxiety disorders, alcohol or other substance abuse, and physical or sexual abuse is especially meaningful to the care of patients. A self-administered form of the genogram (Rogers) can save the physician time. However, because much of the value of the genogram derives from the doctor–patient communication process it fosters, the self-administered genogram is weaker in terms of its ability to help the physician generate hypotheses and therapeutic attitudes. This disadvantage can be partially overcome if the physician conducts a focused personal follow-up discussion.

Many primary care patients would benefit from discussing family or work problems with their physician, but they seldom bring these problems up spontaneously. Screening for patient dissatisfaction with family and work can be done efficiently by including the five questions from the Family System APGAR test (Smilkstein) on the intake questionnaire, along with similar questions about work (Figs. 4–2 and 4–3). Although some individuals minimize or deny their problems, those under severe stress usually acknowledge their difficulties and discuss them.

TIME-EFFECTIVE FAMILY-ORIENTED MEDICAL COUNSELING

The BATHE Technique

The busy physician can help many patients by applying Stuart and Lieberman's "15-minute hour" method

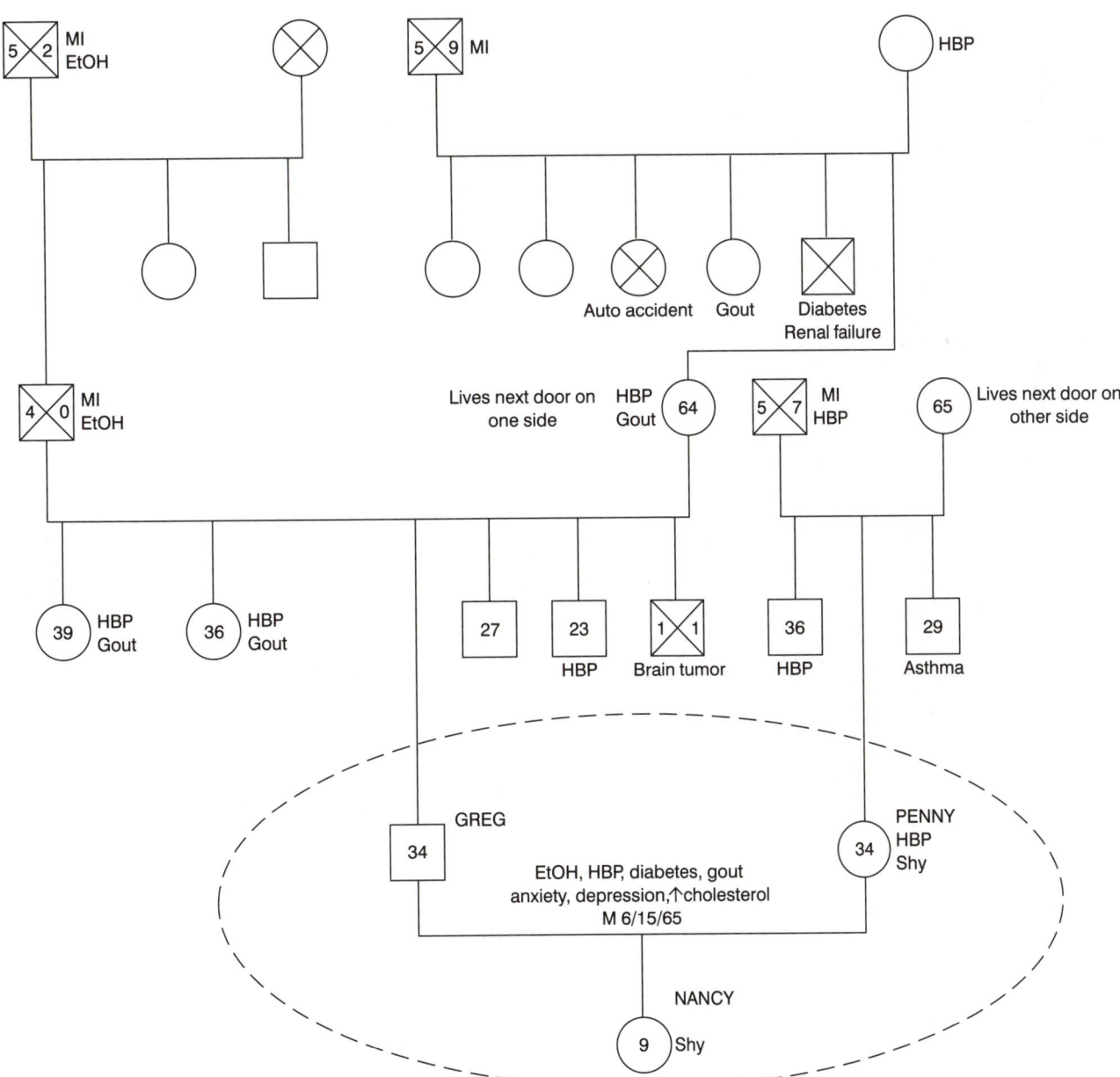

Figure 4–1. Family illness patterns. HBP = high blood pressure; MI = myocardial infarction; EtOH = alcoholism.

FIGURE 4–2. SMILKSTEIN'S FAMILY SYSTEM APGAR ITEMS

	ALMOST ALWAYS	SOME OF THE TIME	HARDLY EVER
1. I am satisfied that I can turn to my family for help when something is troubling me.	_____	_____	_____
2. I am satisfied with the way my family talks over things with me and shares problems with me.	_____	_____	_____
3. I am satisfied that my family accepts and supports my wishes to take on new activities or directions.	_____	_____	_____
4. I am satisfied with the way my family expresses affection and responds to my emotions, such as anger, sorrow, and love.	_____	_____	_____
5. I am satisfied with the way my family and I share time together.	_____	_____	_____

Figure 4–2. Smilkstein's Family System APGAR Items. *Source:* Smilkstein G, Ashworth C, Montano D. Validity and reliability of the Family APGAR as a test of family function. J Fam Pract 1982; 15:303–311. (From Smilkstein G, Ashworth C, Montano D. Validity and reliability of a family APGAR as a test of family function. J Fam Pract 1982; 15:303–311, with permission.)

of primary care counseling. The acronym BATHE (background, affect, trouble, handling, empathy) summarizes the method as follows:

Background: Ask about likely areas of psychosocial problems:

"How are things at *home?*" "At *work?*"
"What's *different* in your life between now and before you got sick?"
"Is anything that hasn't really changed getting to you more lately?"

Affect (Anxiety): Ask about common areas generating strong feelings:

"How do you *feel* about your home life?"
"How do you *feel* about your work/school?"
"How do you *feel* about your life in general?"

Trouble: Ask how much the patient's problems bother him or her:

"What most *worries* you about your life?"
"How *stressed* are you by this problem?"

The symbolic meaning of a symptom is important, so ask:

"What do you think this problem means to you?"

Handling: Problems are often mishandled life difficulties:

"How are you handling the problems in your life?"
"What have you tried to solve the difficulty?"

"How much support are you getting at home/work?"
"Who gives you support for dealing with problems?"

Empathy: Express understanding of the patient's distress:

"That sounds very difficult."
"Terrific!" or "Oh, great!" (empathetic sarcasm)

Using SOAP to BATHE

Physicians can further help patients with emotional and psychological problems by talking in therapeutic ways, summarized by the acronym SOAP (support, objectivity, acceptance, present focus):

Support: Normalize problems as common dilemmas:

"Lots of people struggle with similar problems."

Consider selective physician self-disclosure:

"I've had that problem myself." (Tell brief story.)

Help the patient focus on strengths:

"What resources could you use to deal with this?"

Objectivity: Monitor your emotional responses to patients. Minimize your own reactivity to patient issues. Maintain appropriate professional boundaries (avoiding nontherapeutic self-disclosures). Encourage patients to ask themselves how realistic their thoughts and feelings are (reality test). Elicit their worst fears and put them into perspective:

FIGURE 4–3. SMILKSTEIN'S WORK SYSTEM APGAR ITEMS

	ALMOST ALWAYS	SOME OF THE TIME	HARDLY EVER
1. I am satisfied that I can turn to a fellow worker for help when something is troubling me.	_____	_____	_____
2. I am satisfied with the way my fellow workers talk over things with me and share problems with me.	_____	_____	_____
3. I am satisfied that my fellow workers accept and support my new ideas or thoughts.	_____	_____	_____
4. I am satisfied with the way my fellow workers respond to my emotions, such as anger, sorrow, or laughter.	_____	_____	_____
5. I am satisfied with the way my fellow workers and I share time together.	_____	_____	_____
6. I am satisfied with the way I get along with the person who is my closest or immediate supervisor.	_____	_____	_____
7. I am satisfied with the work I do at my place of employment.	_____	_____	_____

Figure 4–3. Smilkstein's Work System APGAR Items. *Source:* Smilkstein G, Ashworth C, Montano D. Validity and reliability of the Family APGAR as a test of family function. J Fam Pract 1982; 15:303–311. (From Smilkstein G, Ashworth C, Montano D. Validity and reliabililty of the family APGAR as a test of family function. J Fam Pract 1982; 15–303–311, with permission.)

"What's the worst thing that could happen?"
"How likely is that?"

Acceptance: Be as nonjudgmental and accepting as possible:

"That's an understandable way to feel."

Encourage patients to feel better about themselves, their parents, and other family members:

"I think you've done real well considering all the stress."
"Sounds like your parents did the best they could under tough circumstances that were hard for them to survive."

Coach patients to think differently about themselves—more realistically, if they are overly self-critical:

"I wonder if you are being too hard on yourself."
"How much time and energy are you putting into worrying about this?"
"What else could you do with all that time and energy?"

Urge patients to develop more of a sense of humor about their issues:

"I wonder if you could learn to see the humor in this sometimes."

Acknowledge the patient's values and priorities:

"It sounds like family is more important than work to you."

Acknowledge the patient's readiness for change:

"Sounds like you are not quite ready to change."

Acknowledge the difficulty of making changes:

"Change is real hard, and usually pretty scary."

Present Focus: Encourage focusing more on the present, less on the past and future. Help patients identify, explore, and evaluate different attitudinal and behavioral options (including doing nothing):

"How could you cope better?" (reframe problem)
"What could you do different?" (leave or change the situation)
"What are the likely consequences of A versus B?"

Express guarded optimism that the patient can and will do better. Try to set up a positive self-fulfilling prophecy for the immediate future:

"My guess is that if you set your mind to it now, you

can do much better and feel a lot better, and I think you might just do that."

Negotiate a problem-oriented contract for behavioral change; for example, with suicidal patients:

"Would you be willing to repeat this phrase exactly, word for word:
'I promise not to harm myself in any way whatsoever, either accidentally or on purpose, between now and the next time I see you'?"

Suggest a "homework assignment" for the patient to carry out; for example:

a. Practice sending "I" messages:

"I think our vacation plans are too hectic."

b. Practice asking for what you want, rather than just hoping for it:

"I would like more help with the children."

c. Practice telling others how you are responding to their behavior:

"I feel very angry when you go on trips by yourself so often."

COMMUNICATING EXPECTATIONS AND CONDITIONS

It is useful to specify the amount of time you have available for each visit when you are doing brief office counseling. A practical duration is 15 minutes in a busy primary-care practice. Once the time limit has been defined, it is important to stick to it unless the patient is in severe crisis (e.g., suicidal). Try hard not to interrupt a counseling visit for phone calls and beeper messages. Focus on only one or two problems during each visit, and encourage the patient to prioritize multiple problems by asking such questions as:

"What would you like to focus on in our 15 minutes today?"
"If I had a magic wand that I could wave and get rid of one problem, which one would you want it to be?"
"If you could change one thing about your marriage, what would that be?"
"If you family could change in only one way, what would you like that to be?"

Negotiate the frequency and expected number of medical counseling visits based on the nature and severity of the patient's problem. Brief counseling often accomplishes its purpose in as few as two to six visits. Meeting once or twice a week is reasonable for a patient in crisis, whereas once every 2 to 4 weeks is appropriate when the patient's psychosocial problems are less urgent but still serious. Some patients prefer to come in for intermittent counseling when they get "stressed out" or when they are motivated to work on particular issues in their lives. Occasionally, indefinite monthly vis-

its are indicated for patients with chronic, severe, or multiple issues and an ongoing need for therapeutic partnership. Most physicians who do extended counseling or psychotherapy obtain extra training in psychotherapy, family therapy, or both at some point. Such physicians often choose to improve their effectiveness by working in collaboration with a mental health professional, seeing patients together or discussing them in consultation. Such consultations can be a source of catharsis and emotional support for both professionals, especially when they are dealing with unusually difficult patients.

Unless the physician has formal training in psychotherapy or family therapy, he or she should refer patients with severe emotional or psychiatric problems to a mental health professional for evaluation and more intense therapy. Such a referral must be done in a careful, caring manner so that the patient does not feel rejected or labeled as "crazy." The primary-care physician should stay in active contact with the process, however. Ideally, this work is seen as an extension of the family physician's care of the family.

UNDERSTANDING YOUR OWN FAMILY DYNAMICS

Everyone is an expert on at least one family—his or her own. It is more interesting and quite useful, professionally as well as personally, to contemplate your own family patterns (Crouch). You can start by doing your own genogram and looking for patterns of relationship, functioning, and illness. If you can learn to observe yourself in relation to your family patterns and history you can develop strategies for better understanding yourself and changing in response to problematic family issues.

By increasing your awareness of your own dynamic family patterns, you can develop a sense of humor about "losing it" and behaving counterproductively at times. You also can develop new patterns and avoid repeating old ones so frequently or intensely when under greater stress. You can catch yourself sooner and recover more quickly when you do repeat an old pattern. You can develop strategies such as taking a "time out" to ease your anxiety when you sense it escalating. You can improve almost all your relationships with other people by responding more and reacting less in difficult situations.

Every physician can benefit from discussing his or her most difficult patients with a relatively objective colleague. One format for this on a regular, structured basis is a group process named for the British psychiatrist who pioneered the idea (Balint). The most difficult patients discussed in Balint groups are generally the ones who most strongly reactivate parts of family patterns that are most touchy. Such patients can give valuable clues to the issues physicians might most benefit from examining and working on. Physicians with personal problems or problematic family patterns often benefit greatly from getting individual or family therapy themselves.

FAMILY DYNAMICS AND MEDICINE

The infinite variety of family relationships, strengths, and problems adds spice to the practice of medicine. To the experienced clinician, the bare biomedical facts of routine health problems are straightforward and uninteresting. People are seldom simple or dull, however. If you pause long enough to enjoy the uniqueness of each person and each family, you will greatly enhance the help you give and the joy you receive as a physician.

REFERENCES

Balint M. The Doctor, His Patient, and the Illness. New York, International Universities Press, 1957.

Bowen M. Family Therapy in Clinical Practice. New York, Jason Aronson, 1978, pp. 337–387, 461–547.

Crouch MA. Using the genogram clinically. In Crouch MA. and Roberts L (Eds.): The Family in Medical Practice: A Family Systems Primer. New York, Springer-Verlag, 1987.

Crouch MA. Working with one's own family issues. In The Family in Medical Practice: A Family Systems Primer. New York, Springer-Verlag, 1987.

Kerr M. Family Evaluation: An Approach Based on Bowen Theory. New York, Norton, 1988.

Montagu A. Green and black rocks. In Howard J (Ed.): *Families*. New York, Simon and Schuster, 1978, p. 63.

Nabokov V. Ada (or Ardor: A Family Chronicle). New York, McGraw-Hill, 1969, part 1, chap. 1.

Nisbet R. Twilight of authority. In Howard J (Ed.): Families. New York, Simon and Schuster, 1978, p. 11.

Ramsey CN Jr, Lewis JM. Family structure and functioning. In Rakel RE (Ed.): Textbook of Family Practice. Philadelphia, W.B. Saunders, 1990, p. 23.

Ransom DC, Vandervoort HE. The development of family medicine: Problematic trends. JAMA 1973; 225:1098–1102.

Rogers J. The self-administered genogram. In Rakel RE (Ed.): Textbook of Family Practice. Philadelphia, W.B.Saunders, 1991, pp. 1732–1735.

Smilkstein G, Ashworth C, Montano D. Validity and reliability of the Family APGAR as a test of family function. J Fam Pract 1982; 15:303–311.

Stuart MR, Lieberman JA III. The 15-Minute Hour: Applied Psychotherapy for the Primary Care Physician. New York, Praeger, 1986.

Tolstoy LN. Anna Karenina. New York, Dodd, Mead, 1966.

QUESTIONS

1. Which of the following would *not* be considerd a manifestation of chronic family anxiety by the family therapist Bowen?
   a. Mother and father engaging in frequent nonproductive conflict
   b. Mother with frequent "tension" headaches
   c. Father overinvolved in work and underinvolved in family
   d. Parents blaming a hyperactive child for family problems
   e. Mother and father having differing opinions about child rearing

2. Which one of the following is *not* probed by Smilkstein's Family APGAR?
   a. Satisfaction with how the family adapts to stress
   b. Satisfaction with how the family respects members' privacy
   c. Satisfaction with how the family encourages personal growth
   d. Satisfaction with how the family expresses affection
   e. Satisfaction with the sense of committment by the spouse

3. The letters in the BATHE acronym stand for
   a. Biologic, affective, therapeutic, holistic, emotional.
   b. Background, affect, trouble, handling, empathy.
   c. Biochemical, affective, therapeutic, holistic, emotional.
   d. Biologic, affective, therapeutic, holistic, emotional.
   e. Biopsychosocial, affective, therapeutic, holistic, emotional.

4. Which of the following physician roles is *least* conducive to being therapeutic when relating to patients?
   a. Calm, minimally anxious presence
   b. Nonreactive, nonjudgmental listener
   c. Caring, concerned advocate
   d. Emotionally connected, relatively objective "coach"
   e. Emotionally detached, completely objective medical scientist

5. In conjunction with the BATHE technique, SOAP stands for
   a. Subjective, objective, assessment, plan.
   b. Sympathy, objectivity, alliance, palliation.
   c. Support, options, acceptance, present focus.
   d. Sympathy, objectivity, alliance, patient education.

6. How long, on average, should it take to use the BATHE technique to probe a patient's psychosocial situation, identify issues that might be affecting the patient's health, and briefly deal with the main issue?
   a. 5 minutes
   b. 15 minutes
   c. 30 minutes
   d. 45 minutes
   e. 60 minutes

Answers appear on page 445.

5

THE FAMILY'S INFLUENCE ON HEALTH

THOMAS L. CAMPBELL, JAMES H. BRAY, and SUSAN SCHOOLEY

The specialty of family practice is unique in its emphasis on the health care of families over extended periods of time. Despite the changing demographics of the American family, most patients live with other family members and are strongly influenced by family relationships. The family remains the most basic relational unit and intimate social environment in our society. As such, the family has a major influence on the physical and mental health of its members. By understanding how the family influences health, the family physician has the opportunity to anticipate and reduce the adverse effects of family stress and utilize the family as a resource in the care of patients.

A family-oriented approach to health care (McDaniel, Campbell, and Seaburn) is based on the biopsychosocial model, which emphasizes the interrelationships among biologic, interpersonal, and social factors in health. The focus of family practice is on the patient in the context of the family, broadly defined as "any group of people related either biologically, emotionally, or legally." Family physicians recognize that the family is the primary source of health beliefs, health-related behaviors, stress, and emotional support.

FAMILY STRESS AND HEALTH

Although the idea that stress can cause illness is widely accepted by the lay public, it is difficult to demonstrate empirically. Stress is hard to define and study. "Stress" may refer to any of the three components of what has been called the "stress process": (1) the stressors (environmental events experienced by an individual), (2) the physiologic response to the stressors, or (3) the health consequences of the stressors. The most successful method for studying stress and health has been to examine stressors, particularly the relationship of stressful life events to illness. Holmes and Rahe developed their life-event scale by asking a random sample of the population to rank how stressful they perceived each of 43 common life events to be. Many retrospective and pro-

spective studies using this scale have shown that an increase in stressful life events precedes the development of a wide range of different diseases. Life events that are perceived negatively or are not under the individual's control have the most adverse effect on health.

Most of the events on the Holmes and Rahe scale occur within the family, and 10 of the 15 most stressful events are family events. Since children are likely to be affected by this stress, a number of studies have looked at the relationship of family life events and child health. Meyer and Haggerty found that chronic stress was associated with higher rates of streptococcal pharyngitis and that 30% of the infections were preceded by a stressful family event. Beautrais and associates' prospective study of over 1000 preschoolers found that family life events were strongly correlated with subsequent visits to the physician and hospital admissions for a wide range of conditions. Children from families with more than 12 of the stressful life events during the 4-year study period were six times more likely to be hospitalized. Research in psychoimmunology has shown how stress can decrease immunity and make individuals more susceptible to a host of different diseases, including infections.

Several of the most stressful life events on the Holmes and Rahe scale represent major transitions in the family life cycle. These normative life events have powerful influences on physical and mental health and can result in symptoms that bring the individual to the physicians office. The impact of bereavement on health is reviewed in Chapter 7, along with an approach for helping families coping with death. We will focus here on divorce and remarriage, two common and very stressful family life-cycle transitions.

FAMILY SUPPORT AND HEALTH

Because of medicine's emphasis on pathology and disease, physicians tend to focus on problems and dysfunction within families and have more difficulty recognizing family strengths and resources. However, most families cope with significant stresses and major illness without serious difficulties. This is due in part to the emotional and physical support families provide their members. An understanding of how family support promotes health and buffers the effects of stress can help the family physician to utilize these resources in patient care.

A large body of research has shown a strong and consistent relationship between social relationships, especially the perception of social support, and overall morbidity and mortality. In a review of this literature, House and colleagues state:

> The evidence regarding social relationships and health increasingly approximates the evidence in the 1964 Surgeon General's report that established cigarette smoking as a cause or risk factor for mortality and morbidity from a range of diseases. The age-adjusted relative risk ratios are stronger than the relative risks for all cause mortality reported for cigarette smoking [p. 543].

Family members, particularly the spouse, appear to be the most important source of social support and account for most of the association between social support and health. There is evidence that support from sources outside the family cannot compensate for what is missing from within the family.

Social support has been conceptualized in terms of its structure and function. Berkman defines "structural social supports" or "social networks" as "the web of social ties that surrounds an individual" and "functional social supports" as "the emotional, instrumental and financial aid that is obtained from one's social network." The structural components of social support (e.g., marital status, number of children) appear to have a direct effect on health, and functional or perceived social support (e.g., quality of relationships) indirectly affect health by buffering stress.

In a seminal study of over 6000 adults, Berkman and Syme showed that social networks were a major predictor of mortality over a 9-year period, independent of socioeconomic status, previous health status, or health practices. The most socially isolated adults had more than twice the death rate of the least-isolated group. Marital status and contacts with relatives and friends were the most powerful predictors of health.

Studies of social supports in the elderly have shown that the relative importance of different components of family support may change over the life span. Older persons with impaired social supports have two to three times the death rate of those with good supports. Unlike studies of younger populations, marital status was not associated with mortality. The presence and number of living children were the most powerful predictors of survival. This finding suggests that adult children become the most important source of social support in the elderly.

HEALTH PROMOTION AND DISEASE PREVENTION

The family is the primary social context in which health promotion and disease prevention take place.

The World Health Organization characterizes the family as the "primary social agent in the promotion of health and well-being." Research on families and health demonstrates that the family strongly influences most health behaviors and that a family-oriented approach is the most effective and efficient way to prevent disease and promote health. A healthy lifestyle is usually developed, maintained, or changed within the family setting.

A major challenge for medicine for the 1990s and beyond is the prevention of chronic illness. Most chronic illnesses result in part from unhealthy behaviors or risk factors that are difficult to change. This is particularly true for coronary heart disease, the leading cause of death in the United States. Most cardiac risk behaviors, including diet, smoking, and exercise are strongly influenced by the family.

Cardiovascular Risk Factors

Cardiovascular and other health risk factors tend to cluster within families. Family members are more likely to share the same risk factors than would be expected by chance, including smoking, obesity, hypercholesterolemia, lack of exercise, and hypertension. This sharing of risk factors occurs both between spouses and among parents and their children. For example, the Framingham heart study found a higher than expected concordance between spouses for blood pressure, cholesterol, triglyceride, blood sugar, smoking, and lung function. Parent–child blood pressure, body fat, and cholesterol are significantly correlated.

Shared risk factors within families can be explained by several mechanisms. Family members can influence each other's lifestyle and health habits. Adolescents are more likely to smoke if either of their parents or an older sibling smokes. A teenager who has a parent and an older sibling who smoke is five times more likely to smoke than is a teenager from a nonsmoking family. Families usually eat a similar diet and therefore ingest similar amounts of salt, calories, cholesterol, and saturated fats. An emphasis on physical fitness and maintaining ideal body weight is often a shared family value. Parents' exercise habits and attitudes have a strong influence on their children's levels of physical activity.

Since genetics influence some of these risk factors, similarities between parents and children may be inherited. Studies of adopted children suggest that childhood obesity is influenced by both genetics and the family environment. However, the similarity or concordance of cholesterol levels in twins has been shown to be largely due to similar diets rather than heredity.

MATE SELECTION. Spouses may share cardiovascular risk factors because they married someone with similar habits. This tendency to marry someone with the same traits or behaviors, called "assortative mating," is quite common. Smokers tend to marry other smokers, and couples tend to smoke the same number of cigarettes per day. Obese men tend to marry obese women. Marital partners may even choose each other (consciously or unconsciously) based on their dietary or exercise habits.

In the Framingham study, the concordance of risk factors between spouses did not increase over time, suggesting that these similarities existed at the time of marriage.

Whatever the cause of this phenomenon, it has major implications for health care providers. If one family member has a particular cardiovascular risk factor, it is likely to be more difficult to change if the behavior is shared by other members of the family. Smokers are more likely to stop smoking if no one else in the family is a smoker and remain abstinent longer if their spouse or friends do not smoke. Changing one member's risk factor may have a ripple effect and influence the entire family. For example, if one family member starts an exercise program, other family members may join in. Smoking couples tend to quit smoking at the same time. An intervention designed to change the risk factors within the family rather than in only one individual may be more successful, time efficient, and cost-effective.

The ability of an individual to make lifestyle changes and reduce the risk of cardiovascular disease is strongly influenced by the support of family members. Men who have multiple cardiac risk factors are much more likely to participate in supervised exercise programs if their wives have positive attitudes about the program. Support from the spouse is associated with successful smoking cessation. Smokers who have the cooperation and reinforcement of their partner have lower relapse rates, whereas critical behaviors such as "nagging" and "policing" by the partner have the opposite effect.

CHOLESTEROL. The family's health beliefs about prevention influence their support for changing risk factors. As part of a cholesterol-reduction study, Doherty and colleagues examined the relationship of spouses' support and health beliefs to compliance with medication. The wife's beliefs regarding how susceptible she thought her husband was to elevated cholesterol were correlated with both her support and her husband's compliance with a cholesterol-lowering drug. In addition, the wife's "interest in the program" and "reminding him about medicine or diet" correlated with compliance, whereas "nagging about medicine" was negatively correlated with compliance.

EATING HABITS AND OBESITY. An unhealthy behavior sometimes plays a role within a family that can hinder attempts to change the behavior. For example, eating behavior and obesity itself can play an important homeostatic function within families. In a survey of eating behavior within families, 25% of mothers reported that they used food as a reward for their children, and 10% used it as punishment (Bryan and Lowenberg). Parents' encouragement to eat is associated with obesity in children. In one weight-reduction program, 91% of the spouses of obese women reported that they wished their wives would lose weight, but only 49% were willing to help (Stuart and Davis). Fifty-three percent of the men anticipated that weight loss would have an adverse effect on the marriage owing to loss of eating as a shared activity, loss of power in marital conflicts, and concern over marital commitment and sexual fidelity. During recorded mealtime conversations, these husbands were 7 times more likely to talk about food than were their dieting wives and 4 times more likely to offer food to the other. The men criticized their dieting wives 12 times more often than they praised them. When health-related behaviors such as eating serve important functions in the family, changes in these behaviors may be resisted unless attention is paid to how changing the behavior will affect the family.

The family can have a significant effect on the treatment of obesity. Involvement of the spouse or partner in weight-reduction programs has been shown to improve weight loss significantly. Using a behavioral approach, family members provide immediate and long-term reinforcement for weight loss or dieting. When the partner participates in the weight-reduction program, the obese individual is not only able to reduce more weight but maintains the weight loss as well.

HYPERTENSION. Despite the fact that hypertension is relatively easy to identify and treat and that adequate treatment significantly lowers the risk of heart attacks and strokes, only one-fourth of all hypertensive individuals are under treatment and only one-half of those under treatment have their blood pressure adequately controlled. Compliance with medication is a major problem in the treatment of hypertension and reduction of cardiovascular disease. In a randomized, controlled study, Morisky and colleagues demonstrated a dramatic effect of family involvement on hypertension compliance and overall mortality. They studied the impact of three different educational interventions (brief individual counseling, instructing the spouse or significant other during a home visit, and small patient group sessions) on appointment keeping, weight control, and medication compliance. Involving the spouse not only improved overall compliance but also resulted in a significant reduction in blood pressure and overall mortality. Overall, the experimental groups had a 57% reduction in mortality compared with the controls, and those groups which received family education tended to do the best. The family intervention was included in this study after a survey indicated that 70% of the clinic's hypertensive patients wished that family members knew more about hypertension. Based on this and other studies of the role of social supports in improving compliance, the National Heart, Lung, and Blood Institute has stressed the importance of "the help that patients receive from their family and friends to carry on with their treatments" (Haynes et al.).

There is strong evidence for both the healthy and unhealthy influences of families on cardiovascular risk factors. Numerous randomized, controlled trials have demonstrated that family involvement improves the results of weight reduction, and one study shows a similar result for hypertension control. Similar studies are needed for exercise programs, smoking cessation, and dietary changes (low salt and cholesterol). Despite the proven efficacy of a family approach to prevention, health care providers remain focused on the individual. A major challenge to the health profession is to become more effective in health promotion and to incorporate a family approach to prevention.

FAMILIES AND CHRONIC ILLNESS

Most families must face chronic illness in a family member during the life cycle. Chronic illness is increasing in prevalence and has replaced acute illness as the major cause of morbidity and mortality in the United States. Families, not health care providers, are the primary caretakers for patients with chronic illness. They are the ones who help with most of the physical demands of the illness, ranging from preparing special meals for a family member with heart disease, to assisting with insulin injections for a diabetic, to running a home dialysis machine. How well the family copes with and adapts to a chronic illness will have a major influence on the course of the illness.

Research on families and chronic illness is gradually moving from looking for how families "cause" illness (a pathogenic model) to examining ways in which families influence, positively or negatively, the course of chronic illness. The success of this latter approach is best demonstrated by the research on schizophrenia, where the concept of the "schizophrenogenic" family has been largely abandoned, and numerous well-designed, prospective studies have demonstrated how the emotional climate and patterns of communication powerfully affect relapse. Randomized, controlled trials of clinical interventions derived from these studies have shown that family psychoeducation dramatically improves the course of schizophrenia. As a result of this work, family interventions have become a standard part of the treatment of schizophrenia.

The Psychosomatic Family

No such persuasive line of research exists in the work on families and chronic physical illness, where the predominant clinical model remains a pathogenic one—that of the "psychosomatic" family. The concept of psychosomatic families was developed by Salvador Minuchin and colleagues at the Philadelphia Child Guidance Center from their experiences with the families of children with brittle diabetes, severe asthma, or anorexia nervosa. They observed a specific pattern of family interaction, characterized by enmeshment (high cohesion), overprotectiveness, rigidity, and conflict avoidance.

To determine how these family interactions can affect chronic illness, Minuchin and colleagues studied the physiologic responses of diabetic children to a stressful family interview. During the interview, the children from psychosomatic families had a rapid rise in free fatty acids (a precursor to diabetic ketoacidosis) that persisted beyond the interview. The parents of these children exhibited an initial rise in free fatty acid levels that fell to normal levels when the diabetic child entered the room. Minuchin and colleagues hypothesized that in psychosomatic families, parental conflict is detoured or defused through the chronically ill child, and the resulting stress leads to exacerbations of the illness. Minuchin and colleagues also reported the successful treatment of brittle diabetes, severe asthma, and anorexia nervosa

using structural family therapy to help establish more appropriate family boundaries. In all the treated cases there was a dramatic improvement in the illness, with fewer hospitalizations and less need for medication.

Minuchin's work on psychosomatic families has been criticized for conceptual and methodologic reasons. Problems include a lack of clear definitions of the central concepts, small number of subjects, lack of control groups, observer biases, and the absence of statistical analyses. Research on diabetic children with their families demonstrates that poor diabetic control is associated with family dysfunction, but it is not known whether this is a cause or an effect. Most of the families of 30 poorly controlled diabetic children studied by White et al. had numerous "dysfunctional" psychosocial factors, including absent fathers, poor living conditions, inadequate parental functioning, chronic family conflict, and lack of family involvement with the diabetes. On the other hand, clear organization in the family has been associated with good metabolic control.

DIABETES MELLITUS. How emotionally close or cohesive a family is seems to be particularly important for the care of diabetes. Both low cohesion (disengagement) and high cohesion (enmeshment) have been associated with poor blood sugar control. In a carefully controlled study, Anderson and colleagues found that low cohesion and high conflict were associated with poor diabetic control. Parental indifference can result in the worst diabetic control and lead to depression in the diabetic child. Thus, in emotionally distant or disengaged families, inadequate supervision and parental support result in noncompliance with insulin and diet and poor diabetic control.

These studies suggest that the mechanisms by which the family influences diabetic control may depend on the style of family functioning, especially its cohesion. Both high and low cohesion are associated with poor diabetic control. In enmeshed families, diabetic control may be physiologically linked to emotional processes within the family. In disengaged families, inadequate family structure and support may result in noncompliance. Optimal management of diabetes requires the support and supervision of the family, along with respect for individuality and age-appropriate autonomy. While these results suggest specific clinical interventions with each type of family, no controlled studies have been conducted yet.

ASTHMA. Studies of families with an asthmatic child have been too few to determine whether the illness is associated with family dysfunction or any family characteristic. In general, studies have failed to find any relationship between the quality of family life and severity of asthma. Two randomized, controlled trials of family psychotherapy, however, have demonstrated a beneficial effect on the course of asthma. Lask and Matthew randomly assigned 33 families with 37 asthmatic children to experimental and control groups. The experimental groups received 6 hours of family therapy designed to improve the families' coping skills in dealing with acute attacks. At the end of 1 year, the children who received family therapy reported less wheezing and slightly improved pulmonary function tests. In a similar study, Gustafsson and colleagues found that children with severe asthma who received family therapy improved significantly on several measures, while those who received conventional treatment did not improve. These two studies are the only randomized, controlled trials of family therapy for a physical illness in the literature.

Clinical Implications

This research on family support and health has important implications for the assessment of patients and their families and the choice of interventions. When interviewing one or more members of a family, the family physician should determine the amount of stress the family is experiencing, including any recent deaths, divorces, or separations and any current illnesses, marital difficulties, or sexual dysfunctions. When the patient or family is experiencing a high level of stress, an assessment of coping mechanisms should include both how the family is coping with the current stressors and how they have dealt with crises in the past. Social and family supports are an important resource when a patient or family is in crisis and should be assessed. It is useful to know not only the availability and utilization of supports but also how helpful the patient or family perceives the supports to be.

Because health risk factors tend to run in families, the entire family should be screened when an unhealthy behavior is detected in an individual. These include smoking, excess alcohol consumption, hypercholesterolemia, obesity, and hypertension. Education about such risk factors should include the entire family, not just the individual patient. Whenever possible, the intervention should be at a family level. For example, the family physician can encourage both members of a couple to quit smoking or all members of a family to reduce their cholesterol intake. The physician should try to get the patient's spouse to support recommended lifestyle changes or compliance with medication. On the other hand, it is important to block any tendencies for a family member to "nag" or "police" the patient.

Based on rigorous studies of the influences of social support on compliance, the Working Group on Health Education and High Blood Pressure Control of the National Heart, Lung, and Blood Institute has recommended that all physicians use the following as one of three basic strategies for increasing adherence to prescribed antihypertensive regimes:

> *Enhance support from family members—identifying and involving one influential person, preferably someone living with the patient, who can provide encouragement, help support the behavior change, and, if necessary, remind the patient about the specifics of the regimen.*

This government guide, sent to all physicians in the United States, gives specific suggestions on how to enhance family support for each of the five most frequent behavior changes recommended for hypertensive changes: taking medication daily, maintaining desirable weight, reducing dietary sodium, increasing vigorous exercise, and moderating alcohol consumption.

When working with patients who have a chronic illness, the family physician should encourage the family to be involved in the management of illness while supporting the patient's autonomy and ultimate responsibility for care. For distant or disengaged family members, this may involve asking them to accompany the patient for appointments and finding specific ways in which they can assist the patient. For enmeshed families, it is often necessary to help the patient and family negotiate which responsibilities will be the patient's and which will be the family's. Severely dysfunctional families with chronic illness should be referred to a family therapist and cared for jointly with the therapist's assistance. It is important not to blame family members for medical problems. Referrals should be presented as helping the family cope with the chronic illness.

IMPACT OF DIVORCE ON THE FAMILY

Separation and divorce have a major impact on the health and well-being of all family members. Divorce is best understood not as a single event, but as a process of transition that continues for many years. Millions of children and adults are directly involved in the stresses and changes caused by their family's moving from a nuclear family to a postdivorce family to a stepfamily. Some will face even more changes because of the multiple divorces and remarriages of one or more parents.

Divorce and remarriage involve a complex series of changes that often affect every aspect of family functioning: parent–child relationships, parenting practices and effectiveness, family conflict, family income and residence, extended family relationships, and peer and social relationships. These changes may produce both short-term crises and long-term effects on individual family members (Bray; Hetherington and Camara; Kelly).

Individuals within a family may have very different *experiences* of a divorce, and these differences are important in understanding and helping them through this process. For example, a woman may be very unhappy in a marriage and may have been psychologically divorcing her husband for years, yet the husband may be generally satisfied with the marriage and "shocked and surprised" when his wife tells him she wants a divorce. Each child may have different reactions and align with mother or father during the process. By the time of the actual legal divorce, the wife may have resolved much of her grief and negative feelings, but the husband and some of the children may be in the middle of the emotional turmoil of the divorce process. The family physician needs to understand these differences to treat the individual family members and help the family through this process most effectively.

Divorce is not necessarily "bad" for family members. Staying together in an unhappy, conflict-ridden marriage for the "children's sake" or any other reason may not be in a family's best interests. Children actually adjust better in a stable divorced home than in an unhappy, highly conflictual intact home (Hetherington et al.). Hetherington et al. stated, "Our study and previous research show that a conflict-ridden intact family is more deleterious to family members than a stable home situation in which parents are divorced. Divorce is often a positive solution to destructive family functioning" (p. 34). This is not to say that divorce is always good or that it is to be recommended in all cases. In fact, most research indicates that, in general, being married is associated with better outcomes and fewer health problems than being divorced or single (Somers).

Process of Separation and Divorce

The decision by adults to separate and ultimately divorce results in a high degree of emotional distress. During the deliberation period, prior to the separation, partners often quarrel; confront each other with their unhappiness; and seek outside assistance from friends, ministers, primary care physicians, and marital counselors. Many families turn to their family physician for support and assistance because the family physician is seen as someone who has unique knowledge of families. The physician's role is to decrease the psychologic risk of patients, to promote healthy methods of coping with stress, to teach parents ways of relating to their children that maximize their coping, and to make appropriate referrals for additional help.

During the early stages of marital distress, patients may present with anxiety, depression, impotence, ulcers, migraines, or other psychosomatic symptoms related to the stress of living in an unhappy relationship. Common feelings include disillusionment, alienation, anger, and general dissatisfaction. Conflict may escalate between the spouses, and children may become involved as a way of deflecting the marital conflict. Later, there is likely to be withdrawal, both emotional and physical, and a "yo-yo" effect in which partners may attempt to alternately deny problems and win the other back. Physicians should be prepared to recommend marriage counseling if patients present evidence of marital distress. In its early stages, deterioration of the relationship may be reversible. Early assessment, intervention, and, if necessary, referral to a marriage and family therapist can short-circuit the difficulty of a marital separation and help save the marriage. If reconciliation is not possible, counseling may allow the couple to negotiate the separation process with less distress for themselves and any children involved. It should be noted that many couples reconcile after a separation period, and the physician can help the family through this process with support and early intervention.

Postdivorce Families

Following the legal divorce, the family enters a phase in which they attempt to achieve a new equilibrium and stability. There are two basic child custody arrangements following a divorce: sole custody and joint custody. Sole custody is by far the most common custodial pattern following a divorce. In the sole-custody arrangement, the custodial parent retains custody of the children and the noncustodial parent has visitation rights with the children. There are many types of joint custody. In discussing this area it is important to distinguish between joint legal custody and joint physical custody. The common element of the two types is that both parents retain the rights of a parent and have equal power and authority over their children's general welfare, education, and upbringing. With joint physical custody, both parents retain the rights, privileges, and duties of a parent, and the child lives with both parents on a shared basis. It is important to note that usually the custodial parent has the exclusive right to seek medical treatment for the children. This means that without the permission of the custodial parent, the noncustodial parent can only seek medical treatment under emergency situations.

Adults' Reactions to Divorce

The first year after divorce is highly stressful for adults. Both men and women report decreases in self-esteem and feelings of loss of control, loneliness, and isolation. Adults come to physicians with complaints of fatigue, depression, and general somatic problems. These are signs that the person is having difficulty coping with the family changes.

Marital disruption is the single most powerful sociodemographic predictor of stress-related physical illness. Separated individuals have 30% more acute illnesses and physician visits than married adults (Somers). Separated and divorced adults have the highest rates of acute medical problems, chronic medical conditions that interfere with social activity, and disability, even when age, race, and income are controlled (Verbrugge). Divorced men have increased rates of suicide, admissions to mental hospitals, and vulnerability to minor and major physical illness and an increased risk of being victims of violence. Marital separation is associated with reduced qualitative and quantitative immune functioning in men and women compared with their married counterparts (Kiecolt-Glaser et al.), which may explain their increased risk of illness.

Within approximately 2 years after the divorce, most adults have adjusted to the marital breakup and have developed a new stability in their lives (Hetherington et al.; Wallerstein and Kelly). Many people, however, expect to recover from the effects of divorce much faster than is realistic. The physician can advise the patient to set goals for recovery that are achievable rather than overwhelming. With time, feelings of well-being increase, and most adults experience more internal control and satisfaction in life.

Effects of Divorce on Children

The process of divorce has far-reaching influences on children. The effects vary depending on a number of factors, including sex of the child, age of the child, length of time since the divorce, postdivorce family relationships, and socioeconomic status (Hetherington and Camara; Kelly; Wallerstein and Kelly). Many studies have found that divorce is more difficult and traumatic for boys than for girls and that boys have more severe and enduring negative reactions to divorce than girls. Boys tend to develop more behavior, sex-role adjustment, and academic problems than girls, and these problems often persist for 4 to 7 years after the divorce, particularly if the custodial mother remains single.

Children's ages at the time of the divorce influence the type and quality of reactions they have to their parents' divorce. Table 5–1 presents children's reactions based on age groups found by various studies. It is important to point out that an individual child may have a wide range of reactions that include some or all of those problems listed in Table 5–1.

Very young children, 3 years old and below, are likely to regress in their behavior (e.g., bed wetting) and experience developmental delays (e.g., difficulty in toilet training). They are also likely to experience intensified separation anxiety when leaving the custodial parent or primary caretaker. Children at this age are highly influenced by their custodial parent and may respond to that parent's anxiety and fear in certain situations by becom-

TABLE 5–1. CHILDREN'S REACTIONS TO DIVORCE

AGE OF CHILD	REACTION OF CHILD	EXPECTED PROBLEMS	RISK FACTORS	ADVICE TO PARENTS
Infancy (0–3)	Perceives loss of parent	Regression and developmental delays Problems with feeding, sleeping, and toileting Irritability, excessive crying Apathy, withdrawal	Loss of caregiver Diminished capacity of custodial parent Psychologic disturbance of custodial parent	Maintain predictable routines Expect normal separation anxiety to be exaggerated Support for parent caring for herself and baby Substitute care for infant if parent is seriously depressed
Preschool (3–5)	Fears of abandonment Fears loss of custodial parent Confusion	Whining, clinging, and fearful behavior Regression and developmental delays Nightmares, bewilderment, confusion, aggression Sadness, neediness, low self-esteem Denial, perfect behavior	Persistent or severe regression, nightmares, or separation anxiety Persistent encopresis with smearing Refusal of nonresident parent to visit or of resident parent to allow visits Inability of parent to enforce discipline	Both parents should tell children about divorce and what is occurring Establish daily routine Maintain consistent discipline Emphasize that children are not responsible for divorce Encourage involvement of both parents in children's lives
Early school age (6–8)	Guilt, self-blame for divorce Sense of loss Feels betrayed, rejected Confusion	Sadness, crying, depression Longing for absent parent Anger, tantrums, acting out Asks for reconciliation Increased behavior problems	Developmental arrest, no new learning Loss of interest in peers and activities Other losses—friends, pet, relatives Changes in school or teacher	Regular frequent visits by noncustodial parent Shielding from parental hostility Involvement of both parents in child's care Consistent discipline Regular school attendance
Older school age (9–11)	Can view divorce as parents' problem but needs to find blame or reason Feels shame, rejection, resentment, loneliness	Conflicting loyalties between parents Worry about custody Hostility toward one or both parents Dependency School problems Increased behavior problems	Ongoing hostility between parents Complete rejection of one parent Parents pressure child to take sides Decrease in school performance	Involvement of both parents Parents avoid blaming each other Parental honesty Defuse child's anger
Adolescence (12–18)	Concern about loss of family life Concern about own future Feels responsible for family members Anger, hostility	Immature behavior Early or late development of independence Overcloseness or competition with same-sex parent Worry about own role as sexual or marital partner	Persistent academic failure Depression and suicide threats Delinquency or promiscuity Substance abuse	Maintain parent role with child Limit involvement in parent worries Child needs peer support Maintain consistent discipline Be aware of emotional ups and downs of adolescence—may be aggravated by stress of divorce

Source: Adapted from Rhyne MC. Nurs Practitioner 1986; 11(12):37–46; Rae-Grant Q, Robson BE. Can J Psychiatry 1988; 33(6):443–452; Ansett R, Lewis B. Postgrad Med 1986; 80(2):137–140; Hetherington EM, Camara K. In Parke RD (ed.): Review of Child Development Research, vol. 7: The Family. Chicago, University of Chicago Press, 1984; and Wallerstein JS, Kelly J. Surviving the Break-Up: How Children and Parents Cope with Divorce. New York. Basic Books, 1980. *(Used by permission.)*

ing upset and anxious, particularly when such children are left at day-care centers and when the noncustodial parent visits.

Preschool children, ages 4 to 6, are also likely to exhibit regressive behavior and have some developmental delays. They may be whiny and clinging. They will be more aware of and upset by the absence of a parent. Children's anxiety is influenced by their parents' feelings, and they will often respond to a parent's distress rather than to other situational factors. Parents often will assume that the child's distress is caused by visitation of the noncustodial parent, but if the child calms down rapidly (5 to 10 minutes) after the transition from one parent to the other, then the child is most likely responding to the parents' tension and anxiety around the transition.

School-aged children, ages 6 to 11, are likely to respond to divorce with sadness and upset. Younger children, ages 6 to 8, are usually unable to completely understand the divorce process or separate themselves psychologically from their parents' influences and wishes. Thus they may feel responsible for the divorce and blame themselves for the breakup of the family. Older children can understand more about the divorce process. Children at these ages often report frequent reconciliation fantasies. Boys are likely to have increased behavior problems and adjustment difficulties, whereas girls are likely to internalize their feelings and be sad and withdrawn. However, girls also may have an increase in behavior problems.

Adolescents, ages 12 to 18, are usually able to separate themselves from their parents' divorce and not blame themselves for the breakup of the family. Anger, resentment, and hostility are common reactions to the divorce. Both boys and girls are likely to have more behavior problems and adjustment difficulties.

It takes about 2 years for the postdivorce family to stabilize and readjust to the disruption caused by divorce (Hetherington and Camara). This is a time of great change, upheaval, and opportunity for the family. The first year after the divorce is characterized as a crisis period in which the family undergoes major changes and restructuring. Parenting practices change, and children respond differently to their parents as the family struggles to find a new equilibrium. Parenting methods that worked prior to the divorce may not be effective after the divorce. Children, especially boys, are less compliant to their parents' discipline and parenting. Parents are less effective in their discipline, particularly custodial mothers with their sons. Parents are less effective for many reasons, including changes in their parenting practices, guilt over the divorce, less structure and routine for the family, trouble coping with their own feelings over the divorce, and role overload. Between the first and second year after divorce, the family usually settles down and becomes stabilized in new patterns and roles. Parenting often improves, and children respond more to their custodial parent's discipline. The family physician can help with a number of potential problem areas that remain for the binuclear family throughout this process.

Role of the Family Physician

The concerned physician can offer a great deal to the divorcing family in the form of support and concern. To do this, the physician not only must have a general understanding of the situation, but also must understand its particular significance to the individual. As noted before, people can have dramatically different *experiences* of a divorce process. Patients may not volunteer the information that they are contemplating or are involved in a divorce. They may wish to avoid embarrassment or protect their privacy, or they may assume that such information is irrelevant to their care. Inquiry by the physician opens the door and makes it clear that such changes are important to the ongoing care of the patient. Open-ended inquiry, such as "How have things been since our last appointment?" or "How are things going at home?" are good ways to elicit information about such psychosocial changes. Once divorce has been identified, it should be noted in the chart either in the problem list or in the family genogram. If a patient presents who is already a single parent, it is important to ascertain if the patient is a single parent by choice and whether this came about by divorce, death, or other means (Anstett and Lewis). It is also important to know if the patient sees the transition to single parenthood as a positive or negative one. Questions such as "People have many reactions to a divorce, what has it been like for you and your children?" provide a way to elicit information without making biased assumptions about individual experiences.

Adults may seek medical evaluation at the time of separation and want medication for their anxiety, depression, or sleep difficulties. Physicians can assist patients going through this process by considering the role of stress and grief in their problems and by making patients aware of their vulnerability during this time. Educating them about the effects of stress and negative life events can normalize their experiences and help them cope with some of the physical and emotional effects of divorce.

Anstett and Lewis found that single parents unanimously agreed that physicians gave advice *without* first learning about single parenthood and frequently *ignored* the problem altogether. The majority of single parents in Anstett and Lewis's practice preferred that the physician just listen empathically rather than give advice concerning the problems of single parenthood. Most advice was seen as superficial and not really responsive to the particular needs of the individual. A more effective approach is to be an empathic listener and to reassure patients that their feelings are a normal part of a grief process and that this process is temporary and *will change* over time.

Children may be brought to the family physician for behavior and academic problems and stress-related somatic complaints. Parents may or may not recognize the possibility that divorce-related stress is involved. The family physician has the opportunity here to act as the child's advocate. As with other family members, it is important to determine the child's unique perception of events. How the child has been informed about the divorce and what it means is critical. Wallerstein and Kelly noted that less than 10% of children had any adult talk to them about the divorce. Parents may even present unrealistic stories about why one parent has left the household. Physicians should ask parents about how the divorce was presented to the children. This also will give information about how the parents are handling the divorce themselves.

Ideally, both parents should tell the children about the divorce and where the departing parent will be living in terms the children can understand. It should be emphasized that the parents are divorcing each other, not the children. All children should be reassured that they were not the cause of the divorce. Books about divorce are helpful for both older and younger children. Reassurances about continuity of the parent-child relationship and blamelessness of the children should be reiterated throughout the divorce process.

The physician needs to be alert to signs that a child is at risk for emotional and developmental damage. Suspicion should be aroused by depression, anxiety, vague somatic complaints, fatigue and boredom, a drop in school performance, irritability, and withdrawal from parents, friends, and usual social activities. More severe problems such as running away, promiscuity, and alcohol and drug abuse also may indicate problems with adjusting to divorce that need professional intervention.

The physician can assist in prevention and management of problems by suggesting ways for parents to deal with their children during and after the divorce. Consistent parenting, maintaining discipline, and allowing children to express feelings should be encouraged. It should be acknowledged that effective parenting and emotional support of the children may be difficult when the parent feels emotionally overwhelmed and drained, since role overload is a major stress. Supportive encouragement should always include praise for the parents' concern and efforts. Patterns of behavior that suggest blurring of generational boundaries or inappropriate dependency between parent and child should be identified and discouraged. Both parents should be urged to stay involved with monitoring the children's well-being and planning for the future. The physician should discourage actions that force a child to take sides between parents or require the child to be a message bearer between parents.

The physician can assist the child directly during office visits. The child should be allowed to express his or her feelings and perceptions about the divorce. The physician can assist this process by asking how the child feels about his or her parents' divorce and how life has been affected by it. If misperceptions and fears are revealed, the physician can act as the child's advocate and help the parents interpret the divorce more appropriately to the child.

If the child becomes seriously ill during the divorce, the physician should encourage both parents to provide support to the child. Divorced parents of hospitalized children have been shown to need more reassurance from the hospital staff because they often feel that they or the divorce contributed to the child's illness or accident. Divorced couples may carry their interpersonal hostility into the hospital to the detriment of the child's interests. The physician may have to take responsibility for coordinating communication between the parents and encourage them to acknowledge their feelings so that they do not subvert efforts to care for the child.

Children also can develop physical and emotional problems as a way to keep their parents together. If the custodial parent calls the noncustodial parent because she or he cannot handle the child's problems, this reinforces the child's desire to be sick or to create a problem. This indicates a lack of emotional divorce for the family. The family physician has a unique opportunity and authority to promote change in these situations through direct intervention.

IMPACT OF REMARRIAGE ON THE FAMILY

Stepfamilies are quite diverse in their structure and membership. A "stepfamily" is formed when an adult with children from a previous relationship remarries. The adult with children may have been divorced, widowed, or never married. The new spouse, or stepparent, may or may not have been married previously and may or may not have children. The term "step" comes from an Anglo-Saxon term "steop," which means "to make orphan or bereave." Prior to the turn of the century, most children entered a stepfamily as a result of the death of a parent (usually their mother), whereas most children now enter a stepfamily as a result of the breakup of their parents' marriage. Thus stepfamilies are "born out of loss" (Visher and Visher) as a result of the death of a parent or parental marriage and are also "instantly formed families" because of the presence of children from the beginning of the marriage.

Stepfamilies also go through a process that has predictable and unpredictable changes and stresses. Three major tasks are required for stepfamilies during the first years of remarriage: (1) integrating the stepparent into the new family and negotiating parenting for the children, (2) developing a good marital bond and relationship, and (3) integrating the noncustodial parent and his or her kinship system into the stepfamily (Bray et al.; Visher and Visher). Parenting stepchildren is a major task and stress for new stepfamilies (Bray). It is usually best if the stepparent plays a secondary parental role and supports the biologic parent in disciplining the children rather than trying to move in and take over the parental and disciplinary functions early in the remarriage (Bray). It may take from 2 to 4 years for the stepparent to be accepted as a parental figure by the children in a stepfamily. This is likely to occur faster with younger children than with older children and adolescents. Boys seem to accept a stepfather faster and more easily than girls. Girls often have more conflict with their stepparent and have more negative relationships with their stepfathers.

It is important to understand that stepfamilies are much more complex, undergo more changes, and are fundamentally different from nondivorced intact families. Accepting this continuing change, much of which is unpredictable, is one of the most difficult developmental tasks for stepfamilies (Visher and Visher). For example, it is common for remarried couples to have their weekend plans disrupted because the noncustodial parent does not pick the children up for a visitation. This type of change is a reminder that a stepfamily is not a nuclear family and that trying to mold a stepfamily into one is like trying to "force a square peg into a round hole"—it just does not fit.

Effects of Remarriage on Adults and Children

Early during the remarriage there is considerable stress for parents and female children (Bray). The stresses are both positive and negative. The remarriage starts a series of changes for family members. For example, positive stresses often include moving to a new and better home, having more income, and having two adults to help with the children and household. However, moves are often negatively stressful in that they require developing new friends, going to new schools, and losing old friends and familiar surroundings for children. And there is often conflict over parenting and deciding on household routines for the adults. These stresses appears to decrease after 2 years, however, as the family integrates and develops its own routines.

Children in stepfamilies have more behavior problems and adjustment difficulties than children in nuclear families. These problems vary with the age of the child. It appears that both boys and girls below age 9 have increased behavior problems, but these problems decrease after about 2 years of remarriage (Bray). Children between the ages 9 and 13 in stepfamilies also have more behavior problems than children in nondivorced families, but girls have the most difficult time adjusting and their problems persist for longer periods after remarriage (Hetherington et al.). The problems are somewhat different after a remarriage than after a divorce. Children tend to "act out" and, have more behavioral problems and conflicts with parents after a remarriage.

Role of the Family Physician

Family physicians can provide help to stepfamilies by anticipating problems and providing preventive guidance and counseling. A genogram is a good way for the physician to understand the new family relationships, and it will contribute to a thorough history (Wood and Poole). The physician should inquire about behavioral changes and symptoms in each family member, including their temporal relationship to family transitions. Because remarriage entails great change for a family, including further alteration of social and lifestyle patterns, previous adjustment problems may reemerge or intensify after the remarriage. Family members, especially children, may experience new grief because the new marriage underscores the permanence of the divorce (Visher and Visher).

As in the case of divorce, the physician can provide support and guidance to ease the impact of these stressors. An important aspect of this guidance is to debunk some of the myths about stepfamily formation that cause families distress (Visher and Visher; Wood and Poole). These include the belief that formation of a stepfamily will bring an immediate increase in stability. Families also may believe that affection, respect, and love will occur instantly among new members, resulting in guilt, anger, and confusion when this does not occur.

The family physician also can recommend activities that will ease the transition into the new family and encourage the formation of appropriate bonds among its members. Validating and normalizing conflicting feelings will help family members accept that they may feel grief, sadness, and anxiety in addition to such positive feelings as hope, joy, and excitement at the new opportunities. Helping parents negotiate parenting and household responsibilities and helping the family develop its own rituals and rules can greatly facilitate adjustment within a stepfamily. The physician should encourage open communication about these feelings with patients and family members during office visits.

New emotional bonds can be supported by having the family identify common interests and shared goals or values (Wood and Poole). New and old sources of social support should be fostered by adults and children. Younger children may need help from their parents to achieve this. The physician also can provide important assistance by paying attention to the often overlooked marriage bond. The new marriage is the basis of the new family, and its importance can become overshadowed by the stresses of family formation. Couples should be encouraged to take time for themselves without the children in order to renew their commitment to each other.

In the case of severe or long-standing adjustment problems, the family physician may choose to refer the family to a professional counselor. Physicians are advised to refer if there are multiple problems in the family, if there has been marital separation or family violence, if a child has repeatedly run away, or if any family members feel that the situation is hopeless. It is important to refer to a counselor who has specific experience with the problems encountered by stepfamilies.

Conclusion

In conclusion, the process of separation, divorce, and remarriage is replete with potential pitfalls, stresses, problems, *and opportunities* to make positive changes in family members' lives. Understanding the unique experiences of each family member, providing an empathic listening ear, and acknowledging the stresses and problems they are experiencing can contribute greatly to helping family members cope with these life transitions. The family physician has an important role in this process by helping family members focus on the opportunities and options available to make a positive difference in their current lives and for their future health and well-being.

CHILD ABUSE AND THE FAMILY

The problem of child abuse has received dramatically increased attention, both medically and socially, in the last three decades. It is a major cause of morbidity and mortality in childhood and has devastating consequences for its victims, and even the generations that follow, throughout their lives. Most physical and sexual abuse of children occurs within the home by family members and other caregivers. The prevalence of child abuse and the magnitude of its ill effects oblige family physicians to become adept at its recognition, treatment, and prevention.

Inadequate recognition and underreporting of child abuse are well-documented problems ascribed to medical professions, family physicians among them. Reasons for this phenomenon include inexperience at eliciting or identifying clinical presentations, discomfort and denial on the part of the professional, mistaken assumptions about who may be at risk, discomfort at reporting incompletely substantiated suspicions, and lack of confidence in the child protective system. Family physicians may face some unique disincentives in that long-term relationships with families may mitigate their ability to recognize abuse or to function clearly as a child advocate when they also feel bound by an implicit contract to care for the abuser. In all states, physicians are mandated by law to report situations in which they suspect child abuse to the proper authorities. The physician may fear a disruption in his or her relationship with the family as a consequence of reporting, but families can often be convinced of the physician's professional and legal obligation and the nonadversarial nature of the subsequent investigation. The physician can offer continued support to the entire family throughout this difficult time while maintaining a primary posture of child advocacy. The horrible nature of child victimization, the grief and anger of families, and unfamiliarity with the forensic aspects of child abuse, such as testifying in court, make this particularly difficult clinical work. The consequences of failing to recognize or treat abuse, however, must persuade physicians to overcome these barriers through continuing education, frank discussions with colleagues, and personal commitment.

Physical Abuse of Children

Estimating the prevalence of nonaccidental injury to children is problematic. Reported cases may represent only a fraction of the total incidence of actual abuse, and the volume of reports increases annually. Nonaccidental injury is responsible for 3% of all deaths in children aged 1 to 4 years and most often results from violence in the family. Infants are at particular risk for severe injury by virtue of their physical vulnerability.

Abusive caretakers are most likely to exhibit poor self-esteem, a perception of parental deprivation or actual abuse in their own childhoods, and unrealistic expectations about early child development, for example, ascribing aggressive motives to crying infants. Physicians may witness evidence of poor impulse control, unmet dependency needs, or substance abuse that may put a parent at greater risk. Characteristics of child victims also may be risk factors, such as low birth weight and prematurity, congenital problems, or chronic illness. In addition, twins are at greater risk.

Family and social factors that the physician can use to predict risk include isolation, stress, and even cultural attitudes toward violence. Identification of such risk factors during routine care offers the possibility of increased surveillance for abuse. Self-esteem, stress reduction, problem-solving skills, and social support can be enhanced by means of the relationship with the family physician and appropriate community referrals.

IDENTIFICATION OF PHYSICAL ABUSE. Lines between socially acceptable forms of child discipline and child abuse have changed over time but continue to be indistinct. Differentiating nonaccidental trauma from normal childhood accidents also confounds the problem of diagnosis. When the history offered as to how an injury occurred is incompatible with the injury, or when the stories of different witnesses are variable, suspicion should be aroused. Likewise, an injured child accompanied by a hostile, defensive, or unusually anxious parent may be suspect. The victim also may show evidence of abnormal behavior, such as overt fear of adults or caretakers or extreme passivity or inappropriate physical affection with strangers.

Physicians can enhance their ability to make the diagnosis by taking careful, nonjudgmental histories of the injury from the parents or other adults and the child in separate interviews. Avoidance, delay, or discontinuity of medical attention or a previous history of other "accidents" can be important data.

THE PHYSICAL EXAMINATION IN CHILD ABUSE (Table 5–2). Head trauma is common in child abuse, ranging from superficial injuries of the mouth and face from striking blows to severe intracerebral injury from blows or shaking. Infants are particularly vulnerable to severe head trauma and may not show obvious external signs. Their lack of independent mobility makes all such trauma suspect. Computed tomography (CT) of the head may be an appropriate screening tool if another inflicted injury is documented.

Blunt abdominal trauma may be exhibited as internal bleeding, nonspecific pain, vomiting, or obstruction. Visceral injuries are associated with a high mortality rate and must be evaluated with appropriate thoroughness.

Fractures of the extremities are the most common form of bone injury in abuse, followed in order of occurrence by skull, rib, and clavicular fractures. Half the skeletal injuries in abuse occur in infants less than 1 year old.

Dermatologic abnormalities are among the most common findings in physical abuse. Burns purposefully inflicted from lighted cigarettes as a form of punishment are common and leave round, bullous, scabbed, or scarred lesions. Immersion burns take on a stocking and glove shape, with symmetry, involving palms and soles, unlike most accidental burns. Dunking of the trunk causes burns to the buttocks and genitals, sparing protected areas of skin in folds or centrally (donut-shaped)

TABLE 5–2. PHYSICAL MANIFESTATIONS OF PHYSICAL CHILD ABUSE

Skin Findings

Bruises and Welts
Face, lips, mouth
Back, buttocks, thighs, torso
Clusters or regular patterns
Different stages of healing

Burns
Soles, palms, back, buttocks
Stocking and glove distribution
Donut-shaped areas
Unusual areas
Rope burns

Alopecia
Hair pulling
Occipital (infant neglect)

Lacerations
Back of arms, legs, torso
Genitalia
Mouth, lips, gums, eyes
Human bites

Fractures
Epiphyseal-metaphyseal fractures, especially in infants
Diaphyseal fractures, either spiral or oblique
Skull fractures in infants
Rib fractures
Multiple fractures of different ages
Skeletal trauma in combination with other injury

Head Trauma
Skull fracture, linear
Subdural hemorrhage
Epidural hemorrhage (less common)
Retinal hemorrhage, detachment
Hyphema, dislocated lens
Cerebral edema
Cerebral contusion, hematoma

Blunt Abdominal Trauma
Duodenal hematoma (x-ray study with contrast medium shows intramural mass, "coiled spring" mucosa)
Pancreatitis, pancreatic pseudocyst
Hepatic injury—lacerations

Source: From Rakel RE. Textbook of Family Practices, 4th ed. Philadelphia, W.B. Saunders, 1990. *(Reprinted with permission.)*

where the skin contacts the cool tub. Forcible placing of a child against hot objects can leave symmetrical patterns in unusual places, such as buttocks or back. Restraint or gagging can leave marks at the wrists, ankles, and corners of the mouth.

ACUTE MANAGEMENT OF PHYSICAL ABUSE. The family physician has three compelling objectives in the initial response to suspected child abuse. First, the specific injuries must be assessed and treated. Second, the child must be protected from further harm. The child protective system in most areas offers 24-hour availability for prompt notification and initiation of services. When the immediate protection of a child cannot be ensured in the care of his or her usual guardians or another family member, the child can be remanded into temporary custody of the state, and emergency foster placement can be arranged through court order by the department of

social services. Sometimes admission to the hospital is warranted, either because of the severity of the child's condition or until appropriate investigations or alternative placement arrangements can be made. This can be accomplished even against the parents' will through the hospital administrator and a judge by court order. Having to deal with extremely hostile parents may require assistance from the police or hospital security staff.

The third objective in the acute management of child abuse is careful documentation of the medical record. Ultimate protection of the child from further harm often depends on the legal system to intervene in defining the abuse as criminal. This can serve to limit access to the child by the abusing adult and often can help pay for treatment for the family. The thoroughness and specificity of the physician's account of the history and physical examination may be instrumental in helping agencies to document the nature and severity of abuse and succeed in the child's behalf.

LONG-TERM ROLE OF THE PHYSICIAN IN CHILD ABUSE. The family physician who participates in the acute diagnosis and management of child abuse also can become part of the therapeutic process for the child victim and family through the continuity of the physician–patient relationship. A child facing the turmoil of investigative procedures, court processes, and the temporary or permanent loss of an abusing parent can be soothed by ongoing contact with a familiar, caring person. The focus of helping agencies on their role as child advocates may mean that other family members, including the abuser, are neglected and must face the crisis on their own. The physician can lend support and legitimacy to the helping process. Some families are successfully rehabilitated, and the physician can be a member of the team that nurtures and monitors that process along with social workers, home health workers, counselors, and so on.

Sexual Abuse of Children

The sexual abuse of children represents an entity distinct from physical abuse. In the last decade, sexual abuse of children has evolved from a hidden problem to a subject of tremendous social, legal, scientific, and media concern. Reports of sexual abuse now exceed those of physical abuse in many departments of social service. Despite this increased attention, sexual abuse remains cloaked in secrecy, denial, and taboo, and much of it goes undetected and unreported. Confusion as to what constitutes sexual abuse also compounds this problem. The range of exploitative sexual acts perpetrated on children is broad, including forcible violent rape; coercive, nonviolent anogenital penetration; orogenital contact; sexualized fondling and touching; and even noncontact exploitation. The use of children for prostitution or pornography is also a concern. Child-abuse offenders may be strangers but more often are intimate acquaintances and family members, compounding the betrayal and confusion experienced by their victims. The consequences of sexual victimization in childhood are often devastating, with suicide, chronic mental illness, criminal behavior, substance abuse, sexual dysfunction, and incapacity for intimacy among its long-term sequelae. Sexually transmitted diseases and unwanted pregnancies are potential short-term outcomes. Although sexual abuse is rarely associated with life-threatening harm or violence, it may result in even more damage to the victim's self-concept and ability to reach full adult potential.

EPIDEMIOLOGY OF SEXUAL ABUSE. Since only a small percentage of incidents of sexual abuse are reported, estimating the prevalence of such abuse is extremely difficult. Profiles of victims of reported cases demonstrate a bimodal age distribution, with a large proportion of victims being under 6 years of age. A second peak occurs for adolescent victims. Many more female victims are diagnosed than male victims, but this may represent an artifact of silent suffering and nondetection rather than an actual contrast in incidence. Male victims tend to have younger abusers, and those victims who present for treatment have more frequently been sodomized and exposed to threats or violence. Child victims of both sexes often know their perpetrators, who are almost always men, with the majority being either biologic fathers or stepfathers and most of the others being other close relatives or acquaintances. Vaginal or anal intercourse accounts for only a small portion of sexual abuse. The harmful consequences of sexual exploitation do not correlate well with the seriousness of the abusive act, and inappropriate touching or fondling can be as much a betrayal of trust as more invasive forms of abuse.

IDENTIFYING SEXUAL ABUSE. Some victims of sexual abuse present for evaluation after having made specific disclosures about abusive events to a trusted adult. More commonly, however, such presentations may be masked, with disclosures from the child victim elicited with much difficulty. Shame, fear of reprisals, threats of family disruption, and promises of secrecy to the perpetrator may all contribute to a reluctance to tell on the part of the child. This behooves the family physicians and others in the lives of children to be alert to more subtle clues to the occurrence of sexual abuse (Table 5–3).

Sexual abuse shares behavioral features with other forms of psychologic stress and should be considered as part of the differential diagnosis in nonspecific abnormal presentations. Sexual abuse victims, including very young ones, are more likely than other children to demonstrate age-inappropriate, abnormal sexualized activities, with a precocious understanding or role playing of sexual acts with playmates or other adults. Alertness to masked presentations makes it possible for physicians to explore more carefully for the presence of abuse in such cases.

Genital complaints, an abnormal genital or rectal examination, or the presence of sexually transmitted diseases also can alert the physician to the existence of sexual abuse and are discussed later.

INTERVIEWING POTENTIAL VICTIMS OF SEXUAL ABUSE. Children are often reluctant to tell about sexual encounters, fearing punishment, retribution, disapproval, or abandonment. These obstacles pose a challenge to

TABLE 5–3. POSSIBLE CLUES TO THE PRESENCE OF SEXUAL ABUSE

Infants and Toddlers
Intense fear of a person or place
Abrupt change in behavior
Sleep disturbances (bedwetting, insomnia, nightmares)
Withdrawal or depression
Developmental delays

Physical signs and symptoms
Genital, rectal, or oral trauma or irritation
Urinary tract infection
Foreign bodies in the vagina, urethra, or rectum
Other bruises, burns, or injuries
Vaginitis, unusual vaginal odor or discharge
Complaints of genital or rectal discomfort
Excessive masturbation

Preschool Children
All the signs already listed
A direct or coded statement indicating sexual hurt
Sexual acting out with peers or adults
Precocious knowledge of sexual activities
Excessive sexual curiosity

Physical signs and symptoms
Enuresis, encopresis
Regressive behavior
Hyperactivity
Somatic complaints—headache, abdominal pain, constipation

School-Aged Children
All the signs already listed
Disturbed peer interactions
Change in school performance
Mistrust of adults in general
Depression, withdrawal, sadness
Aggression, rage
Sleeping disorders—nightmares, insomnia
Avoidance of physical activity and undressing

Adolescents
All the signs already listed
Self-destructive activity or suicidal thoughts, gestures
Eating disorders (especially binging and purging)
Delinquent behavior or running away
Drug and alcohol use
Early pregnancy
Prostitution, promiscuous behavior, or other unusual sexual
  behavior

Source: From Rakel RE. Textbook of Family Practice, 4th ed. Philadelphia, W.B. Saunders, 1990. *(Reprinted with permission.)*

history taking in suspected cases. Young children may not have an adequate understanding of what has happened to them to be able to provide coherent details, and some victims are too young to communicate verbally at all. As if these problems were not enough, the interviewing process is also subjected to strict requirements of technique, since such disclosures to the physician are often part of crucial legal testimony for use in protection of the child, and the physician's interview must be free of coercion or leading questions.

Sexually abused children have already had the boundaries of their privacy invaded by someone in authority. In such cases, the medical evaluation must balance the needs of the child for control with the need to gather information for the child's protection. The experience can be extremely anxiety-producing for the victim and must be performed with extreme care and gentleness. In addition, the gender of the examiner sometimes makes a significant difference to the child.

If possible, the child should be interviewed alone. The physician can create an atmosphere of acceptance and calm. The child's verbal and cognitive maturity must guide the line of questioning, and when some kind of sexual contact is suspected, one of the first steps at eliciting information is discovery and use of the child's own vocabulary for body parts. Children can be given specific reassurance that the physician will not be angry with them no matter what they say, that they have done nothing wrong, and that the physician wants to help the child. In situations in which abuse is suspected but not corroborated by the child, disclosure to the physician may not occur during the first visit.

Children can be encouraged to say if they have had any problem with an adult in which the adult has touched them or hurt them or asked them to do something they did not want to do. The use of anatomically correct dolls has facilitated such interviews with young children, who may be more comfortable showing what happened using the dolls. Such children can then be asked several questions: "Did someone do that to you?" "Who was that?" "What else did he [or she] do?" "Where were you when this happened?" "Where was your mommy [or daddy]?" "What did he [or she] tell you?" "Did that happen any other time?" This approach avoids complex questions, uses the child's own words, and does not lead the child with closed questions. Specialists in child sexual abuse are experienced and painstaking in this process and can be called on as consultants.

THE PHYSICAL EXAMINATION IN SEXUAL ABUSE. The physician must perform a detailed physical examination, with special attention to the genital and rectal areas for evidence of sexual trauma or infection. This examination can provoke anxiety in the child and in rare extreme cases needs to be performed under sedation. To lessen the possibility of discomfort, the physician should attend to reassuring and informing the child about the examination, attend to the child's modesty, and invite a trusted companion to accompany the child. Inspection of a female child's vulvar area can be accomplished in either the lithotomy or the knee-chest position, with gentle lateral traction of the adjacent buttocks. The child can participate by performing this traction herself. Evidence of trauma or discharge should be sought and detailed (Table 5–4). The transverse diameter of the vaginal orifice should be measured in millimeters, since an opening of greater than 4 mm in prepubertal girls is associated with sexual abuse at least 85% of the time (Cantwell). Physicians must become familiar with the varied appearance of the normal prepubertal hymen in order to identify abnormalities and should make this inspection a routine part of all well-child examinations. The anus also should be inspected for dilation, laxity, and trauma.

LABORATORY EVALUATION IN SEXUAL ABUSE. Adjunctive laboratory examination can assist in documenting the existence of sexual contact and can determine po-

TABLE 5–4. PHYSICAL FINDINGS IN SEXUAL ABUSE OF CHILDREN

Genital Fondling or Manipulation
Erythema
Perihymenal neovascularization
Hymenal rounding, microscarring
Clitoral hood hypertrophy
Introital synechiae
Hymenal or labial trauma above three o'clock and nine o'clock positions

Vulvar Coitus
As listed earlier plus:
Perihymenal abrasions
Laceration or scarring of posterior fourchette

Vaginal Penetration—Acute
As listed earlier plus:
Labial contusion, ecchymosis
Introital abrasions
Vaginal abrasions
Fourchette or hymenal transection
Pubococcygeal spasm

Chronic Genital Sexual Abuse
Vulvar hypopigmentation, hyperpigmentation
Clitoral hood cutaneous hypertrophy
Introital scarring, neovascularization, synechiae
Fourchette scarring, deformity
Enlarged hymenal diameter
Vaginitis

Anal Penetration
Perianal edema, abrasions, petechiae
Acute anal fissures
Acute anal spasm
Chronic fissures with induration
Venous dilation
Pigmentation changes
Perianal hyperkeratosis
Scarring, anal deformity
Skin tags
Funnel anus with laxity
Reflex dilatation of anal sphincter

Source: From Rakel RE. Textbook of Family Practice, 4th ed. Philadelphia, W.B. Saunders, 1990. *(Reprinted with permission.)*

tential harmful consequences of such contact, such as pregnancy or infection. A pubertal victim should have a sensitive urine pregnancy test. Three orifices—mouth, rectum, and vagina (or urethra in males)—should be cultured for *Neisseria gonorrhoeae* and *Chlamydia trachomatis*. The presence of either of these infections in children can be considered presumptive evidence of sexual abuse. Collections of vaginal secretions in saline to reveal *Trichomonas* or *Gardnerella* infections should be done, if indicated.

PSYCHOLOGIC TREATMENT OF INCESTUOUS FAMILIES AND SEXUAL ABUSE VICTIMS. Once sexual abuse is documented and the victim is protected from further exploitation, the healing process can begin. Single assaults in the context of a supportive family environment are rarely damaging to the developing child. Chronic sexual abuse by a family member is more insidious. Victims often have ambivalent feelings about the abuse itself, since there may be aspects of the close relationship with the abuser and the physical contact itself that may be associated with positive feelings for the child. Through treatment, it is hoped that victims gain insight into their lack of culpability despite their ambivalence; integrate ambivalent feelings for the abuser, including resolution of rage; and gradually gain confidence in their ability to control interpersonal boundaries in their lives while risking the loss of trust and intimacy with others.

Offenders have varying rates of rehabilitative success depending on the etiology and nature of their disorders. Those who are compulsive child molesters, with multiple victims, and who demonstrate a persistent sexual orientation toward children are refractory to most treatment. Others who revert to child partners under times of stress but who have the capacity to relate to adults normally may be treatable.

ADULT VICTIMS OF PREVIOUS CHILD ABUSE. Among the adult patients of the family physician are likely to be many persons who were victimized in their childhood, physically, sexually, or both, and who were never identified or treated. Some of the same behavioral indicators used as clues for the identification of child victims are pertinent for adults as well. Chronic somatic complaints with an unclear etiology, depression, substance abuse, and poor self-esteem are all clues to prompt the physician to inquire about a history of abuse. Until victims acknowledge their childhood wounds, it is unlikely that they will be able to function in fully satisfied lives. Former victims can be found among populations of physicians as well, and their histories may handicap them even further in their response to this important clinical situation. Once previous abuse is diagnosed, however, treatment can begin, with supportive listening, individual psychotherapy, and group work with other survivors of incest and sexual abuse.

REFERENCES

Anderson BJ, Miller JP, Auslander WF, Santiago JV. Family characteristics of diabetic adolescents: Relationship to metabolic control. Diabetes Care 1981; 4:586–594.

Anstett R, Lewis B. The single parent family: How an understanding physician can help. Postgrad Med 1986; 80(2):137–140.

Beautrais AL, Fergusson DM, Shannon FT. Life events and childhood morbidity: A prospective study. Pediatrics 1982; 70:935–940.

Berkman LF, Syme SL. Social networks, host resistance and mortality: A nine-year follow-up study of Alameda County residents. Am J Epidemiol 1979; 109:186–204.

Berkman LF. Assessing the physical health effects of social networks and social supports. Annu Rev Public Health 1984; 5:413–432.

Bray JH. Children's development during early remarriage. In Hetherington EM, Arasteh J (eds.): The Impact of Divorce, Single-parenting and Step-Parenting on Children. Hillsdale, N.J., Lawrence Erlbaum Associates, 1988.

Bray JH, Berger SH, Silverblatt A, Hollier A. Family process and organization during early remarriage: A preliminary analysis. In Vincent JP (ed.): Advances in Family Intervention, Assessment, and Theory, vol. 4. Greenwich, Conn., JAI Press, 1987.

Bryan MS, Lowenberg ME. The father's influence on young children's food preferences. J Am Diet Assoc 1958; 34:30–35.

Cantwell HB. Update of vaginal inspection as it relates to child sexual abuse in girls under thirteen. Child Abuse Neglect 1987; 11:545–546.

Doherty WJ, Schrott HG, Metcalf L, Iassiello-Vailas L. Effect of spouse support and health beliefs on medication adherence. J Fam Pract 1983; 17:837–841.

Gustafsson PA, Kjellman NM, Cederblad M. Family therapy in the treatment of severe childhood asthma. J Psychosom Res 1986; 30:369–374.

Haynes RB, Mattson ME, Chobanian AV, et al. Management of patient compliance in the treatment of hypertension: Report of the NHLBI working group. Hypertension 1982; 4:415–423.

Hetherington EM, Cox M, Cox R. Long-term effects of divorce and remarriage on the adjustment of children. J Am Acad Child Psychiatry 1985; 24:518–530.

Hetherington EM, Cox M, Cox R. Effects of divorce on parents and children. In Lamb, ME (ed.): Nontraditional Families: Parenting and Child Development. Hillsdale, N.J., Lawrence Erlbaum Associates, 1982.

Hetherington EM, Cox M, Cox R. The aftermath of divorce. In Stevens JH, Mathews M (eds.): Mother–Child, Father–Child Relations. Washington, NAEYC, 1978.

Hetherington EM, Camara K. Families in transition: The processes of dissolution and reconstitution. In Parke RD (ed.): Review of Child Development Research, vol. 7: The Family. Chicago, University of Chicago Press, 1984.

Holmes TH, Rahe RH. The social readjustment scale. J Psychosom Res 1967; 39:413–431.

House JS, Landis KR, Umberson D. Social relationships and health. Science 1988; 241:540–545.

Kelly JB. Longer-term adjustment in children of divorce. J Fam Psychol 1988; 2:119–140.

Kiecolt-Glaser JK, Fisher LD, Ogrocki P, et al. Marital quality, marital disruption, and immune function. Psychosom Med 1987; 49:1:13–34.

Lask B, Matthew D. Childhood asthma: A controlled trial of family psychotherapy. Arch Dis Child 1979; 54:116–119.

McDaniel SH, Campbell TL, Seaburn D. Family-Oriented Primary Care: A Manual for Medical Providers. New York, Springer-Verlag, 1989.

Meyer RJ, Haggerty RJ. Streptococcal infections in families: Factors altering individual susceptibility. Pediatrics 1962; 29:539–549.

Minuchin S, Rosman BL, Baker L. Psychosomatic Families. Cambridge, Harvard University Press, 1978.

Minuchin S, Baker L, Rosman BL, et al. A conceptual model of psychosomatic illness in children: Family organization and family therapy. Arch Gen Psychiatry 1975; 32:1031–1038.

Morisky DE, Levine DM, Green LW, et al. Five-year blood pressure control and mortality following health education for hypertensive patients. Am J Public Health 1983; 73:153–162.

Somers AR. Marital status, health, and the use of health services. JAMA 1979; 241:1818–1822.

Stuart RB, Davis B. Slim Chance in a Fat World: Behavioral Control Obesity. Champaign, Ill., Research Press, 1972.

Verbrugge LM. Marital status and health. J Marr Fam 1979; 41:267–285.

Visher EB, Visher JS. Stepfamilies. New York, Brunner/Mazel, 1979.

Visher EB, Visher JS. Old Loyalties, New Ties: Therapeutic Strategies with Stepfamilies. New York, Brunner/Mazel, 1988.

Wallerstein JS, Kelly J. Surviving the Break-Up: How Children and Parents Cope with Divorce. New York, Basic Books, 1980.

White K, Kolman ML, Wexler P, et al. Unstable diabetes and unstable families: A psychosocial evaluation of diabetic children with recurrent ketoacidosis. Pediatrics 1984; 73:749–755.

Wood LE, Poole SR. Stepfamilies in family practice. J Fam Pract 1983; 16(4):739–744.

Working Group on Health Education and High Blood Pressure Control, National Institute of Heart, Lung, and Blood. The Physician's Guide: Improving Adherence among Hypertensive Patients. Washington, U.S. Government Printing Office, 1987.

World Health Organization. Statistical Indices of Family Health 1976; 589:17.

QUESTIONS

1. Chronic family stress has been associated with more frequent occurrence of which of the following?
   a. Spontaneous abortions
   b. Streptococcal pharyngitis
   c. Alzheimer's disease
   d. Myocardial infarction
   e. Head injuries

2. Which of the following is the most important source of social support for adults?
   a. Parents
   b. Close friends
   c. Co-workers
   d. Children
   e. Spouse

3. The clustering or concordance of cardiovascular risk factors between spouses is best explained by which of the following?
   a. Genetics
   b. Shared environment
   c. Assortative mating
   d. Influence of one spouse on the others behavior
   e. Chance

4. Which of the following has *not* been associated with successful smoking cessation?
   a. Being married to a nonsmoker
   b. Having a partner who has quit smoking
   c. Reinforcement of quitting by spouse
   d. Having no other smokers in the family
   e. "Policing" of smoking by partner

5. Which of the following is *not* a characteristic of psychosomatic families, as described by Minuchin et al.?
   a. Enmeshment
   b. Expressed hostility
   c. Overprotectiveness
   d. Rigidity
   e. Conflict avoidance

6. Good blood sugar control in diabetes has been associated with which of the following family characteristics?
   a. High cohesion (enmeshment)
   b. Low cohesion (disengagement)
   c. Absence of family conflict
   d. Clear organization
   e. Open communication

7. Family therapy has been shown to improve the outcome of which of the following childhood diseases?
   a. Asthma
   b. Diabetes mellitus
   c. Hypercholesterolemia
   d. Cystic fibrosis
   e. Atopic dermatitis

8. The experience of divorce is
   a. Always bad for family members.
   b. Varies in its impact and duration of effects.
   c. Is more extensive and harder for adult women.
   d. Is easiest for boys.

9. Children's reactions to their parents' divorce varies according to their
   a. Gender.
   b. Genotype.
   c. Intelligence.
   d. Children's reactions are all basically the same.

10. Which of the following has the most *negative* impact on children following divorce?
    a. Living only with their mothers
    b. Living only with their fathers
    c. Exposure to high levels of interparental conflict
    d. Being labeled from a "broken home"

11. Family physicians can best help their patients who are undergoing a divorce by
    a. Reassuring them that everything will be better in a year or two.
    b. Telling them that divorce is not all bad anymore and not to worry.
    c. Not talking to patients about these issues.
    d. Listening emphatically and providing emotional support.

12. Young children (ages 2 to 4 years) are more likely to respond to their parents' separation and divorce by
    a. Blaming the parent who leaves for all the problems.
    b. Regressing and being more whiney and clingy.
    c. Becoming depressed.
    d. Children this age are not likely to have any particularly negative response to their parents' separation and divorce.

13. Marital disruption
    a. Is unrelated to an individual's health and adjustment.
    b. Causes minimal damage to a person's health.
    c. Is a powerful predictor of stress-related physical illness.
    d. Only affects an individual's health if he or she is above the age of 40.

14. Options for physicians who suspect that a child may be a victim of abuse include all the following *except*
    a. Careful physical examination.

b. Admitting the child to a hospital against the parents' wishes.
c. Radiologic examination to look for previous trauma.
d. Documenting current findings and waiting for more definitive evidence.
e. Interviewing the child without caretakers present.

15. Which of the following is definitive evidence that sexual abuse *did not* take place?
a. Denial by the child of sexual abuse
b. Normal physical examination
c. Close relationships with family members
d. Unfamiliarity with the names of genital parts
e. None of the above.

16. The most common fractures resulting from physical abuse of children are
a. Skull fractures.
b. Fractures of the extremities.
c. Clavicular fractures.
d. Rib fractures.
e. Fractures of the nasal bones.

17. Behavior in a preschool child that is *least likely* to arouse suspicion about possible sexual abuse is
a. Excessive sexual curiosity.
b. Anxiety in the presence of men.
c. Sleep problems.
d. Hitting younger siblings.
e. Regressive behavior.

18. The most common perpetrators of child sexual abuse are
a. Women.
b. Strangers.
c. Fathers or stepfathers.
d. Older siblings.
e. Male neighbors.

Answers appear on page 445.

THE FAMILY IMPACT OF ILLNESS AND DISABILITY

JOHN S. ROLLAND

This chapter provides a family systems–oriented model for clinical practice with chronic and life-threatening illness. At the heart of all systems–oriented inquiry is the focus on *interaction*. In the arena of physical illness, particularly chronic disease, the focus is the systemic interaction of a disease with an individual, family, and other biopsychosocial systems (Engel). This chapter centers on the family level in recognition that the family is a system influenced heavily by a range of social, economic, institutional, and political forces in the larger environment. A scheme of the systemic interaction of family and illness might look like the diagram in Figure 6–1.

This diagram illustrates the three central constructs of the family systems–illness model that will be described: (1) psychosocial typology and key time phases in the natural history of illnesses; (2) interface of illness, individual, and family development; and (3) family health/illness belief system (Rolland).

PSYCHOSOCIAL TYPOLOGY OF ILLNESS

In order to think in an interactive or systemic manner about illness, individual and family, we need a way to characterize the illness in psychosocial terms over time. The standard disease classification is based on purely biologic criteria that are clustered in ways to establish a medical diagnosis and treatment plan rather than the psychosocial demands on patients and their families. A schema that conceptualizes chronic diseases is required that remains simultaneously relevant to both the psychosocial and biologic worlds and provides a common language that transforms or reclassifies our usual medical terminology. Better linkage of these two worlds will help to clarify the relationship between long-term illnesses and the family. There have been two major impediments to progress in this area. First, insufficient attention has been paid to the areas of diversity and commonality inherent in different chronic illnesses. Second, there has been a glossing over of the qualitative and quantitative differences in how various diseases are manifest over the course of an illness. Chronic illnesses need to be conceptualized in a manner that organizes these similarities and differences over the disease course so that the type and degree of demands relevant to clinical practice are highlighted in a more useful way.

The psychosocial importance of different time phases of an illness is poorly understood. Clinicians often become involved in the care of an individual or family coping with a chronic illness at different points in the "illness life cycle." Understanding the evolution of a long-term illness is hindered because clinicians rarely follow the family through the complete life history of a disease. For example, a longitudinal framework will help clarify the adaptive versus harmful effects of denial over the course of an illness. For parents of a child with leukemia, denial may enable them adaptively to perform necessary duties during earlier phases of the illness but might lead to devastating consequences for the family if maintained during the terminal phase. Likewise, denial may be functional for recovery on a coronary care unit after a myocardial infarction but harmful if this translates into ignoring medical advice vis-à-vis diet, exercise, and work stress over the long term.

The problems of illness variability and time phases are addressed in two separate dimensions: (1) chronic illnesses are grouped according to key biologic similarities and differences that dictate significantly distinct psychosocial demands for the ill individual and his or her family, and (2) the prime developmental time phases in the natural evolution of chronic disease are identified.

Psychosocial Types of Illness

The goal of a psychosocial typology is to facilitate the creation of categories with similar psychosocial demands for a wide array of chronic illnesses. This typology is not intended for traditional medical purposes but

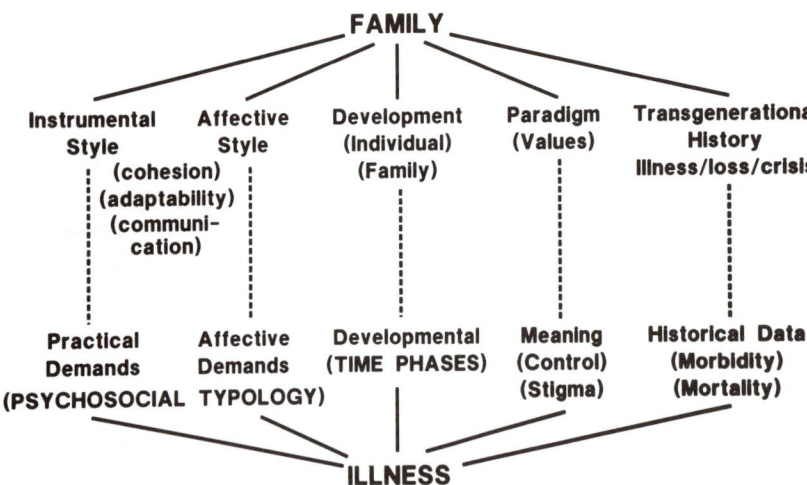

Figure 6–1. Interface of chronic illness and the family. (Modified from Rolland, J.S.: Family systems and chronic illness: A typological model. J. Psychother. Fam., 3(3):143–168, 1987, with permission.)

to examine the relationship between family dynamics and chronic disease. It conceptualizes broad distinctions of (1) onset, (2) course, (3) outcome, and (4) degree of incapacitation of illness. For a broad range of diseases, these categories are hypothesized to be the most psychosocially significant. Although each variable is actually a continuum, it will be described here by the selection of key anchor points along the continuum.

ONSET. Illnesses can be divided into those which have either an acute onset, such as strokes, or a gradual such as Parkinson's disease. Although the total amount of family adaptation might be the same for both types of illness, for acute onset illnesses these affective and practical changes are compressed into a short time. This will require that the family more rapidly mobilize crisis management skills. Families able to tolerate highly charged affective states, exchange clearly defined roles flexibly, solve problems efficiently, and utilize outside resources have an advantage in managing acute-onset illnesses. The rate of family change required to cope with gradual-onset diseases allows for a more protracted period of adjustment.

COURSE. The course of chronic diseases can take three general forms: progressive, constant, or relapsing/episodic. A "progressive" disease (e.g., Alzheimer's disease, emphysema) is one that is continually or generally symptomatic and progresses in severity. The individual and family are faced with the effects of a perpetually symptomatic family member, in whom disability increases in a stepwise fashion. This means that a family must live with the prospect of continual role change and adaptation as the disease progresses. Periods of relief from the demands of the illness tend to be minimal. Increasing strain on family caretakers is caused by both exhaustion and the continual addition of new caretaking tasks over time.

A "constant" course in illness is one in which, typically, an initial event occurs and then the biologic course stabilizes. A single-episode myocardial infarction or spinal cord injury are two examples. Typically, after an initial period of recovery, the chronic phase is characterized by some clear-cut deficit or residual functional

limitation. Recurrences can occur, but the individual or family is faced with a semipermanent change that is stable and predictable over a considerable time span. The potential for family exhaustion exists without the strain of new role demands over time.

A "relapsing" or "episodic" course in illnesses such as ulcerative colitis and asthma is distinguished by the alternation of stable periods of varying length, characterized by a low level or absence of symptoms, with periods of flare-up or exacerbation. Strain on the family system is caused by both the frequency of transitions between crisis and noncrisis and the ongoing uncertainty of *when* a recurrence will occur. This requires a family flexibility for alternation between two forms of family organization. Also, the wide psychologic discrepancy between periods of normalcy versus illness is a particularly taxing feature unique to relapsing diseases.

OUTCOME. The extent to which a chronic illness is a likely cause of death and the degree to which it can shorten one's life span are critical features with profound psychosocial impact. The most crucial factor is the *initial expectation* of whether a disease is a likely cause of death. At one end of the continuum are illnesses that do not typically affect the life span, such as lumbosacral disc disease or arthritis. At the other extreme are illnesses that are clearly progressive and usually fatal, such as metastatic cancer or acquired immune deficiency syndrome (AIDS). There is also an intermediate, and more unpredictable, category, including both illnesses that shorten the life span, such as cardiovascular disease, and those with the possibility of sudden death, such as hemophilia. Perhaps the major difference between these kinds of outcomes is the degree to which the family experiences anticipatory loss and its pervasive effects on family life (Rolland).

When loss is less imminent or certain an outcome, illnesses that may shorten life or cause sudden death provide a fertile ground for idiosyncratic family interpretations. The "it could happen" nature of these illnesses creates a nidus for both overprotection by the family and powerful secondary gains for the ill member. This is particularly relevant to childhood illnesses, such as hemophilia, juvenile-onset diabetes, and asthma (Herz; Minuchin et al.).

INCAPACITATION. Incapacitation can result from impairment of cognition (e.g., Alzheimer's disease), sensation (e.g., blindness), movement (e.g., stroke with paralysis, multiple sclerosis), energy production (e.g., cardiovascular disease), and disfiguring (e.g., severe burns) diseases associated with social stigma (e.g., AIDS).

The extent, type, and timing of incapacitation imply sharp differences in the degree of stress facing a family. For instance, the combined cognitive and motor deficits of a person with a stroke necessitate greater family role reallocation than for a spinal cord–injured person who

retains his or her cognitive abilities. For some illnesses, such as stroke, incapacitation is often worst at the time of onset and would magnify family coping issues related to onset, expected course, and outcome. For progressive diseases, such as Alzheimer's disease, disability looms as an increasing problem in later phases of the illness, allowing a family more time to prepare for anticipated changes. It provides an opportunity for the ill member to participate in disease-related family planning.

By combining the kinds of onset, course, outcome, and incapacitation into a grid format, we generate a typology with 32 potential psychosocial types of illness (Table 6–1).

TABLE 6–1. CATEGORIZATION OF CHRONIC ILLNESSES BY PSYCHOSOCIAL TYPE

		INCAPACITATING		NONINCAPACITATING	
		Acute	Gradual	Acute	Gradual
Progressive	F a t a l		Lung cancer with CNS metastases AIDS Bone marrow failure Amyotrophic lateral sclerosis	Acute leukemia Pancreatic cancer Metastatic breast cancer Malignant melanoma Lung cancer Liver cancer, etc.	Cystic fibrosis*
Relapsing				Cancers in remission	
Progressive	P o s s i b l y	S h o r t e n e d		Emphysema Alzheimer's disease Multi-infarct dementia Multiple sclerosis (late) Chronic alcoholism Huntington's chorea Scleroderma		Juveniel diabetes* Malignant hypertension Insulin-dependent adult-onset diabetes
Relapsing		L i f e	Angina	Early multiple sclerosis Episodic alcoholism	Sickel cell disease* Hemophilia*	Systemic lupus erythematosus*
Constant	F a t a l	S p a n	Stroke Moderate severe myocardial infarction	PKU and other inborn errors of metabolism	Mild myocardial infarction Cardiac arrhythmia	Hemodialysis treated renal failure Hodgkin's disease
Progressive				Parkinson's disease Rheumatoid arthritis Osteoarthritis		Non-insulin-dependent adult-onset diabetes
Relapsing	N o n f a t a l		Lumbosacral disc disease		Kidney stones Gout Migraine Seasonal allergy Asthma Epilepsy	Peptic ulcer Ulcerative colitis Chronic bronchitis Othr inflammatory bowel diseases Psoriasis
Constant			Congenital malformations Spinal cord injury Acute blindness Acute deafness Survived severe trauma and burns Posthypoxic syndrome	Nonprogressive mental retardation Cerebral palsy	Benign arrhythmia Congenital heart disease	Malabsorption syndromes Hyper-/hypothyroidism Pernicious anemia Controlled hypertension Controlled glaucoma

Source: From Rolland JS, Toward a psychosocial typology of chronic and life-threatening illness. Fam Systems Med 1984; 2(3):245–263. (Reprinted with permission.)
*Early.

The predictability of an illness and the degree of uncertainty about the specific way or rate at which it unfolds overlay and color the other attributes: onset, course, outcome, and incapacitation. For illnesses with highly unpredictable courses, such as multiple sclerosis, family coping and adaptation, especially future planning, are hindered by anticipatory anxiety and ambiguity about what they will actually have to deal with. Families unable to put long-term uncertainty into perspective are at high risk of exhaustion and dysfunction.

The complexity, frequency, and efficacy of a treatment regimen, the amount of home- versus hospital-based care required by the disease, and the frequency and intensity of symptoms vary widely across illnesses with important implications for individual and family adaptation. Some regimens require significant financial resources and caregiving time and energy (e.g., home kidney dialysis, cystic fibrosis). Treatments least likely to be adhered to are those which have a high impact on lifestyles, are difficult to accomplish, and have minimal effects on the level of symptoms or prognosis (Strauss). Although they reduce time-consuming dependence on medical centers, home-based treatments place heavier responsibility on patient and family. Therefore, the degree of family emotional support, role flexibility, effective problem solving, and communication in relation to these treatment factors will be crucial predictors of long-term treatment compliance.

It is important to consider the likelihood and severity of disease-related crises (Strauss) and associated family anxiety. A clinician should assess the family's understanding about the possibility, frequency, and lethality of a medical crisis. How congruent is the family's understanding with that of the medical team? Are their expectations catastrophic, or do they minimize real dangers? Are there clear warning signs that the patient or family can recognize? Can a medical crisis be prevented or mitigated by detection of early warning signs or institution of prompt treatment? When a patient or family heeds the early warning signs of a diabetes insulin reaction or asthma attack, a full-blown crisis can usually be averted. How complex are the rescue operations? Do they require simple measures carried out at home (e.g., medication, bed rest), or do they necessitate outside assistance or hospitalization? How long can crises last before a family can resume "day-to-day" functioning? It is essential to ask a family about its planning for such crises and the extent and accuracy of their medical knowledge. How clearly has leadership, role reallocation, emotional support, and use of resources outside the family been formulated? If an illness began with an acute crisis (e.g., stroke), then assessment of that event provides useful information as to how that family handles *unexpected* crises. Evaluating the overall viability of the family's crisis planning is crucial.

Time Phases of Illness

In this psychosocial schema of chronic diseases, the developmental time phases of illness is a second dimension. The concept of time phases provides a way for the clinician to think longitudinally and to reach a fuller understanding of chronic illness as an ongoing process with landmarks, transitions, and changing demands. Each phase has its own unique psychosocial developmental tasks that require significantly different strengths, attitudes, or changes from a family. To capture the core psychosocial themes in the natural history of chronic disease, three major phases can be described: (1) crisis, (2) chronic, and (3) terminal. The relationship between a more detailed chronic disease time line and one grouped into broad time phases is diagrammed in Figure 6–2.

The "crisis" phase includes any symptomatic period before diagnosis and the initial period of readjustment and coping after the problem has been clarified through a diagnosis and initial treatment plan. This period holds a number of key tasks for the ill member and family. Moos describes certain universal practical illness-related tasks, including (1) learning to deal with pain, incapacitation, or other illness-related symptoms, (2) learning to deal with the hospital environment and any disease-related treatment procedures, and (3) establishing and maintaining workable relationships with the health care team. In addition, there are critical tasks of a more general, sometimes existential, nature. The family needs to (1) create a meaning for the illness event that maximizes a preservation of a sense of mastery and competency, (2) grieve for the loss of the preillness family identity, (3) gradually accept the illness as permanent while maintaining a sense of continuity between their past and future, (4) pull together to undergo short-term crisis reorganization, and (5) in the face of uncertainty, develop a systemic flexibility toward future goals.

During this initial crisis period, health care providers have enormous influence over a family's sense of competence and the methods devised to accomplish these developmental tasks. The initial meetings and advice

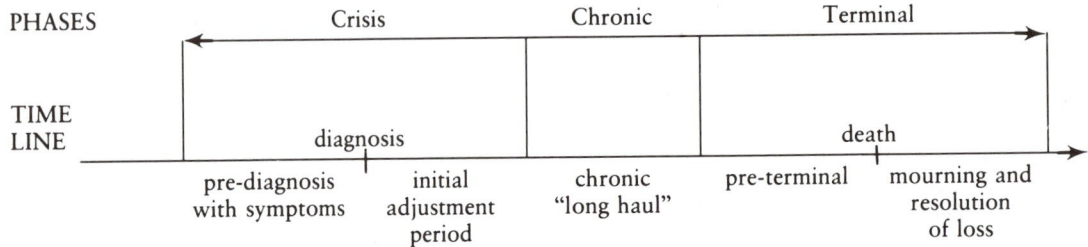

Figure 6–2. Psychosocial time phases of illness. (From Rolland, J.S.: Toward a psychosocial typology of chronic and life-threatening illness. Fam. Systems Med., 2(3):245–263, 1984, with permission.)

given by providers at the time of diagnosis can be thought of as a "framing event." Because families are so vulnerable at this point, clinicians need to be extremely sensitive to their interactions with family members. Who is included or excluded (e.g., patient) from a discussion can be interpreted by the family as a message of how a family should plan their communication for the duration of the illness. One family, accustomed to open, frank discussion, described how the physician came to the mother's hospital room and took the family members to a separate room to inform them that the mother had cancer and to discuss the diagnosis. At this vulnerable moment, the family felt that they were being instructed implicitly to exclude the mother in any discussion of her cancer. Providers who—in some fashion—blame the patient, a family member, or the whole family for an illness (e.g., delay in seeking an appointment, negligence by parents, poor health habits) or distance themselves from a family may undercut a family's attempt to sustain a sense of competence.

The "chronic" phase, whether long or short, is the time span between the initial diagnosis and readjustment period and the third phase when issues of death and terminal illness predominate. This phase can be marked by constancy, progression, or episodic change. Thus its meaning cannot be grasped by simply knowing the biologic behavior of an illness. Rather, it has been referred to as "the long haul," or "day-to-day living with chronic illness," phase. Often the individual and family have come to grips psychologically and organizationally with the permanent changes presented by a chronic illness and have devised an ongoing modus operandi. The ability of the family to maintain the semblance of a normal life with a chronic illness and heightened uncertainty is a key task of this period. If the illness is potentially fatal, this is a time of "living in limbo." For certain highly debilitating but not clearly fatal illnesses, such as a massive stroke or dementia, the family can become saddled with an exhausting problem seemingly without end. Paradoxically, a family's hope to resume a normal life cycle might only be realized after the death of their ill member. This highlights another crucial task of this phase: the maintenance of maximal autonomy for *all* family members.

For long-term disorders, customary patterns of intimacy for couples become skewed by discrepancies between the ill member and well spouse/caretaker. Emotions often remain underground and contribute to "survivor guilt." As one young husband lamented about his wife's cancer, "It was hard enough 2 years ago to absorb that, even if Ann was cured, her radiation treatment would make pregnancy impossible. Now I find it unbearable that her continued slow, losing battle with cancer makes it impossible to go for our dreams like other couples our age." Psychoeducational family interventions that normalize such emotions related to threatened loss can help prevent cycles of blame, shame, and guilt.

Medical care for chronic illnesses is often provided in specialty clinics, where patients and families dealing with similar disorders may develop significant relationships, even in the clinic waiting area. Progression, relapse, or death of another patient can trigger fears of "Will I [we] be next" and deflate family morale. It is useful for clinicians to inquire about such contacts and offer family consultations.

The last or "terminal" phase includes the preterminal stage of an illness, where the inevitability of death becomes apparent and dominates family life. This phase is distinguished by issues surrounding separation, death, grief, resolution of mourning, and resumption of normal family life beyond the loss.

Critical transition periods link the three time phases. Carter and McGoldrick and Levinson have clarified the importance of transition periods in the family and adult life-cycle literature. Transitions in the illness life cycle are times when families reevaluate the appropriateness of their previous life structure in the face of new illness-related developmental demands. Unfinished business from the previous phase can complicate or block movement through the transitions. Families can become permanently frozen in an adaptive structure that has outlived its utility (Penn). For example, the usefulness of pulling together in the crisis period can become a maladaptive and stifling prison for all family members in the chronic phase. Enmeshed families would have difficulty negotiating this delicate transition.

The interaction of the time phases and typology of illness provides a framework for a chronic disease psychosocial developmental model that resembles models for human development. The time phases (crisis, chronic, and terminal) can be considered broad developmental periods in the natural history of chronic disease. Each period has certain basic tasks independent of the type of illness. Each "type" of illness has specific supplementary tasks. The basic tasks of the three illness phases and transitions recapitulate in many respects the unfolding of human development. For example, the crisis phase is similar in certain fundamental ways to the period of childhood and adolescence. Child development involves a prolonged period during which the child learns the fundamentals of life as parents temper other developmental plans (e.g., career) to accommodate raising children. In an analogous way, the crisis phase is a period of socialization to the basics of living with chronic disease, when other life plans are frequently put on hold by the family to accommodate to the illness. Just as the transition from adolescence to adulthood is marked by the relinquishing of a moratorium in order to assume adult identity and responsibilities (Erikson), the transition to the chronic phase of illness emphasizes autonomy and the creation of a viable, ongoing life given the realities of the illness. In the transition to the chronic phase, a "hold" or moratorium on other developmental tasks that served to protect the initial period of socialization/adaptation to life with chronic disease is reevaluated. The separate developmental tasks of "living with chronic illness" and "living out the other parts of one's life" must be brought together.

The psychosocial types and phases of illness can be combined into a typology so that each "psychosocial type" of illness can be thought about in relation to each

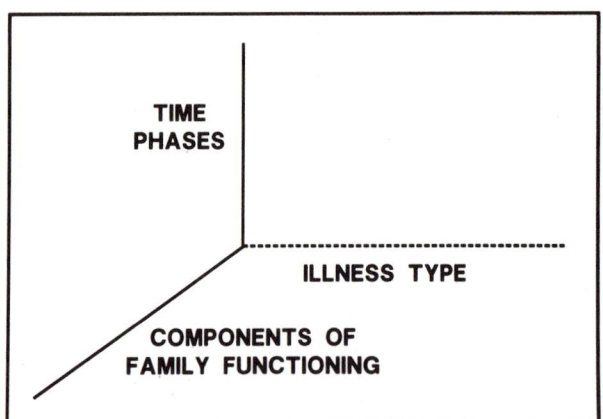

Figure 6–3. Three-dimensional model representing the relationship between illness type, time phases, and family functioning. (Modified from Rolland, J.S.: Chronic illness and the life cycle: A conceptual framework. Fam. Proc., 26(2):203–221, 1987, with permission.)

of the time phases. The addition of a family systems model creates a three-dimensional family systems–illness model (Fig. 6–3). Psychosocial illness types, illness time phases, and key family systems variables constitute the three dimensions. This model allows consideration of the importance of strengths and weaknesses in various components of family functioning in relation to different types of disease at different illness phases.

Clinical Implications

By facilitating a clinician's grasp of chronic illness and disability in psychosocial terms, this model provides a framework for assessment and clinical intervention with a family facing a chronic or life-threatening illness. Attention to features of onset, course, outcome, and incapacitation provide markers that focus a clinician's questioning of a family. For instance, acute-onset illnesses demand high levels of adaptability, problem solving, role reallocation, and balanced cohesion. A high degree of family enmeshment might make a family less likely to be able to cope with these demands. Forethought on this issue would cue a clinician toward a more appropriate family evaluation.

An illness time line delineates psychosocial developmental stages of an illness, each phase with its own unique developmental tasks. It is important for families to solve phase-related tasks within the time limits set by the duration of each successive developmental phase of an illness. The failure to resolve issues in this sequential manner can jeopardize the total coping process of the family. Therefore, attention to time allows the clinician to assess a family's strengths and vulnerabilities in relation to the present and future phases of the illness.

The model clarifies treatment planning. Taken together, the psychosocial types and the time phases provide a context to integrate other aspects of a comprehensive family assessment (described in the next section) (Chilman et al.). Awareness of the components of family functioning most relevant to particular types or phases of an illness guides goal setting. Sharing this information with the family and deciding on specific goals will provide a better sense of control and realistic hope to the family. This knowledge educates the family about warning signs that should alert them to call on a family therapist at appropriate times for brief goal-oriented treatment.

Clinical Applications

Using the psychosocial typology and time phases of illness as a reference point has important implications both for the patient's/family's relationship to health professionals and for the organization of health services. Helping professionals need to be included in the conceptualization of any therapeutic treatment system with a family. Application of this idea in the medical world has led to various descriptions of the "therapeutic triangle in medicine" (Doherty and Baird). This triangle includes the patient, his or her family, and the physician (health care team).

Including the concept of types of psychosocial illnesses into the scheme creates a four-sided diagram (Fig. 6–4). It is easier to conceptualize the illness as a fourth member if one pictures each illness type as having a personality (which includes the kind of onset, course, outcome, degree of incapacitation, and predictability) and particular developmental life course.

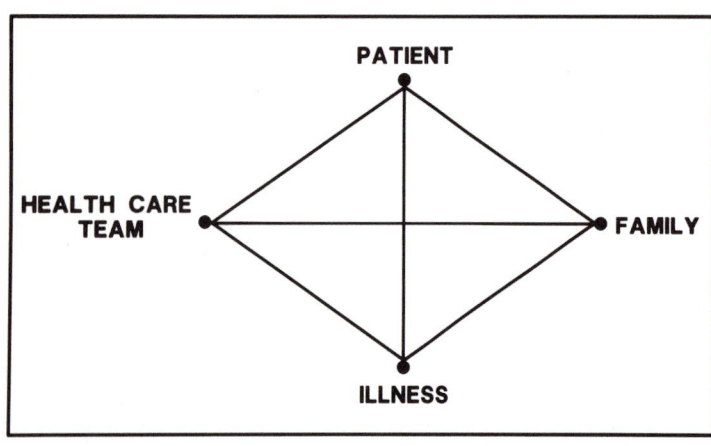

Figure 6–4. The therapeutic quadrangle. (Modified from Rolland, J. S.: A conceptual model of chronic and life-threatening illness and its impact on the family. *In* Chilman, C., Nunnanlly E., and Cox, F. (Eds.): Chronic Illness and Disability: Families in Trouble. Beverly Hills, CA, Sage Productions, 1988, with permission.)

Using this four-sided diagram, one can see how the original therapeutic triangle is colored by different types of illness. For instance, consider the concept of locus of control in relation to disease. This concept refers to how much an individual or family sees outcomes as being influenced by their own efforts. A family's beliefs about the potential to control biologic processes can vary along a continuum from an internal to an external orientation. A certain minimal level of agreement concerning this kind of health belief is critical to the establishment of a viable therapeutic relationship between the patient, his or her family, and the health care team. The degree of consensus concerning locus of control can vary dramatically for this triad depending on the type of chronic disease. A particular family physician may have had a good working relationship with a family that had presented over the years with non-life-threatening and nonincapacitating illnesses. If the father suffers a serious heart attack and there are differences in beliefs about control that surface in relation to this more life-threatening and incapacitating illness, the stability of the long-standing therapeutic triangle might be threatened. If the physician checked his or her own beliefs and questioned the family about theirs in relation to a life-threatening, incapacitating disease, a potential serious rift in this therapeutic system might be averted.

The illness time phases offer a framework for timing family psychosocial checkups to coincide with key transition points in the illness life cycle. The typology facilitates the development of various preventively oriented psychoeducational or support groups for patients and their families (Gonzales et al.). For example, groups could be designed to meet the needs of patients dealing with progressive, life-threatening diseases; relapsing disorders; acute-onset, incapacitating illnesses; or the chronic phase of disabling diseases. Sometimes there are not enough families involved with any particular disease to form such groups, particularly in more rural settings or for less common illnesses. Organizing group-oriented services in terms of illness types overcomes these obstacles while maintaining the groups' thematic coherence. Also, packaging brief psychoeducational modules, timed for critical phases of particular "types" of diseases, enables families to digest manageable portions of a long-term coping process. Each module could be tailored to the particular phase of the illness life cycle and family coping skills necessary to confront disease-related demands. This would provide a cost-effective preventive service that also could aid in the detection of families at high risk for maladaptation to chronic illness.

FAMILY ASSESSMENT

This section centers on illness-oriented family dynamics that concern belief systems and the dimension of time, and these dynamics are used to illustrate how one can apply the psychosocial typology of illness to family assessment more generally. This includes inquiry about family communication, problem solving, hierarchy, roles, affective involvement, information gathering, so-cial support, utilization of community resources, mastery of home-based medical care, medical crisis planning, and maintenance of self-esteem. This discussion will pay particular attention to (1) the family transgenerational history of coping with illness, loss, and crisis, (2) the interface of the illness with the individual and family life cycles, and (3) the family illness/health belief system.

Transgenerational History of Illness, Loss, and Crisis

Many systems-oriented practitioners have emphasized that a family's present behavior cannot be adequately comprehended apart from its history (Boszormenyi-Nagy; Bowen; Carter and McGoldrick; Framo; Walsh and McGoldrick). Historical questioning is a way to track key events and transitions to gain an understanding of a family's organizational shifts and coping strategies *as a system* in response to past stressors. This is not a cause-and-effect model but reflects a belief that such a historical search may help explain the family's current style of coping and adaptation. A historical systemic perspective involves more than simply deciphering how a family organized itself around past stressors; it also tracks the evolution of family adaptation over time. Patterns of adaptation, replications, discontinuities, shifts in relationships (i.e., alliances, triangles, cutoffs), and sense of competence are important considerations. These patterns are transmitted across generations as family myths, taboos, catastrophic expectations, and belief systems. By gathering this information, a clinician can create a family genogram (McGoldrick and Gerson). A chronic illness–oriented genogram focuses on how a family organized itself as an evolving system specifically around previous illnesses and unexpected crises in the current and previous generations. A central goal is to bring to light the adults' "learned differences around illness" (Penn).

The psychosocial types and phases of illness are useful concepts in the family evaluation. Although a family may have certain standard ways of coping with any illness, there may be critical differences in their style and success in adaptation to different types of diseases. If the clinician inquires about different types of illnesses (e.g., relapsing versus progressive, life-threatening versus non-life-threatening), he or she will make better use of historical data. For instance, a family may have consistently organized itself successfully around non-life-threatening illnesses but reeled under the weight of metastatic cancer. This family might be particularly vulnerable if another life-threatening illness were to occur. A different family may only have had experience with non-life-threatening illnesses and be ignorant of how to cope with the uncertainties particular to life-threatening diseases. Cognizance of these facts will draw attention to areas of strength and vulnerability for a family facing cancer. A recent family consultation highlights the importance of tracking prior family illnesses:

Joe, his wife Ann, and their three teenage children presented for a family evaluation 10 months after Joe's diagnosis with moderate–severe asthma. Joe, age 44, had been successfully employed for many years as a spray painter. Apparently, exposure to a new chemical triggered the onset of asthmatic attacks that necessitated hospitalization and occupational disability. Although somewhat improved, he continued to have persistent and moderate respiratory symptoms. Initially, his physicians had predicted that improvement would occur but remained noncommittal as to the level of chronicity. Continued breathing difficulties contributed to increased symptoms of depression, uncharacteristic temperamental outbursts, alcohol abuse, and family discord.

In the initial assessment, I inquired as to their prior illness experience. This was the nuclear family's first encounter with chronic illness, and their families of origin had limited experience. Ann's father had died 7 years earlier of a sudden and unexpected heart attack. Joe's brother had died in an accidental drowning. Neither had experience with disease as an ongoing process. Joe had assumed that improvement meant "cure." Illness for both had meant either death or recovery. The physician/family system was not attuned to the hidden risks for this family coping with the transition from the crisis to chronic phase of his asthma—the juncture where the permanency of the disease needed to be addressed.

Tracking a family's coping capabilities in the crisis, chronic, and terminal phases of previous chronic illnesses highlights complications in adaptation related to different points in the "illness life cycle." A family may have adapted well in the crisis phase of living with a spinal cord injury but failed to navigate the transition to a family organization consistent with long-haul adaptation. A rigidly enmeshed family may have become frozen in a crisis structure and may have been unable to deal appropriately with issues of maximizing individual and collective autonomy in the chronic phase. Another family with a member with chronic kidney failure may have functioned very well in handling the practicalities of home dialysis. However, in the terminal phase, their limitations around affective expression may have left a legacy of unresolved grief. A history of phase-specific difficulties can alert a clinician to potentially vulnerable periods for a family over the course of the current chronic illness. The following case illustrates the interplay of problems coping with a current illness, fueled by unresolved issues related to a particular type and/or phase of disease in a family of origin:

Mary, her husband Bill, and their son Jim sought treatment 4 months after Mary had sustained a serious concussion in a life-threatening head-on auto collision caused by the driver of another vehicle. Initially, there was some concern by the medical team that she might have suffered a cerebral hemorrhage. Ultimately, it was clarified that this had not occurred. Despite strong reassurance, Mary became increasingly depressed and continued to believe she had a life-threatening condition and would die from a brain hemorrhage.

In the initial evaluation, she revealed that she was experiencing vivid dreams of meeting her deceased father. Apparently, her father, with whom she had been extremely close, had died from a cerebral hemorrhage after a 4-year history of a progressive debilitating brain tumor, marked by progressive and uncontrolled epileptic seizures. Mary, 14 at the time, was the "baby" in the family; her two siblings were much older. The family had shielded her from his illness, culminating in her mother's decision that she not attend either the wake or the funeral. This event galvanized her position as the "child in need of protection"—a dynamic that carried over into her marriage. Despite her hurt, anger, and lack of acceptance of the death, she had avoided dealing with her feelings with her mother for over 20 years. Other family history revealed that her maternal grandfather had died when her mother was 7 years old. The mother had had to endure an open-casket wake at home. This traumatic experience was a major factor in her mother's attempt to protect her daughter from the same kind of memory.

Mary's own life-threatening head injury had triggered a catastrophic reaction and dramatic resurfacing of previous losses involving similar types of illness and injury. Therapy focused on a series of tasks and rituals that involved her initiating conversations with her mother and visits to her father's gravesite.

The family's history of coping with crises in general, especially unanticipated ones, should be explored. Illnesses with acute onset (i.e., heart attack), moderate–severe sudden incapacitation (i.e., stroke), or rapid relapse (i.e., ulcerative colitis, diabetic insulin reaction, disc disease) demand in various ways rapid crisis mobilization skills. In these situations, the family needs to reorganize quickly and efficiently, shifting from its usual organization to a crisis structure. Other illnesses can create a crisis because of the continual demand for family stamina (i.e., spinal cord injury, rheumatoid arthritis, emphysema). The family history of coping with moderate–severe ongoing stressors is a good predictor of adjustment to these types of illness.

For any significant chronic illness in either adult's family of origin, a clinician should try to get a picture of how those families organized to handle the range of disease-related affective and practical tasks. Also, it is important to find out what role each played in handling these emotional or practical tasks. Whether the parents (as children) were given too much responsibility (parentified) or shielded from involvement is of particular note. What did they learn from those experiences that influences how they think about the current illness? Whether they emerge with a strong sense of competence or failure is essential information. In one particular case involving a family with three generations of hemophilia transmitted through the mother's side, the father had been shielded from the knowledge that his older brother who died in adolescence had had a terminal form of kidney disease. Also, this man had not been allowed to attend his brother's funeral. From that trauma, he made a strong commitment to openness about disease-related issues with his two sons with hemophilia and his daughters who were genetic carriers.

By collecting such information about each adult's family of origin, one can anticipate areas of conflict and consensus. Unresolved issues related to illness and loss can remain dormant in a marriage and suddenly reemerge triggered by a chronic illness in the current nuclear family (Penn; Walker). Penn describes how particular coalitions that emerge in the context of a chronic illness are replications of those which existed in each adult's family of origin, as in the following vignette:

If a mother has been the long-time rescuer of her mother from a tyrannical husband, and then in her own family bears a son with hemophilia, she will become his rescuer, often against his father. In this manner she continues to rescue her mother but, oddly enough, now from her husband rather than from her own father. . . . In this family with a hemophiliac son, the father's father had been ill for a long period and had received all the mother's attention. In his present family, this father, though outwardly objecting to the coalition between his wife and son, honored that relationship, as if he hoped it would make up for the one he had once forfeited with his own mother. The coalition in the nuclear family looks open and adaptational (mother and son), but is fueled by coalitions in the past (mother with her mother, and father with his mother).

The reenactment of previous system configurations around illness can occur largely as an unconscious, automatic process. Further, this kind of dysfunctional complementarity for couples can emerge specifically within the context of a chronic disease. On detailed inquiry, couples frequently reveal a tacit unspoken understanding that if an illness occurred they would reorganize to reenact "unfinished business" from their families of origin. Typically, the role chosen represents a repetition or opposite role played by themselves or the same-sex parent. A clinician needs to maintain some distinction between functional family process with and without chronic disease. For families that present in this manner, placing a primary therapeutic emphasis on the resolution of family-of-origin issues might be the best approach to prevent or rectify an unhealthy triangle.

Families like those just described with encapsulated illness "time bombs" need to be distinguished from families with more pervasive, long-standing dysfunctional patterns, where illnesses can become embedded in a web of preexisting fused family transactions. In the traditional sense of psychosomatic, a severely dysfunctional family often has a greater level of baseline reactivity such that when an illness enters their system, this reactivity is expressed somatically through a poor medical course and/or treatment noncompliance. These families lack the foundation of a functional nonillness system. The initial focus of therapeutic intervention may need to be targeted more on pragmatic immediate help rather than on family-of-origin work, with more limited therapeutic aims.

A third group of symptomatic families facing chronic disease are those without significant intra- or intergenerational family dysfunctional patterns. Any family may falter in the face of multiple superimposed disease and nondisease stressors that occur over a relatively short time. With progressive, incapacitating diseases or the concurrence of illnesses in several family members, a pragmatic approach that focuses on expanded or creative use of supports and resources outside the family is most productive.

Interface of the Illness, Individual, and Family Life Cycles

To place the unfolding of chronic disease into a developmental context, it is crucial to understand the intertwining of three evolutionary threads: the illness, individual, and family life cycles (Rolland). The psychosocial typology offers a language to characterize diseases in psychosocial and longitudinal terms—each illness having a particular pattern and expected developmental life course. Since an illness *is* part of an individual, it is essential to think simultaneously about the interaction of individual and family development.

The "life cycle" is a central concept for both family and individual development. "Life cycle" means there is a basic sequence and unfolding of the life course within which individual, family, or illness uniqueness occurs. A second key concept is the human "life structure." Levinson described "life structure" to mean the design of a person's life at any given point in the life cycle. This design is made up of an individual's various commitments (e.g., work, family, religious affiliation, hobbies) and the relative importance of each commitment. The life structure mediates transactions between the individual/family and the environment. Although Levinson described the individual adult male life cycle, his concepts can be applied to the family as a unit.

Illness, individual, and family development have in common the notion of periods marked by the alternation of life structure–building/maintaining and life structure–changing (transitional) periods linking developmental periods. The primary goal of a life structure–building/maintaining period is to form a life structure and enrich life within it based on the key choices an individual/family made during the preceding transition period. The delineation of separate periods derives from a set of developmental tasks associated with each. Transition periods are potentially the most vulnerable because previous individual, family, and illness life structures are reappraised in the face of new developmental tasks that may require major, discontinuous change rather than minor alterations. Levinson has described four major periods in individual life structure development: childhood and adolescence, and early, middle, and late adulthood. Each period lasts approximately 20 years. Carter and McGoldrick have delineated the following six family life-cycle stages: (1) the unattached young adult, (2) the newly married couple, (3) the family with young children, (4) the family with adolescents, (5) launching children and moving on, and (6) the family in later life.

The concept of centripetal versus centrifugal family styles and phases in the family life cycle is particularly useful to the task of integrating illness, individual, and family development (Beavers). Combrinck-Graham describes a family life spiral model where she envisions a three-generational family system oscillating through time between periods of family closeness (centripetal) and periods of family disengagement (centrifugal). These periods coincide with shifts between family developmental tasks that require intense bonding or high cohesion, such as early childrearing, and tasks that emphasize personal identity and autonomy, such as adolescence. In a literal sense, "centripetal" and "centrifugal" describe a tendency to move, respectively, toward and away from a center. In life-cycle terms, they connote a fit between family developmental tasks and the relative need for family members to direct their energies inside the family and work together to accomplish those tasks. During a centripetal period, both the individual member's and family unit's life structures emphasize internal family life. External boundaries around the family are tightened, while personal boundaries between members are somewhat diffused to enhance family teamwork. In the transition to a centrifugal period, the family life structure shifts to accommodate goals that emphasize an individual family member's life outside the family. The external family boundary is loosened, while separateness between some family members increases.

From this brief overview of life-cycle models, we can

cull out several key concepts that provide a foundation for discussion of chronic disease. The life cycle contains alternating transition and life structure–building/maintaining periods. Further, particular periods can be characterized as either centripetal or centrifugal in nature (Fig. 6–5).

The notion of centripetal and centrifugal modes is useful in linking the illness life cycle to the individual and family life cycles. In general, chronic disease exerts a centripetal pull on the family system. In family developmental models, centripetal periods begin with the addition of a new family member (infant) that propels the family into a prolonged period of socialization of children. In an analogous way, the occurrence of chronic illness in a family resembles the addition of a new member, which sets in motion for the family a process of socialization to illness. Symptoms, loss of function, the demands of shifting or new illness-related practical and affective roles, and the fear of loss through death all refocus a family inward.

If the onset of an illness coincides with a centrifugal period for the family, it can derail the family from its natural momentum. If a young adult becomes ill, he or she may need to return to the family of origin for caretaking. Each member's autonomy and individuation are at risk. The young adult's ability to establish a life away from home is threatened either temporarily or permanently. Both parents may have to relinquish interests outside the family. Family dynamics as well as disease severity will influence whether the family's reversion to a centripetal life structure is a temporary detour within their general movement outward or a permanent involutional shift. A highly cohesive or enmeshed family frequently faces the transition to a more autonomous period with trepidation. A chronic illness provides a sanctioned reason to return to the "safety" of the prior centripetal period. For some family members, the giving

up of the building of a new life structure already in progress can be more devastating than when the family is still in a more centripetal period with more preliminary future plans. An analogy would be the difference between a couple discovering that they do not have enough money to build a house versus being forced to abandon their building project with the foundation already completed.

Disease onset that coincides with a centripetal period in the family life cycle (e.g., early childrearing) can have several important consequences. At minimum, it can foster a prolongation of this period. At worst, the family can become permanently stuck at this phase of development, when the inward pull of the illness and the phase of the life cycle coincide. The risk here is their tendency to amplify one another. For families that function marginally before an illness onset, this kind of mutual reinforcement can trigger a runaway process leading to overt family dysfunction. Minuchin's and colleagues' research of "psychosomatic" families has documented this process in several common childhood illnesses.

When a parent develops a chronic disease during this centripetal childrearing phase of development, a family's ability to stay on course is severely taxed. The impact of the illness is like the addition of a new infant member with "special needs" competing for potentially scarce family resources. For psychosocially milder diseases, efficient role reallocation may suffice, as in the following case:

Tom and his wife Sally presented for treatment 6 months after Tom had sustained a severe burn injury to both hands that required skin grafting. A year of recuperation was necessary before Tom would be able to return to his job, which required physical labor and full use of his hands. Prior to this injury, his wife had been at home full time raising their two children, ages 3 and 5. Although Tom was temporarily handicapped in terms of his career, he was physically fit to assume the role of househusband. Initially, both Tom and Sally remained at home using his disability income to "get by." When Sally expressed an interest in

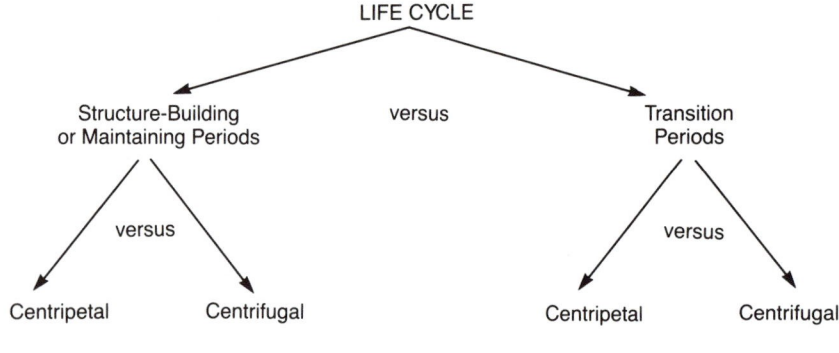

Figure 6–5. Periods in the family and individual life cycle. (Modified from Rolland, J. S.: Chronic illness and the life cycle: A conceptual framework. Fam. Proc., *26*(2):203–221, 1987, with permission.)

finding a job to relieve financial pressures, Tom resisted and marital strain caused by his injury flared into dysfunctional conflict.

Sufficient resources were available in the system to accommodate the illness and ongoing childrearing tasks. Their definition of marriage lacked the necessary role flexibility to master the problem. Treatment focused on rethinking his masculine and monolithic definition of "family provider," a definition that had, in fact, emerged in full force during this centripetal phase of the family life cycle.

If the disease affecting a parent is more debilitating (e.g., traumatic brain injury, cervical spinal cord injury), its impact on the childrearing family is twofold. A "new" family member is added, a parent is "lost," and the semblance of a single-parent family with an added special needs child is created. For acute-onset illnesses, when both events occur simultaneously, family resources may be inadequate to meet the combined childrearing and caretaking demands. This situation is ripe for the emergence of a "parentified" child or the reenlistment into active parenting of a grandparent. These forms of family adaptation are not inherently dysfunctional. A clinician needs to assess these structural realignments. Are certain individuals assigned rigid caretaking roles, or are they flexible and shared? Are caretaking roles viewed flexibly from a developmental vantage point? For an adolescent caretaker, this means the family being mindful of the approaching developmental transition to an independent life separate from the family. For grandparent caretakers, it means sensitivity to their increasing physical limitations or need to assist their own spouse.

The degree of centripetal/centrifugal pull varies enormously in different types and phases of illness. The tendency for a disease to pull a family inward increases with the level of incapacitation or risk of death. Progressive diseases over time are inherently more centripetal than constant-course illnesses. The ongoing addition of new demands as an illness progresses keeps a family's energy focused inward. After a modus operandi has been forged, a constant-course disease (excluding those with severe incapacitation) permits a family to enter or resume a more centrifugal phase of the life cycle. The added inward pull exerted by a progressive disease increases the risk of reversing normal family disengagement or freezing a family into a permanently fused state.

Mr. L., age 54, had become increasingly depressed as a result of severe and progressive complications of his adult-onset diabetes that had emerged over the past 5 years. These complications included a leg amputation and renal failure that recently required the instituting of home dialysis on a four times daily basis. For 20 years, Mr. L. had had an uncomplicated constant course, allowing him to lead a full active life. An excellent athlete, he engaged in a number of recreational group sports. Short- and long-term family planning had never focused around his illness. This optimistic attitude was reinforced by the fact that two people in Mrs. L.'s family of origin had had diabetes without complications. Their only child, a son age 26, had uneventfully left home after high school and had recently married. Mr. and Mrs. L. had a stable marriage, where both maintained many outside independent interests. In short, the family had moved smoothly through the transition to a more centrifugal phase of the family's life cycle.

His disease's transformation to a progressive course coupled with the incapacitating and life-shortening nature of his complications had reversed the normal process of family disengagement. His wife took a second job that necessitated her quitting her hobbies and civic involvements. Their son moved back home to help his mother take care of his father and the house. Mr. L., disabled from work and his athletic social network, felt a burden to everyone and blocked in his own midlife development.

The essential goal of family treatment in developmental terms centered around reversing some of the system's centripetal overreaction back to a more realistic balance. For Mr. L., this meant a reworking of his life structure to accommodate his real limitations while maximizing a return to his more independent style. For Mrs. L. and her son, this meant developing realistic expectations for Mr. L. and reestablishing key aspects of their autonomy within an illness/family system.

Relapsing illnesses alternate between periods of drawing a family inward and periods of release from the immediate demands of disease. However, the on-call state of preparedness dictated by many such illnesses keeps some part of the family in a centripetal mode despite medically asymptomatic periods, hindering the natural flow between phases of the family life cycle.

One way to think about the phases of illness is that they represent to the family a progression from a centripetal crisis phase to a more centrifugal chronic phase. The terminal phase, if it occurs, forces most families back into a more inward mode. The so-called illness life structure, developed by a family to accommodate each phase in the illness life cycle, is colored by these tendencies. For example, in a family where illness onset has coincided with a centrifugal phase of development, the transition to the chronic phase permits a family to resume more of its momentum.

Clinicians need to be mindful of the timing of the illness onset with individual/family transition and life structure–building/maintaining periods of development. All *transitions* involve the basic processes of beginnings and endings. Arrivals, departures, and losses are common life events, generating an undercurrent of preoccupation with death and finiteness (Levinson). Chronic and life-threatening illness means the loss of preillness life for a family. It forces the family into a transition in which one of the family's main tasks is to accommodate the anticipation of further loss and possibly untimely death. When the onset of a chronic illness coincides with a transition in the individual or family life cycle, issues related to previous, current, and anticipated loss will likely be magnified. Transition periods are often characterized by upheaval, rethinking of prior commitments, and openness to change. As a result, such times hold a greater risk for the illness to become unnecessarily embedded or inappropriately ignored in planning for the next developmental period. During a transition period, the very process of loosening prior commitments creates a context for emergence of family rules regarding loyalty through sacrifice and caretaking. Indecision about one's future can be resolved by excessive focus on a family member's physical problems. This can be a major precursor of family dysfunction in the context of chronic disease. By adopting a longitudinal developmental perspective, a clinician will stay attuned to future transitions and their overlap.

An example can highlight the importance of the illness in relation to future developmental transitions. Imagine a family in which the father—a carpenter and primary financial provider—develops multiple sclerosis. At first, his level of impairment is mild and stabilized, allowing him to continue part-time work. Because their children are all teenagers, his wife is able to undertake part-time work to help maintain financial stability. The oldest son, age 15, seems relatively unaffected. Two years later, the father experiences a rapid progression of his illness that leaves him totally disabled. His son, now 17, has dreams of going away to college to prepare for a science career. The specter of financial hardship and the perceived need for a "man in the family" create a serious dilemma of choice for the son and the family. In this case, there is a fundamental clash between developmental issues of separation/individuation and the ongoing demands of progressive chronic disability on the family. This vignette demonstrates the potential clash between simultaneous transition periods: the illness transition to a more incapacitating and progressive course, the adolescent son's transition to early adulthood, and the family's transition from the "living with teenagers" to "launching young adults" stage. Also, this example illustrates the significance of the type of illness. A less incapacitating or a relapsing illness (as opposed to a progressive or constant-course disease) might interfere less with this young man's separation from his family. If his father had an intermittently incapacitating illness, such as disc disease, the son might have moved out but tailored his choices to remain close by and thus available during acute flare-ups.

Illness onset may cause a different kind of disruption if it coincides with a *life structure–building/maintaining period* in individual or family development. These periods are characterized by the living out of choices made during the preceding transition period. Relative to transition periods, family members try to protect their own and their family unit's current life structure. Diseases with only a mild level of psychosocial severity (e.g., nonfatal, mild incapacitation, nonprogressive) may require some revision of individual/family life structure but not a radical restructuring that would necessitate a return to a transitional phase of development. A chronic illness with a critical threshold of psychosocial severity will demand the reestablishment of a transitional form of life, at a time when individual/family inertia is to preserve the momentum of a stable period. An individual's or family's level of adaptability is a prime factor determining the successful navigation of this kind of crisis. In this context, family adaptability involves the ability to transform its entire life structure to a prolonged transitional state.

For instance, in the previous example, the father's multiple sclerosis rapidly progressed while the oldest son was in a transition period in his own development. The nature of the strain in developmental terms would be quite different if the father's disease progression had occurred when this young man was 26, had already left home, had finished college and secured a first job, and had married and had a child. In the latter scenario, the oldest son's life structure is in a centripetal, structure-maintaining period within his newly formed nuclear family. To fully accommodate the needs of his family of origin could require a monumental shift of his developmental priorities. When this illness crisis coincided with a developmental transition period (age 17), al-though a dilemma of choice existed, the son was available and less fettered by commitments in progress. Later, at age 26, he has made commitments and is in the process of living them out with his newly formed family. To serve the demands of an illness transition, the son might need to shift his previously stable life structure back to a transitional state. And the shift would happen "out of phase" with the flow of his individual and nuclear family's development. One way to resolve this dilemma of divided loyalties might be the merging of the two households.

This discussion raises several key clinical points. From a systems viewpoint, at the time of diagnosis it is important to know the phase of the family life cycle and the stage of individual development of all family members, not just the ill member. This is important information for several reasons. First, chronic disease in one family member can profoundly affect developmental goals of another member. For instance, a disabled infant can be a serious roadblock to a mother's mastery of childrearing, or a life-threatening illness in a young adult can interfere with the spouse's task of beginning the phase of parenthood. Second, family members frequently do not adapt equally to chronic illness. Each member's ability to adapt and the rate at which he or she does so is related to the individual's own developmental stage and role in the family (Eisenberg et al.). The oldest son in the previous example illustrates this point.

There exists a normative and nonnormative timing of chronic illness in the life cycle. Coping with chronic illness and death is considered a normally anticipated task in late adulthood. On the other hand, illnesses and losses that occur earlier are "out of phase" and tend to be developmentally more disruptive (Herz; Neugarten). As untimely events, chronic diseases can severely disrupt the usual sense of continuity and rhythm of the life cycle. The timing in the life cycle of an unexpected event, such as a chronic illness, will shape the form of adaptation and the event's influence on subsequent development (Levinson).

The notion of "out of phase" illnesses can be conceptualized in a more refined way. First, since diseases have a centripetal influence on most families, they can be more disruptive to families in a centrifugal phase of development. Second, the onset of chronic disease tends to create a period of transition, the length or intensity of which depends on the psychosocial type and phase of the illness. This forced transition is particularly "out of phase" if it coincides with a life structure–building/maintaining period in the individual's or family's life cycle. Third, if the particular illness is progressive, relapsing, increasingly incapacitating, and/or life threatening, then the phases in the unfolding of the disease will be punctuated by numerous transitions. Under these conditions, a family will need to alter their illness life structure more frequently to accommodate the shifting and often increasing demands of the disease. This level of demand and uncertainty keeps the illness in the forefront of a family's consciousness, constantly impinging on their attempts to get back "in phase" developmentally. Finally, the transition from the crisis to the chronic phase of the illness life cycle is often the key juncture where the intensity of the family's socialization to living with chronic disease can be relaxed. In this sense, it offers a "window of opportunity" for the family to recover its developmental course.

Chronic diseases that occur for adults in the child-rearing period can be more devastating because of their potential impact on family financial and childrearing responsibilities (Herz). Again, the actual impact will depend on the "type" of illness and preillness family roles. Families governed by rigid gender-defined roles as to who should be the primary financial provider and caretaker of children will potentially have the greatest problems with adjustment and need to be coached toward a more flexible view about role interchange.

In the face of chronic disease, an overarching goal is for a family to deal with the developmental demands presented by the illness without family members completely sacrificing their own or the family's development as a system. Therefore, it is vital to ask about what life plans had to be canceled, postponed, or altered as a result of the diagnosis. It is also useful to know whose plans are most and least affected. By asking a family when and under what conditions they will resume plans, put on hold, or address future developmental tasks, a clinician can anticipate developmental crises related to "independence from" versus "subjugation to" the chronic illness. Family members can be helped to resume their life plans, at least to some extent, by helping them to resolve feelings of guilt, overresponsibility, and hopelessness and to find resources that are internal and external to the family for more freedom, both to pursue their own goals and to provide needed care for the ill member.

HEALTH/ILLNESS BELIEF SYSTEM

Each of us as an individual and as part of larger systems adopts a value orientation, belief system, or philosophy that shapes our patterns of behavior toward the common problems of daily life in society (Kluckhohn). Beliefs lend coherence to cognitive and affective dimensions of family life and temporal continuity to past, present, and future. Values provide a mode of approaching new and ambiguous situations. Depending on which system we are speaking of, this phenomenon can be labeled as values, culture, religion, belief system, world view, or family paradigm.

Reiss has argued that families as a unit develop paradigms for how the world operates. These models dictate how families interpret events and behaviors in their environment. One component of the family's overall construction of reality is their set of health/illness beliefs that will determine how they interpret illness events and guide their health-seeking behavior (Rolland). Although individual family members can hold different beliefs, the values operative at the level of the whole family may be the most significant.

At the time of a medical diagnosis, a primary devel-opmental task for the family is to create a meaning for the illness event that preserves a sense of competency and mastery in the context of partial loss, possible further physical compromise, and/or death. Chronic illness is a betrayal of both our fundamental trust in our bodies and our belief in our invulnerability and immortality (Kleinman). At an existential level, family health beliefs are designed to grapple with dilemmas of our (1) universal fear of finiteness and mortality, (2) attempts to sustain our denial of death, and (3) attempts to reassert control over unjust suffering and untimely death. At a practical level, belief systems serve as a cognitive map guiding decisions and action.

It is essential for clinicians to inquire about a family's health beliefs as part of a routine evaluation, focusing on the following key components (Rolland). First, one needs to ascertain the specific values to which a family adheres. These include assessment of (1) a family's basic belief about the relationship between mind and body, control and mastery, and change, (2) the meanings attached by a family, ethnic group, religion, or the wider culture to certain symptoms (e.g., chronic pain), types or time phases of illness (e.g., life-threatening disorders), or specific diseases, (3) the family's assumptions about what caused an illness and what will influence its course and outcome, (4) family-of-origin or nuclear family historical factors related to illness, loss, adversity, and crisis that have shaped a family's health beliefs, and (5) anticipated nodal points in the unfolding of the illness, individual, and family life cycle where health beliefs will be strained or need to shift. Second, a clinician needs to assess the fit of health beliefs (1) within the family and its various subsystems (e.g., spouse, parental, extended family), (2) between the family and provider system, and (3) between the family and wider culture.

The Family's Sense of Mastery In Relation to an Illness

A clinician needs to determine a family's beliefs about their competence to master health and illness from a biologic, psychologic, and social perspective. "Mastery" is similar to the concept of "health locus of control" (Lefcourt; Dohrenwend), which can be defined as the belief an individual or family has about their influence over the course/outcome of an illness. It is critical to distinguish whether a family's belief system is based on the premise of internal control, external control by chance, or external control by powerful others.

An "internal" locus of control orientation means that there is a belief that an individual/family can affect the outcome of a situation. Families with such a belief about their health will endorse such statements as "I am directly responsible for my health" or "If I become sick, I have the power to make myself well again."

An "external" orientation entails a belief that outcomes are noncontingent on the individual's or family's behavior. Families that view illness in terms of chance will agree with such statements as "Luck plays a big part in determining how soon my family member will recover from an illness" or "When I become ill, it's a matter of fate." Individuals who see health control as in the hands of powerful others will see health professionals, God, or sometimes "powerful" family members, rather than themselves, as exerting control over their bodies. They will endorse statements such as "Regarding my health, I can only do what my doctor tells me to do" or "My family has a lot to do with my becoming sick or staying healthy."

A family may adhere to a different set of values concerning control when dealing with a *biologic* process as opposed to other day-to-day types of problem solving. Therefore, it is important to assess a family's basic value system first, and then, with increasing specificity, assess notions about control for illnesses in general, chronic and life-threatening illness, and finally, the specific disease facing the family. A family guided normally by an internal locus of control may switch to an external viewpoint when a member develops any chronic illness, or perhaps only in the case of a life-threatening disease. Such a change might occur in a family with a strong need to remain in accord with society's values, a particular ethnic background, or a specific cross-generational experience with life-threatening diseases. One can inquire as to whether a family has any particular beliefs surrounding specific types of illnesses. Regardless of the actual severity in a particular instance, cancer may be equated with death or loss of control because of medical statistics, cultural myth, or prior family history. For many, certain types of heart disease with a similar life expectancy as certain forms of cancer could be seen as more manageable because of prevailing cultural beliefs. Imagine a family traditionally guided by a strong sense of personal control. If the paternal grandfather, the powerful patriarch of the family, died at midlife because of a rapidly progressive and painful form of cancer, the family may develop an encapsulated exception to their views about control that is specific for cancer or generalized to include all life-threatening illnesses.

A family's value orientation about mastery strongly affects the nature of its relationship to an illness and to the health care system. A family's beliefs about control are a predictor of certain health behaviors, particularly treatment compliance, and suggest the family's preferences about participation in their family member's treatment and healing. In my experience, families that view disease course/outcome as a matter of chance tend to establish marginal relationships with health professionals largely because their belief system minimizes the importance of their own or a health professional's relationship to a disease process. Just as any psychotherapeutic relationship depends on a shared belief system about what is therapeutic, a "fit" between the patient, his or her family, and the health care team in terms of these fundamental values is essential. Families that express feelings of being misunderstood by health professionals are often referring directly or indirectly to a lack of joining at this basic value level.

A family's beliefs about mastery can change or vary in terms of goodness of fit depending on the time phase of the illness. For some illnesses, the crisis phase involves a lot of involvement outside the family. For instance, the crisis phase after a stroke may begin with an intensive care unit and months of extended care at a rehabilitation facility. This kind of protracted care outside the family's direct control may be stressful for a family that prefers to tackle its own problems with a minimum of outside leadership. For this family, the patient's return home may increase the workload but allow members to reestablish more fully their values concerning control. A family guided more by a preference for external control by experts will have greater difficulty when their family member returns home. For this family, leaving the rehabilitation hospital means the loss of their locus of competency—the professionals. Health providers' cognizance about this basic difference in belief about control can guide a psychosocial treatment plan tailored to each family's needs.

In the terminal phase of an illness, a family may feel least in control of the biologic course of the disease and the decision making regarding the overall care of their ill member. Families with a strong need to sustain their centrality may need to assert themselves more vigorously with health providers. Effective decision making regarding the extent of heroic medical efforts or whether a patient will die at home or in an institution or hospice requires an effective family/provider relationship that respects the family's basic beliefs.

The Family's Beliefs about the Etiology of an Illness

The context within which an illness event occurs is a very powerful organizer and mirror of a family's belief system. The limits of current medical knowledge mean that tremendous uncertainties persist about the relative importance of a myriad of biopsychosocial factors in disease onset. This fact allows individuals and families to make highly idiosyncratic attributions about what caused their family member's illness. Therefore, a family's beliefs about the etiology of an illness need to be assessed separately from its beliefs about control once an illness is present. One way to gather this information is to ask *each* family member for his or her explanation of the existence of the disease. Responses will reflect a combination of the current level of medical knowledge about the particular disease in concert with family mythology. This mythology might include punishment for prior misdeeds (e.g., an affair), blame of a particular family member ("Your drinking made me sick"), a sense of injustice ("Why am I being punished, I have been a good person"), genetics (e.g., cancer runs on one side of the family), negligence by the patient or parents (e.g., sudden infant death syndrome), or bad luck. Asking this question can function as an effective family Rorschach, bringing to light unresolved family conflicts.

Attributions about the cause of an illness that invoke blame, shame, or guilt are particularly important to uncover. Beliefs of this nature make it extremely difficult for a family to establish functional coping and adaptation to an illness. In the context of a life-threatening illness, the blamed family member is held accountable for potential murder if the patient dies. Decisions about treatment can become confounded and filled with tension. A mother who feels blamed by her husband for their son's leukemia may be less able to accept stopping a low-probability experimental treatment than the angry, blaming husband. A husband who believes his drinking caused his wife's coronary and subsequent death may have a pathologic grief reaction and may increase his drinking to mask his profound guilt.

In my clinical experience, families with the strongest, at times extreme, beliefs about personal responsibility and those with the most severely dysfunctional patterns will be those most likely to attribute the cause of an illness to a psychosocial factor. For high internal locus of control families, an ethos of personal responsibility guides all facets of life, including the etiology of an illness. For these families, a relative lack of acknowledgment of "outrageous fortune" as a factor in illness events can create for these families a nidus for blame, shame, and guilt. For highly dysfunctional families, characterized by unresolved conflicts and intense blaming, attributions of what or who is responsible for an illness often becomes ammunition in long-term family power struggles.

It is difficult to characterize an "ideal" family health belief about mastery or control. On one hand, a major thesis of systems-oriented medicine is that there is always an interplay between disease and other levels of the system. On the other hand, illnesses and phases in the course of disease may vary considerably in their responsiveness to psychosocial factors versus their inherent nature. Distinctions need to be made between a family's beliefs about their overall participation in a long-term disease process, their beliefs about their ability to control the biologic unfolding of an illness, and the flexibility with which they can apply these beliefs. An optimal expression of family competence or mastery would seem to depend on their grasp of these distinctions.

A family's belief in their participation in the total illness process can be thought of as independent from whether a disease is stable, improving, or in a terminal phase. Sometimes, mastery and the attempt to control biologic processes coincide. A family coping with a member who has cancer in remission may tailor its behavior to help maintain health. This might include changes in family roles, communication, diet, exercise, and balance between work and recreation. Suppose the ill family member loses remission and vigorous efforts to reestablish a remission fail. As the family enters the terminal phase of the illness, participation as an expression of mastery must now be transposed for a successful process of letting go.

The difference between a family experiencing a loss with a sense of competency versus profound failure is intimately connected to this kind of flexible use of their belief system. For instance, it can be helpful if clinicians recognize that the death of a patient whose long debilitating illness has heavily burdened others can be a matter of relief as well as sadness to some or all family members. Since a sense of relief over death goes against most conventions in our society, it can trigger massive guilt reactions that may be expressed tangentially through such symptoms as depression and negative family interactions. Clinicians will need to help family members accept, with a minimum of guilt and defensiveness, the naturalness of ambivalent feelings they may have for their deceased member.

Thus flexibility within the family and the health provider system may be the key variable in optimal family functioning. Families can view mastery in a rigid, circumscribed way that sees biologic outcome as the sole determinant of success, or families can define control in a more "holistic" sense where involvement and participation in the overall process are the main criteria defining success. This is analogous to the distinction between healing the system and curing the disease. Healing the system may influence the course/outcome of an illness, but disease outcome is not necessary to a family's feeling successful. This flexible definition of mastery permits the quality of relations within the family or between the family and health providers to become more central to criteria of success. It permits the health provider's competence to be viewed from both a technical and caregiving perspective (Reiss) that is not linked only to the biologic course of the disorder.

The Family's Ethnic, Religious, and Cultural Beliefs

Ethnicity, race, and religion are major determinants of a family's belief concerning health and illness (McGoldrick et al.; Zborowski). There are cultural differences in definitions of what constitutes a family in different ethnic, racial, and religious groups; what the responsibility of families is for the care of ill members; who in the family is chiefly responsible for this care (usually the wife/mother/daughter in traditional cultures); what the role of the extended family is in patient care; and so on. Health professionals need to familiarize themselves with belief systems of various ethnic, racial, and religious groups in their community, particularly as these translate into different behavioral patterns with regard to illness. For instance, it is customary for Italians and Jews to describe physical symptoms freely and in detail, whereas individuals of Irish or white Anglo-Saxon descent tend to deny or conceal ailments. One can surmise about the potential for misunderstanding and tension that could develop between Italian or Jewish health providers working with Irish or white Anglo-Saxon patients and their families. A mutually frustrating cycle of health providers pursuing a distancing family could develop. At minimum, dissatisfaction would ensue; at worst, a family might leave treatment, their negative experience reinforcing its alienation and isolation from adequate care. Clinicians need to be mindful of the cultural differences between themselves, the patient, and the family. Deference to these distinctions is a necessary step to forging a workable provider–patient–family alliance that can endure a long-term illness. Disregarding these issues can lead families to wall themselves off from health providers and available community resources—a major cause of noncompliance and treatment failure.

Family and Family–Provider Health Belief Congruence

As family illness beliefs are articulated, a clinician should inquire about the degree of family consensus or congruence concerning a particular value, such as health locus of control. This is important because it is a common, but unfortunate, error to regard "the family" as a monolithic unit that feels, thinks, believes, and behaves as an undifferentiated whole.

In assessing the family's level of agreement, one should learn about the family's general tolerance for differences. What is the family rule? "We must agree on all/some values," or "diversity and different viewpoints are acceptable." Further, clinicians should determine whether the family policy about consensus is adhered to in relation to the prevailing cultural or societal beliefs. Can the family hold values that differ from the wider culture? The family's general rule has multiple determinants that include cultural norms, historical context (era of "family consensus" versus each member "doing his or her own thing"), and the beliefs of the adults' families of origin.

A family's rules about consensus can have profound implications for permissible options when a family faces chronic illness. If consensus is the rule, then individual differentiation implies deviance. If the guiding principle is "We can hold different viewponts," then diversity is allowed. When working with illness-related values in a family where consensus is the rule, attention to the entire family is mandatory. One treatment goal can be to help families negotiate their differences and support the separate identity, needs, and goals of each member. In a family where diversity is permitted, there may be greater latitude to work on certain disease-related psychosocial issues with the ill member alone or with particular members of the family without mobilizing family resistance.

Next, it is important to look into the *actual* level of agreement with regard to health beliefs both within the family and between the family and the medical system. How congruent are the family's basic beliefs about control with their health belief system? A family that is uniformly external will generally adapt best if psychosocial interventions are tailored to that fact. On the other hand, a family that generally adheres to an internal locus of control but feels the opposite with a particular disease may, through exploration of underlying issues, be able to change its beliefs about illness. It is critical to keep in mind that beliefs about control refer to a family's beliefs about the importance of their *participation in the total illness process* rather than just their beliefs about a disease's curability.

It is important to analyze differences among family members in terms of illness values. Disparities in two- and three-person relationships involving the ill member are particularly significant. Consider a common situation in which there is a long-standing loyalty conflict for a man caught between his spouse and his mother. Both women vie for his devotion, while he is unable to define boundaries between his family of origin and nuclear family. This dysfunctional triangle may have smoldered for years in a precarious balance when the man develops a slowly progressive and debilitating illness, such as multiple sclerosis. If the man and his mother share a strong sense of internal control while his spouse grew up in a family that saw chronic illness as a matter of fate, an unbalancing of this triangle is likely to occur. The smoldering mother–son coalition now reemerges in full force fueled by shared basic beliefs concerning mastery, while the marital couple is driven apart.

The different ethnic backgrounds of the adults in a family may be a primary reason for the kind of discrepancies about illness beliefs that emerge at the time of a major illness. Differences may occur in such areas as the definition of the appropriate sick role for the patient; the kind and degree of open communication about the disease; who should be included in the illness caretaking system (e.g., extended family, friends, professionals); and the kind of rituals viewed as normative (Wolin and Bennett) at different stages of an illness (e.g., hospital bedside vigils, healing and funeral rituals). In families of mixed ethnic heritage, clinicians should assess these areas for consensus, disagreement, and negotiation.

It is common for differences in beliefs or attitudes between family members to erupt at major transition points in the treatment or disease course. For instance, in situations of severe disability or terminal illness, one member may want the patient to return home while another prefers extended hospitalization or transfer to an extended-care facility. Since the chief task of patient caretaking is usually assigned to the wife/mother, she is the one most apt to bear the chief burdens in this regard. If this family also operates under the constraint of traditional role assignments where the wife/mother defers to her spouse as the family decision maker, she may not make her true feelings known and may become the family martyr, taking on the home nursing tasks without overt disagreement at the time critical decisions are made with health professionals. Clinicians can be misled by a family that presents this kind of united front. A careful and perceptive assessment can help avert the long-term consequences to such a family of role overload, resentment, and deteriorating family relationships.

It is essential to assess the fit between the belief systems of the family and the health care team. The same questions asked of the family are relevant to the medical team. What is the attitude of the health care team about their and the family's ability to influence the course/outcome of the disease? How does the health team see the balance between theirs versus the family's participation in the treatment and control of the disease? If basic differences in beliefs about health locus of control exist, it is critical to assess how to reconcile these differences. Because of the tendency of most health facilities to disempower individuals and thereby foster dependence, utmost sensitivity to family values is needed to create a therapeutic system. Many breakdowns in relationships between "noncompliant" or marginal patients and their health care providers are related to lack of agreement at this basic level.

The relative need for consensus will vary according to the illness phase. One point where a good fit of values is usually needed is during the initial crisis period when health providers engage in much high-technology medicine and rapid decision making and exchange of information, especially if life-threatening circumstances prevail. Teamwork is particularly important. Illnesses characterized by recurrent crises or key transitions have nodal points of stress where consensus will again become important.

One major transition is the often murky junction between the chronic and terminal phases of an illness. The attitudes and behaviors of the medical team can have a major influence in either facilitating or hindering this process for a family. A medical team that maintains heroic efforts to control the terminal phase of an illness can convey confusing messages. Families may not know how to interpret continued lifesaving efforts. Is there still real hope that should be taken by families as a message to redouble their faith in and support of medical improvement? Do the physicians feel bound to a technologic imperative that requires them to exhaust *all* possibilities at their disposal, regardless of the odds of success? Often physicians feel committed to this course for ethical reasons, a "leave no stone unturned" philosophy, or because of fears concerning legal liability. Is the medical team having its own difficulties letting go? Strong relationships with certain patients can be fueled by identifications with losses, often unresolved, in the health providers' own lives. Health care professionals and institutions can collude in a pervasive societal wish to deny death as a natural process truly beyond technologic control (Becker). Endless treatment can represent the medical team's inability to separate a general value placed on controlling diseases from their beliefs about participation (separate from cure) in a patient's total care. Professionals need to closely examine their own motives for treatments geared toward cure rather than palliation, particularly when a patient may be entering a terminal phase. Professionals' self-examination need to be done in concert with a careful understanding of the family's belief system.

Because information about and linkage to community resources and services is frequently valuable, the clinician must assess how family health beliefs influence their overall illness behavior within a community (Mechanic; Kleinman). Clinicians need to know the availability of and access to community resources relevant to the management of long-term illnesses. This includes a range of primary and tertiary medical, rehabilitation, respite, transportation, housing, institutional, and financial entitlement services. Also, it includes potential psychosocial support from friends, neighbors, self-help groups, and religious, ethnic/cultural, or other group affiliations. On the family side, one must inquire about a family's prior experience using such resources. Have these experiences been affirming or alienating? To what extent is the family adequately informed about potential outside sources of help? Ignorance may reflect family isolation from the community due to such things as geographic distance in a rural setting, lack of education (e.g., literacy), language barrier, poverty, race, and ethnic or religious distinctions from the wider culture. On the other side, a family's willingness to use outside resources may be limited by ethnic/cultural values, certain family dynamics, and their own illness paradigms.

For example, rigidly enmeshed families tend to view the world as dangerous and threatening to their fragile sense of autonomy. Individual autonomy is sacrificed to keep the family system intact. Their beliefs about control will need to be defined within a framework of family exclusiveness that minimizes the role of outsiders. The occurrence of a chronic illness presents a powerful dilemma for these families. The illness may necessitate frequent excursions beyond the family borders or require the inclusion of outside professionals in disease management. Any hope of establishing a viable family health care team relationship depends on exquisite sensitivity to this interplay of dysfunctional family dynamics and their belief system.

REFERENCES

Beavers WR. Healthy, midrange, and severely dysfunctional families. In Walsh F (ed.): Normal Family Processes. New York, Guilford Press, 1982.

Becker E. The Denial of Death. New York, Free Press, 1973.

Boszormenyi-Nagy I, Spark G. Invisible Loyalties. New York, Harper and Row, 1973.

Bowen M. Theory in the practice of psychotherapy. In Bowen M (ed.): Family Therapy in Clinical Practice. New York, Jason Aronson, 1978.

Carter EA, McGoldrick M (eds). The Changing Family Life Cycle: A Framework for Family Therapy, 2d ed. New York, Gardner Press, 1988.

Chilman CS, Nunnally EW, Cox FM (eds.). Chronic Illness and Disability: Families in Trouble Series. Beverly Hills, Calif., Sage Publications, 1988.

Combrinck-Graham L. A developmental model for family systems. Family Process 1985; 24(2):139–150.

Doherty WJ, Baird MA. Family Therapy and Family Medicine: Toward the Primary Care of Families. New York, Guilford Press, 1983.

Doherty WJ, Baird MA (eds.). Family-Centered Medical Care: A Clinical Casebook. New York, Guilford Press, 1987.

Dohrenwend BS, Dohrenwend BP (eds.). Stressful Life Events and Their Contexts, New York, Prodist, 1981.

Engel GH. The need for a new medical model: a challenge for biomedicine. Science 1977; 196:129–136.

Engel GH. The clinical application of the biopsychosocial model. Am. J. Psychiatry 1980; 137:535–544.

Eisenberg MG, Sutkin LC, Jansen MA (eds.). Chronic Illness and Disability Through the Life Span: Effects on Self and Family. New York, Springer, 1984.

Erikson EH. Childhood and Society. New York, Norton, 1950.

Framo J. Family of origin as therapeutic resource for adults in marital and family therapy. Family Process 1976; 15:193–210.

Gonzales S, Steinglass P, Reiss D. Putting the illness in its place: Discussion groups for families with chronic medical illnesses. Fam Proc 1989; 28(1):69–89.

Herz F. The impact of death and serious illness on the family life cycle. In Carter EA, McGoldrick M (eds.): The Changing Family Life

Cycle: A Framework for Family Therapy, 2d ed. New York, Gardner Press, 1988.

Kleinman AM. The Illness Narratives: Suffering, Healing and the Human Condition. New York, Basic Books, 1988.

Kluckhohn FR. Variations in the basic values of family systems. In Bell NW, Vogel EF (eds.): A Modern Introduction to the Family, Glencoe, Ill., Free Press, 1960.

Lefcourt HM. Locus of Control, 2d ed. Hillsdale, N.J.: Lawrence Erlbaum Associates, 1982.

Levinson DJ. The Seasons of a Man's Life. New York, Knopf, 1978.

Levinson DJ. A conception of adult development. Am Psychol. 1986; 41(1):3–13.

McGoldrick M, Gerson R. Genograms in Family Assessment. New York, Norton, 1985.

McGoldrick M, Pearce JK, Giordano J. Ethnicity and Family Therapy. New York, Guilford Press, 1982.

Mechanic D. Medical Sociology, 2d ed. New York, Free Press, 1978.

Minuchin S, Rosman BL, Baker L. Psychosomatic Families. Cambridge, Harvard University Press, 1978.

Minuchin S, Baker L, Rosman B, et al. A conceptual model of psychosomatic illness in children: family organization and family therapy. Arch Gen Psychiatry 1975; 32:1031–1038.

Moos RH (ed.). Coping with Physical Illness, vol. 2: New Perspectives. New York, Plenum, 1984.

Neugarten B. Adaptation and the life cycle. The Counselling Psychologist 1976; 6(1):16–20.

Penn P. Coalitions and binding interactions in families with chronic illness. Fam Systems Med 1983; 1(2):16–25.

Reiss D. The Family's Construction of Reality. Cambridge, Harvard University Press, 1981.

Reiss D. The family and medical team in chronic illness: A transactional and developmental perspective. In Ramsey CN Jr (ed.): Family Systems in Family Medicine. New York, Guilford Press, 1989.

Rolland JS. Toward a psychosocial typology of chronic and life-threatening illness. Fam Systems Med 1984; 2(3):245–263.

Rolland JS. Chronic illness and the life cycle: A conceptual framework. Family Process 1987; 26(2):203–221.

Rolland JS. Family illness paradigms: evolution and significance. Fam Systems Med 1987; 5(4):467–486.

Rolland JS. Family systems and chronic illness: A typological model. J Psychother Fam 1987; 3(3):143–168.

Rolland JS. Helping Families with Chronic and Life-Threatening Disorders. New York, Basic Books, in press.

Rolland JS. Anticipatory loss: A family systems developmental framework. Fam Proc 1990; 29(3):229–244.

Strauss AL. Chronic Illness and the Quality of Life. St. Louis, Mosby, 1975.

Walker G. The pact: the caretaker–parent/ill-child coalition in families with chronic illness. Fam Systems Med 1983; 1(4):6–30.

Walsh F, McGoldrick H (eds.). Living Beyond Loss: Death in the Family. New York, Norton, 1991.

Wolin SJ, Bennett LA. Family rituals. Fam Proc 1984; 23(3):401–420.

Zborowski M. People in Pain. San Francisco, Jossey-Bass, 1969.

QUESTIONS

1. Which of the following are core variables of the "psychosocial typology" of illness?
   a. Disease outcome
   b. Genetics
   c. Degree of incapacitation
   d. Disease onset
   e. Child versus adult onset

2. Which of the following are core developmental time phases in chronic illness?
   a. Chronic
   b. Terminal
   c. Bereavement
   d. Postdiagnosis

3. How many valences of health locus of control are described?
   a. 4
   b. 2
   c. 3
   d. 5

4. According to the family systems–illness model, at what point in the illness life cycle would an "overly cohesive or enmeshed" family be most vulnerable?
   a. At the time of diagnosis
   b. Bereavement
   c. Transition to terminal phase
   d. Transition to chronic phase

5. Which of the following describe common patterns of disease course in the family systems–illness model?
   a. Spiraling
   b. Progressive
   c. Relapsing
   d. Complex
   e. Constant

6. The "therapeutic triangle" in medicine refers to which of the following?
   a. Patient, health care team, community
   b. Patient/family, health care institution, health care team
   c. Patient/family, friends/extended family, health care team
   d. Patient, family, health care team

7. Which of the following questions best acts like a family Rorschach about unresolved conflict related to blame, shame, or guilt?
   a. Ask about each family member's explanation for the illness
   b. Ask about how the family has decided caretaking roles
   c. Ask the family about their religious beliefs and views about sin
   d. Ask the family to describe a recent family argument

8. Families in which stage of family development are very vulnerable when a young-adult member has a serious traumatic brain injury?
   a. Transitional
   b. Centrifugal
   c. Centripetal

9. True or false, life-threatening diseases are most likely to cause feelings of blame, shame, or guilt?

10. What are the three dimensions of the family systems–illness model?
    a. Time phase or illness
    b. Stage of family life cycle
    c. Components of family functioning
    d. Stage of individual development
    e. Psychosocial type of illness

Answers appear on page 446.

Short essay: Using this model, describe four to five ways that your work as a clinician with families facing illness, disability, and threatened loss is influenced by your own family's transgenerational and developmental experience with illness/loss/adversity. Emphasize effects on your belief system.

7

CARE OF THE DYING PATIENT

ROBERT E. RAKEL and PORTER STOREY

Informed physicians, family, and friends can do much to help the terminal patient die with integrity and dignity. However, if dying is really to be accepted as a normal component of the life cycle, then reintegration of the dying patient into the routine course of living is necessary.

> The concept of quality care does not always demand that death be regarded as an enemy to be fought with every weapon at a physician's disposal. An obsession with quantity of life can adversely affect its quality . . . there are times when graceful death with dignity is preferable to lingering torment.
>
> LORAN COMMISSION REPORT

Too often, care of a terminally ill patient centers primarily on the disease, and the patient as a whole person is neglected. The value of treatment must be interpreted on the basis of its net value to the individual. When additional treatments no longer provide benefits, the patient then needs concerned care from someone who provides personalized care with attention to the patient's emotional as well as physical comfort. The dying person is often physically and emotionally isolated from familiar surroundings and placed in a social setting that gives very low priority to individual personality, fears, and past experiences.

It is not surprising for an empathic family physician who has enjoyed a long and close relationship with a patient to be uncomfortable in dealing with the patient's impending death. While expressing concern and compassion for a terminal patient, the family physician must still maintain composure and objectivity to remain effective. Osler refers to this as "calm equanimity" and adds, "Our equanimity is chiefly exercised in enabling us to bear with composure the misfortunes of our neighbors." Medicine has long emphasized the need for physicians to remain objective and deal with problems factually, but if a physician is unable to do so effectively, attempts to hide emotion may lead the physician to adopt a fascade that appears unsympathetic and insensitive to the patient's needs. Such a physician fears rejection and alienation. During the terminal stages of a fatal illness, it is vital to the dying patient that the family physician maintain a warm and caring relationship and through the strength of the physician–patient bond provide support for the patient.

Physicians are most uncomfortable when they feel helpless. Unfortunately, this leads to withdrawal from the patient who is terminally ill because the physician inappropriately feels helpless and impotent when in fact a great deal of comfort and help can be provided. Physicians sometimes lose enthusiasm for care once an illness has been recognized as incurable and inevitably fatal. If this occurs, interaction with the patient diminishes at the very time emotional support is needed most and the patient's fear of abandonment is greatest. Time-and-motion studies indicate that nurses and other ward personnel also spend less time with the terminally ill patient when giving baths and providing routine care.

The physician who is uncomfortable discussing impending death can discourage conversation in many subtle ways. Hospital rounds are made rapidly, perhaps in a superficial, lighthearted manner, never pausing long enough to give the patient an opportunity to express fears and concerns. Comments such as "Everything will be all right" effectively close lines of communication with an intelligent patient who is fully aware of the seriousness of the situation. When the physician tells a patient, "Don't worry," the patient interprets this as, "Don't bother me." Patients are unlikely to initiate discussions regarding their fears of death or feelings of helplessness under such circumstances and will remain silent or avoid these issues unless they feel the physician is willing to listen and is interested in them. The physician can easily squelch such conversation, but a slight indication of willingness to discuss the problems disturbing the patient often results in frank conversations, which relieve much of the patient's anxiety and bring into the open concerns that can be shared with no one other than the physician.

THE "RIGHT TIME" TO DIE

Simpson describes the "how dare you die on me" syndrome, in which the patient has the effrontery to die before medical and nursing staff have used all the treatments in their repertoire. The patient is supposed to die "at the right time," neither before all potential effective therapies have been tried nor too long after all palliative procedures have been utilized. Health professionals often have a need to feel that everything possible was done for the patient prior to death. These attitudes have developed because the health care process too often focuses more on the health professionals' expectations than on the patients' needs.

We might consider what we have done to the patient who dies in the isolation of a laminar flow room, without having been able to touch another person's hand during his last few weeks of life. Such treatment is a false-positive, a treatment inappropriate to the real needs of the patient.

SAUNDERS

It is impossible, however, for physicians to provide adequate support during this difficult time unless they have come to terms with their own mortality.

Studies by the Group for the Advancement of Psychiatry have revealed that physicians are afraid of death in greater proportion than controls of patients.

ARING

COMMUNICATION: WHEN TO TELL THE PATIENT

The issue today is not so much whether or not to tell patients they have a terminal illness, but how to share this information with them—since most patients know the nature of their disease process to some degree. Because family physicians know their patients well, they should be able to gauge the patients' desire to be told and their capacity to withstand the shock of disclosure.

A frank discussion of death or of how long the patient is expected to live may not be necessary or even indicated. A good understanding between doctor and patient may make open disclosure unnecessary. The physician's role may be primarily one of supporting patients during the progressive terminal course of their illness. Such a situation should not be used by the physician who is uncomfortable with the subject as an excuse to avoid discussing the issue, however. The family physician's primary responsibility is to take the time to evaluate the situation, make sure the patient's true desires have been assessed correctly, and provide whatever support is needed, based on the patient's concepts and needs rather than on those of the physician.

The physician who can deal with death honestly is able to focus more attention on the patient and can determine the patient's level of awareness by listening and observing nonverbal cues. Clues to the patient's wish to discuss his or her condition may be nothing more than a deep sigh, a tear, or a shaky voice. The physician must be alert during busy hospital rounds for these or similar signs. If time permits, the physician can pause to sit and encourage conversation or return later when more time is available. Whenever possible, however, the response should be at that moment, since the patient is more likely to communicate freely in a spontaneous situation. A physician who is uncomfortable in this situation may check every inch of the IV tubing for air bubbles or otherwise direct attention away from the patient, effectively ignoring overt as well as subtle clues to the patient's needs.

When the patient is ready to discuss impending death, physician and patient are probably past the most difficult stage and the physician needs merely to listen, accept the patient's feelings, and respond to questions honestly.

Most patients will raise questions that indicate how much they wish to know, provided the physician gives them the opportunity. These openings or invitations may take the form of the physician asking, "Do you have any questions or worries?"

Patients also will usually indicate when they would like to discuss their prognosis and also will let the physician know when they would like to avoid the subject altogether and focus on more pleasant topics. Even patients who have reached a full level of acceptance of their terminal illness cannot remain constantly focused on that subject and must divert their attention to more satisfying issues from time to time. Physicians should honor and respond to this need, just as they would respond to a desire to discuss pain or other problems.

What physicians say to dying patients is not nearly as important as physicians' willingness to listen. One of the most comforting steps physicians can take in caring for the dying is to allow them to talk about their fears, frustrations, hopes, needs and desires. *Talking about problems can be very therapeutic.* Patients who are permitted to examine and discuss their feelings about death and dying are grateful for the opportunity and usually become less anxious, experience less pain, and accept their situation more easily. If they are denied this opportunity, especially when the terminal process is obvious, they may be convinced that the time remaining is too terrible to be discussed and their anxiety will be significantly increased.

Often, the terminally ill are more fearful of the manner in which their death will occur (e.g., painful, alone and abandoned, weak and helpless) than they are of death itself.

Do all patients wish to be told of their fatal illness, however? Surveys indicate that 80% to 90% of patients say they wish to be told, whereas many physicians prefer not to tell a patient that he or she is dying. A study by Ward revealed that family physicians are more likely to discuss a fatal diagnosis with women than with men (22% versus 7.5%) and more often with patients in the upper social class than the lower social class (24% versus 5% for men and 30% versus 26% for women). Many physicians who state they theoretically believe in telling patients of the terminal nature of their illness employ evasion in their actual practice as often as most other physicians.

Most physicians will tell a patient about terminal cancer if the patient asks a direct question but otherwise will evade the issue and discuss it openly only with the family. There are many occasions when this is the most appropriate course of action; patients are not infrequently encountered who clearly indicate they cannot and do not wish to face the fact that they have an incurable disease. It is essential, however, that the physician evaluate the true nature of the patient's desire in the matter and neither avoid the issue when the patient wishes to discuss it or force a discussion on an unwilling individual.

Patients should be given adequate time to absorb the knowledge of the terminal nature of their illness and the opportunity to react appropriately before death intervenes. This is not possible if the physician procrastinates or rationalizes that it is better not to inform the patient. The process should not be allowed to advance to so final a stage that there is inadequate time remaining for the individual to react appropriately and put his or her affairs in order.

There is no need to answer questions the patient has not yet asked. One way to approach the subject is to ask patients their perception of the problem or how sick they think they really are. The response may be straightforward "I think I have cancer"; or the patient may indicate a wish to avoid the issue by saying, "I hope it's nothing serious." The patient's condition can be revealed gradually or in stages, such as telling him or her following surgery that there is a suspicion of cancer but that further information will have to wait for the pathology report. Observe the patient's response to this initial hint, and based on that reaction, choose a method for presenting subsequent information. Tumulty supports the concept of gradualism in informing a patient and the family of the terminal nature of the illness:

The total truth is revealed in small doses as the illness unfolds, affording the family the opportunity to get its feet under itself before another blow falls. . . . The patient and the family need to be eased into the truth . . . not slugged with it.

Such a gradual disclosure is likely to lead to acceptance, whereas a harsh, sudden, or abrupt disclosure is likely to result in denial or severe depression. If the patient appears reluctant to accept the information, do not push the issue; merely make sure that openings for discussion are periodically made available and that further information is provided when the patient is ready.

When sharing information regarding a fatal diagnosis with a patient, eye contact, touch, and personal closeness are important. If possible, sit with patients and hold their hands or touch their forearms. Such gestures convey a sense of support, closeness, and compassion, reinforcing verbal assurance that the patient will not be abandoned during the difficult time remaining. Sitting with the patient on the bed or at the bedside rather than standing puts the physician on the same level and conveys in a clear, nonverbal manner a willingness to talk and listen. A study was done in which physicians visited with hospitalized patients for exactly 3 minutes. Half the time they sat down, and the other half they remained standing, a little removed from the bed.

Every one of the patients where the physician had sat down thought the physician had stayed at least 10 minutes. None of the ones where the physician remained standing estimated that it was as long.

KÜBLER-ROSS

CONSPIRACY OF SILENCE

Honesty with the terminal patient will provide the greatest benefits. However, the physician is frequently torn between patient and family, with the patient saying, "Don't tell my wife because she can't handle it," while simultaneously the wife is saying, "Don't tell my husband because he can't handle it." Although the wishes and desires of the family must be considered when deciding how to care for a dying patient, the physician's primary obligation is to the patient. The method of management must be based on the physician's knowledge of the patient and insight into his or her desires, feelings, and approach to life. Despite all efforts at deception, the patient knows or will soon learn about the condition anyway.

By cooperating with the family in a conspiracy of silence, information that really belongs to the patient is withheld. Only if the physician believes the patient is not yet ready to cope with the information or sincerely wishes not to be told should the information be withheld. This is more often the exception than the rule, however. One patient said, "I knew it was cancer from the moment they started lying to me" (Lamerton). Simpson describes a 63-year-old woman whose family insisted she knew nothing of her inoperable gastric carcinoma. When visited by the physician, "She gave a dry chuckle: 'Only a little ulcer . . . and my relatives down from Wales to see me for the first time in 15 years, and the priest here at 6 in the morning?'" Obviously, the patient knew the seriousness of her condition, and the mutual deception was nothing more than a charade. When such a game continues, terminally ill patients become more and more isolated because they are unable to communicate honestly and openly with those closest to them about their concerns and fears. The elaborate schemes some families and physicians develop to "protect" the patient lead to a great deal of tension within the family as everyone attempts to perpetuate the lie while continuing to interact with the patient.

Similarly, failure to provide the information to the patient's family can lead to a decrease in the quality of their relationship in the time remaining, since tensions and fears felt by the patient are not understood by those close to him or her. Dunphy describes an incident in which a patient with terminal cancer asked that his wife not be told. He then quickly planned a world cruise, which they had wanted to take for some time. The wife, unaware of the reason for the hasty departure, was unhappy and complaining throughout the trip, while the husband saw himself as a silent martyr, trying to provide a final measure of happiness for his wife. Only after returning home and reminiscing on this miserable cruise was his wife told the truth and the reason for the precipitous departure. Had she been told earlier, each one of their final days together could have been a pleasant and memorable experience.

DENIAL

Most patients tend to deny the reality of their situation after being made aware of the terminal nature of their illness. Denial is one way of coping with or protecting oneself against overwhelming anxiety, which could otherwise be incapacitating. This reaction is more marked in the patient who is told abruptly without being adequately prepared beforehand. Although denial is noted primarily when the patient first learns of his or her impending death, it can appear in different degrees at different times. Even patients who have accepted the terminal nature of their illness will need to employ denial periodically to avoid feelings of hopelessness. The mental burden of impending death is too heavy to carry all the time, and periodic relief is necessary in order to carry on customary activities and enjoy the limited time left. As Aring notes, La Rochefoucauld said, "Neither the sun nor death can be looked at steadily."

A patient who avoids asking about his or her illness or prognosis when the physician offers every opportunity to do so is normally experiencing denial. Excessive denial usually means that the patient subconsciously knows the truth but wishes to avoid facing it consciously. Even when repeatedly given the accurate diagnosis, some patients deny ever having been told. This denial provides constant emotional protection until the patient is ready to face the truth.

WATCH WITH ME

The greatest fear of the dying patient is that of suffering alone and being deserted. There is less fear of a painful death than of the loneliness and alienation that may accompany it. A patient particularly dreads being abandoned by the physician in the face of death and may need increasing levels of professional support as the illness progresses. This is particularly true if family and friends are not able to cope with the deteriorating condition and begin to avoid contact, thus contributing further to the patient's feelings of loneliness and abandonment. If the patient feels there is no one with whom to discuss a condition or to relate in an open and honest fashion, despair is likely to ensue. The patient's fear of the unknown is easier to cope with if the apprehension can be shared with a caring physician who provides comfort, support, encouragement, and even a modicum of hope.

Each new problem of the dying patient should be viewed as a nuisance requiring relief or removal and approached with the vigor that one would devote to an acute, short-term illness. Whenever a fresh complaint arises, the patient should be reexamined and attempts made to relieve the symptom so the patient will not feel unworthy of further attention. If everyday nuisances can be controlled or lessened, the patient will feel that there is sincere concern for making his or her remaining life pleasant. The physician should give attention to details such as improving the taste of food by fixing or replacing dentures, stimulating the patient's appetite, eliminating foul odors, or suggesting occupational therapy in an attempt to avoid boredom. The physician should take advantage of every opportunity to touch and examine the patient rather than standing apart. Gentle palpation of areas of pain or merely taking a pulse can convey a sense of concern and warmth and provide comfort for an apprehensive and lonely patient. The physician and other health professionals can

provide a great deal of support merely through conversation. The tendency to withdraw and reduce conversation contributes to the patient's sense of loneliness. Silence is an enemy of the dying and serves to widen their separation from society. Conversation is a social bond that affirms life and reduces anxiety by providing a means of catharsis. Saunders sums up the need of a dying patient with the words of one patient, "Watch with me," asking that he not be abandoned in his final days. The readiness to listen and the personal caring contact are a comfort that cannot be matched by our modern wonder drugs and procedures.

When dying patients notice that people are avoiding them, they may interpret it as rejection because they have failed to get better or see it as the loss of love from family and friends. The last-mentioned situation is particularly traumatic, since it tends to negate relationships the patient has cherished throughout life. The pleasures and joys of a rewarding life can suddenly appear to lose their value as the dying patient reflects over past events if he or she is ignored or avoided during these final days. The dying patient's contentment is dependent on maintaining warm relationships with loved ones as well as continuing other satisfying interpersonal relationships—such as with the physician. If physicians and others withdraw from interaction with the terminally ill patient, much of the motivation for living disappears and is replaced by despair or terminal depressions. The following plea to fellow health professionals is from a young student nurse who is terminally ill:

> *I know you feel insecure, don't know what to say, don't know what to do. But please believe me, if you care, you can't go wrong. Just admit that you care. . . . All I want to know is that there will be someone to hold my hand when I need it. I am afraid. Death may get to be a routine to you, but it is new to me. You may not see me as unique! . . . If only we could be honest, both admit of our fears, touch one another. If you really care, would you lose so much of your valuable professionalism if you even cried with me? Just person to person? Then, it might not be so hard to die—in a hospital—with friends close by.*
>
> KÜBLER-ROSS

PATIENT CONTROL

Terminally ill patients have a need to believe that they are still in control of their affairs as far as possible, even though they have lost control of their bodies. They should be given the freedom to make choices and assume responsibility over as many aspects of their existence as possible. For many individuals, this is an essential part of living, and its loss may destroy their motivation to live. A terminally ill patient should be helped to focus on and cope with the realities of daily living, since these problems remain very real and can serve as a diversion from constant preoccupation with the prospect of death. When patients have understanding and insight into the treatment and feels they still have some control over the decision-making process regarding their lives, they are more likely to cooperate with prescribed treatment regimens. It is often fear of the unknown that makes a patient suspicious and resistant to therapy. The patient also should be given the opportunity to settle his or her affairs. Concentration on preparing his or her financial business and putting the house in order is a pragmatic approach to active participation in the decision-making process. Some patients may have a burning desire to complete a cherished project, reconcile an estranged relationship, or visit particular places before they die. Positive motivation can be maintained by assisting them to focus on and deal with these issues.

A sense of control is more possible for the patient if pain is controlled and he or she is made comfortable. Sleep should not be forced with medication, because some patients resist going to sleep fearing they may never awaken, whereas others frequently have terrifying dreams.

HOPE

Hope is one of the essential ingredients of human existence, without which life is dark and cold and frustrating. It maintains strength and gives substance to courage. In the presence of hope, suffering of all sorts still has some positive qualities. In its absence, suffering is a completely negative experience.

TUMULTY

The physician should not raise false hopes or be overly aggressive in treating a terminal illness to help the patient maintain hope. Advanced cancer patients can, however, maintain a positive outlook.

Hope increases when honest information is provided, and it is reduced when information is withheld.

Even when death is near, the patient can hope for a measure of happiness during the amount of time remaining. The physician can support the patient's hope for a good quality of life in the remaining time, for spiritual healing, and for a final phase of life that has integrity and dignity.

PROLONGING LIVING OR PROLONGING DYING?

It has been a long time since pneumonia was accepted as "the old man's friend." As one organic system after another slowed to a halt, the aged person was released from nausea, pain, delirium, and the degradation of lingering deterioration by finally developing pneumonia and dying. The family doctor merely showed concern and support; before antibiotics, there was not much to do but stand by and "let nature take its course." With improved medical care, it is possible that a person whose dying process might have taken only a few days in previous years can now have the unrewarding dying experience dragged out for months (Veatch). Modern technology makes it possible to carry the benefits of improved medical care to unrealistic extremes; one person was kept alive in a vegetative state for over 37 years (LORAN Commission Report).

Protraction of the dying process is a modern epidemic. Some physicians seem to forget that their primary responsibility is to relieve suffering, not to prolong it. Greater clinical skill is often required to provide daily supportive care than to cure acute illness. Tenderness and caring must be included in the protocols of the terminally ill so that the ravaged patient is allowed to die peacefully, without tubing and respirators. Patients should

be allowed to experience those waning moments unencumbered by high-tech devices that serve only to impede their capacity for human interaction. Here it is the patient's comfort, not the caregiver's need "to do something" that should prevail.

LORAN COMMISSION REPORT

Sometimes therapeutic restraint is necessary to permit a patient to die with dignity. When a cure is no longer possible, care should focus on the comfort of patient and family. At St. Christopher's Hospice in London, medical equipment is shunned, and feeding is provided by human hands instead of nasogastric or intravenous tubes—"even if the patient does not get enough physical nourishment, he or she gets what is more important—the personal nourishment of someone who cares enough to sit by the bed several hours each day" (Nelson and Rohricht).

MANAGEMENT OF SYMPTOMS

A great deal can be done to help a patient whose disease is incurable. The family physician can help alleviate the fear, symptoms, and family stress that so often make this a distressing time. Care of the dying patient can be one of the most rewarding aspects of the family physician's practice. Yet too often the physician's discomfort with this stage of life contributes to the isolation and discouragement of the terminally ill patient. Unwarranted fears of respiratory depression, addiction, or tolerance prevent the prescribing of adequate amounts of analgesics. The resulting uncontrolled pain makes those final weeks a nightmare for all. Families may disintegrate as a result of the sleepless nights, fears, and guilt that come from trying to cope with the uncontrolled symptoms.

Good control of pain, nausea, and dyspnea can enable patients to die in the place of their choosing with comfort and dignity. Families can cope with their responsibilities and carry good memories of their loved one's final weeks. Physicians can feel gratified at the excellent relief from distress they can provide in this trying time.

The keys to symptom control, as in all areas of medicine, are a careful history and physical examination to determine the various causes of discomfort and a broad knowledge of the therapeutic agents available.

Pain Control

Chronic pain is influenced by memories of past pain and by the anticipation of pain yet to come. The fear of worsening pain may color the present perception of discomfort. Frustration and anxiety may accentuate the pain. All these factors can lower the patient's pain threshold so that even minor disturbances take on immense proportions (Twycross).

Failure to treat the whole person often results in inadequate pain control for patients with terminal cancer. Fatigue, insomnia, anxiety, boredom, and anger all contribute to a lower threshold of pain. Rest, sleep, diversion, and companionship all help to increase the patient's tolerance to pain.

Analgesics should be given in adequate amounts to provide comfort (Angell). The approach to analgesic medication in which doses are given as needed should be abandoned in the treatment of dying patients, since it contributes to a lower pain threshold and a need for increasing doses of medication to relieve the pain. When medication is given regularly in adequate doses, the anxiety and fear that accentuate pain are avoided and lower doses of the drug are effective, since the patient no longer fears recurrence or "breakthrough" of the pain.

High doses of narcotics may be necessary to obtain initial pain control in a patient with severe pain. Dependence is rarely a problem in patients who receive appropriate narcotic doses for chronic severe cancer pain. When medication is given *prior* to the recurrence of pain, craving for medication does not occur. After several weeks of freedom from chronic pain, the dose of medication can be reduced in a stepwise fashion without the appearance of withdrawal phenomena. There should be no more than a 20% reduction in dosage in any 2-day period; otherwise, withdrawal symptoms may occur.

Narcotics. A symptom-oriented history and careful examination may reveal a number of different sources of pain. Oral candidiasis, decubitus ulcers, constipation, and infected wounds all have specific remedies. Most patients with pain from cancer (and many patients with pain from nonneoplastic illnesses) will require a narcotic analgesic. Narcotics are often the safest analgesics available, usually causing only temporary sedation and increased need for laxatives.

Concerns about addiction, respiratory depression, and tolerance are usually unwarranted in these patients. If the dose is carefully titrated, the patient's pain (or dyspnea) can usually be completely controlled, and the patient can still be alert and mentally clear on even hundreds of milligrams of oral morphine given every 4 hours. Underprescribing, however, remains extremely common.

A number of effective oral narcotic preparations are available (Table 7–1). If codeine 30 to 60 mg every 4 hours is not adequate, oxycodone 5 to 10 mg every 4 hours should be used. Oral morphine, beginning with 10 to 15 mg every 4 hours, is usually the next step. The morphine dose should be titrated upward until analgesia lasts the full 4 hours, even if a dose of 200 mg every 4 hours is required.

WEEKLY MEDICATION RECORD

NAME OF DRUG/DOSE/TIME	MON	TUES	WED	THURS	FRI	SAT	SUN
6-7AM							
MORPHINE 2	✓						
SENOKOT 1	✓						
NAPROSYN 1	✓						
CYTOTEC 1	✓						
10AM							
MORPHINE 2	✓						
2PM							
MORPHINE 2							
NAPROSYN 1							
CYTOTEC 1							
6PM							
MORPHINE 2							
SENOKOT 1							
10PM							
MORPHINE 4							
NAPROSYN 1							
CYTOTEC 1							

IF NEEDED FOR PAIN – EXTRA MORPHINE 1 EVERY 2HRS
CONSTIPATION – DULCOLAX SUPP 1-2 DAILY

Figure 7–1. Weekly medication record.

TABLE 7–1. SELECTED ORAL NARCOTICS

	ORAL MORPHINE EQUIVALENT (mg)
Codeine 30 mg and acetaminophen 300 mg (Tylenol #3)	1–2
Hydrocodone 5 mg + homatropine (Hycodan)	1–2
Hydrocodone 5 mg + acetaminophen 500 mg (Vicodin)	1–2
Oxycodone 5 mg + aspirin 325 mg (Percodan)	5
Oxycodone 5 mg + acetaminophen 325 mg (Percocet)	5
Oxycodone 5 mg/5 ml (Roxicodone)	5 mg/5 ml
Hydromorphone 2 mg (Dilaudid)	10
Morphine slow release 30 mg (M S Contin 30 mg, Roxanol SR)	10 mg q4h × 3
Morphine	
Tablets (Lilly, Roxane, Purdue-Frederick)	10, 15, or 30 mg
Syrup (Roxane, Purdue-Frederick)	10 or 20 mg/5 ml
Solution (Roxane, Purdue-Frederick)	20 mg/ml

Source: From Rakel RE. Textbook of Family Practice, 4th ed. Philadelphia, W.B. Saunders, 1990. *(Reprinted with permission.)*

The particular drug used is less important than the method of administration. In order to *prevent* pain and end the cycle of uncontrolled pain followed by oversedation, an oral narcotic should be administered on a regular schedule around the clock. "Booster" doses equal to about half the regular 4-hour dose can be used as needed for breakthrough pain. Long-acting drugs such as methadone (half-life 48 to 72 hours) can be prescribed every 6 to 8 hours but are unsuitable for "booster" doses. They will accumulate over several days and are difficult to titrate, especially in patients who have fluctuating levels of pain or deteriorating renal or hepatic function. Slow-release morphine preparations such as MS Contin and Roxanol SR can provide excellent analgesia for 8 to 12 hours but are expensive and unsuitable for "booster" doses. These tablets are also useless when the patient cannot swallow because they must not be crushed. Small soluble tablets or concentrated solutions of morphine or hydromorphone can be given sublingually when the patient is too weak to swallow and can be used for both 4-hour and "booster" doses. There is no need to use injections when an adequate dose by mouth will work as well. Table 7–2 provides a checklist of items to remember when prescribing a narcotic.

Two narcotic agents that are also available orally are not recommended for cancer pain. Meperidine (Demerol) has a very low oral potency, a short duration of action, and a toxic metabolite that can cause tremors or even seizures (Kaiko et al.). Pentazocine (Talwin, Talacen) is an agonist–antagonist agent that is no more potent than aspirin with codeine and has a high incidence of psychotomimetic effects (hallucinations, confusion) in cancer patients.

Co-Analgesics. "Co-analgesics" are drugs that potentiate the analgesic effects of narcotics for particular types of pain (Table 7–3). Nonsteroidal anti-inflammatory drugs are quite helpful in the alleviation of pain

TABLE 7–2. PHYSICIAN'S CHECKLIST WHEN PRESCRIBING NARCOTICS

1. Has an appropriate starting dose been determined?
2. Is a co-analgesic needed?
3. Is an antiemetic needed?
4. Has a laxative been prescribed?
5. Is the drug regimen written out in sufficient detail?
6. Has the patient been warned about possible side effects that might occur initially?
7. Do the patient and family know what to do if the pain remains uncontrolled?
8. Have arrangements been made for follow-up after 1, 3, and 7 days—either by the physician or a trained hospice nurse?
9. Does the patient know what to do if he or she needs help or advice before the next follow-up visit?
10. Is the patient confident that the pain will improve considerably, probably within a few days, certainly within 1 or 2 weeks?

Source: Modified from Twycross RG, Lack SA. Symptoms Control in Far Advanced Cancer: Pain Relief. London, Pitman, 1983. *(Reprinted with permission.)*

from lesions in bones or skeletal muscles. The nonacetylated salicylates [e.g., salsalate (Disalcid), choline magnesium trisalicylate (Trilisate)] are less toxic to the gastric mucosa and do not inhibit platelet function (Zucker and Rothwell) but are less potent analgesics. The newer nonsalicylate nonsteroidal anti-inflammatory drugs are more potent, more convenient, more expensive, and less toxic than aspirin. Although no single agent has been shown to be consistently more efficacious, particular patients do seem to favor one drug over another. If swallowing large tablets becomes a problem, piroxicam (Feldene) capsules, naproxen (Naprosyn) suspension, or indomethacin (Indocin) rectal suppositories may be used.

For the burning, stabbing, or shooting pain caused by nerve damage, a tricyclic antidepressant or an anticonvulsant may be a useful addition. Amitriptyline, in doses smaller than those used to treat depression (10 to 50 mg at bedtime), is often effective. If swallowing problems arise, doxepin (Sinequan) solution should be used. The addition of carbamazepine (200 mg three times daily) should be considered if the tricyclic agent alone is not adequate. A short course of steroids also has been helpful in treating difficult, narcotic-resistant pain.

Visceral or Bladder Spasms

These spasms are best treated with an anticholinergic agent such as dicyclomine (Bentyl) or oxybutynin (Ditropan). If only small doses are needed, Transderm Scop patches may be useful. For more severe cases, the addition of 0.8 to 2.0 mg of scopolamine to a 24-hour subcutaneous infusion of a narcotic should be used.

Anxiety

Gentle, open discussion with the physician, social worker, or chaplain is often effective for anxiety. If anxiety is severe enough to require drug therapy, consider hydroxyzine (Atarax or Vistaril) 10 to 50 mg orally every 4 to 8 hours. This drug also has been shown to potentiate morphine in large doses. If a parenteral agent is

TABLE 7–3. CO-ANALGESICS

PAIN SOURCE	PAIN CHARACTER	DRUG CLASS	EXAMPLES	
Bone or soft tissue	Tenderness over bone or joint	NSAID	Ibuprofen 400 mg q4 h	Inexpensive, *big* pills
	Pain on movement		Sulindac (Clinoril) 200 mg q12h	Well tolerated, preferred in renal impairment
			Naproxen (Naprosyn susp) 125 mg per 5 ml, 15 ml q8h	Liquid preparation
			Indomethacin (Indocin 50 mg) caps *or* supp. q8h	Suppository, more gastritis?
			Piroxicam (Feldene 20 mg) capsules, 1qd	Easiest to swallow, more gastritis?
			Choline Mg Trisalicylate (Trilisate susp) 500 mg per 5 ml, 15 ml q12h	No platelet dysfunction, less problem with gastritis, less effective
Nerve damage or dysaesthesia	Burning or shooting pain radiating from plexis or spinal root	Tricyclic antidepressant	Amitriptyline (Elavil 10 to 50 mg qhs)	Best studied, sedating, start with low dose
		Alone or with	*or* Doxepin (Sinequan 10–50 mg qhs)	10 mg/ml susp. available
			or Trazodone (Desyrel 25–150 mg qhs)	Less anticholinergic effect, ⅛ as potent as amitriptyline
		Anticonvulsant	Carbamazepine (Tegretol 200 mg q6–12 h)	Absorbed from rectum, unlike phenytoin
Smooth-muscle spasms	Colic—cramping abdominal pain bladder spasms	Anticholinergic	Scopolamine (Transderm-Scōp 1 to 2 patches q3d)	May also be mixed with narcotic in SQ infusion, 0.8–2.0 mg/day
			Dicyclomine (Bentyl 10 mg q4–8h)	Capsules
			Oxybutynin (Ditropan 5–10 mg q8h)	Tablets
Anxiety	Generalized restlessness and discomfort	Antihistamine	Hydroxyzine (Atarax or Vistaril 10 to 50 mg q4hrs)	PO or by SQ infusion
		Phenothiazine	Methotrimeprazine (Levoprome 50–300 mg/day)	IM or SQ infusion only

Source: From Rakel RE. Textbook of Family Practice, 4th ed. Philadelphia, W.B. Saunders, 1990. *(Reprinted with permission.)*

needed, use methotrimeprazine (Levoprome). This is the only phenothiazine with analgesic activity, and it is a potent sedative and antiemetic as well. An intramuscular injection of 20 to 30 mg will usually calm a crisis, and 50 to 300 mg per day can be given by subcutaneous infusion. Orthostatic hypotension and irritation at the injection site are possible side effects.

Dyspnea

Like pain, dyspnea can have a multitude of causes. When anemia, bronchospasm, and heart failure have been excluded or treated, the focus should be on symptom control. Oxygen can be helpful but is much less effective than narcotics for controlling this distressing symptom. When the dose of narcotic is carefully titrated to control the pain and the narcotic is administered on a regular schedule with "booster" doses available, the patient can experience excellent relief without significant respiratory depression (Twycross and Lack; Walsh et al.). Careful consideration should be given to the use

of antibiotics for pneumonia in the terminally ill patient. Since dyspnea can be well controlled without antibiotics, the physician must decide whether the antibiotics will improve the quality of life or just prolong dying.

Constipation

When mobility and oral intake decrease and narcotic analgesics are required, virtually every patient will require regular doses of laxatives to avoid distressing constipation. The laxative should be given once or twice *every* day, and the amount should be increased until an effective dose is found. Bulk laxatives are poorly tolerated and are rarely adequate for such patients. If docusate (Colace) 100 to 200 mg twice daily is not effective, add senna (Senokot) or bisacodyl (Dulcolax) 1 to 4 tablets twice daily. Lactulose (Chronulac) should be added in doses of 15 to 45 ml two or three times per day if the tablets are inadequate or cause excessive cramping. If a patient has gone several days without a bowel movement or is having small, frequent, liquid stools, an impaction may require manual removal. Bisacodyl suppositories or enemas may be needed occasionally until an effective oral regimen is found.

Nausea and Vomiting

In patients with nausea and vomiting, first look for a reversible cause such as constipation or gastritis from nonsteroidal anti-inflammatory drugs. If increased intracranial pressure is the cause, then the patient may require steroids. Overfeeding may be the problem if a nasogastric or gastrostomy tube is in place. Metoclopramide (Reglan) is the agent of choice when an enormous liver limits gastric emptying. Many patients whose nausea and vomiting have not responded to prochlorperazine (Compazine) or promethazine (Phenergan) will be relieved by haloperidol (Haldol) 0.5 to 2 mg every 8 hours.

Like persistent pain, persistent nausea should be treated with regularly scheduled doses. Combinations of antiemetics that have different modes of action may be needed. A combination of haloperidol with metoclopramide or cyclizine (Marezine) is effective. When oral antiemetics cannot be tolerated, rectal suppositories can be tried but rarely provide adequate control for persistent nausea and vomiting. Continuous subcutaneous infusions of metaclopramide, haloperidol, or methotrimeprazine (Levoprome) are more effective (Baines). Even vomiting associated with complete bowel obstruction can be controlled *without* a nasogastric tube or gastrostomy with a continuous subcutaneous infusion of narcotics, antiemetics, and anticholinergic agents (Baines et al.).

Hiccup

Persistent hiccuping can be caused by any lesion affecting the phrenic nerve and by gastric distension or systemic problems such as uremia. Treatment can consist of chlorpromazine (Thorazine) 25 to 50 mg orally every 4 to 6 hours, metoclopromide (Reglan) 10 to 20 mg orally every 6 to 8 hours, or haloperidol (Haldol) 1 to 2 mg orally every 4 to 6 hours.

NUTRITION

Although uncontrolled pain is the principal complaint of many patients, their family's principal concern is often how little they are eating. The causes of cancer cachexia are still unknown. Since patients seem to stop eating, lose weight, and eventually die, the natural assumption has been made that even if we cannot effectively treat the cancer, we can at least treat malnutrition and thereby delay death.

The problem is that more harm than good can come from aggressive dietary therapy. Families are sometimes referred to aggressive dietitians who emphasize the need for multiple cans of supplement each day so strongly that the family feels responsible if the patient loses weight and dies. Unfortunately, the patient's final weeks become a struggle with the family over how much they have eaten. One patient said, "Tell her to stop pushing that spoon into my face, I don't want any more!" This can be carried to extremes, such as inserting nasogastric tubes in patients who "do not cooperate." Their hands are even tied to bed rails if the tube is tugged on. A study of tube feedings in elderly patients revealed that within 2 weeks, 67% of patients with nasogastric tubes had attempted self-extubation and 43% had aspiration pneumonia. Gastric or jejunal tubes had a lower self-extubation rate (44%), but 56% of the patients had aspiration pneumonia, 31% had a leak or infection at the insertion site, and 50% had a clogged or kinked tube (Ciocion et al.). Large volumes of supplemental feeding can cause painful gastric distension, nausea, diarrhea, and copious pulmonary secretions.

There is no evidence that forced feeding really prolongs life. Careful metabolic studies on force-fed cancer patients at the University of Rochester showed irreversibly increased metabolic rates from force feeding. It was speculated that tumor growth was accelerated (Terepka and Waterhouse). Animal experiments have shown that growth rates of a variety of different cancers are nutrient dependent—the growth rate slows down with fasting or protein-free diets and speeds up with total parenteral nutrition (Buzby et al.; Stragand et al.). Several trials have been conducted in which patients receiving total parenteral nutrition plus chemotherapy were compared with those receiving chemotherapy alone. The group receiving total parenteral nutrition died faster. This was especially true for patients with adenocarcinoma of the lung (Jordan et al.), colorectal cancer (Nixon et al.), and small-cell lung cancer (Shike et al.). When Klein and associates pooled the data from papers written on total parenteral nutrition and cancer through 1985, they found that infections were more common in patients receiving total parenteral nutrition and that these patients were less responsive to chemotherapy and had shortened survival times.

After reviewing all the clinical trials of parenteral nutrition in patients receiving cancer chemotherapy, the American College of Physicians concluded:

> *The evidence suggests that parenteral nutritional support was associated with net harm, and no conditions could be defined in which such treatment appeared to be of benefit. Thus, the routine use of parenteral nutrition for patients undergoing chemotherapy should be strongly discouraged.*

What should be done to relieve the anorexia of advanced cancer? Table 7–4 lists a number of treatable causes of anorexia. Uncontrolled pain blunts anyone's appetite and can be alleviated. Low-level nausea, oral candidiasis, and constipation can certainly interfere with eating, and all are easily treated. Families can be taught how to relieve xerostomia (dry mouth) with a small syringe filled with water or juice and how to prepare soft foods. Corticosteroids have been beneficial to some. The most important service the family physician can provide is to allay guilt. An appropriate statement would be "I do *not* feel that how much time your husband has or how comfortable he is depends on how much he eats."

TABLE 7-4. MANAGEMENT OF ANOREXIA

Treat "anorexia"
   Aches and pains
   Nausea
   Oral candidiasis
   Reactive depression
   Evacuation problems (constipation)
   Xerostomia (dry mouth)
   Iatrogenic problems (from chemotherapy or radiation therapy)
   Acid problems (gastric, ulcers)
Teach the family to prepare soft, easy-to-swallow foods
Consider steroids
Avoid nasogastric or gastrostomy tubes or hyperalimentation
Allay guilt

Source: From Rakel RE. Textbook of Family Practice, 4th ed. Philadelphia, W.B. Saunders, 1990. *(Reprinted with permission.)*

WHERE TO DIE

Death with dignity is easiest to accomplish when the patient dies amid the surroundings that gave meaning to his or her life and in the company of those whose companionship provided most of the rewards of living. Physicians too often deny this, however, in the medically conditioned struggle to prolong life. Medical technology has advanced to the point that few patients are permitted to die at home, even though improved diagnostic techniques identify the irreversible nature of a terminal process at an earlier stage. A sorry commentary, reflecting the abuse of technology, is the case of a man who had built his house with his own hands and wanted to die there but was prevented from doing so while physicians exhausted their therapeutic armamentarium in an attempt to prolong his life a few days or weeks longer.

Charles Lindberg is an excellent example of an individual who insisted on designing his final days in a manner that would preserve dignity and allow him to die as comfortably as possible. When dying of lymphoma, he refused to remain in a medical center on the East Coast and returned to his home in Hawaii, where he made final arrangements regarding his estate and discussed with friends and family the details of his memorial service and burial site. His death was as he preferred— quiet, dignified, private, and in the company of family and friends—a striking contrast to what it would have been had he not insisted on leaving the medical center.

HOSPICE CARE

A "hospice" program consists of palliative and supportive services that provide physical, psychologic, social, and spiritual care for dying persons and their families. Services are provided by a medically supervised interdisciplinary team of professionals and volunteers and are available both in the home and in an inpatient setting. Home care is provided as necessary—on a part-time, intermittent, regularly scheduled, or around-the-clock on-call basis. The hospice concept is directed toward providing

. . . support and care for persons in the last phases of incurable diseases so that they might live as fully and as comfortably as possible . . . [and] that, through appropriate care the promotion of a caring community sensitive to their needs, patients and families may be free to attain a degree of mental and spiritual preparation for death that is satisfactory to them.

NATIONAL HOSPICE ORGANIZATION

Hospice care is not focused only on the patient; the unit of care is the patient and family. The physical, psychologic, and interpersonal needs of both the patient and the family are addressed.

Admission to a hospice program requires that a person have an inevitably fatal illness with a prognosis of weeks or months, that a request be made for the services, and that the attending physician consent to and cooperate with the hospice care. Table 7–5 lists the stan-

TABLE 7-5. NHO STANDARDS OF HOSPICE PROGRAM OF CARE

1. Appropriate therapy is the goal of hospice care.
2. Palliative care is the most appropriate form of care when cure is no longer possible.
3. The goal of palliative care is the prevention of distress from chronic signs and symptoms.
4. Admission to a hospice program of care is dependent on patient and family needs and their expressed request for care.
5. Hospice care consists of a blending of professional and nonprofessional services.
6. Hospice care considers all aspects of the lives of patients and their families as valid areas of therapeutic concern.
7. Hospice care is respectful of all patient and family belief systems, and will employ resources to meet the personal philosophic, moral, and religious needs of patients and their families.
8. Hospice care provides continuity of care.
9. The hospice care program considers the patient and the family together as the unit of care.
10. The patient's family is considered to be a central part of the hospice care team.
11. Hospice care programs seek to identify, coordinate, and supervise persons who can give care to patients who do not have a family member available to take on the responsibility of giving care.
12. Hospice care for the family continues into the bereavement period.
13. Hospice care is available 24 hours a day, 7 days a week.
14. Hospice care is provided by an interdisciplinary team.
15. Hospice programs will have structured and informal means of providing support to staff.
16. Hospice programs will be in compliance with the Standards of the National Hospice Organization and the applicable laws and regulations governing the organization and delivery of care to patients and families.
17. The services of the hospice program are coordinated under a central administration.
18. The optimal control of distressful symptoms is an essential part of the hospice care program requiring medical, nursing, and other services of the interdisciplinary team.
19. The hospice care team will have:
   a. a medical director on staff
   b. physicians on staff
   c. a working relationship with the patient's physician
20. Based on the patient's needs and preferences as determining factors in the setting and location for care, a hospice program provides inpatient care and care in the home setting.
21. Education, training, and evaluation of hospice services in an ongoing activity of a hospice care program.
22. Accurate and current records are kept on all patients.

Source: From the NHO Standards Document, National Hospice Organization. *(Reprinted with permission.)*

dards of a hospice program as developed by the National Hospice Organization.

The interdisciplinary hospice team consists of a patient care coordinator, a nurse, a physician, a counselor, a volunteer coordinator, and spiritual support. Medical services are on call 24 hours a day, 7 days a week. Continuity of care by the same group of team members provides a familiarity that is comforting to the patient. Volunteers are an integral part of the program and provide many helpful services.

Support for the Family

Following a patient's death, family members experience increased morbidity and mortality, emphasizing the need for greater family support from the physician. Unfortunately, most physicians do not routinely contact the family following a patient's death, so this need often goes unrecognized (Tolle et al.).

The hospice team provides follow-up bereavement care to the family for up to 1 year after the patient's death. Family members who experience grief following the death of a loved one are more vulnerable to physical and other emotional disturbances than at any other time in their lives. They need help dealing with the grief, guilt, and the symptoms associated with this emotional turmoil. The bereavement services of a hospice team can minimize these problems and can help family members cope with the pain of memories that arise from time to time, especially at holidays, birthdays, and other stressful occasions.

The most remarkable contribution of the hospice movement is not that it provides a special and compassionate setting in which terminally ill persons can die without heroic measures being applied to them, but that the family becomes involved and comfortable in caring for the ill member.

With the rapid increase of scientific and technologic competence in the field of medicine, families feel increasingly incompetent and impotent to deal with dying. The hospice movement has reversed this trend and helps family members to work with community support services to provide home care for many of these patients. When symptoms cannot be controlled at home, the hospice inpatient unit can provide medical and nursing expertise in a "homelike" setting.

The hospice concept can benefit patients and families wherever death takes place. What is important is a network of support for all concerned. However, there should not be an arbitrary judgment as to what is best for all people. Some patients do not want to be a burden to their family and pride themselves on being able to afford hospitalization or nursing home care. For some of these patients, the gradual withdrawal from family may be an emotional "letting go" that is necessary for all concerned in their particular family and circumstances. On the other hand, there may be a spouse of a perfectly good marriage who is simply not equipped either physically or psychologically to deal with the loved one dying right there in the house over a 2-month period. The family physician will be sensitive to the style of living and the style of dying that seems most appropriate in a given case once the options have been explained to the family.

EUTHANASIA OR ASSISTED SUICIDE

Virtually every dying patient thinks about suicide, and many ask their physician to help them. The greatest difficulties in dying are sometimes seen in patients who linger much longer than expected—so-called postmature deaths. How should the caring physician respond?

In any areas in which medicine intersects moral codes, there are bound to be diverse opinions and heated debate. The distinction between "active" and "passive" euthanasia should be kept in mind. Active euthanasia involves the purposeful administration of drugs to end life. It is common practice in Holland but unlawful in the United States. "Passive" euthanasia involves the withholding of drugs and permitting the disease to run its course. "Assisted suicide" involves the prescribing of large quantities of sedatives for the purpose of empowering a patient to take his or her own life.

The principal reason for most patients wanting to end their lives is the high degree of suffering—usually because of uncontrolled pain or intolerable debilitation. However, much can be done to relieve pain, and support systems can be devised to provide the necessary care for an incapacitated patient. One experience of being thanked for *not* agreeing to assist in suicide by a patient whose pain was previously intolerable but is now well controlled makes any physician hesitate before agreeing to participate in assisted suicide. Permanent solutions to temporary problems should be avoided.

The notion that any treatable complication of a terminal illness *must* be treated because it *can* be treated is also wrong. Most patients do not want to die, but they are just as concerned about the *quality* of their time remaining as they are about the *quantity*. The physician may rescue an advanced cancer patient from one potentially lethal complication only to find that another, which may cause much worse suffering, will end the person's life. Hippocrates' admonition, *"primum non nocere"* (first do no harm), may apply to treatments that are often helpful, such as antibiotics and percutaneous ureterostomies.

"Do Not Resuscitate" Orders

Obviously, one will die if the heart stops working; yet cardiac arrest happens in persons who need not die, because the incident is a temporary crisis and is reversible, sometimes even by the intervention of a lay person trained in cardiopulmonary resuscitation. At the other end of the spectrum, it is technically possible with heart–lung machinery and a pacemaker to keep a heart stimulated or keep the blood circulating in a body to which, according to consensus, consciousness will never return. Neither of these extremes presents a major problem in medical ethics. Decision making is more difficult in the gray area between these two extremes. There are complex moral and legal issues involved in decisions not to treat or not to resuscitate or in so-called no code orders (Wong and Swazey).

The physician should be acquainted with any policy statement or guidelines that have been developed by the hospital. In or out of the hospital, persons with unexpected cardiac arrest should be resuscitated because it is an emergency and there is no time to assess the cause or attendant circumstances. It is not wise to allow age, mental retardation, or other "quality of life" issues to enter at this time. In the case of a patient with no response on an electroencephalogram, the physician should be alert to the possibility that drug overdose, hypothermia, or barbiturate therapy may be responsible. It is entirely within the physician's prerogative to determine the care that is medically appropriate for a patient. An attending physician may determine that a patient is irreversibly terminally ill and that no course of therapy offers any reasonable expectation of remission or cure of the terminal condition. Once this determination has been made, then the decision not to resuscitate may be appropriate. The essence of terminal illness is the expectation that death is imminent "within a short time." Since it is not possible to predict the time of death precisely, the decision is based on medical judgment. Consultation with a medical colleague should be sought if there is any doubt about the status of the patient. This consultation also may provide reassurance for the family.

The patient may request that no cardiopulmonary resuscitation be initiated in case of an arrest, raising the issue of "voluntary informed consent" and the patient's rights. The physician needs to assess the mental status of the patient to ascertain that there are no extenuating circumstances such as disorientation due to chemotherapy, metabolic abnormalities, or psychosocial factors. (One patient developed a sudden loss of interest in living when served with divorce papers while receiving treatment in the hospital.)

It is not pleasant to talk about dying. If one perseveres and overrides the initial reticence, however, the rewards of this kind of interaction are great. Many physicians report that their most meaningful relationships with patients have been precisely those which involved deep and personal sharing about the meaning of life that was allowed to surface by facing death together. There are issues to be considered other than pleasure and the avoidance of pain. Being truly human means being open to all the meanings of existence.

CASE STUDY

Bob E. is a hard-driving, successful attorney. He remained in active practice despite his age of 68 years and only sought medical attention when he became unable to urinate. The rectal examination suggested, and transurethral resection confirmed, the diagnosis of adenocarcinoma of the prostate. His serum acid phosphatase and prostate specific antigen levels were high, and the bone scan strongly suggested metastatic disease throughout his pelvis and spine. He was not compliant with the prescribed estrogen therapy because of the impotence and gynecomastia it caused. Orchiectomy or chemotherapy was suggested, and he flatly refused, despite increasing amounts of low back pain. Radiation therapy was somewhat helpful, and he returned to work a little. The pain increased, however, and his wife became concerned about his obvious depression and increasing immobility. The oxycodone with aspirin (Percodan) his urologist prescribed helped for a month or two, but his increasing requirements caused anxiety on the part of the physician, who again recommended bilateral orchiectomy. Bob said he would rather die. He did not tell his doctor about the increasing dyspepsia from the Percodan. Bob began to talk openly about euthanasia and suicide. His wife heard about hospice from a friend and asked his doctor to refer him.

The hospice nurse and physician visited Bob and his wife Janet in their beautifully furnished townhouse in early June. Bob was bitter and angry. He was in severe pain but insisted on getting to his feet to shake hands with the visitors. His pain and Janet's anxiety were obvious. They all sat down in the formal living room, and Janet fixed them coffee. The doctor took a medical history. When Bob asked for euthanasia and declared, "Holland is the only civilized country," Janet left and went to the kitchen.

The hospice physician listened attentively. He let Bob spout all that anger and bitterness and then confidently stated that much more could be done to relieve Bob's pain. Bob agreed that he would have no interest in being euthanized if he could get relief from his pain. The doctor explained that hospice is a team approach to the problems that come with advanced cancer. He said that there would not be a lot of tests or hospitalizations, but that the focus of attention would be on Bob's comfort and Janet's ability to care for him. "How much will this cost me?" Bob inquired. The nurse explained that the Medicare Hospice Benefit paid for all the visits, his medications, and any equipment or supplies needed. Janet was concerned that Bob had to waive his right to further hospital care. The hospice nurse started to explain about the hospice inpatient unit, but Bob interrupted with "I'm not going back to any hospital so you can forget about that!"

The hospice physician asked to examine Bob and said the living-room couch would be adequate. Bob insisted on climbing the stairs to his bedroom. It took nearly 5 minutes of slow, painful effort for Bob to get up those stairs.

The physical examination revealed diffuse tenderness in Bob's back and pelvis. He also had abdominal distension and tenderness with no palpable masses. Bob admitted to taking 10 to 12 Percodan tablets each day, and since each one contains both a narcotic analgesic and 325 mg uncoated aspirin, this explained the dyspepsia and epigastric tenderness. The physician inquired further into Bob's bowel habits and learned that Bob was quite constipated. He had avoided laxatives for fear of not being able to get to the toilet in time. Bob refused a rectal examination.

Meanwhile, the nurse was talking with Janet about how to reach the hospice and what services were available. Janet shared her anxieties about the possibility that Bob would commit suicide if he did not get some relief of his pain. He had not discussed a plan for this, and they had no firearms in the house. Janet also looked exhausted and admitted to getting very little sleep, since Bob was up and down all night. She gratefully accepted the services of the social worker and volunteers. She was relieved that help was on the way and felt reassured by the doctor's confidence that something could be done for Bob's pain.

The hospice doctor calculated that (since each Percodan contains the narcotic equivalent of 5 mg oral morphine) Bob had been taking the equivalent of 50 to 60 mg oral morphine each day. He wanted to double this amount, so he prescribed 20 mg oral morphine (two 10-mg tablets) every 4 hours. He explained to Bob and Janet that Bob would be a bit drowsy for a day or two, but that he would soon adjust to the medication and feel as alert as ever. He also prescribed bisacodyl (Dulcolax) suppositories to remedy Bob's present constipation and then recommended senna (Senokot), one tablet twice daily, to prevent recurrent constipation. The doctor also felt a nonsteroidal anti-inflammatory drug would be helpful with the bone pain and prescribed a naproxen (Naprosyn) 375-mg tablet every 8 hours. He also added misoprostel (Cytotec) 200 μg every 8 hours to prevent gastric ulcers. Finally, he told Bob and Janet that Bob could have an extra 10-mg morphine tablet every 2 hours as needed for breakthrough pain, but that if he required more than three of these "boosters" each day, he should call the hospice for a dosage adjustment. He also suggested that Bob take a double dose (40 mg) of morphine at bedtime to last for 8 hours of better sleep. He wrote all this down on a medication schedule listing which pills to take and when (see Fig. 7–1). He strongly encouraged Bob to take the medications at the designated hours even if he was not hurting. He explained that the most effective method of controlling cancer pain was to "stay ahead of it." He wrote the triplicate prescription while the nurse found a drugstore that carried the medications and gave Janet directions. Finally, he encouraged Bob and Janet to call the hospice for any questions or problems and put a sticker with the hospice phone number on their phone. Bob and Janet thanked them, and Janet said she would look forward to seeing the social worker the next day.

The on-call nurse did not hear from them that night, and the social worker arrived the next morning. Janet was less frantic after a good night's sleep, and Bob had eaten a little breakfast and gone back to bed. He was glad the social worker had come "to help Janet" but did not have anything to say himself. Janet said, in private, that she was not only concerned about Bob's suicide risk, but also about their finances. Bob had always handled all the money, and she had no idea how much they had and what she would do when Bob died. They had "lost a lot, like everyone else" in the oil bust of the mid-1980s and had moved from their large colonial home into this townhouse 3 years ago. Janet had lost touch with many of their friends, and their grown children rarely visited. Bob was not very pleasant to be around when he was in pain. Janet's health was generally good, but she had not returned to her physician in several months and she was almost out of her heart medication. She also was very worried about the pile of official-looking statements and IRS inquiries that Bob had not quite "gotten around to." She used to be a regular church member of the local Methodist church but had not attended in some months because she worried about leaving Bob. He had never attended church.

The social worker listened attentively and made a few notes. She suggested that they hire a bookkeeper of Bob's choosing to straighten out their finances and teach Janet about their financial situation. She also suggested that a volunteer might stay with Bob while Janet went to church, visited her doctor, and renewed the social contacts that sustained her. She felt that it was too early to mention funeral arrangements and that the hospice chaplain would not be helpful. Janet seemed notably relieved to get her concerns out in the open, and they agreed to meet again the following week.

At the hospice team meeting the next morning, Bob's case was presented by the doctor, nurse, and social worker. The volunteer coordinator agreed to visit later in the week to line them up with the right volunteer. The chaplain mentioned that often nonchurch members have deep questions that they want to talk about once the physical and social problems are addressed. He asked that the team stay alert to this possibility. The team agreed that with no plan, family history of suicide, or firearm present, Bob's suicide risk did not seem too high—if the pain was controlled. There also was a hope expressed that his mobility would improve with better pain control, so the physical therapist and home health aide decided that they were not needed right now.

A registered nurse from the hospice, Betty, visited later that afternoon. She found a different Bob than the team described that morning.

Bob was much more comfortable and mobile than before. He complained of some lethargy and poor appetite, but the pain was markedly improved and his bowels were moving. Since he had required bisacodyl (Ducolax) suppositories both days to have a bowel movement, she increased his senna (Senokot) dose to two tablets twice daily. Bob was worried about "getting hooked on this dope," but Betty reassured him that normal people are not turned into addicts by taking pain medications prescribed to them for cancer pain and that if the pain went away, she felt certain that he could taper off the medications without difficulty. Janet had not had the courage to discuss the bookkeeper idea with Bob, but with Betty's help, his hesitation was overcome and a commitment was made to hire a person Bob knew from the office. Betty promised to visit again in the next week.

Bob's pain remained under control, although his morphine requirement gradually increased from 20 to 60 mg every 4 hours. Suicide or euthanasia was never mentioned again. His strength and appetite steadily declined, however, and Betty and the hospice team did a lot to help Janet cope. Bob finally agreed to a hospital bed in the downstairs den when he could not climb the stairs anymore. A bedside commode and home health aide visits to bathe Bob made it possible for Janet to care for him there. Bob did discuss his long-standing guilt feelings and anger against God with the hospice chaplain. The social worker helped with Janet's anxiety and the need for funeral arrangements. When Bob became totally bedbound, Betty inserted a Foley catheter.

In mid-September Bob began having periods of confusion. They were particularly bad at night. Haloperidol (Haldol) was helpful at first, but when he began insisting that he "had to go" and climbed over the bedrails a couple of times, it was more than Janet could handle. Betty mentioned the possibility of private-duty nurses, but their insurance and finances would not cover the costs. Janet also knew she would not sleep with a restless husband at night no matter who was there to help. Bob was transferred by ambulance to the hospice inpatient unit.

Bob was not very willing (able?) to swallow medications from the inpatient nurses, and he seemed restless and uncomfortable. The hospice doctor had the nurses start a continuous subcutaneous infusion of morphine and haloperidol. This seemed quite helpful. Janet liked the homelike environment and calm, unhurried manner of the hospice nurses. When their daughter flew into town and got very upset that "everything" was not being done for (to) Bob, the doctor and social worker explained that CT scans and IV fluids would not get rid of the cancer, which was Bob's main problem. The daughter was finally able to see her guilt over not visiting much the last few years.

Bob quietly stopped breathing the next night with his wife and the hospice nurse at the bedside. Janet asked that in lieu of flowers, donations be sent to the hospice. Betty attended the funeral, and the bereavement coordinator checked with Janet regularly over the next year. It was hard for her, yet she was glad she had been able, with the help of the hospice, to care for Bob at home—where he wanted to be.

REFERENCES

American College of Physicians Position Paper. Parenteral nutrition in patients receiving cancer chemotherapy. Ann Intern Med 1989; 110(9):734–736.

Angell M. The quality of mercy. N Engl J Med 1982; 306:98.

Aring CD. The Understanding Physician. Detroit, Wayne State University Press, 1971.

Baines M. Nausea and vomiting in the patient with advanced cancer. J Pain Symptoms Manage 1988; 3:81–85.

Baines M, Oliver DJ, Carter RL. Medical management of intestinal obstruction in patients with advanced malignant disease. Lancet 1985; 2(8462):990–993.

Buzby GP, Mullen JL, Stein TP, et al. Host–tumor interaction and nutrient supply. Cancer 1980; 45:2940–2948.

Ciocon JO, Silverstone FA, Grouer M, et al. Tube feedings in elderly patients. Arch Intern Med 1988; 148:429–433.

Coping with Cancer: A Resource for the Health Professional. Prepared by the Office of Cancer Communication. Bethesda, Md., National Cancer Institute, September 1980 (NIH Pub. No. 80–2080).

Davidson GW. Living with Dying. Minneapolis, Augsburg Publishing House, 1975.

Driscoll CE. Pain management. Prim Care 1987; 14(2):337–352.

Driscoll CE. Symptom control in terminal illness. Prim Care 1987; 14(2):353–363.

Dunphy JE. On caring for the patient with cancer. N Engl J Med 1976; 295:313.

Graham J. In the Company of Others. New York. Harcourt Brace Jovanovich, 1982.

Hively J (ed.). Hospice of Marin Information Handbook, 2nd ed. San Rafael, Calif., Hospice of Marin, November 1981.

Jordan WM, Valdivreso M, Frankmann C, et al. Treatment of advanced adenocarcinoma of the lungs with ftoratur, doxorubicin, cyclophosphamide and cisplatin (FACP) and intensive I.V. hyperalimentation. Cancer Treat Rep 1981; 65:197–205.

Kaiko RF, Foley KM, Gravinsky PLJ, et al. Central nervous system excitatory effects of meperidine in cancer patients. Ann Neurol 1983; 13:180–185.

Kelly OE, Murray WC. Make Today Count. New York, Delacorte Press, 1975.

Klein S, Simes J, Blackburn GL. Total parenteral nutrition and cancer clinical trials. Cancer 1986; 58:1378–1386.

Kübler-Ross E. Death: The Final Satge of Growth. Englewood Cliffs, N.J., Prentice-Hall, 1975.

Kübler-Ross E. On Death and Dying. New York, Macmillan, 1969.

Kushner HS. When Bad Things Happen to Good People. New York, Schocken Books, 1981.

Lamerton R. Care of the Dying. Westport, Conn., Technomic Publishing Co., 1976.

Lindemann E. Symptomatology and management of acute grief. Am J Psychol 1944; 101:141.

Lipman AG. Drug therapy in cancer pain. Cancer Nurs 1980; 3:39.

LORAN Commission. A Report to the Community. Brookline, Mass, Harvard Community Health Plan, 1989.

National Hospice Organization. Hospice Principles and Standards, 6th ed. Vienna, Va., National Hospice Organization, 1979.

Nelson JB. Human Medicine: Ethical Perspectives on New Medical Issues. Minneapolis, Augsburg Publishing House, 1973.

Nelson JB, Rohricht JS. Human Medicine: Ethical Perspectives on Today's Medical Issues. Minneapolis, Augsburg Publishing House, 1984.

Nixon DW, Moffit S, Lawson DH, et al. Total parenteral nutrition as an adjunct to chemotherapy of metastatic colorectal cancer. Cancer Treat Rep 1981; 65(suppl. 5):121–128.

Osler W. Aequanimitas. Philadelphia, Blakiston's, 1904.

Pearson L. (ed.). Death and Dying. Cleveland, The Press of Case Western Reserve University, 1969.

Saunders C. Living with dying. Man Med 1976; 1:227.

Shike M, Russell DMcR, Detsky AS, et al. Changes in body composition in patients with small-cell lung cancer—The effects of TPN as an adjunct to chemotherapy. Ann Intern Med 1984; 101:303–309.

Shimm DS, Logue GL, Maltie AA, et al. Medical management of chronic cancer pain. JAMA 1979; 241:2408.

Simpson MA. The Facts of Death. Englewood Cliffs, N.J., Prentice-Hall, 1979.

Simpson MA. Planning for terminal care. Lancet 1976; 2:192.

Snow LW. A Death with Dignity: When the Chinese Came. New York, Random House, 1974.

Stedeford A. Couples facing death: II. Unsatisfactory communication. Br Med J 1981; 238:1098.

Stragand JJ, Braunschweiger PG, Pollice AA, et al. Cell kinetic alterations in marine mammary tumors following fasting and refeeding. Eur J Cancer 1979; 15:218–286.

Switzer DK. The Dynamics of Death. New York, Abingdon Press, 1970.

Terepka AR, Waterhouse C. Metabolic observations during forced feedings of patients with cancer. Am J Med 1956; 20:225.

Tolle SW, Elliot DL, Hickam DH. Physician attitudes and practices at the time of patient death. Arch Intern Med 1984; 144:2389–2391.

Tumulty PA. The Effective Clinician. Philadelphia, W. B. Saunders, 1973.

Twycross RG. Principles and practice of pain relief in terminal cancer. In Corr CA (ed.): Hospice Care—Principles and Practice. New York, Springer, 1983.

Twycross RG. The assessment of pain in advanced cancer. J Med Ethics 1978; 4:112.

Twycross RG, Lack SA. Symptoms Control in Far Advanced Cancer: Pain Relief. London, Pitman, 1983.

Veatch RM. Choosing not to prolong dying. Med Dimensions, December 1972.

Volkan V. Typical findings in pathological grief. Psychiatr Q 1970; 44:231.

Walsh TD, Baxter R, Bowman K, et al. High-dose morphine and respiratory function in chronic cancer pain. Pain 1981; 1(Suppl.):39.

Ward A. Telling the patient. J R Coll Gen Pract 1974; 24:465.

Weisman A, Brettell HR. The preterminal and terminal patient. In Rakel RE, Conn H (eds.): Family Practice, 2nd ed. Philadelphia, W. B. Saunders, 1978.

White RB, Gathman LT. The syndrome of ordinary grief. Am Fam Physician 1973; 8:96.

Wong CB, Swazey JP (eds.). Dilemmas of Dying: Policies and Procedures for Decisions Not to Treat. Boston, G. K. Hall, 1981.

Zucker MB, Rothwell KG. Differential influences of salicylate compounds on platelet aggregation and serotonin release. Curr Ther Res 1978; 23:194–199.

QUESTIONS

1. Which of the following are true regarding the use of morphine in a terminally ill patient?
   a. Tolerance develops rapidly.
   b. It causes respiratory depression and should be avoided.
   c. It is effective when given orally.
   d. It can contribute to the drug culture when stolen and should be avoided.

2. Sources of pain in a dying patient are
   a. Anxiety.
   b. Interpersonal problems.
   c. Physical problems.
   d. Nonacceptance.

3. Which of the following are true regarding hospice care?
   a. The patient and the family are the unit of care.
   b. Hospice care is available 24 hours a day, 7 days a week.
   c. Care is provided by an interdisciplinary team.
   d. Care continues after the patient dies.

Answers appear on page 446.

8

HOME CARE

ROBERT E. RAKEL and WARREN L. HOLLEMAN

Home care is playing an increasingly important role in health care delivery as hospital care becomes more oriented toward the care of critically ill patients and third-party payers encourage less expensive care in the home. This is facilitated by advancing technology that makes possible the home care of serious problems that previously required hospitalization. For many patients, home health care is a viable alternative to extended hospital care. It allows the patient to recover in the comfort and security of the home.

Home care has always been an important part of family practice, and although today house calls are made more frequently in other countries, especially Great Britain, home care is experiencing a renaissance in the United States. This rebirth is made possible by more home-specific technology and new types of health care professionals.

Although home care is best suited to the needs of older persons and those with chronic illnesses and AIDS, it can manage a growing number of acute problems and those which have first been stabilized in the hospital. Although the incentive is often cost containment (overall cost of home care is close to half that of hospital care), it is actually more expensive for the family. While home care is more pleasant and comfortable for the patient, it places considerable stress on family members.

Home care is currently one of the most rapidly growing sectors of our health care system, and this will certainly increase as our population ages. The old old (over age 85) are currently the fastest growing segment of the population and by the year 2040 will consume 50% of the long-term care dollars spent on the elderly (Collopy et al).

HOME CARE SERVICES

The services provided by a home health agency include skilled nursing care, physical therapy, occupational therapy, speech therapy, home health aides, social services, respiratory therapy, pharmacy services, durable medical equipment, homemaker assistance, meals-on-wheels, transportation, and shopping assistance.

Most patients will require multiple services and products. Skilled nursing care includes the administration of intravenous and intramuscular injections, the care of drainage tubes and Foley catheters, wound care and dressing changes, ostomy care, and the care of central venous catheters involved in providing total parenteral nutrition (TPN).

TPN is the intravenous infusion of nutrients into a central vein such as the subclavian. It includes all necessary nutrients: carbohydrates, fats, amino acids, vitamins, electrolytes, and minerals. The most common candidates for TPN are patients who have a nonfunctioning gastrointestinal tract caused by obstruction (e.g., cancer) or inflammation, those with pancreatitis requiring a period of bowel rest, and malnourished patients who are under stress from burns, trauma, or sepsis. Infection of the catheter site is a potential problem, and dressings should be changed by a nurse two to three times a week. TPN in the home has the advantage of avoiding the risk of nosocomial infections. In addition, most patients are happier at home and recover more quickly.

Home pain management also can permit terminally ill patients or those suffering from chronic pain to resume a more normal lifestyle (see Chap. 7). This is made possible by portable intravenous patient-controlled analgesia (PCA) pumps and portable subcutaneous infusion (SCI) pumps that give the patient greater mobility and control.

Intravenous antibiotic therapy has allowed many patients who previously required extensive periods of hospitalization to now be cared for in the home. The best candidates are those with bone and joint infections, such as osteomyelitis, or intravascular infections, such as bacterial endocarditis. More than 50% of the patients receiving home intravenous antibiotic therapy have osteomyelitis, septic arthritis, or infected devices (joint prostheses and intravenous catheters). The complication rate is no different at home than in the hospital, and patients appear to recover more rapidly. The physician establishes a treatment plan and supervises the patient's care just as in the hospital. A peripheral long-line catheter (or central line) with a heparin lock is usually needed; regular inspection and dressing changes by a nurse are needed to prevent complications.

The American Medical Association has recognized the need for physicians to be adequately trained to practice effective home care. The following goals are recommended to prepare physicians to manage patients in the home. The physician should

1. Acquire appropriate home care assessment skills.
2. Be able to assess the adequacy of family caregivers and informal care resources.
3. Be able to evaluate the efficacy of home care efforts.
4. Be able to apply home care principles and guidelines appropriately.
5. Know community resources.
6. Be knowledgeable about cost reimbursement policies in home care.
7. Be knowledgeable about home care technology.
8. Be able to integrate home, office, and hospital care for patients.
9. Be a leader of the home care team.

Most home care will be provided by health professionals other than the physician, and although it is a collaborative, team effort, the physician will often be expected to be a knowledgeable team leader.

THE HOUSE CALL

The house call is a powerful statement of the physician's commitment to the patient's well-being and comfort. It does much to counteract claims that medicine has become too remote and impersonal.

Some 2400 years ago, Hippocrates advised the physician to study the patient and his or her environment. Assessment of a patient in the home provides additional insight and improved understanding of the influence that environmental, familial, and social factors play in a patient's health. It is much easier for a physician to evaluate a patient's functional and psychosocial status in the home than in the office. It is also important to monitor the emotional status of the caregivers. Burnout can be a significant problem as a result of the tremendous strain placed on family members who bear the primary burden (80%) of home care. One-third of the family caregivers also work outside the home. The primary caregiver is usually an adult child, followed by spouse, sibling, and other relatives. Most will provide care for 1 to 4 years, and 20% will do so for 5 years or more. The potential for burnout, anger, and guilt are obvious (Collopy et al).

House calls not only enhance rapport between physician and family, they also provide an opportunity to evaluate the home environment, family dynamics, and medications in a way that is not possible in the office. One family physician usually asks to use the bathroom and takes that opportunity to observe the medications in the medicine cabinet.

PROBLEMS TO OVERCOME

One problem with home health care that must be addressed is the frequent lack of communication between the physician and home care nurses and other health professionals. This lack of coordination can result in treatment failures, since many chronically ill patients cared for in the home are perpetually on the brink of a crisis that requires emergency hospital treatment. Too often the physician who should be coordinating the care is outside the communication loop. The visiting nurse, respiratory therapist, meal supplier, and home health aide may all work for different agencies, and none of them has the whole picture or appreciation of the overall plan of the physician.

CASE STUDY
Pamela M. Kircher

Marjorie Brown is a 65-year-old Caucasian woman with chronic obstructive pulmonary disease (COPD) and acute respiratory distress. When she was first seen in the emergency room by the family physician on call, Dr. Jones, she was unable to give much history because of her extreme shortness of breath. Blood studies revealed an elevated white blood cell count, no theophyllin in her system, and profound hypoxemia. After treatment with oxygen, intravenous theophyllin, steroids, antibiotics, and respiratory therapy treatments with albuterol, she became more comfortable and the next day was able to give her history.

Ms. Brown had been living in another state until about 1 month previously. At that time, her daughter visited her when she was hospitalized with pneumonia. It was her third hospitalization in the past year. At the insistence of the doctor and her daughter, she had moved in with her daughter. Because of Marjorie's recent illness, her daughter had disposed of her property and completed her business affairs while she was recuperating from the pneumonia in the hospital. When Marjorie was discharged, she moved directly to her daughter's home. The doctor had given her several prescriptions upon discharge, but in the haste of the move, she had misplaced them.

Upon moving in with her daughter, Marjorie had become quite depressed. She had her own room, but she had none of her own belongings from her previous home. Her daughter worked all day. Marjorie had no transportation, knew no one in the city, and did not feel well enough to get out anyway. When the teenagers, Mark and Bill, got home from school in the afternoon, it seemed as though the phone rang and music blared for the next 9 hours. Marjorie had lived alone for the past 25 years and was having a hard time adjusting to her new life. She did not talk about this with her daughter, however, because she did not wish to appear ungrateful and knew that this was a strain on her daughter too.

Since moving in with her daughter, Marjorie had been taking some of her old medicine, but she was not sure what or how much she had been taking. She used an inhaler when she felt especially short of breath, but otherwise, she did not take medications. Since her move, she had found herself increasingly short of breath. She had essentially stopped eating, except for pieces of candy. She had not stopped smoking, however. She found that as her stress increased, her smoking increased as well. She had begun coughing up yellow mucus 4 days ago. Her experience in the past had been that when she went to the doctor with these symptoms, she was hospitalized, frequently for weeks at a time. She just did not want to start the cycle again, so she ignored the symptoms, except to use her inhaler more often, sometimes every hour, if necessary. On the day of admission, she had been unable to get a breath at all, and it had been necessary to call the paramedics to get her to the emergency room.

On physical examination, Marjorie was markedly short of breath and appeared depressed. Her blood pressure was 100/60, with a heart rate of 120. She was emaciated. Her lungs revealed decreased breath sounds throughout, with rales on the right side. Scattered rhonchi and wheezes were heard throughout. The remainder of the physical examination was unremarkable.

Dr. Jones requested her permission to have a family conference.

The next day Dr. Jones sat down with Mrs. Susan Anderson (Marjorie's daughter), Marjorie, Mr. John Anderson (Susan's husband), and Mark and Bill (Susan and John's teenage sons). The social worker was invited to the meeting to facilitate the discussion. Dr. Jones had discussed the situation with the director of the home care program and had asked her to be present in order to tell the family what kind of help might be available at home upon discharge.

Dr. Jones explained to Marjorie and her family that hospitalizations could be decreased dramatically by careful adherence to a good pulmonary regime between exacerbations. Susan talked about how upset and inadequate she felt that her mother had only become sicker since moving in with her. She had thought that it would be so good to be able to help her mother, but she felt that the move had put a wedge between them. The social worker encouraged everyone in the family to talk about their hopes and frustrations about the situation. For the first time since the move, Marjorie grieved aloud for the loss of her life in the other state. Susan understood this and grieved herself for the childhood memories that had been lost in the sale of the property. Mark and Bill talked about their ambivalence about having Marjorie live with them. They wanted to know their grandmother better. She had been a business executive until last year and had always been too busy to do ordinary grandmother activities. On the other hand, they knew that their high level of energy made their grandmother more nervous and short of breath. John wanted to be helpful but felt lonely and confused in the intense unexpressed emotions that had permeated the house since Marjorie had moved in.

After everyone had been encouraged to openly express their feelings and concerns, there was a much calmer feeling in the group. Marjorie turned to Dr. Jones and asked where they should go from there.

In this more open atmosphere, Dr. Jones suggested that Marjorie participate in the pulmonary rehabilitation program. It could be initiated during the current hospitalization and continued upon discharge. She explained the multifaceted program. The respiratory therapist is a specialist in teaching pursed-lip breathing, the use of respiratory equipment in the home, relaxation techniques to assist in control of shortness of breath, and cupping and clapping maneuvers to alleviate excess mucus production. The nutritionist helps develop a diet that is easily digested but provides adequate nutrition. She also helps create a dietary program that takes into account other medical problems as well as personal preferences. The physical therapist assists with an exercise program. People who develop a sensible program, usually involving primarily walking, have fewer exacerbations. It is important, however, to develop a program that is specific for one's ventilatory capacity. The occupational therapist helps with maintaining the activities of daily living. He or she works with individual tasks to make modifications in them to make them easier. Pacing oneself is also emphasized. Finally, a psychologist is on the team to direct the smoking cessation program and to provide psychologic support for working through the problems associated with having chronic obstructive pulmonary disease. A smoking cessation program involves relaxation techniques. The period just after an exacerbation is an excellent time to begin the program, since oxygen cannot be used in the presence of smoking because of the explosive potential.

Having begun these programs in the hospital, they can be followed up by home health care. The director of home health care explained that a visiting nurse could visit weekly to follow up the various aspects of the pulmonary rehabilitation program. The nurse would discuss the medications and see if there were any side effects. If blood level determinations of medications were required, the nurse could draw these at home. The nurse would encourage the routine use of relaxation techniques with increased frequency during periods of increased shortness of breath and would monitor the nutrition and exercise programs as well and be available for discussions of any problems that arise. When problems were identified, the nurse would call the doctor, who would request that the appropriate team member visit. Respiratory therapy treatments at home frequently prevent trips to the emergency room. Home oxygen can be used on a regular basis or during acute exacerbations. Oxygen concentrators and portable oxygen tanks are both available. Portable oxygen tanks allow a person to leave home and still have oxygen.

Marjorie was pleased to learn about all the areas that she could work on and all the support that was available. She had gained some sense of control over her life again. The rest of the family felt better to have some direction. They all knew that there would be tough times ahead, but it all seemed more manageable with the addition of the home health care team.

THE MEDICAL STUDENT HOME VISIT

Objectives of Home Visits (Table 8–1)

VISITS TO HOMEBOUND PATIENTS. Many patients suffer from impaired mobility, and the most widely recognized purpose of the home visit is to provide a service for these patients, their families, and their caregivers. Elderly patients, patients with debilitating illnesses, severely handicapped patients, and some postoperative patients have difficulty traveling to the doctor's office and might not receive the medical care they need unless physicians visit them in their homes.

In addition to addressing the medical and psychologic needs of the homebound patient, the physician should evaluate the quality of home care being provided by family, friends, and nursing personnel. Adequacy of nursing skills, availability of supplies, atmosphere and layout of the home, compatibility of patients and caregivers, and access to social services all should be scrutinized. Physicians also should address the medical and psychologic needs of the caregivers. Caregivers often lack access to physicians; many are themselves homebound by old age, illness, or the need to stay with the patient. Physicians should look for signs of caregiver stress and should support caregivers through encouragement, advice, education, and training.

Home visits to very elderly, debilitated, or handicapped patients provide medical students the opportu-

---

TABLE 8–1. OBJECTIVES OF THE HOME VISIT

VISITS TO ELDERLY, HOMEBOUND PATIENTS

Medical Objective: To provide a service for patients, family, and caregivers
- Address medical and psychosocial needs of patients
- Evaluate quality of home care
- Address medical and psychosocial needs of family and caregivers

Educational Objective To learn about the mechanics and dynamics of home care
- Learn the economics of geriatric and home care
- Learn how to utilize and coordinate home care services
- Learn about the benefits available through Medicare and third-party insurers
- Learn about the difficulties of negotiating the social services bureaucracies
- Learn about the emotional stresses of living with a serious illness

VISITS TO PATIENTS WHO ARE NOT HOMEBOUND

Medical Objective: To observe patients in the context of their family and living environment
- Identify hidden medical and psychosocial problems
- Detect ways that illness affects the family, and vice versa
- Assess patient's resources for dealing with medical and psychosocial problems

Educational Objective: Recognize the psychological, familial, cultural, and ethical dimensions of illness
- Learn to treat patients in the context of their families, culture, and values

nity not only to render a service to patients and their caregivers, but also to learn about the mechanics and dynamics of home care. On their hospital rotations, many student–clinicians "discharge to home" their patients, unaware of the type of home to which the patient is being discharged, unaware of the economic and family resources necessary to make the transition successful, unaware of the persistence, patience, and savvy necessary to obtain the social services to which one may be entitled, and unaware of the patient's emotional preparation to face these challenges.

Students should view the home visit as an opportunity to study the economics of geriatric care, home care, and long-term care, and they should learn how to utilize and coordinate the various services available to these patients. Students should observe economic barriers, bureaucratic time lags, and other hassles facing elderly and homebound patients. Students should learn the extent to which Medicare, private insurers, and other third-party payers currently reimburse home care services and how to file for them.

Students also should view the home visit as an opportunity to explore the emotional stresses—for patients, family, and caregivers—of living with a terminal or debilitating chronic illness. Students train mostly in hospitals where the atmosphere is not always conducive to conversations about deeply personal and sensitive topics such as disability, dying, death. Many patients—and many physicians, too—feel more comfortable discussing these matters in the relaxed atmosphere of the home. Most students feel uneasy in this area, and home visits provide them with an opportunity to gain experience and skills that will prove useful in future encounters with patients in hospital and clinical settings.

VISITS TO PATIENTS WHO ARE NOT HOMEBOUND. Few would dispute the need to provide medical care for homebound patients in their homes. Less widely established is the need to visit all patients, not merely those homebound, in order to observe them in the context of their family and living environment. Visiting patients in their homes enables physicians to identify and address many medical, psychosocial, and family problems that might otherwise remain hidden during clinic visits. It also enables physicians to assess the patient's resources for addressing these problems and to design strategies for ameliorating them.

Visiting patients in their homes, out of choice and not necessity, is integral to the nature and ideals of family medicine. The many recent innovations in medical technology have not obviated this need. In fact, the need may be greater now than ever.

In the old days and in country practice especially, it was doubtless possible for the doctor to follow the lives of his patients individually as acquaintances, and through many years, to watch the growth and development of families, to know their members as a friend and not merely in a professional capacity. He would meet them as a neighbor, in church, in town meetings, in agricultural fairs, in village sports and holidays. Thus he would touch the lives of his fellow citizens on many sides, and when he came to their aid in his narrower professional capacity he could supplement his diagnostic findings

and his therapeutic resources out of the wealth of knowledge which years of association with them outside the sick-room had furnished him.

RICHARD CABOT, CITED BY YOUNG ET AL.

If these words rang true in 1919, when Richard Cabot penned them, how much more empty today must be the reservoir from which many physicians draw knowledge of their patients. Because of the growth, pace, and transience of urban society, most physicians today have little or no personal knowledge of patients with which to supplement their diagnostic findings and therapeutic resources. This problem is magnified for medical students who train in large medical centers and who rotate constantly from one service to another. The home visit provides an excellent means of compensation.

Many medical schools have shown an increasing interest in training students to recognize the psychologic, familial, cultural, and ethical dimensions of illness. The home visit provides an excellent stage from which to observe these dimensions, and follow-up discussions with supervising faculty and fellow students can illumine, clarify, and connect them. Of particular value is the opportunity to observe the dynamics of family interactions and the family's role in the illness and healing of the patient. The home visit should make the student more aware of the inextricable relation of patient and family, better able to recognize the impact of family function on a patient's well-being, and better able to treat patients in the context of their family environment.

The Value of Longitudinal Visits

Ideally, students should have the opportunity to follow at least one family throughout their 4 years of medical school. In addition to seeing family members in the clinical setting, the students would see the family once per year in their home, under the close supervision of a faculty mentor. Such an approach is commensurate with family medicine's concern for continuous, comprehensive, context-sensitive care. It requires a significant commitment on behalf of the supervising faculty, but the fruits of such labor make the effort worthwhile, both for the students and for family medicine as a discipline. Instead of viewing medicine as the "tuning up" of an organ system or a battle against a disease process, as is the current tendency, students experience an ongoing, healing relationship with patients. Students also learn to care for patients in the context of the family and social environment.

Most medical schools are not prepared at this time to make such an ambitious commitment. Typically, they require only one home visit to an elderly or homebound patient, and typically this is not a patient with whom the student has an ongoing physician–patient relationship. Even though this is not the ideal, such a visit can still achieve many of the objectives outlined above. The following guidelines have been developed with the one-time-only visit in mind, but they must be adapted to each situation. The success of the visit is contingent on thorough preparation and intelligent supervision. It also helps if the medical student has already encountered the patient in the clinical setting. Attention can then be focused on areas that can best be explored in the home setting, and the student is better able to appreciate the particular advantages of the home visit.

Guidelines for Students Doing Home Visits
(Table 8–2)

Phase 1:   Preparation

STEP 1:   SELECT A PATIENT.   The student should contact a family physician or home nursing agency, explain the nature of the home visit assignment (including its emphasis on psychosocial as well as medical concerns), and ask for permission to visit one of their patients. The student should ask the physician or nurse to identify a good candidate and should ask for advice regarding areas to be addressed during the visit. The student also should ask the physician or nurse to identify any sensitive areas for the patient, any potential boundary problems, any dangers or risks of performing the visit, and the names of any relatives or caregivers who ought or ought not to be present during the visit. Finally, the student should ask for permission to visit the patient, to review the chart, and to call for further questions and follow-up.

STEP 2:   SCHEDULE THE VISIT.   Many students feel anxious about calling the patient to schedule a home visit, fearing that the patient will be embarrassed or offended or will misunderstand the student's motives. Experience indicates that most patients are not nearly as intimidated as the students and that the best way to justify the home visit to the patient is by being completely honest about the educational objectives of the visit (Young et al.).

> "Hello. I'm _____, a student at _____ Medical School. As part of my medical school training, I'm required to make a home visit, and Dr./ Nurse _____ suggested your name. I wondered if you would be willing to have me come and interview you at home?"

TABLE 8–2.   GUIDELINES FOR STUDENTS DOING HOME VISITS

PHASE 1:   PREPARATION
Step 1:   Select a patient
Step 2:   Schedule the visit
Step 3:   Review the medical record
Step 4:   Background research
Step 5:   Devise a plan
Step 6:   Consult with supervisor

PHASE 2:   THE VISIT
Step 1:   Pay attention to details
Step 2:   What to look for and ask about
Step 3:   Problem areas

PHASE 3:   POSTVISIT EVALUATION AND FOLLOW-UP
Step 1:   Write a report of the visit
Step 2:   Follow-up consultation with supervisor
Step 3:   Other follow-up consultations

If the patient expresses genuine reservations, which is rare, the student should not press for an affirmative answer. Otherwise, the student should schedule the visit at a time convenient to the patient, family, and caregivers; get good directions to the home; and express appreciation for their willingness to participate in this exercise. Sometimes the patient will not be able to speak on the phone, and the permission must be gained through the caregiver. Even so, it is important to ask for the patient's permission, via the proxy, and the caregiver's as well.

STEP 3:   REVIEW THE MEDICAL RECORD.   It is important to learn as much as possible through reading the patient's medical record; otherwise, much of the home visit will be squandered on superficial introductory discussion. The student should read the record four times. The first reading provides a general overview of the patient's medical history and current illness(es), and the second reading should focus on family history and genogram. The focus of the third reading should be psychosocial issues. These are not always explicit in the medical record but can be detected simply by asking, "What issues might I be dealing with if I had the same illness and life situation as this patient?" During the fourth reading, the student should focus on the areas of concern identified by the physician or nurse in the initial conversation. At this point students should be taking notes, forming questions, and making hypotheses.

STEP 4:   BACKGROUND RESEARCH.   The student may feel woefully inadequate to address the needs of the patient, so time should be set aside for study. Textbook chapters will be useful in providing general information about the illnesses and psychosocial situations confronting the patient. Journal articles should be consulted for the latest research findings. Medical specialists, nurses, social workers, psychologists, medical anthropologists, ethicists, and others can provide additional information and insights as needed.

STEP 5:   DEVISE A PLAN.   Based on the information and impressions gained from the previous steps, it is now time to develop a strategy for achieving the objectives of the visit. One should write a list of questions to be asked of the patient and caregivers and a tentative order in which to do so. One must consider whether to visit alone or with another individual, based on an assessment of the risks and benefits of each option as well as the availability of others. Careful consideration should be given to patients with borderline personality disorders or histories of violence or crime, patients who live in unsafe neighborhoods, and teenage and young-adult patients who might misinterpret the visit as a sexual ploy. The student also should consider the tone and pace appropriate for this home visit. Generally, it is best to be professional but not stiff, respectful but not servile, a good listener but not passive or boring, friendly but not presumptive, caring but not sentimental, and inquisitive but not nosy or voyeuristic.

STEP 6:   CONSULT WITH SUPERVISOR.   In some situations, the patient's physician or nurse will serve as supervisor; in others, a faculty member from the medical school will serve in this capacity. The student and supervisor should (1) review the patient's medical history, psychosocial issues, and family and caregiver situation, (2) discuss initial impressions of the patient and hunches concerning the emotional issues facing the patient, (3) agree on the concerns to be addressed by the visit, (4) evaluate the strategy for approaching these issues, (5) discuss expectations of the visit and attitudes toward the visit, and (6) identify any areas requiring further study or preparation.

Phase 2: The Visit

STEP 1: PAY ATTENTION TO DETAILS. Seemingly minor matters can derail a home visit. Therefore, it is important to pay appropriate attention to details. To avoid getting lost or being late, one should review a map before leaving and should leave in plenty of time to make the appointment. Last-minute preparations should include care in bringing the appropriate medical instruments and supplies, along with notes, pen, and paper. It is also useful to review one's notes and to spend a few minutes visualizing the interview. One should dress professionally.

STEP 2: WHAT TO LOOK FOR AND ASK ABOUT. This will be based on the plan devised in phase 1, but a generally successful approach (see Table 8–3) is to begin with a brief review of the patient's medical history, including not only the history of present illness(es) but also questions regarding pain, diet, sleep, and exercise. This should be followed by an exploration of psychosocial issues, such as the effect of the illness on the patient's emotional well-being; quality and access to support systems; frequency of contact with friends, relatives, and neighbors; social and other activities, and values and religious beliefs. Discussion of the latter is particularly relevant in helping to clarify the patient's wishes concerning aggressiveness of care during the last stage of life. It is also important to obtain a thorough description of the current activities of the patient. One method is to ask the patient to describe a typical day.

Another area to examine is the patient's family. Topics include family medical history and identification of family health risks; household responsibilities of each family member; quality of interpersonal relationships and communications skills within the family; impact of the illness on the family; impact of the family on the illness; economic, cultural, and occupational characteristics of family members; and tobacco, alcohol, and drug use within the family.

When evaluating the living conditions of the patient, special attention should be paid to the cleanliness, comfort, stability, and security of the home. When observing the neighborhood, such factors as safety, stability, and friendliness of neighbors ought to be considered. Other important issues include access to transportation, shopping, recreation, and health services.

It is important to appraise the skill level of the caregivers and to discern the patient's attitude toward the care he or she is receiving from family caregivers and health professionals. Attention should be paid to the medical and psychosocial health of caregivers, whose job can be quite stressful. Students should identify sources of stress and should explore ways to accommodate the needs of caregivers and family members, as well

TABLE 8–3. ITEMS TO BE INCLUDED IN THE HOME VISIT REPORT

BRIEF MEDICAL HISTORY
History of present illness(es)
Pain
Diet
Sleep
Exercise
Interventions and recommendations
Questions

PSYCHOSOCIAL ISSUES
Impact of the illness on emotional well-being
Support systems
Contact with friends and relatives
Social and other activities
Values and religious beliefs
Descriptions of a typical day
Interventions and recommendations
Questions

FAMILY ISSUES
Family medical history (genogram)
Health risks
Household responsibilities
Compatibility of family members
Family communication
Impact of illness on the family
Impact of the family on the illness
Economic, cultural, and occupational characteristics
Use of tobacco, alcohol, and drugs
Interventions and recommendations
Questions

LIVING CONDITIONS
Comfort and safety of home environment
Condition of the home
Privacy of home environment
Pets
Comfort and safety of neighborhood
Access to transportation, health services, and favorite activities
Interventions and recommendations
Questions

QUALITY OF HOME CARE
Skill level of caregivers
Patient's attitude toward caregivers
Caregivers' attitudes toward patient
Medical and psychosocial health of caregivers
Dental care
Preventive measures
Use of folk remedies and alternative healers
Interventions and recommendations
Questions

"COMPLIANCE" QUESTIONS
Is patient following physician's advice?
Why or why not?
Interventions and recommendations
Questions

OTHER ISSUES
Patient's perception of illness
Patient's preferences regarding end-of-life decisions
Interventions and recommendations
Questions

as those of the patient. Caregiver stress is characterized by fatigue, anxiety, depression, and low morale and is one cause of "elder abuse," which occurs in 3% of the population over age 65. Students should note signs of caregiver stress or a history of family violence.

Another aspect of home care that must not be neglected is the tendency of many patients to rely on folk remedies and alternative healers. Physicians and patients often feel nervous discussing this issue. The home visit provides an excellent setting for exploring this subject. The student doing the home visit should encourage openness regarding these practices and coordination of the care between the parties involved.

Particular attention should be paid to the so-called compliance questions: Is the patient following the physician's recommendations regarding exercise, diet, and smoking, and is the patient taking the medications in the manner prescribed? If problems are detected, the student should ask why and then should address misconceptions, motivational problems, differences in values, concerns regarding side effects or costs of medications, and disagreements with the judgment of the physician.

Other areas deserving attention include the patient's perception of the implications of his or her disease and the patient's preferences regarding how aggressively to be treated at the end of life.

STEP 3: PROBLEM AREAS. Two errors commonly committed by students are spending too much time socializing at the beginning of the interview and conducting the interview in an informal, conversational style. Students do this in an effort to "set the patient at ease," but it is usually the student who is uneasy and who procrastinates by engaging in "small talk." Much time is wasted in the process, and sometimes the circumlocution becomes a source of anxiety for the patient. Since many patients do not have the energy for long interviews and most are not offended by—and may prefer—a more formal, efficient interview, and since most medical students are inexperienced at patient interviews in general and home visits in particular, it is generally best to conduct the interview simply by reading the questions straight off the prepared list. The structured approach helps set everyone at ease because it enables one to ask difficult questions without their being taken personally.

It is also important to recognize the special problems created by the fact that the student–clinician is practicing medicine on the patient's home turf. Some physicians feel uncomfortable with the loss of control inherent in this situation, and this is one of the reasons that physicians do not perform home visits as often as they should. What these physicians fail to appreciate are the many therapeutic advantages to being "on the patient's turf" and in a more nonthreatening, egalitarian relation with the patient. Such a situation is conducive to nurturance of the friendship role that physicians should play in addition to the more comfortable roles of healer, teacher, and priest. Such a setting, in which the locus of control shifts toward the patient and in which the atmosphere is generally more familiar and comfortable to the patient, often empowers the patient to truly "tell his or her story" for the first time.

The shifting locus of control can create problems for the student–clinician. Offers of alcoholic refreshments should almost always be refused, but other situations must be evaluated on a case-by-case basis. On occasion, hospitality will be offered with strings subconsciously attached. Sometimes patients will misinterpret motives or misunderstand the student–clinician's role on the health care team. Generally, however, such visits are overwhelmingly successful, both as medical interventions and as educational experiences.

Phase 3: Postvisit Evaluation and Follow-Up

STEP 1: WRITE A REPORT OF THE VISIT. The first part of the report should follow the outline of the interview (see Table 8–3). Every topic should be commented on, but particular attention should be devoted to those areas most pertinent to the patient's ongoing medical care.

The second part of the report consists of a problem list, a summary of the most important findings. In addition to writing a problem list for the patient, the student may wish to write a problem list for the family and other caregivers.

The third part of the report comprises interventions made and interventions recommended. The student should document any advice, education, training, or referrals given during the visit. The student also should indicate further recommendations for interventions by the student, physician, or nurse.

STEP 2: FOLLOW-UP CONSULTATION WITH SUPERVISOR. The purposes of the consultation are to review the report, to discuss the needs of the patient, and to evaluate the effectiveness of the visit. The student should be prepared to discuss how knowledge gained from the visit should be utilized in the management of the patient. The student also should bring to the consultation unanswered questions regarding the patient's condition and any difficulties encountered in the visit. The supervisor may wish to recommend additional reading in these areas of difficulty. The student and supervisor should consider whether the patient would benefit from further consultations with medical specialists, social workers, social services agencies, ministers, or others. The student also should compare his or her initial attitudes toward and expectations of the home visit with postvisit impressions and should consider which goals of the visit were met and why others were not met.

STEP 3: OTHER FOLLOW-UP CONSULTATIONS. If the supervisor is not involved in the ongoing care of the patient, the student should report major findings, interventions, and recommendations to the patient's physician or nurse. If it is agreed that the patient would benefit from further consultations or the involvement of social service agencies or other third parties, the student should make those arrangements. Finally, the student should be given the opportunity to discuss the visit with his or her classmates. This amplifies the educational value of the visit and enhances student appreciation of the home visit as an important means of patient care.

Housecalls*

Some would call it work,
this drive through the countryside
on a Sunday afternoon

       to visit friends.

---

*From Dimensions. J Fam Pract 1991; 32:535. (Reprinted with permission.)

The mud season of early spring
is here. Tufts of green grass and
robins poking amid the brown.
Johnny Paycheck on the radio ironically singing
"Take this job and shove it."

Of course, the friends are all sick, bent and
crippled. One with a stroke, one with liver failure,
one with arthritis and old age. They have run out of
springs—almost. But they are still friends—each with
a spark and a smile.

They complain a lot: about dizziness, fatigue,
joints that don't work, limbs that don't work,
bowels that don't work.

We both know I am impotent . . . no match for the
problems at hand. What counts is I am here.
We are here—together.

Like doctors in olden days, before antibiotics.

PAUL S. FRAME, M.D.

REFERENCES

American Academy of Family Physicians, Society of Teachers of Family Medicine, and American Geriatrics Society. Recommended Core Curriculum Guidelines on Aging and Care of the Aged for Family Practice Residents (AAFP Reprint No. 264). Kansas City, Mo., American Academy of Family Physicians, 1987.

Collopy B, Dubler N, Zuckerman C. The ethics of home care: Autonomy and accommodation. Hastings Center Report 1990; 20 (Suppl):1–16.

Frame PS. Dimensions "Housecalls." J Fam Pract 1991; 32:535.

Gjerdingen DK, Fontaine P. Family-centered postpartum care. Fam Med 1991; 23:189–193.

Huston PG. Family care of the elderly and caregiver stress. Am Fam Physician 1990; 42:671–676.

Knight AL, Adelman AM, Sobal J. The house call in residency training and its relationship to future practice. Fam Med 1991; 23:57–59.

Neale AV, Hodgkins BJ, Demers RY. The home visit in resident education: Program description and evaluation. Fam Med 1992; 24:36–40.

Rakel RE (ed.). Textbook of Family Practice, 4th ed. Philadelphia, W.B. Saunders, 1990.

Sadovsky R, Brecher D. Structuring a home visit program for residents. Fam Med 1986; 18:361–362.

Spiegel AD. Home Health Care, 2nd ed. Owings Mills, Md., National Health Publishing, 1987.

Warburton SW, Sadler GR. House call training in the family practice curriculum. J Med Ed 1977; 52:768–770.

Young R, Freiberg E, Stringham P. The home visit in the multidisciplinary teaching of primary care physicians. J Med Ed 1981; 56:341–346.

QUESTIONS

1. Total parenteral nutrition (TPN) includes the IV infusion of
   a. Minerals.
   b. Fats.
   c. Amino acids.
   d. Carbohydrates.
   e. Vitamins.

2. Physicians managing patients in the home should
   a. Assess the adequacy of the family members to provide care.
   b. Know community resources.
   c. Have hospital privileges in the ICU.
   d. Be a leader of the health care team.
   e. Know each of the caregivers by name.

3. Which of the following are true regarding caregivers of homebound patients?
   a. The primary caregiver is usually an adult child.
   b. Most primary caregivers provide care for 5 or more years.
   c. Family members provide 40% to 50% of the home care.
   d. One-third of primary caregivers work outside the home.
   e. Burnout is a rare problem.

4. Home visits enable the medical student to
   a. Evaluate the quality of home care provided by family, friends, and nursing personnel.
   b. Learn about the economics of geriatric care and home care.
   c. Explore the emotional stresses of living with a debilitating illness.
   d. Observe how family function affects medical and emotional well-being.

5. The most important indicators of "elder abuse" are
   a. A reliance on folk remedies or alternative healers.
   b. A failure to take prescribed medications.
   c. A history of family violence.
   d. Caregiver stress.

Answers appear on page 446.

9

DEVELOPING COMMUNICATION SKILLS

ROBERT E. RAKEL

Effective communication between doctor and patient is essential to good medical care. It serves as the basis for rapport, understanding, confidence, and patient compliance. The interview, our most powerful tool, strengthens our alliance with the patient by convincing him or her that we understand the patient's feelings and will do our utmost to help. It is this capacity for understanding another person's feelings that serves as the foundation of the doctor–patient relationship.

Poor communication, on the other hand, is the most common cause of malpractice suits. When there is good rapport, the physician is less likely to get defensive and withdraw if there is a problem, and will be able to discuss a bad outcome in a nondefensive manner. An explanation is much more effective in building and maintaining patient rapport than is an apology. A patient is less likely to consider a physician negligent if he or she feels the physician is not trying to hide something. A reluctance to communicate openly can be interpreted as an attempt to cover up something.

Effective communication depends much more on one's ability to be a good listener than on what one says to a patient. Most physicians mistakenly feel they listen more than is actually the case when recordings are made of their patient interviews. Epictetus said 2000 years ago, "We have two ears and one mouth and should use them in that proportion" and Will Rogers said, "Be a good listener because you never learn much from talking."

Compassion, interest, and thoroughness are essential components of successful patient care. These features have been traditionally embodied in the term "bedside manner," which also connotes qualities of concern, kindness, friendliness, wit, and cheerfulness, all of which result in an atmosphere of trust and confidence between physician and patient. The physician with the best bedside manner may actually be the one who makes no special effort to communicate these feelings but simply acts in a concerned, natural, and comfortable manner.

Since the health care relationship involves trust and a certain degree of control over another person, the provider must be skilled and effective in the requisite technical services. Charm, a warm bedside manner, or a pleasant personality, in the absence of skill, sound judgment, and knowledge, is hollow. On the other hand, competence of the highest level, in the absence of rapport, results in less than optimal clinical outcome.

A good first impression is a great help in establishing rapport. The physician should approach the patient in an assured, confident (but not cocky or arrogant) manner, and present a personal appearance that is acceptable to the patient. Patients consider house staff who wear white coats with conventional street clothes as more competent than those who wear scrub suits. Negative attitudes toward physicians are associated with casual clothing (such as blue jeans, athletic shoes, and clogs), with overly feminine items such as prominent ruffles and dangling earrings, and with temporarily fashionable items (such as long hair on men, male earrings, and patterned hose on women) (Gjerdingen et al.).

A genuine smile can be helpful in quickly establishing a friendly atmosphere and developing a warm interpersonal relationship. A grin can be the physician's most effective weapon for breaking down resistance or apprehension in patients, especially children or young adults. Posture is also important in conveying an image of confidence and competence. Standing erect, moving briskly with head up and stomach in, is better than slouching. Energetic people seldom slump; they sit upright and appear alert. A listless or lethargic appearance can be interpreted as lack of concern.

Before entering the examining room or hospital room to see a patient, review the chart briefly and become familiar with the patient's name and its proper pronunciation. If the pronunciation is either unusual or difficult, place phonetic markings on the chart as a reminder for future use. Review the chart also for particular aspects of the previous visit that should be remembered and commented upon, such as the illness treated at that time, family conditions, or other personal problems. Patients will feel that the well-informed physician is truly interested in them. Additional courtesy, such as opening the door and assisting patients with their coats, especially an elderly patient, shows a consideration that aids in establishing and maintaining rapport.

RESPECT

The greatest deterrent to establishing patient rapport is an attitude of indifference or lack of interest by the physician. Patients should feel that their comments are being listened to, carefully considered, and taken seriously. They must feel that the physician values their comments and opinions before trusting him or her with information of a more personal nature. As long as the physician's attitude toward the patient embodies respect, concern, and kindness and a sincere effort is made to understand the patient's difficulties, the patient will overlook or forgive a myriad of other problems.

Oliver Wendell Holmes advised patients to

choose a man who is personally agreeable, for a daily visit from a intelligent, amiable, pleasant, sympathetic person will cost you no more than one from a sloven or a boor, and his presence will do more for you than any prescription the other will order.

Ideally, there will be a bond of mutual respect between physician and patient. A physician can show respect for patients, and accept their respect, only insofar as respect is an integral part of his or her personality. There must be a concept of self-respect before one can respect others. When one is secure and satisfied with one's self, one is then able to relate comfortably with warmth and feeling to another person.

It may be that it is the lack of this security rather than an excess of it that leads physicians to appear aloof and unconcerned. Too often physicians feel that a godlike image of omnipotence is necessary for the maintenance of patient respect and confidence. It is usually a lack of self-confidence that causes physicians to retreat behind this protective image, which in turn limits their ability to help. Secure physicians are more free to establish close personal relationships with patients without fearing their position will be threatened. A physician with a positive self-image is also willing to recognize and admit the limits of personal competence and feels comfortable seeking help from a colleague when such consultation is of value to the patient's care.

The bond of mutual respect is enhanced if the physician makes positive statements about other people. Patients find it difficult to respect a physician who is regularly detractive, making negative statements about other people or other physicians. Any comments that can be interpreted as "building yourself up by tearing someone else down" merely accomplish the reverse.

The effectiveness of physicians depends upon the degree of their insight into the limitations of their personalities and the psychologic defenses that distort their perceptions of patients. Physicians must recognize those situations or patients that make them unreasonably angry or provoked (for example, a whining, complaining individual who shows no interest in being rehabilitated, preferring a role of social dependency). Obviously, the physician's emotions, if they go unrecognized, can serve as a barrier to the development of mutual respect. If the physician is aware of negative feelings toward a patient, an effort can be made to avoid showing signs of irritation or anger. It has been said that clenching of the physician's fist is a clinical sign of the hysterical patient. The physician should attempt to remain objective and analyze the situation for its diagnostic value.

DEVELOPING COMMUNICATION SKILLS

Even the most knowledgeable and skilled physician will have limited effectiveness if unable to develop rapport with patients. Rapport is not easily analyzed within any one body of knowledge. Yet it is fair to say that the basis of rapport is the development of communication skills that instill in patients a sense of confidence and trust by conveying sincerity and an interest in their care and well-being. The patient's satisfaction and compliance with the physician's instructions (both measures of rapport, so to speak) depend upon the ability of the physician to communicate understanding, compassion, and genuine interest in the patient and to display a thorough approach to solving the patient's problems. Patient satisfaction is also related to the physician's talent for educating patients regarding the disease process and for motivating them to participate in their treatment.

A common error of communication is to assume that patients are not interested in knowing more than we have told them, especially if they are among the poorly educated. Although patients with less education ask fewer questions, it is not true that they have less desire for information. There is no difference in the desire for information between poorly educated, lower-class patients and better-educated, upper-class patients (Waitzkin).

Patients want to be knowledgeable about their medical care but are not so interested in being responsible for making medical decisions. They prefer to leave the decision making in the hands of their physician. The paradox is that patients almost always want more information, but physicians do not recognize this because patients usually do not express this desire openly (Beisecker and Beisecker).

The majority of complaints against physicians—and those that all too frequently lead to legal action—are simply the result of a lack of communication between doctor and patient. The potential for a serious problem always exists when a patient is inadequately informed regarding a diagnostic procedure, treatment, prognosis, or anticipated cost. The misunderstandings that result cause a great deal of unnecessary expense and grief for both parties.

Similarly, the worries that result from distorted information can severely jeopardize the doctor–patient relationship. When a patient is discussed on hospital rounds or with a colleague in the office, take care that the discussion is not within the patient's hearing distance or within that of other patients. Another patient, overhearing the conversation, may believe that the comments apply to him, or he may know the patient involved and relay the information in a distorted manner. Fragments of such conversations, overheard by the patient or others, are too easily taken out of context and can become the focus of fearful fantasies that only serve to increase uneasiness and apprehension.

Failure of communication between physician and patient can also affect the outcome of treatment, often as seriously as can an error in treatment. More complaints against physicians result from a breakdown of the caring aspect of the doctor–patient relationship than from the technical quality of treatment.

Unfortunately, there are no criteria for the establishment of rapport, as there are criteria for the diagnosis of this or that disease. Each physician must develop his or her own unique style.

Establishing an open channel is the first element of the communication process and influences all that follows. In the clinical setting, the channel is the face-to-face conversation of patient and clinician in the interview or examination; the telephone is an important secondary channel.

Establishing communication means that the patient can gain access to the clinician—on the phone or by an early appointment—without having to run an obstacle course created by an overly protective staff. Delay in returning a phone call may result in a patient remaining home all day waiting; if the call is not returned at all, the negative effect on rapport is great.

Unwillingness to make communication convenient for the patient usually results in a spiral of increasingly frequent attempts to reach the physician and mounting frustration for everyone. On the other hand, physicians who give a high priority to communicating discover that most patients are considerate and even protective of the physician's time. At the beginning of a practice, a certain amount of testing is done by patients to determine how accessible a physician is; those who pass the test find that they are rarely inconvenienced by unnecessary calls or visits.

In any face-to-face encounter, communication is both intended and unintended, and the distinction is important. *Intended* messages are verbal statements that transmit fact and nonverbal messages that the sender hopes will elicit predictable responses from the receiver. One patient, for example, may enact by a sophisticated blend of verbal and nonverbal communications the role of "strong, brave, unafraid, and willing to face reality." Another patient (or, indeed, the same patient in another setting) may communicate verbally and nonverbally a message of "weak, helpless, needing support and sympathy." Such a performance is not the result of a well-thought-out, conscious decision; it results mostly from learned processes that are unconscious but accessible to scientific analysis.

Unintended communication refers to messages that are given off by individuals beyond their awareness. Subtle clues are, however, perceptible to the astute ob-

server. The patient who wishes to create an impression of bravery, for example, may contradict the intended message by a slight hand tremor, a barely noticeable weakness of the voice, or beads of perspiration on the forehead. In clinical practice, the recognition of the patient's true thoughts and feelings is a central skill in establishing and maintaining rapport.

Verbal Communication

Much of the communication process in the clinical interview centers on verbal interchange. Symptoms, past medical history, family medical history, and psychosocial data are transmitted primarily by verbal means. Some aspects of verbal communication play an important role in establishing and maintaining rapport. Slips of the tongue or major areas of omission (for example, a married person who never mentions a spouse) may signify problem areas that, when explored, help establish the interviewer as a perceptive person who understands what lies beneath the surface. The interviewer must constantly consider: Why is the patient telling me that? Even simple, casual remarks may be the patient's way of sending up a trial balloon about issues of great concern—for example, the patient who says, "Oh, by the way, a friend of mine has been having some chest pain when he walks upstairs—do you think that sounds serious?" may be actually talking about a concern of his own that he is unable to face directly. Or, a child may be brought to the office with a trivial problem in order that the mother might have a chance to discuss with the physician something that is troubling her; the child is a calling card, signaling the need to open the communication channel. The physician who is sensitive to these subtle clues and encourages the patient to discuss what is actually troublesome will find that the rapport thus established allows future interviews to be much more open and direct.

Physicians in practice who have established rapport during an ongoing relationship with patients communicate more easily than do physicians seeing a patient for the first time in an emergency department. Studies by Korsch and Negrete showed that doctors in an emergency room did more talking than the patients, although their perception was just the opposite. This was attributed to interaction with unfamiliar patients by house staff in a setting in which the stress level is high and the orientation therapeutic.

Vocabulary

The use of appropriate vocabulary assists in establishing rapport by ensuring easy and accurate communication. Phrasing questions in simple language appropriate to the patient's level of understanding and avoidance of medical jargon help establish a sense of working together. The patient's cultural background and educational level should be considered, and the physician should avoid using slang (or a contrived accent), since the patient will detect the artificiality and consider this patronizing. However, a language style can easily be assumed that is different from the physician's normal speech yet natural and comfortable for both physician and patient (see Mirroring).

Medical terminology should be avoided unless it is familiar to the patient. No longer does the physician gain a therapeutic advantage by writing prescriptions in Latin or impressing the patient with medical words. Today's patients prefer to be enlightened and demand maximum insight into their care. It is best to start all explanations at a basic level and proceed only as rapidly as patient understanding permits.

Physicians should also be sure of what patients mean to convey by their word selection and make certain that they are operating at a common level of understanding. When the patient says he "drinks a little," inquire further to find out what is meant by a little; or if he "spits up blood," determine whether he is truly spitting or vomiting. A major barrier to accurate interpersonal communication is the tendency of people to react to a statement from their own points of view, rather than attempting to interpret it from the speaker's vantage point. If a question exists regarding the clarity of the interpretation, it is best to repeat it to the speaker's satisfaction. Contract negotiators have found that when parties in a dispute realize that they are being understood and each party sees how the situation appears to the other, there is less need to exaggerate and act defensively.

Korsch and Negrete found that some of the longest interviews between physician and patient were due to failures in communication; the doctor and patient had to spend considerable time trying to get on the same wavelength. An analysis of the conversations revealed that less than 5% of the physician's conversation was personal or friendly in nature and that although most of the physicians believed that they had been friendly, fewer than half of the patients had this impression. The following partial transcript of an interview from Korsch and Negrete is a vivid illustration of failure to communicate because of inappropriate vocabulary and lack of attention to patient understanding.

Father: How does his heart sound?

Doctor: Sounds pretty good. He's got a little murmur there. I'm not sure what it is. It's . . . it uh . . . could just be a little hole in his heart.

Mother: Is that very dangerous when you have a hole in your heart?

Doctor: No, because I think it's the upper chamber, and if it's the upper chamber then it means nothing.

Mother: Oh.

Doctor: Otherwise they just grow up and they repair them.

Mother: What would cause the hole in his heart?

Doctor: H'm?

Mother: What was it that caused the hole in his heart?

Doctor: It's 'cause . . . uh . . . just developmental, when their uh . . .

Mother: M-h'm.

Doctor: There's a little membrane that comes down, and if it's the upper chamber, there's a membrane that comes down, one from each direction. And sometimes they don't quite meet, and so there's either a hole at the top or a hole at the bottom and then . . . it's really . . . uh . . . almost never causes any trouble.

Mother: Oh.

Doctor: It's uh . . . one thing that they never get SBE from . . . it's the only heart lesion in which they don't.

Mother: Uh-huh.

Doctor: And uh . . . they grow up to be normal.

Mother: Oh, good.

Doctor: And uh . . . if anything happens they can always catheterize them and make sure that's what it is, or do heart surgery.

Mother: Yeah.

Doctor: Really no problem with it. They almost never get into trouble so . . .

Mother: Do you think he might have developed the murmur being that my husband and I both have a murmur?

Doctor: No.

Mother: No. Oh, it's not hereditary, then?

Doctor: No.

Mother: Oh, I see. (Someone whistling in the room)

Doctor: It is true that certain people . . . tendency to rheumatic fever, for instance.

Mother: H'mm.

Doctor: There is a tendency for the abnormal antigen–antibody reaction to be inherited, and therefore they can sometimes be more susceptible.

Mother: Oh, I see. That wouldn't mean anything if uh . . . I would . . . I'm Rh negative and he's positive. It wouldn't mean anything in that line, would it?

Doctor: Uh-huh.

Mother: No? Okay.

Doctor: No. The only thing you have to worry about is other babies.

Mother: M'h'm.

Doctor: Watch your Coombs' and things.

Mother: Watch my what?

Doctor: Watch your Coombs' and things.

Mother: Oh, yeah.

Doctor: Your titers, Coombs' titers.

Nonverbal Communication

Verbal communication occupies so much of daily social interaction that nonverbal communication is often ignored. However, much that is said is unspoken. Communication specialists have convincingly demonstrated the major importance nonverbal messages have in validating or contradicting verbal messages, and their enormous influence as communication symbols in their own right.

Communication between two people is usually one-third nonverbal. What is said verbally is often emphasized nonverbally, and personal attitudes and emotions are usually communicated at the nonverbal level. Since nonverbal communicative signals are under less censorship from conscious control than are verbal messages, they are likely to be more genuine.

Charles Darwin held that there is a unique pattern of nonverbal actions for each emotion. In *The Expression of the Emotions in Man and Animals* Darwin suggested that emotional expressions are evolutionary remnants of previous adaptive behavior that persist even though currently useless. Snarling as a sign of aggression is one example.

Paralanguage

Paralanguage is the voice effect that accompanies or modifies talking and often communicates meaning. It includes velocity of speech (fast, slow, hesitant), tone and volume of voice, sighs and grunts, pauses, and inflections. Urgency, sincerity, confidence, hesitation, thoughtfulness, gaiety, sadness, and apprehension are all conveyed by qualities of voice. McCaskey believes that the literal interpretation (definition) of words accounts for only 10% of communication between two people, while facial expression and tone of voice account for up to 90% of the communication.

Certainly there is a real difference between verbal and vocal information. The verbal message refers to the words literally transmitted. The vocal message includes the emotional quality, the tone of voice, and the frequency and length of pauses—information that is lost when the words are written. Tone of voice, for example, can actually reverse the meaning of words. Comparative studies have shown that when the vocal and verbal messages transmit contradictory information, the vocal is more accurate. Sarcasm is a common example of a contradiction between vocal and verbal messages.

Physicians should be alert to subtle changes of tone, such as when patients ask whether everything will be all right. Are they asking for reassurance, showing fear, or doubting the diagnosis? Rather than concentrate exclusively on *what* patients are saying, the astute physician will concentrate on *how* they are saying it.

Touch

A close personal interest in the patient can be communicated by the appropriate use of touch. The most socially acceptable method in this country is a handshake, enabling the physician to establish early contact with the patient. The handshake, properly used, can convey to the patient sincerity and interest as well as security and poise. It is an inoffensive intrusion into the other person's area of privacy and can be extended under certain circumstances to include the application of the left hand to the upper or lower arm. This technique is often used by politicians to emphasize sincerity and concern.

The handshake as a traditional greeting of friendship began by the raising of exposed hands by two approaching individuals to give evidence that they held no weapons. This proceeded to the grasping of hands, or in Roman society, the forearms. In the United States, a firm handshake is most acceptable. Usually, the limp or "wet dishrag" handshake indicates lack of interest or insincerity, especially if it is rapidly withdrawn. A moist palm is a sign of nervousness or apprehension, and the "halfway-there," fingers-only handshake indicates reluctance or indecision. But the handshake continues to be culturally modified, and one should be extremely wary of misinterpreting another person's handshake without understanding his or her cultural background.

In China, the Confucian code of etiquette dictated that there should never be a touching of persons, and even today Chinese officials may appear reluctant to grasp an extended hand (a Chinese formerly shook his own hand) (Butterfield).

Touching can be an effective method for communicating concern or compassion and can break down some of the defensive barriers to communication. Caution should be exercised, however, not to use it excessively or earlier than is socially permissible. If used without adequate preparation, touch can be interpreted as an invasion of privacy and a forward and inconsiderate act. Touch by a physician can be viewed as aggressive behavior if it is used before rapport is established. During the physical examination, it is best to talk before touching by explaining to the patient what will be done next. Studies of primates have shown that touching gestures are usually considered nonaggressive and calming in nature. When used properly by the physician, touch can be facilitative and welcome.

The tremendous symbolic value of touch as a healing power was demonstrated during the Middle Ages when people sought relief from scrofula (tuberculous lymphadenitis) through the King's touch, or royal touch, in spite of the notoriously low cure rates. This power has been transferred to physicians, and patients often feel better after a routine physical examination. Friedman states that 85% of patients leaving a physician's office feel better even if they have not received medication or treatment, and 50% of patients in the waiting room feel better in anticipation of the help they will receive.

Touch, or laying on of the hands, may indeed promote healing, especially if it is imbued by the patient with a special symbolic value. Franz Mesmer (1734–1815) was among the first to emphasize the medical importance of "laying on of the hands." Mesmer, however, believed that there was a magnetic power in his hands, which he called animal magnetism and which he applied to ailing individuals. His theory was unscientific, and although he became famous for successfully treating a number of hysterical patients, he was finally discredited by a committee that included Benjamin Franklin and Antoine Lavoisier. They found his treatments to be without magnetism and essentially useless. They did agree, however, that he had helped many people and had brought about many cures. They attributed these cures to as yet unknown factors rather than to the animal magnetism he claimed. Incidentally, mesmerism was the forerunner of hypnosis (initially called artificial somnambulism), which was developed by Puysegur, a disciple of Mesmer.

The magic of touch can be good medicine, especially when combined with concern, support, and reassurance. Stroking, a special kind of touching, describes a physical or symbolic recognition of a person's finer attributes. A stroke may be a kind word, a warm gesture, or a simple touch of the hand. Infants deprived of touch and stroking suffer mental and physical deterioration. Adults also require stroking to maintain a healthy emotional state. Stroking occurs whenever an interchange between two people leaves one or both with a good, or fulfilled, feeling.

Body Language

The astute physician will cultivate observational skills that enable the detection of hidden or subtle clues to diagnosis contained in the patient's nonverbal behavior. It is essential to remember that specific gestures and their interpretation are of importance only when judged in the context of the circumstances surrounding them. Body language alone does not reveal the entire behavioral image any more than does verbal language alone. Just as one word does not make a sentence or even have much meaning without the sentence, a single gesture has clinical relevance only as part of a sequence of actions. Although individual signs have significance, they are not reliable when they stand alone; they are meaningful only when considered in the context of a person's total behavioral pattern.

A clue that there is "more going on than meets the eye" is a mismatch between the verbal and nonverbal messages called *cognitive dissonance*. The physician is given information that just does not "add up." For example, a patient may respond that everything is fine at home while at the same time rubbing his nose and looking down and away. When such cognitive dissonance occurs, it means something "doesn't fit," and an attempt should be made to determine which portion of the message was incorrect. In this illustration, as is usually the case, the nonverbal is more likely to be correct than the verbal.

Attempts by the patient to mask feelings can be readily detected by observing body behavior. True feelings are more likely to leak through conscious efforts to conceal one's feelings. Likewise, a physician's attempt at deception will be detected by patients and can destroy confidence and damage rapport. Positive verbal communication such as "You're looking better today" when accompanied by negative nonverbal cues will be interpreted by the patient as insincere. For example, a patient who is not told the true nature of a terminal illness usually knows it anyway and may distrust family, friends, and physician if they persist in the charade.

Reassuring a patient that "nothing is wrong," rather than putting the patient at ease because the physician found nothing abnormal, may instead be interpreted as "the doctor is unable to make me better." Premature reassurance may be interpreted as rejection. If reassurance is used, it must be genuine and realistic and given only after a thorough evaluation of the problem.

Alan Alda, in a medical school commencement address, challenged new physicians to learn to read patients' involuntary muscles as well as their x-ray studies. He said, "Can you see the fear and uncertainty in my face? If I tell you where it hurts, can you hear in my voice where I ache? I show you my body, but I bring you my person. Will you tell me what you are doing and in words I can understand? Will you tell me when you don't know what to do?" The physician will see the fear and uncertainty in the patient's face only if he or she is looking at the patient rather than the medical record. Alda's statement reflects the concern and compassion that patients desire. By using appropriate body language, the physician can convey this attention and concern in the most effective manner possible.

BODY POSITION. The body position when sitting can show varying degrees of tension or relaxation. The tense person sits erect with a fairly rigid posture. One who is moderately relaxed has a forward lean of approximately 20 degrees and a side lean of up to 10 degrees. A very relaxed position (usually too relaxed for physicians interacting with patients) is a backward lean (recline) of 20 degrees and a sideways lean of over 10 degrees.

Higher patient satisfaction is associated with forward body lean and rotation of the torso toward the patient. Larsen and Smith found that "the patient also responds more favorably to the physician who relaxes his chin in his hands and gazes directly at the patient, rather than a physician who elevates his chin (unsupported) as if to imply a more superior status." Physicians whose communication styles have been considered patient-oriented have been noted to change body position more frequently than physicians whose conversations were physician-centered.

An attempt should be made, whenever possible, to sit rather than stand when interviewing a patient. Rapport is improved if the physician does not intimidate patients by placing them in a submissive position. Patients feel more comfortable, and less helpless, speaking in a sitting position rather than prone. Sitting on the patient's bed has been frowned upon, but for some patients it is an effective means of establishing closeness and conveying warmth in a relaxed yet attentive manner.

MIRRORING. When good rapport exists between two people, each will mirror the other's movements. Some people consciously try to establish rapport with another by mirroring that person's body posture. Disruptions in this mirroring may signal that one member disagrees with what the other has said or feels betrayed or insulted but cannot express this verbally. If the physician notices this sudden disruption of mirroring activity by the patient, more attention should be focused on the comment that led to the change of position. Renegotiation or further explanation may be indicated.

Another subtle yet effective way to use mirroring to establish rapport is to compliment the person by following his or her actions. The patient feels secure and reassured as you reflect what is comfortable and familiar to him or her. The outstanding family therapist Virginia Satir would breathe along with the person, assume a similar body position, and use the person's preferred words.

People usually prefer to think and speak in one of three sensory-based categories: visual, auditory, or kinesthetic. This is reflected in the verbs they use. Those who are auditory oriented will use "listen" or "hear" frequently; if visually oriented they will use "see," "observe," or "recognize"; and if kinesthetic they will use "feel" or "turn."

Patients who feel the physician is "in sync" with them and understands how they feel are less likely to be defensive and will be less anxious.

NEUROLINGUISTIC PROGRAMMING. The use of verbs described above is an effective way to build rapport because it matches the representational system being used by the speaker. Another way to identify a person's favorite representational system is to observe his or her "eye-accessing cues," the direction of gaze. The direction a person is looking has been shown by Bandler and Grinder to correlate with thinking process. The basis of neurolinguistic programming (NLP) is that one's eyes move differently when remembering than when creating. Most right-handed people look up to the right when creating a visual image and up to the left when recalling something visual. Similarly, when someone is listening to a conversation or recalling sounds or words, the eyes will usually move from side to side, as when someone is on the telephone. When thinking about experiences or feelings, gaze is likely to be down toward the dominant hand.

The validity of NLP is currently being debated and further research is needed. Many times no eye movements are detectable, and when they do occur they may not consistently reflect the above. Although most studies do show that upward eye movements accompany attempts to recall visual information, these movements, as with all forms of body language, should be considered clues, not pathognomonic signs.

HEAD POSITION. Typically, the head is held forward in anger and back in defiance, anxiety, or fear. It is down or bowed in sadness, submissiveness, shame, or guilt. The head tilted to one side indicates interest and attention, and when circumstances are appropriate, it can be a flirtation. The head erect indicates self-confidence and maturity.

When listening to a patient, the physician should show interest and concern by an attentive position—best illustrated by sitting forward in the chair with an interested, attentive facial expression and the head slightly tilted. Darwin was one of the first to note that animals assume a head tilt when listening intently.

FACE. Darwin proposed that cultures throughout the world express similar emotions or states of mind with remarkably uniform body movements. His information was gathered from missionary friends working with aborigines, persons under hypnosis, infants, and the insane. He also studied the blind and deaf, who, without benefit of learning from others, were noted to raise their eyebrows when surprised and shrug their shoulders to indicate helplessness.

Darwin held that the facial expression of emotion when undisguised is independent of culture and is identical throughout the world. Thus, the facial expressions of joy, sadness, and anger are the same in the Australian aborigine, the American farmer, and the Norwegian fisherman. Various cultures, however, do disguise the facial expression in different ways. In the American culture, the mouth is most commonly used to disguise feelings. A person in a social gathering may be smiling, although inwardly sad or angry. The eyebrows, eyes, and forehead are least affected by these cultural disguises and are the most consistently dependable indicators of emotion. As Shakespeare wrote, "I saw his heart in his face" (The Winter's Tale, Act I, Scene II).

Ekman and Friesen found that the facial expressions of fear, disgust, happiness, and anger were the same in countries with widely disparate language and culture. They also found that these expressions involve both sides of the face, but contempt involves only one side, such as tightening one corner of the mouth.

Ekman and Friesen used composite facial photographs to show how each part of the face contributes to the expressions of emotion, especially surprise, fear, disgust, anger, happiness, and sadness.

In our culture when people wish to disguise their true feelings and convey an impression that is more socially acceptable, they do so by smiling. This may be especially true in patients who are sad or depressed.

Formerly, infants were thought to be unable to imitate facial gestures until 8 months of age. Meltzoff and Moore showed that infants 2 to 3 weeks old were able to do this.

MICRO-EXPRESSIONS. Ekman and Friesen also described micro-expressions, a valuable indication of masking or deception. "Micro-expressions are caused by the face's all too rapid efficiency in registering inner feelings" (Morris). Most facial expressions last more than 1 second, but micro-expressions last only one-fifth to one-twenty-fifth of a second. This is approximately the time it takes to blink an eye and can easily be missed if the physician is not carefully observing the patient. Micro-expressions occur when the patient begins to show a true facial expression, senses this, and immediately neutralizes or masks the expression. Some micro-expressions are complete enough to show the true emotion felt, but many times they are squelched to such extent that the physician has only a clue that patients are managing their facial expressions.

EYES. The eyes are probably the principal organs of expression. They are so important to a person's appearance that when anonymity is desired, only the eyes need to be covered. The eyebrows have been shown to have 40 different positions of expression and the eyelids 23. Consider the magnitude of possible combinations when all facial elements are involved as indicators of expression. The message conveyed by each position can be further modified by the length of a glance and its intensity.

The eyes can give more information for some emotions than others. Knapp found that the eyes were better than the brow, forehead, or lower face for the accurate portrayal of fear but were less accurate for anger and disgust.

It has long been known that *pupils* dilate when the person sees something pleasant and contract when he or she sees something unpleasant. This involuntary signal can be a valuable indication of what is really going on. Oriental jade dealers wore dark glasses so that no one could see their pupils dilate when they discovered an especially valuable piece of jade. Likewise, a magician doing card tricks can tell when a preselected card is seen by a subject because of the sudden pupil enlargement. In one experiment (Hess), the pupils of heterosexual males dilated when the men were shown photographs of nude females and constricted for nude males. Homosexual men demonstrated the opposite. Baby pictures produced pupil dilation in both single and married women and in married men with children. The pictures produced pupil constriction in single men and married but childless men. Dilated pupils can also indicate that listeners are interested, while constricted pupils suggest that they do not like what is being said (as well as viewed).

Sincerity is expressed with the eyes. The best method for conveying sincerity is frequent eye contact, a technique most appropriately used when listening to the other person. One trait of good listeners is that they constantly look at the speaker. A listener who does not maintain eye contact, but continues to look down or away from the speaker, may be shy, depressed, or indicating rejection of either the speaker or the comments being made. One patient recently said, "I had one student doctor who looked at his toes instead of me. If he ever opens a practice, I don't believe I would trust him." On the other hand, speakers may frequently break eye contact when talking and are permitted a distant stare when formulating ideas and selecting phrases. But they should still try to make frequent, though less prolonged and intense, eye contact.

A special kind of human-to-human awareness is conveyed by eye contact. Prolonged eye contact, or staring, can be offensive. Monkeys can be provoked to combat by a person staring at them because of the threat of aggression that this represents. Under other circumstances, however, staring can be flirtatious, emphasizing that the meaning of eye behavior depends upon other factors in the situation.

The acceptability of eye contact varies significantly among different cultures. In the United States, focusing one's eyes on the speaker indicates respect and attention regardless of the age of the individuals involved. However, Mexican-Americans and blacks tend not to maintain as much eye contact while listening as do other Americans and may look away from the speaker more often. This is not a sign of disrespect or inattention. In Latin American countries, a younger person may be thought disrespectful if his eyes meet those of the adult who is speaking. A physician could be considered seductive in that culture if he maintained steady eye contact while talking to a patient. In the United States, it is impolite to maintain eye contact with a stranger for more than 3 seconds, but Europeans feel that longer periods of eye contact are perfectly normal. Obviously, then, the physician needs to consider the patient's cultural background when interpreting the meaning of eye contact behavior. Looking away from the speaker from time to time may be a sign of respect and sensitivity rather than the opposite. At the same time, the physician's failure to look a patient in the eye can be dehumanizing and cause the patient to feel more like an object than a person. Patients are most comfortable when the physician looks at them approximately 50% of the time and are uncomfortable when eye contact is avoided.

The frequency of eye contact can also provide clues to whether the patient is anxious or depressed. Waxer demonstrated that both the presence of anxiety and its intensity could be determined on the basis of nonverbal cues alone. Prominent cues involved the hands, mouth, and torso. Anxious patients generated more stroking of themselves, such as hand on hand or hand on face, and had more twitches and tremors. They smiled less, and their torsos were stiff and rigid as though they were afraid to move. They also had a more rapid respiratory rate. The eyes of anxious patients blinked frequently or darted back and forth. They looked at the interviewer as frequently as low-anxiety patients but maintained eye contact for less time on each gaze. (Similarly, the patient may interpret the physician's lack of eye contact as indicative of anxiety or discomfort, even rejection.)

Depressed patients also maintain eye contact only one-fourth of the time of nondepressed patients. Downward contraction of the mouth and a downward angling of the head are also clues to depression. As with the anxious patient, there is no difference in frequency of eye contact in the depressed patient; the difference is only in the duration of contact.

Patients with abdominal pain that is due to organic disease are more likely to keep their eyes open during palpation of the abdomen than those with nonspecific pain (Gray et al.). This may be because the patient with genuine abdominal tenderness apprehensively watches the doctor's hand as it approaches the tender area.

HANDS. The hands will be droopy and flaccid with sadness, fidgety or grasping in anxiety, and—when responding to anger—will form clenched fists, often moving in a pounding fashion.

The hands of an anxious patient can be noted to shake when holding a pen or cigarette, to twitch, or to be braced unnaturally. The white-knuckle pose of tightly locked fingers can be an effort to mask the jitters. Patients with clenched fists, tight masseters, and frowns may be depressed, especially if they show evidence of turning anger upon themselves by scratching the back of their hands.

Hands can also be a subtle indicator of the urge to interrupt. Be alert for this sign in a patient so that important information will not be suppressed, and the patient can be given every opportunity to supply valuable information. Indications of this urge to interrupt are a slight raising of the hand or perhaps the index finger only, pulling at the ear lobe, or raising the index finger to the lips. The latter may also indicate an attempt to suppress a comment and should alert the physician to inquire further and elicit the hidden information. A patient listening in "The Thinker" position, with the index finger across the lips or extended along the cheek, or one sitting with elbows on the table and hands clenched in front of the mouth, although listening intently, may not be buying what the physician is saying. Take additional time to amplify the issue or explain the diagnosis or treatment regimen further.

ARMS. Although folded arms are found in all cultures, this is considered a discovered action rather than an inborn trait, since it is a natural position of comfort that is as easily discovered by the African tribesman as the New York banker. It is the subtle ways in which the arms are held that can give clues to underlying emotions. Crossed arms can be a defensive posture, indicating disagreement with another's view, or it can be a sign of insecurity. It can also be nothing more than a position of comfort and should, as with all other signs, be considered in the context of the individual's total behavior.

Note the manner in which the arms are crossed. Are they relaxed in the normal position of comfort, or are they in a hugging posture, reflecting insecurity or sadness and indicating a need for reassurance? Anger can be seen in clenched fists that are held tightly against the body in a holding-back manner, preventing them from hitting. If the patient has assumed a position of resistance or defensiveness, sitting with arms and legs crossed and perhaps with body turned away, search for the reason for this defensiveness and try to eliminate it. A recommendation that the patient stop smoking may be threatening and difficult to accept. In that case, it is important to make an additional effort to explain the rationale for the recommendation; do not hurry over it with a brief comment or admonition.

LEGS. Although crossing the legs is a common position of comfort, it can also indicate a shutting out of, or protection against, the outside world. If crossed legs in a patient confirm the total kinesic picture of resistance, including crossed arms and other signals discussed earlier, make every effort to identify the reason for the resistance and correct it before proceeding further. Diagnostic information obtained from a resistant patient is likely to be incomplete, and instructions are unlikely to be followed.

Note also the position of the feet and their movement. Just as anxiety is associated with fidgety hand movements, so it is with the fidgety, constantly moving foot. An anxious or scared person may sit forward in the chair with feet placed in the ready-to-run position, one foot in front of the other. The angry person is more likely to place the feet widely apart in a position of stability, while the feet of a sad person tend to move in a slow, circular pattern.

PREENING GESTURES. Preening gestures, such as the male's pulling up socks, adjusting tie, or combing hair, and the female's adjusting clothing or using a mirror to review makeup, may not necessarily be seductive in nature but can be an attempt to establish rapport and good interpersonal relations. If the preening is intended to be flirtatious, however, the woman may cross her legs, place her hand on her hip, caress her leg, or stroke her arm or thigh in some fashion. The flirtatious male will usually utilize gaze holding and head tilt to accentuate normal preening gestures. The physician should remain alert to the accentuation of normal preening gestures into courtship actions in order to identify the seductive patient and deal with the issue early, before unknowingly encouraging the patient to proceed further along this course.

RESPIRATORY AVOIDANCE RESPONSE. The respiratory avoidance response involves a frequent clearing of the throat when no phlegm or mucus is present. All animals exhibit a respiratory avoidance response as a means of clearing something unpleasant or undesirable from the respiratory tract. This action can also be a nonverbal indication of disgust or rejection. When physicians find themselves doing this, they should observe the accompanying circumstances and note whether posterior pharyngeal mucus is truly present.

Another component of the respiratory avoidance syndrome is the nose rub. This involves a light or subtle rub of the nose with the index finger and signals rejection of a statement being made either by the subject or by another individual. The nose rub to relieve an itch is usually vigorous and involves a repeated series of rubs, whereas that of the respiratory avoidance response is soft and consists of one or two light strokes, often involving nothing more than a light flick of the nose.

Morris describes the nose flick as "a reflection of the fact that a split is being forced between inner thoughts and outward action." It can be associated with lying or with the struggle to appear calm while suppressing anger or discomfort.

This sign can be quite useful in patient interviewing. For example, the physician may ask a patient, "How are things at home?" The patient may answer, "Fine," then clear his throat and lightly rub his nose with the index finger. He is actually saying, "I don't like what you are asking me," or "I feel uncomfortable with my answer; things really aren't going very well at home." If there is a cause to pursue the issue further, a simple comment such as "Really?" or "You mean not even an occasional argument?" may lead to a flood of information masked by the previous response.

Another example of a conflict between what a patient is saying and what is being felt is a "verbal-nonverbal mismatch," for example, when the patient answers "Fine" to "How are things between you and your husband?" while looking sad and avoiding eye contact.

Other clues that the patient may not be telling the truth or that there are repressed feelings are asymmetrical facial expressions and a prolonged smile or expression of amazement. Almost all authentic facial expressions fade after 4 or 5 seconds (Ekman).

Hidden (or Masked) Communication

Although the average person has a symptom about every 6 days, he or she visits a physician only once every 4 months. Some people will visit a physician much more frequently than others, for the same symptom. Patients who visit more frequently tend to have a higher level of anxiety, fear, grief, or frustration. It is the physician's responsibility to search for, identify, and treat organic disease if it is present, yet in about half of the cases none will be found. Of course, it is equally important to identify the reason for these visits—the basis for the heightened concern or increased anxiety. A person may see a minor symptom as a potential catastrophe if he or she feels it may be a sign of cancer similar to that which caused a parent's death. In other words, patients may come because of what they imagine is causing the symptoms rather than because of the symptoms themselves. Identifying what patients hope can be done for them— that is, focusing on their expectations for the visit—will often reveal hidden reasons for the visit. The physician should be sure to address the patient's expectations and make certain that the interpretation is correct. Is the patient really there "just for a blood pressure check" or because of concern over the condition of his coronary arteries since a friend recently had an acute myocardial infarction? If the physician deals only with the symptoms, the real concerns may go undetected, and the result will be a dissatisfied and noncompliant patient. Barsky cautions that "patients who express dissatisfaction with their medical care should be questioned about this, as they may be dissatisfied because their real motivation in seeking care has not been illuminated." He also advises the physician to investigate the patient's current life stresses if visits are made when there is no change in clinical status.

HAND ON THE DOORKNOB SYNDROME. The patient's parting phrase is sometimes a clue to the primary reason for the visit, or it may reflect another issue of great concern that is emotionally threatening and could not be voiced until adequate courage was summoned at the moment of departure. It sometimes finally surfaces as a last, desperate attempt to communicate—since, with hand on door, escape is readily accessible if the physician's reaction is unfavorable. Reasons for this hidden communication by the patient are important and must be recognized and dealt with. Because of fear of rejection or humiliation, the patient may test the physician

with minor complaints before mentioning the real reason for the visit. Be alert to any unusual behavior during an interview, such as slips of the tongue, unexpected responses, and overly enthusiastic denials. Search further for the underlying reason for the visit when a patient presents with a trivial complaint that appears inappropriate at that time. It is a good practice to routinely ask the patient at the end of a visit, "Is there anything we have not covered or anything else you would like to ask me?"

Patients with a fear of cancer, for instance, are often unable to voice their concern to the physician. Instead, they present with somatic complaints or contrived reasons that necessitate a complete examination. They hope the examination will allay their fears without their having to express them openly. For example, a female patient presenting for a complete physical examination may actually be concerned over the possibility of a carcinoma of the breast, which her elder sister may have had at the same age or for which a friend recently had surgery. Such situations emphasize the need for a complete family history and a discussion of any patient concerns, in an effort to allow these feelings to surface. Attention should then be paid to alleviating the anxiety. Apprehension regarding cancer is widespread, and often the only cure for this fear is a therapeutic conversation with the physician. It is very likely that most patients harbor some fear of cancer, and, therefore, following a complete history and physical examination, specific mention should be made that no signs of cancer can be detected at this time. If this precaution is not taken, a patient with a hidden anxiety or fear of cancer may remain suspicious that a cancer could be present, since there was no apparent attempt to look specifically for it.

Proxemics (Spatial Factors)

SPACE. Proxemics is the study of how people unconsciously structure the space around them. This structuring varies with every culture. North Americans, for example, maintain a protective "body bubble" of space about 2 feet in diameter around them when they interact with strangers or casual acquaintances. Violators of that space are considered intruders and cause the person to become defensive. In the Middle East, no such bubble exists, and it is proper to invade this area. In fact, not to do so may be interpreted as unfriendly and standoffish. Arabs prefer to stand close enough to touch and smell the other person. Americans, however, if forced to stand close together, as on a crowded subway, will use their eyes (distant gaze) to maintain a more proper distance. An arm's length is a good measure of the appropriate personal distance for most people. A wife can stand inside her husband's bubble, but she will be unhappy if another woman invades this sphere of privacy (and vice versa).

Intimate space has been classified as that ranging from close physical contact to 18 inches, *personal* space from 18 inches to 4 feet, *social* space from 4 feet to 12 feet, and *public* space 12 feet and beyond. Placing a desk between two people shifts personal space to social space.

The office desk can also be a barrier to communication when it is placed between the physician and the patient, thereby emphasizing the illusion of the physician's importance and power. There may be occasions when this is desired, but it usually is not necessary in a family physician's office. Office furniture should be arranged so that a minimum number of obstacles lie between physician and patient. The patient should also be made to feel as comfortable as possible, with a minimum of bright lights, smoke, and other irritating stimuli present in the room.

Listening Well

A good family physician must be a good listener. Of all the communication skills essential to rapport, the ability to listen well is probably the most important. All the information in the world about body language, vocal messages, and nonverbal cues is of limited value unless it helps the family physician be a more astute listener.

Physicians should listen to patients in an alert and uncritical manner. They should appear relaxed yet attentive. They should be nonjudgmental, so as not to inhibit the patient's expression and willingness to relate problems of a sensitive nature.

In general, the less the physician says during an interview, the more the patient will say. Silence can be as effective a means of eliciting further information as direct questions. The timing is important, however, and silence should be used as a technique only when the physician is relatively certain that there is more information to follow the last statement. A shift of position, or a nod and a smile, properly timed and coupled with silence can be more effective than an encouraging comment. Nonverbal encouragement to continue is less distracting and may be more facilitative than the verbal. The patient may be following a line of thought and may be about to open up more but must stop and refocus on the physician if he or she "captures" the patient's attention with a verbal statement. The physician should interrupt a patient's statement only if it is necessary to change the conversation to a new topic, clarify an issue, elicit information not produced spontaneously, offer reassurance, or reduce patient anxiety.

The appearance of readiness to listen is aided by bending forward and maintaining eye contact. The physician can discourage a patient from talking simply by looking away or writing in the medical record. Well-chosen questions can be rendered useless by inappropriate nonverbal behavior.

Interviewing Effectively

The skilled family physician can spend 10 minutes with a patient and the patient will feel it was 20. This is far better than the physician who spends 20 minutes but leaves patients feeling that the physician was in a hurry and that they were encroaching on the physician's precious time every minute of the visit.

Overly brief or abrupt conversations in the office or at the bedside can severely damage rapport. Physicians signal how much time they plan to spend by a variety of nonverbal cues, and patients rarely have the courage to counter this by asking for more time. The physician who hurriedly asks, "How are you?" while flipping through a chart with only a quick glance at the patient destroys communication. Even the busiest physicians can accomplish wonders in a very few minutes by indicating that their full attention is on the patient. Everyone remembers an outstanding physician who, for whatever time was available, would, by a relaxed posture and attentive manner, truly communicate with the patient.

The interesting and revealing study by Korsch and Negrete, involving analysis of taped doctor–patient encounters in a pediatric clinic, revealed that many of the mothers were dissatisfied because the physician paid too little attention to their concern and apprehension about their children. Their attitude had little relationship to the amount of attention that the physician actually paid to the infant, which was usually very adequate.

Even in an established family practice where essentially none of the patients was dissatisfied with the physician, 54% of the patients either forgot to mention something of concern or misunderstood facts about diagnosis or treatment (Snyder et al.). Twenty-nine of the 84 patients forgot to tell the physician something that was bothering them. This illustrates the wisdom of concluding every interview with the statement "Is there anything else bothering you that we haven't discussed?" Snyder suggests that "the physician will be well advised to consciously underestimate his ability to communicate." Rather than assume that patients have understood the instructions, ask them to repeat the instructions as they understand them. Patients with chronic illnesses, and those visiting the physician for the first time, are most likely to misunderstand treatment instructions. When seeing a patient with a chronic illness, assess the patient's understanding of instructions given at a previous visit by asking, "What medications are you taking?" or "How are you taking your medication?" A patient seen for the first time can be asked, "How have you been treating this problem?"

When meeting a new patient, the method used to address the patient during the introduction can help establish rapport by conveying an atmosphere of mutual respect. Use the patient's name during the introduction, during the interview, and upon leaving. An appropriate introduction would be "Good morning, Mrs. Brown, I'm Dr. _____" or "Good morning, Mrs. Brown, I'm _____, a second-year medical student, and I'll be taking your medical history and examining you today."

Rapport can be influenced positively or negatively by how the physician addresses the patient. Although the majority of patients prefer to be addressed by their first name, some may be irritated by this if sufficient familiarity has not been established.

FACILITATING TECHNIQUES. In addition to the nonverbal facilitating techniques of silence and body positioning mentioned previously, patients can be encouraged to talk further with simple comments, such as "And then?" or by repeating a portion of the statement just made. For example:

Patient: I have been very nervous lately.

Doctor: Nervous?

CONFRONTATION. Confrontation, wisely used, can help establish communication and rapport. Statements such as "You look unhappy" or "You appear very anxious" are based on the physician's observation of the patient. If the physician has been unable to establish rapport, it may help to approach the issue openly and frankly: "We don't seem to be communicating very well. Can you tell me what is wrong?" This is also a useful maneuver when a previously good relationship suddenly turns sour.

SUMMARIZATION (OR PARAPHRASING). Summarization is a brief restatement of what the patient has said and gives both the interviewer and the patient a chance to correct errors or misunderstandings. It demonstrates the physician's interest in the patient's history and his or her effort to collect the facts accurately. The physician can restate what the patient has said and emphasize the important points to assure clear understanding. Summarization assures that both parties are using the same definitions and minimizes inappropriate assumptions. "Let me see if I have understood you correctly" or "Am I understanding this correctly?" are good ways to introduce a paraphrase.

CONCLUDING A HISTORY. As mentioned above, in an effort to avoid leaving gaps in the history or allowing patient concerns to go unattended, it is wise to conclude every complete history by asking, "Is there anything else you would like to mention?"

OPEN-ENDED QUESTIONS. Probably the single most valuable rapport-promoting element of verbal communication is the use of open-ended questions at the onset of an interview. "Tell me more about it" is both an interview technique and a state of mind. The physician who understands that no checklist of "yes-no" questions can possibly portray the patient as a unique human being will create an atmosphere of sensitivity and interest that contributes greatly to the early establishment of rapport. Once the broad outlines of the patient's unique situation are indicated, detailed questioning moves along quickly.

Specific questions beget specific answers and rarely anything more. However, the physician may wish to use this technique on occasion, as when dealing with the verbose, rambling patient who refuses to stick to the point or when specific information is needed. When more general or hidden data are sought, however, the physician must choose questions and gestures that offer the maximal potential for obtaining information. In order to be effective, open-ended questioning requires that the physician appear relaxed and ready to listen regardless of the amount of pressure from waiting patients. Once it becomes apparent that more time is needed than is available, a new appointment should be made so that adequate time is assured.

SIGNALS THAT DISCOURAGE COMMUNICATION. While appearing to respond affirmatively and facilitate the conversation, people can in fact turn off the speaker if they frequently comment "Yes" in a manner that conveys disinterest or impatience. Everyone has experienced the person who says "Yes" before the sentence is finished or the point made.

CONFIDENTIALITY. Confidentiality is a cardinal principle of professionalism. Effective communication requires that the patient feel secure in the knowledge that all information will be kept strictly confidential. It is the ethical responsibility of each physician to maintain this bond of confidentiality. The family physician must appreciate this intimate and confidential bond and avoid any threat to its dissolution. Hippocrates said, "And whatever I shall see or hear in the course of my profession, as well as outside my profession in my intercourse with men, if it be what should not be published abroad, I will never divulge, holding such things to be holy secrets."

Assurance that all information and actions will be kept confidential is especially important when dealing with adolescents. They may not be aware of this basic ethical principle in the medical profession or realize that it applies to them. They may be reluctant to share information and trust completely for fear that parents or peers may find out.

CARE WITH CARING

One of the essential qualities of the clinician is interest in humanity, for the secret of the care of the patient is in caring for the patient.

This statement by Francis Peabody in 1923 could well serve as the maxim for establishing patient rapport. While continuing to emphasize the curing aspects of medicine, family medicine places increased emphasis upon its caring aspects. Caring is the opposite of apathy and implies the application of human tenderness and compassion to the curing of individuals. It involves respect for the individual as a human being and enables the physician to motivate patients to participate in their care. Physicians must convince the patient that they care and are sincerely interested in providing help.

Allen Gregg has said that more mistakes in medicine are made by those who do not care than by those who do not know. The caring implies an empathetic relationship between physician and patient. Empathy is the capacity of physicians to participate in the feelings of the patient and is best accomplished if physicians place themselves in the role of patients in an effort to understand their feelings. This does not imply a sharing of feelings with the patient (sympathy), since the physician would then become emotionally affected. Empathy involves only insight into the patient's feelings. It is best that the physician avoid becoming emotionally involved in order to maintain professional equanimity and objectivity when caring for the patient.

Chekov, a physician himself, thought that medical students should spend half of their time learning what it feels like to be ill. Although this may be an extreme method for developing empathy, it is important that the student, before becoming immersed in the technical and cognitive aspects of medicine, be able to identify with the patient's feelings, fears, apprehensions, and expectations so that the knowledge acquired during medical school can be applied meaningfully in the context of these needs. Exposing students to patients in the first year of medical school, before they have been preoccupied with the diagnosis and treatment of disease, offers them an opportunity, under the watchful gaze of an instructor, to focus on the process of communication. Barriers to effective communication can then be identified. For example, a student may have difficulty permitting a patient with terminal cancer to talk about the disease or his impending death. More than one student has been known to convey his discomfort nonverbally by conducting the interview standing at the foot of the hospital bed, adjacent to the door, ready to escape.

Although the physician may be able to cure a disease only occasionally, he or she can always console the patient. An unknown French author has admonished the medical profession "to cure sometimes, to relieve often, to comfort always." The family physician provides personalized patient care and attempts to minimize the often frightening and dehumanizing experience to which patients are subjected in our highly structured modern medical system. The physician must constantly strive to preserve personal dignity for patients, especially when their identities are threatened by a strange and somewhat frightening hospital environment. Care *for* a patient is more personal than care *of* a patient.

REFERENCES

Alda A. Time, May 28, 1979, p. 68

Bandler R, Grinder J. The Structure of Magic I. Palo Alto, Calif., Science & Behavior Books, 1975.

Barsky AJ. Hidden reasons some patients visit doctors. Ann Intern Med 1981; 94:492.

Beisecker AE, Beisecker TD. Patient information-seeking behaviors when communicating with doctors. Med Care 1990; 28:19–28.

Butterfield F. China: Alive in the Bitter Sea. New York, Times Books, 1982.

Darwin C. The Expression of the Emotions in Man and Animals. London, John Murry, 1872.

Ekman P. Telling Lies. New York, W.W. Norton, 1985.

Ekman P, Friesen WV. Unmasking the Face: A Guide to Recognizing Emotions from Facial Clues. Englewood Cliffs, N.J., Prentice-Hall, 1975.

Friedman HS. Nonverbal communication between patients and medical practitioners. J Social Issues 1979; 35:82.

Gjerdingen DK, Simpson DE, Titus SL. Patients' and physicians' attitudes regarding the physicians' professional appearance. Arch Intern Med 1987; 147:1209–1212.

Gray DW, Dixon JM, Collin J. The closed eyes sign: An aid to diagnosing non-specific abdominal pain BMJ 1988; 297(6652):837.

Hess ET. The Telltale Eye. New York, Van Nostrand Reinhold, 1975.

Holmes OW. Medical Essays: 1842–1882. Boston and New York, Houghton Mifflin, 1911.

Knapp ML. Nonverbal Communication in Human Interaction, 2nd ed. New York, Holt, Reinhart and Winston, 1978.

Korsch BM, Negrete V. Doctor-patient communication. Sci Am 1972; 227:66.

Larsen KM, Smith CK. Assessment of nonverbal communication in patient-physician interview. J Fam Pract 1981; 12:481.

McCaskey MB. The hidden messages managers send. Harvard Business Review, Nov.–Dec. 1979, p. 135.

Meltzoff AN, Moore MK. Imitation of facial and manual gestures by human neonates. Science 1977; 198:75–78.

Morris D. Manwatching: A Field Guide to Human Behavior. New York, Abrams, 1977.

Peabody FW. Doctor and Patient. New York, Macmillan, 1930.

Snyder D, Lynch JJ, Gruss L. Doctor-patient communication in a private family practice. J Fam Pract 1976; 3:271.

Waitzkin H. Doctor-patient communication: Clinical implications of social scientific research. JAMA 1984; 252:2441–2446.

Waxer PH. Nonverbal cues for anxiety: An examination of emotional leakage. J Abnorm Psychol 1977; 86:306.

Widmer RB, Cardoret RJ. Depression in primary care: Changes in pattern of patients' visits and complaints during a developing depression. J Fam Pract 1978; 7:293.

QUESTIONS

1. The most useful technique in obtaining a medical history is
   a. Silence.
   b. Specific questions.
   c. Open-ended questions.
   d. Questions requiring a "Yes" or "No" answer.
   e. Humor.

2. Match the following:
   a. Facilitates rapport by imitation
   b. Often used to cover hidden sadness
   c. Uncomfortable with what is being said
   d. Shows true emotion before it is masked
      1. Nose rub
      2. Mirroring
      3. Micro-expression
      4. A smile

3. Which of the following best shows sincerity?
   a. A handshake
   b. The initial greeting
   c. A smile
   d. The eyes
   e. Touch

4. Neurolinguistic Programming (NLP)
   a. Is different for right- and left-handed people.
   b. Builds rapport by matching the patient's use of verbs.
   c. Proposes that right-handed people look up and to the left when recalling a visual image.
   d. Proposes that eyes move from side to side when the person recalls a symphony.

Answers appear on page 446.

INTERVIEWING TECHNIQUES

F. MARIAN BISHOP and ROBERT E. FROELICH

PURPOSE OF THE MEDICAL INTERVIEW. The interview has several purposes. The two most often identified are (1) gathering data from the patient that will lead to an understanding of the disease process and the underlying physiologic status, and (2) establishing a relationship and a treatment contract between the patient, the physician, and the physician's staff. Both are equally important.

ORGANIZING THE MEDICAL INTERVIEW

There are several ways to organize a medical interview. The important thing is to develop a pattern or outline that works for you and is adaptable to the various kinds of patient situations. The following approach has been found to be adaptable to a variety of settings, specialties, and patient problems. This approach emphasizes developing skills in the *process* of gathering information and the process of problem-solving.

1. BE CLEAR ABOUT THE PURPOSE FOR THE VISIT AND THE PATIENT'S WILLINGNESS TO TALK ABOUT PROBLEMS. By seeing the physician, the patient expresses a willingness to talk with the physician about an acute or chronic problem, illness, or discomfort. Occasionally the patient comes for other reasons, such as to get out of work or obtain disability. The session can be frustrating if its purpose is not clear to both the patient and the physician.

By seeing the patient, the physician expresses a willingness to consider and deal with the patient's problems. Some physicians have other reasons, such as earning a living or fulfilling an educational requirement. If one of these other reasons prevails, the session may be very frustrating to the patient.

2. USE THE FIRST 20 SECONDS OF CONTACT WISELY. In the first 20 seconds, visual input dominates the awareness of the two participants. For the patient, the warmth or coldness of the room's decor, the light level, and the privacy or lack of it are important first impressions. Next, the posture, dress, attitude, physical distance, sex, age, and body build of the physician are noted. The physician's voice pitch, volume, and expression are judged by the patient and fitted into prejudices built up by past experiences. What the physician actually says is then judged in this context. Thus, who says it, how it is said, and when it is said play as big a role as what is said.

Similarly, the physician judges the patient's body build, posture, sex, age, dress, and gestures. The physician quickly imagines that the patient is sick, a complainer, an alcoholic, and so on, and guesses the economic resources and type of work the patient does. Based upon past experiences, the physician also stereotypes the patient before a word is spoken. With a new patient, it is probably best for the physician to be quiet for 5 seconds to allow this "sizing-up" process to take place.

3. VERIFY THE MAIN REASON FOR THE PATIENT'S VISIT. The opening of a medical interview varies with the setting and style of the physician. Generally, a nurse, clerk, or secretary obtains descriptive data about a patient, such as name, address, age, other family members, medical insurance, and telephone number before the interview. Some physicians prefer to acquire this information themselves as a way to open an interview on a nonthreatening topic. By gathering this information firsthand, the physician can also observe and obtain information concerning the patient's memory, orientation, and problem relationships.

Once the descriptive data are obtained, the next step is to ask what led the patient to make an appointment. Usually the record will indicate a reason for the visit. Remember that a patient needs an "admission ticket" to see a physician, that is, a socially and medically acceptable excuse for the visit. But it may be just that, an excuse. To find the real reason, it is helpful to ask for the chief complaint, using a facilitation or an open-ended question, not a specific question. For example, "What is the situation that brings you here today?" rather than "The nurse says you have an earache. What seems to be the trouble?"

Once the chief complaint is identified and clarified, the patient and the physician need to agree that both are willing to share information, to explore the complaint, and to do what is necessary to understand, diagnose, and treat it. Ideally the contract also defines the type of relationship they will have, that is, whether they will relate as a superior and an inferior, as two equals, as a teacher and a student, or as two advocates with veto power over each other's decisions.

Most often the contract is understood by behavior and willingness to respond to each other. However, when there is hesitancy to respond, when the patient asks questions of the physician, or when either person is uncomfortable, it is important to define a contract verbally and see if the other will agree. For example, "You seem a bit hesitant to answer my questions. Are you willing to share information with me about this problem?" Such a question will bring out what each expects and is willing to do. If the answer is "No," the next question might be "What are you willing to do?"

The type of relationship is usually established by the style and personality of the physician. But the physician can learn to adapt and modify the approach to meet best the needs of each patient. Sometimes the type of relationship contract is established and agreed to nonverbally through posture, tone of voice, relative physical positions, and the medical problem.

4. DEVELOP A WORKABLE PROCESS FOR DATA GATHERING. Once the chief complaint has been understood and clarified, data concerning the present illness are elicited from the patient. The interview for a simple acute problem is generally limited to specific questions, such as "Where did the fall occur?" or "How did the cut happen?"

The interview for a complex or chronic condition usually follows a guideline to obtain specific details of the present symptoms, diet, exercise, medications, work and home environments, social and financial stresses, emotional and behavioral reactions to the symptoms, and what the patient does to alleviate the symptoms.

One successful, efficient process for the medical interview is to begin with open-ended questions followed by facilitation, reflections, empathic replies, and silences to learn as much as the patient is able to tell without physician suggestion and interference. Once the patient has said as much as he or she can, the patient is facilitated further by so-called laundry-list questions, direct questions, yes-no questions, and summary statements of clarification. The topic is closed and a bridging comment is made to move to the next topic. This process is repeated many times during a medical interview in dealing with each topic.

Relevant data from the past medical, social, work, and family histories are obtained using the same technique and process of opening the topic, assisting the narrative, closing the topic, and bridging to a new topic. Table 10–1 sets out the types of physician interventions most suited for each phase of the medical interview. In addition, a Glossary for defining the various responses of interventions is found at the end of the chapter.

5. ANALYZE THE INFORMATION AND DETERMINE THE PROBLEM. Once the data are obtained, they must be analyzed to give meaning to the symptoms, history, and

TABLE 10–1. PHYSICIAN INTERVENTIONS FOR PHASES OF THE MEDICAL INTERVIEW

I. OPENING A TOPIC
Facilitation
Open-ended question
Bridging phrase

II. ASSISTING THE PATIENT'S NARRATIVE
Support and reassurance
Empathy
Confrontation
Reflection
Interpretation
Silence
Modified laundry-list

III. FOCUSING UPON A TOPIC
Confrontation
Reflection
Probing
Interpretation
Summation

IV. OBTAINING SPECIFIC INFORMATION
Direct question
Yes-no question
Probing
Problem question
Laundry-list

V. CLOSING TOPIC OR INTERVIEW
Summation
Prescription for action

Source: Froelich RE, Bishop FM. Clinical Interviewing Skills. 3rd ed. St. Louis, C. V. Mosby, 1977, with permission.

associated data. This analysis defines the patient's discomforts as a physiologic or disease process. Thus a tentative diagnosis is formed. Though dependent upon the interview, the diagnostic process is related to training, information, and ability to synthesize numerous types of data.

6. VERIFY NONVERBAL CUES. The nonverbal accompaniment to the words (context, voice quality and emphasis, facial expression, body posture, setting, attire, patient's age and culture) helps the physician fill in the unexpressed. However, the only way to be sure that the physician's understanding is accurate is to check out the understanding with the patient. Using summary statements and asking, "What I hear you saying is . . . Am I correct?" is an effective technique to be sure that the patient is being heard correctly.

7. DETERMINE TREATMENT ALTERNATIVES. After the physiologic process is defined, diagnostic or treatment alternatives are considered. In the ideal problem-solving process, the patient has enough understanding to suggest some of the diagnostic or treatment alternatives. The physician presents suggestions and alternatives along with their probable outcomes, cost, and side effects. Ideally this decision is made jointly by the physician and the patient.

8. CARRY OUT THE PLAN AND PROPOSE ACTIONS FOR THE FUTURE: The diagnostic or treatment alternative is instituted and the results are evaluated by both the physician and the patient. If the decision involves a treatment and the treatment solves the problem, this episode of health care for this patient is concluded with questions and suggestions of how to avoid similar illnesses in the future. If the decision is a diagnostic activity or an unsuccessful treatment, the physician and patient return to the interview process to obtain the new data.

NOTHING SUBSTITUTES FOR FACE-TO-FACE INTERACTION

A good interview should result in an accurate and comprehensive story of the patient's situation. This story is sometimes referred to as the medical history. A common phrase is "taking a medical history." But medical histories are not taken. They are developed from oral accounts of the patient's present and past illnesses provided by the patient, family, and friends, as well as from oral and written statements of colleagues, records of previous hospitalizations, and so on. Selection, interpretation, and ordering of information pervade the process of developing the case history.

A written questionnaire or checklist filled out by the patient may result in information. However, there is no relationship established between a patient and a questionnaire or checklist. The questionnaire completed by a patient either on paper or taken by an interviewer is quite different from the personal interview in two major ways. First, the questionnaire lacks the qualities of human interaction—a constantly renegotiated give-and-take. It lacks all the nonverbal aspects of meaningful communication. Second, the questionnaire lacks the ability to make meaning out of the patient's responses. Without meaning, the physician has limited use for the information.

For example, the information that a patient was married at age 15 is of little use in and of itself. However, the circumstances surrounding the decision to get married at age 15 may have profound meaning for understanding the patient's reactions to a present illness. The raw fact "married age 15" is made meaningful and useful in the present context by elaboration in the interview. Since the relationship is important to the treatment of the patient and the patient's cooperation, the human intervention is an essential element of the patient's visit to the physician.

A lot of interest and money has been put into the technology of computerizing patient information and developing machine branching questionnaires that can be entered by the patient. But a machine interaction and a human dialogue are not equivalent. A computer can organize information but it does not understand information. A computer cannot ask the patient for further explanation of the questions in a computerized history. It also cannot ask the patient what he or she meant by a response to a question.

The computer is also unable to understand a patient's communication, since communicating includes verbal and nonverbal messages. The meaning of words is shaded by the nonverbal as well as the linguistic aspects of the message, and the computer is unable to pick up

this meaning. But for storing, organizing, and retrieving information, it can be a valuable tool.

PITFALLS IN INTERVIEWING

The effectiveness of the physician in conducting a medical interview and creating a medical history is dependent in part upon the ability to avoid some common pitfalls.

ONSET OF THE ILLNESS. Once the present condition is defined, the onset of the problem should be dealt with. The physician needs a detailed description of the symptoms, how they were precipitated, how they progressed, and any data associated with each period of symptoms up to the present time.

One of the most common pitfalls is for the physician to deal with the onset of the illness before knowing enough about the patient's present state to have a good idea of the organ of involvement. Without this understanding, the physician does not know where to focus attention in obtaining details of the progression of the present illness. If the physician does not know whether the pain described in the chest is cardiac, esophageal, or chest wall, he or she will not know on which organ to focus the review of the present illness.

DIRECT QUESTIONS. The temptation to resort to direct questions is probably the major pitfall for the inexperienced interviewer and the interviewer who lets skills languish. An interview made up of direct questions gathers little information per unit time, since most of the time is spent by the interviewer framing and asking questions, each of which gives a specific bit of information.

The direct question approach does not permit the patient to give information about his or her experience, and the interviewer may never obtain the piece of information the patient wanted to give unless the interviewer just happens to ask the one specific question that taps the information. Remember the problem of the computer interview noted earlier in the chapter. Computer-generated questions, by necessity, must be direct questions, since the computer is unable to accept dialogue as a response.

"WHY" QUESTIONS. A third pitfall is asking "Why" questions. Questions such as "Why did you take that medicine?" "Why did you leave work?" or "Why did you get a divorce?" call on the patient to account for his or her behavior and encourage him or her to be on the defensive.

"Why" questions imply that the patient did something wrong. Since much of the patient's behavior may be derived from the unconscious or be related to reasons that are not socially acceptable, the patient may be antagonized by this implication. The patient may feel that such a question finds fault with him or her and may thus become irritated or annoyed.

It is difficult to begin a question with "Why" and avoid the overtones of accusation. In addition, "Why" questions come from a whining transactional position on the part of the interviewer. The whining position may be described as a position of helplessness, pleading, or angry frustration. The above questions could be rephrased as "Tell me about taking that medicine," "You needed to leave work?" and "Are you willing to tell me about the divorce?"

SUGGESTIVE QUESTIONS. A fourth pitfall is a question that has within it the answer. This is called a suggestive question. For example: "When you discussed your problem, your breathing was a little rapid. Were you a little nervous at the time?" What choice does the patient have in responding to such a question? Obviously, much misinformation can be obtained by using suggestive questions. This is especially true when the patient feels put down or inferior to the physician and feels a need to be compliant.

"YES" AND "NO" QUESTIONS. With many patients there is a danger in using questions requiring "Yes" or "No" answers. The patient's answer may be more dependent on the immediate milieu than on the facts. When a question is answered with a "Yes," it is not clear what the "Yes" means. Is it given to please, to give the interviewer what the patient thinks he or she wants to hear, to avoid discussing an area that the patient wants to avoid, or is it a factual response?

Similarly, when the question can be answered with a "No," the patient may just wish to disagree, to please, or to avoid discussing a topic rather than to give a factual response. Much inaccurate information can be obtained by using this type of question. An experienced interviewer can get misinformation from any patient by a question that can most appropriately be answered by "Yes" or "No."

UNSIGNALED TOPIC CHANGES. When the physician asks the patient for information and there is a longer than usual pause before answering, the topic has probably been changed without signaling this intention to the patient. This interviewing pitfall slows the interviewing process and, because the topic change is unsignaled, gives the patient the impression the interviewer has no clear plan of action. When it is time to change a topic, it is best to use a bridging phrase, such as "Let's shift to talking about . . . ," to guide the patient in the direction the interview is to go.

LACK OF EYE CONTACT. A pitfall that is sometimes forgotten is that lack of eye contact through concentration on a note pad, a chart, or a referral note will greatly affect the information obtained from a patient. In addition to giving the message that the paper is more important than the patient, the interviewer misses out on all of the gestures, facial expressions, and shifts in position that add so much to the meaning of what is said. At times when listening to only the words, with no eye contact, the interviewer even misses the intonation of the voice, the guttural emphasis, the slight laugh, or the held-back cry.

LACK OF FEEDBACK TO PATIENTS. Giving no feedback to the patient is an interviewing pitfall that will interfere with the doctor–patient relationship. In the extreme, giving no feedback is impossible if both the doctor and the patient are in the same room in view of each other and able to hear each other. As one patient said to her physician, "I knew how you felt about that by your raised eyebrows." The physician, however, had been unaware of any eyebrow movement. Whatever we do is interpreted by the patient as either encouraging or discouraging his or her current responses. With practice and videotape review of interviews, an interviewer can gain increasing conscious control of the nonverbal feedback given to the patient.

While there are other potential interviewing problems that could be reviewed, the ones discussed are some of the more common pitfalls that, with practice and conscious effort, can be avoided.

PROBLEM PATIENTS

The effectiveness of an interviewer, in large part, is dependent upon the number and variety of interviewing techniques the physician can utilize to meet the variety of situations that arise in an interview. For example, the same techniques will not work with the over-talkative and the reticent, the sad and the angry, or the frightened and the stoic patient.

Some of the interviewing literature focuses upon problem patients. While this focus has led to some meaningful understandings, the broader view that the problem patient is a part of an interview system has led to additional insights with a focus on the physician as well as the patient. A problem patient to one physician may be an ideal patient to the next physician. This section will focus on both the patient and the physician, using a personalized approach to attitudes and feelings of the physician in the discussion.

DEFENSIVE PATIENT. Patients are usually defensive because of an expected negative outcome if they were to talk freely about the topic at hand. For instance, the patient may expect anger, rejection, blame, or ridicule, and there is fear or anxiety about the expected outcome. Several techniques may be used to deal with defensiveness and the obstacle it poses to evaluation and diagnosis.

One technique is to ask, "What might happen if you were to talk about . . . ?" The patient's answer is pursued until the physician understands the fear. In rare instances, the physician may agree that the expected outcome is a probable outcome, for example, information used in a pending lawsuit, and that the patient has been advised not to discuss the topic. More likely, once the outcome is discussed, it becomes evident to the patient that nothing bad will happen if the topic is discussed. As the topic is dealt with, the defensiveness begins to melt away.

A second technique is to ask, "What is the worst possible thing that could happen if you talked about . . . ?" Again, the physician may agree that the catastrophe might occur or, as is more often the case, the patient will realize that the catastrophe is unlikely to take place.

A third technique that is especially helpful if the patient is teasing, that is, suggesting there is important information and then withholding it, is to agree not to discuss the topic and to go on to another one. If the patient is teasing, he or she will bring up the topic later in the session or in the next session if it is of great importance to the patient. By not responding, the physician reinforces a straightforward open discussion rather than a continuation of teasing innuendos.

A fourth technique is to comment on the defensiveness: "You seem very reluctant to discuss this topic," followed initially by silence on the physician's part. If the patient does not respond, the physician may proceed with "Is there anything that will make it easier for you to discuss this topic?" or "Are there any questions you want to ask before proceeding?" or "Can you identify your concerns in talking about this topic?" And finally the physician might ask, "Is there something that concerns you about trusting me with the information about this topic?" or "Is there something that concerns you about my reaction to or feelings toward you if we discuss this topic?"

If the physician asks these questions, he or she needs to be prepared to discuss the patient's replies honestly, directly, objectively, and without personal distance, in the sense that the patient is reacting to his own beliefs about the person in the physician role. The first time the relationship between the physician and the patient is focused on the defensiveness, it may be helpful to record the session on tape and review the session with a peer or supervisor who can provide some objective observations on the doctor–patient relationship. Defensiveness is usually a transference problem rather than a reality problem.

FEARFUL PATIENT. One can produce anxiety in oneself with a scary thought and restricted breathing. By doing the opposite, relaxing the breathing and avoiding the fear-producing thoughts, anxiety can be controlled.

A decision needs to be made as to whether the patient's fear is related to a real threat, sometimes referred to as reality fear, or to an imagined threat, referred to as neurotic fear. Fear associated with a real threat is considered healthy. Relaxation techniques, focusing the person's attention away from the threat, and caring support are useful ways to comfort these patients. It is important to let patients experience their real fear and help them through it.

The neurotic fear of an imagined threat should be handled by exploring the threat, the probability that it might actually occur, and the consequences if it did occur. What is the catastrophic fear and how likely is it to happen? The question, "So what if it does happen?" may help. This process confronts the unreality of the fear and the imagined threat.

The next step is to encourage the patient to agree to breathe slowly and deeply and to stop the scary thoughts. The patient should focus on some pleasant thoughts instead. This uses a positive approach, rather than a negative approach.

ANGRY PATIENT. Several issues are raised when dealing with an angry patient: (1) What is the direction and quality of the anger? (2) Can the physician accept or allow the patient to be angry? (3) Is the patient's anger affecting the medical problem? (4) How is the patient justifying the anger? (5) Is the anger due to frustration or is it a cover-up for sadness?

In the normal, healthy person, anger is the natural result of frustration. To overcome the frustration in a socially acceptable manner, the anger takes the form of aggression. Once the anger changes to hostility, it becomes destructive rather than constructive and is considered maladaptive.

Physicians vary widely in their ability to recognize anger and tolerate it in a patient. One physician may enjoy the spunk of the angry patient while another fears, withdraws from, or denies a patient's anger. The issue is, how can the physician be comfortable with an angry patient? Is the physician willing to learn how to be comfortable with an angry patient? Some physicians answer this question with "Yes, if I am sure the patient is in control of himself and will not hurt me." This is a diagnostic decision that needs to be addressed, but not in this chapter.

Whether or not a person is angry at a given moment is under his or her control. A person who chooses not to be angry cannot be made angry. Invitations to be angry may be ignored or viewed as just idiosyncrasies. Also, attention can be focused on what might motivate others to send out such behavioral signals or invitations. Any of these techniques will effectively help a person avoid becoming angry.

Understanding anger as a feeling under the control of the individual suggests a way to manage it. An additional factor to consider is how the person uses anger in the interpersonal process. Anger is frequently used as blackmail: "If you do . . . , I will be angry and when I get angry you'd better watch out!" Anger is also frequently used as an attempt to control the behavior of others. Thus, the treatment of anger is to acknowledge it and then ignore it with a statement such as "You sure are angry. If you want to be angry it's okay with me." And if it fits, "I really think it is kind of dumb to stay angry in this situation."

These statements acknowledge the anger, accept the patient's being angry, and avoid being a part of the game with subsequent payoff. The physician might follow these statements with "If you want to look at how you make yourself so angry, I am willing to look at it with you," or "I will be happy to refer you to someone who will help you find a way to be more comfortable rather than angry."

MANIPULATIVE OR DEMANDING PATIENT. A manipulative patient is skilled in getting something from other people by using a variety of artful maneuvers, such as threats to produce a fit of temper, attempts at suicide that are aimed at influencing others, and behavior that otherwise plays on the guilt of others, such as seduction.

The second issue is, "Can I accept the patient's being manipulative?" or "Can I out-manipulate the patient for his own good?" The issue of manipulation becomes potentially pathologic when the patient becomes dishonest or deceives the physician as a way to obtain more drugs, hospital admission, unwarranted surgery, or some special treatment. At this level of manipulation, consultation with a psychiatrist or someone who knows how to manage such patients may be needed. Most manipulative patients can be managed by the family physician by the use of a very specific contract regarding the issues of discomfort, such as demands to be seen after hours or unnecessary night calls.

MODIFYING PERSONAL REACTIONS TO PROBLEM PATIENTS.   The key to changing behavior is for the physician to ask, "How?" When the process, mechanism, or procedure for the behavior, in this case interview style, is understood, it is possible to change some part or all of the process, mechanism, or procedure to initiate a new behavior.

For example, if a physician becomes angry with a patient and wishes to change this feeling, the question should be asked, "How did I make myself angry?" or "How did I interpret the patient's statements or behavior to make myself angry?" or "What meaning did I assign to the patient's behavior?" Once these "How" and "What" questions are answered, the physician can ask, "Is there another way to interpret the patient's behavior?" or "Would I still be angry if I interpreted the behavior another way and gave it a different meaning?"

The conclusive step to institute change is to decide to interpret the behavior in another way and decide to feel something other than anger the next time the physician is faced with the patient's behavior. This process involves asking: (1) How do the physician's behavior or feelings come about? (2) What meaning is assigned to the patient's behavior? (3) How can the perception of the behavior be interpreted differently? The process also involves (4) deciding on an alternative way to interpret the behavior to initiate change. This process of change is key to improving medical interviewing skills.

CONCLUSION

The medical interview is a key element to success and should be an integral part of the family physician's armamentarium. Though some physicians appear to be natural interviewers, most who are deemed to be skilled developed their art through practice and vigilance.

If medical education does not provide adequate opportunities for developing and practicing the skills of interviewing, the student can learn a great deal by observing skillful interviewers working with patients. However, nothing substitutes for active, "do-it-yourself," hands-on experience with real or programmed patients. The physician who is serious about developing and maintaining his or her interviewing skills will utilize every opportunity to experiment with various responses that enhance the contact with patients and facilitate mutual satisfaction.

GLOSSARY OF TERMS AND INTERVIEW RESPONSES

bridging phrase—a phrase that provides direction and/or continuity. An interview is created from a number of merging topics. The professional guides and directs the selection of topics through many of the interviewer's verbal and nonverbal communications and by deliberately changing (or preventing the patient from changing) the topic. The interviewer may use phrases to tie one topic logically to the next or may specifically state, "Now I want to move to a different topic."

confrontation—a response that points out to the patient his or her feeling, behavior, or previous statement. Confrontations are most effective in focusing the patient's attention upon his or her feeling, behavior, or statement. They may also let the patient know you understand what he or she said. Many times a special inflection or insinuation is made in repeating his or her statement to emphasize a part of it.

direct question—a response that asks for a specific bit of information. A direct question can usually be answered in one word or a brief phrase.

empathy—a response that recognizes or names the patient's feeling and does not in any way criticize it, accepting the feeling in the patient even though the interviewer may believe the feeling to be wrong or uncalled for.

facilitation—a verbal or nonverbal communication that encourages the patient to say more, yet does not specify the area or topic to be discussed.

final statement—a succinct survey of what the interviewer has learned from the interview. It is a summary. It contains information to which the interviewer and patient have already agreed. It is not controversial. The final statement is positive rather than negative. Critical comments or an unfavorable prognosis are avoided.

interpretation—a confrontation that is based upon two or more events presented by the patient in a manner to tie the events together.

laundry-list—a question that gives a patient a list of more than three descriptive words to define his or her sensations, aches, or pains. A modification of the laundry-list question can be used to draw out a patient to tell you more. When the list is limited to two items, both of which are absurd, the patient must then clarify his or her position.

multiple questions—a double or triple question in one phrase. Multiple questions have one specific use and many difficulties. The one specific use is to encourage a quiet patient to take responsibility and talk more freely. By asking multiple questions, the patient (if he or she can remember all of the questions) is encouraged to start talking and to continue talking until all of the questions are answered. This is used to avoid short answers from the patient. When it works it can be very effective; however, the multiple question approach often confuses the patient, who may feel rushed, put down, confused, or pushed. If any of these feelings are present, the patient is NOT likely to give meaningful information.

open-ended question—a question asking for information from the patient and specifying the content in general terms.

patient question—a patient-initiated inquiry. Patients ask questions for many different reasons. When a patient asks a question during data gathering, the patient is occasionally asking for objective information. More often patient questions are asked for other reasons, which are not always clear. It helps to check the question out and understand what information or support the patient is really asking for.

physically parting—a part of closing the interview. How to get out of the room, whether to shake hands, and so forth may be the most awkward and the most difficult part of an interview for both the patient and the interviewer. However, parting is the natural conclusion to the mutually successful experience if the patient's anticipated needs have been met. The physical parting is initiated when the interviewer rises and opens the office door for the patient.

prescription for action—a statement that gives the patient a constructive plan. There is a distinction between a prescription for action and the giving of advice. A prescription for action should be based upon medical knowledge. Advice is often based upon little more than a hunch or a personal feeling.

probing—a response that may restate a question in a different way using different words or may even ask the same question. In telling about their symptoms, patients do not give you all the details you need. Once they have told you about a phase of the illness, it may be necessary to probe for more specific information.

problem question—a response that poses a problem in the form of a question. It requests the patient to use some aspect of his or her mental functions to answer. Examination of the sensorium usually involves problem questions and includes evaluation of the person's mathematical ability, abstract reasoning, orientation, judgment, memory, information, and attention.

reassurance—a response that tends to establish the sense of merit, well-being, or self-reliance in the patient.

reflection—a response that repeats, mirrors, or echoes a portion of what the patient just said. Although it focuses on a particular point, a reflection helps the patient to continue in his or her own style.

silence—a communication, a response. Those scientists who study communication report that we cannot fail to communicate. Silence can show interest or lack of interest; it can also show support or withdrawal. Most useful to the professional are the supportive silence and the interested silence.

suicide—is such an important topic, that it is included in the glossary. The rule is, "If in doubt, ask." Should you have any suspicion that the patient is suicidal, ask about his or her plans for the future, whether or not he or she plans to live, if he or she plans to end his or her life, any way you are able to. If you believe from the patient's answer that he or she may be suicidal, get professional help for the patient.

suggestive questions—questions that give away or suggest to the patient what answer you expect.

summation—a response of an interviewer that reviews information given by the patient. This is useful in closing the interview and/or moving from one topic to another.

support—a response that shows interest in, concern for, or understanding of the patient.

yes-no questions—direct questions that can be answered "Yes" or "No." Their value is extremely limited in obtaining reliable information, and it takes a lot of them to elicit sufficient information to assess the patient's problem.

Why questions—questions that start with the word "Why." A "Why" question has two qualities. First, the receiver of the question is placed on the defensive. Second, the answer to a "Why" question is a "Because." Since we are not always capable of understanding our own behavior, the "Because" answer is the most socially acceptable the patient can provide. It is an alibi, an excuse, or, in professional terms, a rationalization. Rationalizations are of interest to some but are of little or no value in the professional interview or interaction.

QUESTIONS

Pick the one best answer to each question.

1. Once you have learned from the nurse or secretary why the patient has come for the visit, it is best to
   a. Open the interview with a direct question about the problem the patient has previously identified.
   b. Wait for the patient to say something.
   c. Make a comment about a current event in the community to learn how the patient stands on an important issue.
   d. Use an open-ended question that will allow the patient to introduce a different topic from what was previously identified.
   e. Make a summary statement about what you know about the patient from the chart.

2. Of the following interviewing responses, the one most likely to put the patient on the defensive, that is, make the patient feel that his or her problem or behavior must be justified and/or defended is
   a. A laundry-list question.
   b. The use of silence.
   c. Beginning the question with "Why."
   d. A direct question.
   e. An open-ended question.

3. The most important part of a communication between two individuals is thought to be
   a. The speaker's intent.
   b. The choice of words.
   c. The style of the speaker.
   d. The voice quality.
   e. The receiver's understanding.

4. Of the following interviewing responses, the one that does not interfere with the gathering of important information from the defensive patient is
   a. Ignore the defensiveness and proceed with the questions.
   b. Comment on the patient's reluctance to talk about the topic and ask what would help the patient talk about it.
   c. Move forward in your chair and show more interest.
   d. Tell the patient there is nothing to fear in discussing the topic.
   e. Tell the patient that you are a professional and he or she can talk about anything with you.

5. An empathic response is best defined by
   a. A response that shows the interviewer's feeling to be the same as that of the patient.
   b. A response that names the patient's feeling and shows approval that the feeling is a correct one to have in the situation.
   c. A response that recognizes the patient's feeling and allows the patient to have the feeling.

   d. A response that names the patient's feeling and points out the rationale for having the feeling.

   e. A response that ignores the content of what the patient just said and neither criticizes nor accepts the patient's feeling.

6. "And then?" is usually considered to be a(n)

   a. Direct question.

   b. Open-ended question.

   c. Facilitation.

   d. Reflection.

   e. Supportive question.

Match each of the following interviewing responses according to the level of freedom or latitude a patient has in responding.

   a. Patient can initiate a wide variety of topics and various kinds of information.

   b. Patient has some latitude about subject but has been provided some guidance of the subject area the physician wishes to discuss.

   c. Patient is directed to a specific area of information.

7. Direct question

8. Facilitation

9. Open-ended question

10. Reflection

11. Laundry-list

12. Empathic

13. Yes-no question

14. Silence

15. Problem question

16. Summation

Which of the following are true statements?

17. The face-to-face medical interview, while costly and time-consuming when compared with computer programs and questionnaires, persists because

   a. Adequate computer programs have not yet been written.

   b. Patients insist on face-to-face contact.

   c. More reliable information can be obtained from an interview.

   d. A treatment contract is established in the interview.

   e. A relationship is established between the physician and patient.

18. The interview process or the style of the interview affects the

   a. Patient's confidence in the physician.

   b. Patient compliance and outcome in the treatment process.

   c. Efficiency by which meaningful information is obtained.

   d. Types of responses that a physician makes during an interview.

19. When a patient shows a strong emotion such as anger during an interview, the physician can be most effective by:

   a. Telling the patient to get control of his or her emotions.

   b. Allowing the patient to have and to express (within reason, safely) the emotion.

   c. Learning to ignore strong feelings in patients.

   d. Helping the patient recognize, understand, and deal with the emotion.

20. Closing an interview may be uncomfortable because

   a. The patient may ask last-minute questions without time to go into them.

   b. Saying goodbye for many is an uncomfortable activity.

   c. The interviewer may not have a clear understanding of his or her task at that moment.

   d. Clear agreements may not have been reached and leaving business unfinished may be uncomfortable.

   e. Social gestures, embraces, and other parting rituals may not be appropriate in the social setting.

Answers appear on page 446.

PATIENT COMPLIANCE

C. EDWARD EVANS and R. BRIAN HAYNES

Compliance is now becoming an everyday term in medical practice. Fifteen years ago medical students and practising physicians alike would have been more familiar with the term in its engineering context, for example, when referring to *lung compliance* during ventilation in anesthesia. Surprisingly, Hippocrates recognized that patients did not always follow the advice of their physicians: "[The physician] should keep aware of the fact that patients often lie when they state that they have taken certain medicines." More than 90% of the literature on compliance has been published since the early 1970s. Thus, although physicians have dispensed medicines and potions through the centuries in vast quantities, it is only in recent years that there has been systematic examination of whether patients actually take the treatment.

This interest in patient compliance seems to parallel the introduction of more and more efficacious medications. Whether or not this is by chance, it was perhaps to the patient's benefit in the past that little attention was paid to compliance, as poor compliance may well have saved the patient's life on many occasions. Some treatments, especially the massive purges and bleedings of the eighteenth century and the use of arsenic and hydrochloric acid in this century, certainly had more lethal than therapeutic potential. Such lessons of the past should not be forgotten in considering compliance today, as we still prescribe many treatments of dubious value. Nevertheless, our armamentarium of useful treatments is now sizable and continues to expand; low patient compliance stands squarely in the way of achieving the full benefit of modern therapy.

The extent of poor compliance is disquieting. Fifty percent is a representative compliance figure for many classes of long-term therapy. Only about two-thirds of those who continue under care take enough of their prescribed medication to achieve adequate blood pressure control (Haynes, Sackett, et al.). The figures for compliance with diets and lifestyle changes such as stopping smoking are much worse (Best and Block). For example, when asked to give up smoking, only about 4% of patients will be able to do so and remain successful for a year.

Added to this, physicians—even family physicians—are not good at estimating compliance levels in patients (Gilbert et al.). Physicians have a strong tendency to overestimate the compliance of their own patients and are usually unable to predict which patients will comply with treatment.

Fortunately, the story does not end here. There are practical methods of detecting poor compliance and strategies for improving it.

DEFINITIONS

Compliance has been defined as the extent to which a person's behavior (keeping appointments, taking medications, and executing lifestyle changes) coincides with medical advice. Poor compliance is more difficult to define. What percentage of prescribed medication can a patient forget or omit before being classed as a poor complier? How are patients who take too much medication classified? One way of looking at the problem is to use patient outcomes as a guide. For instance, in hypertension studies patients taking 80% or more of prescribed medication were considered compliant because this amount of medication is required to produce systematic blood pressure reduction (Sackett et al.). It makes sense that efforts directed at poor compliers should be concentrated on those not achieving therapeutic goals. This obviously makes for more efficient use of resources. However, this pragmatic approach is not entirely satisfactory, in that some patients who respond to treatment may be doing so because of overprescribing rather than good compliance. In the hospital or in other situations in which compliance may be nearly 100%, they may experience serious effects of overdose.

FACTORS INFLUENCING COMPLIANCE

In looking at the many factors involved in compliance, there is a natural tendency for physicians to feel that poor compliance is the patient's fault. In the final analysis this may be true. After all, it is the patient who must

TABLE 11–1. INFLUENCES ON COMPLIANCE

MAJOR FACTORS INFLUENCING COMPLIANCE	FACTORS NOT AFFECTING COMPLIANCE
Psychiatric diagnosis (−)	Age
Degree of disability (+)	Gender
Amount of supervision (+)	Intelligence/education
Duration of disease/treatment (−)	Economic status
Complexity/demands of treatment (−)	Knowledge (for long-term treatments)
Form of treatment (see text)	
Meeting the patient's expectations (+)	
Patient satisfaction with care (+)	

The sign in the bracket indicates a positive (+) or negative (−) relationship with compliance.

swallow the pill, but there are many other factors leading up to the final act of pill-taking. For instance, what about the disease or condition being treated: Is it symptomatic or asymptomatic? Life-threatening or merely a nuisance? And the treatment: Is it unpleasant, inconvenient, or expensive? Does it work? Is the environment in which the treatment is prescribed conducive to regular follow-up? Does the physician inspire confidence in the treatment? Do his or her attitudes interfere with compliance? All of these factors could have important effects on compliance behavior, but, as we shall see, only some of them do.

The Patient

The sociodemographic characteristics or attitudes of the patient have received a great deal of attention, and such attributes as age, sex, marital status, education, intelligence, and economic status bear no consistent relationship to compliance. Two exceptions, for age, are the very young and the very old, whose compliance characteristics tend to conform to those of their caretakers. Economic status can affect access to medical care, but once a patient is in care it does not consistently affect compliance.

Perhaps the most widely held theory of compliance behavior, probably because of its intuitive appeal, is that of the "communications" approach (Leventhal et al.). In this model it is proposed that patients generally do not know enough about their illness or treatment, and that it is this ignorance that leads to poor compliance. It follows that adequate instruction should result in improved compliance. While it appears that this is true for short-term treatments (less than 2 weeks in duration), knowledge bears little relationship to compliance with chronic disease regimens (Haynes).

Another popular theory looks at patient motivation and beliefs. The Health Belief Model (Becker) argues that the likelihood of an individual's undertaking a recommended health action is dependent on his or her perception of the level of personal susceptibility to the particular illness or condition; the degree of severity of the consequences of contracting the condition; the potential benefits or efficacy of the treatment in preventing or reducing susceptibility and/or severity; and the physical, psychologic, financial, and other barriers or costs involved in initiating or continuing the treatment. The

model also requires a stimulus or "cue to action" to trigger the appropriate behavior. This model has been shown to have predictive value for some preventive and short-term therapeutic health actions, such as immunizations and medical regimens for acute disease, but the extent of its predictive value is modest at best.

Other models have been studied, including the behavioral learning model and the self-regulating model, but as yet no model has been developed that adequately explains a person's compliance behavior or gives a clear rationale for modifying it.

The Disease

With a few exceptions, disease factors are relatively unimportant as determinants of compliance. Psychiatric patients with schizophrenia, paranoid features, and personality disorders are less compliant than other psychiatric patients, a fact that probably accounts for the lower compliance of psychiatric patients compared with patients with nonpsychiatric disorders.

Surprisingly, no relationship has been demonstrated between the severity of symptoms and compliance, but the *more* symptoms a patient reports, the *lower* his or her compliance is likely to be. On the other hand, increasing disability produced by a disease appears to be associated with better compliance. Whether this is a result of increased severity of disease or simply the result of the *increased supervision* that often accompanies increased disability has not been examined directly.

Chronic diseases requiring long-term treatment have been clearly shown to result in increasingly poor compliance. This fact is of great clinical importance in such potentially serious diseases as tuberculosis and hypertension and is more likely to be a function of the duration of the *treatment* regimen than the duration of the *disease* itself.

The Regimen

On the whole, the greater the behavioral demands of a treatment, the poorer the compliance. This means that regimens requiring changes in lifestyle such as dieting, exercising, and stopping bad habits result in much poorer compliance than simply taking pills.

Nevertheless, it is quite clear that the greater the number of drugs or treatments prescribed for a patient, the greater the probability of poor compliance. While the frequency of pill-taking is not so important, it also has an effect in that patients are less likely to comply with a regimen requiring four or more doses a day than with one requiring one or two daily doses.

Although alternative oral medications for the same condition do not appear to result in substantial differences in compliance, there does appear to be a difference between different treatments for different problems. This ranges from 17% compliance with antacids to 89% with cardiac drugs (Closson and Kikugawa).

One form of alternative treatment that has been shown to have a beneficial effect is the injection of long-acting parenteral preparations. Examples of this are the use of benzathine penicillin for acute streptococcal pharyngitis and rheumatic fever prophylaxis and long-acting phenothiazines for schizophrenia, both of which have been shown to be both acceptable to patients and more successful than oral preparations. This has also been demonstrated with twice-weekly injections of streptomycin for tuberculosis. The fact that diabetics comply so poorly with self-injected insulin suggests that the success of long-acting preparations is less likely to be due to their parenteral nature than to the medical supervision necessary to administer them.

Another disappointment for intuitive reasoning is the fact that there is very little evidence that side effects of treatment are a major cause of poor compliance. Studies have shown that there is no difference in the reported frequency of side effects between compliers and noncompliers. In studies in which patients were asked for reasons for their noncompliance, only 5% to 10% implicated side effects (Glick; Rickels et al.).

The cost of treatment is an important barrier to compliance for many people, although the total effect of cost is not as obvious as might first appear. For instance, one study showed that hospital admissions *increased* among psychiatric outpatients given drugs at nominal cost compared to a group paying regular prices (Cody and Robinson).

The Physician

The physician is obviously in a key position to influence compliance. After all, it is the physician who initiates the treatment in the majority of cases. For example, if the frequency of dose affects compliance, then by the very act of prescribing a four-times-a-day regimen the physician is potentially reducing compliance below the level achievable with a prescription requiring a single daily dose.

More complex than the mechanics of prescribing, however, is the interaction between physician and patient. Patients are more likely to comply with treatment if their expectations are met by the visit and if they are well satisfied with their care. The concept of a personal physician or the feeling of knowing a physician well has also been associated with increased compliance. The problem is that dissecting the physician–patient relationship and measuring factors resulting in increased satisfaction are not easy. This is demonstrated in one study in which some patients felt they knew their physician *well* after only one visit, while others felt they still did not know their physicians after as many as *fourteen* visits (Ettlinger and Freeman).

DETECTION OF POOR COMPLIANCE

Clinical Judgment

Most of us would like to believe that a good physician can detect poor compliance in his or her patients; surely this goes along with increasing clinical experience. Unfortunately, studies have shown that this is not the case: using clinical judgment has been shown to be no better than flipping a coin as a detection method. The first studies demonstrating this were carried out in specialty settings and with physicians who did not have an ongoing relationship with patients. Unfortunately, the hope that family physicians with their ongoing relationships with their patients might be in a better position to make predictions has also been dispelled. Family physicians were not only unable to detect poor compliers among their patients, but the length of time they had known their patients had no effect on their ability to predict.

The emphasis on the unreliability of clinical judgment is important in that it serves to direct us to a more systematic approach to detection of poor compliance.

Monitoring Attendance

As referred to previously, over 50% of hypertensives stop visiting their physicians within a year of starting treatment, and patients who do not keep follow-up appointments are unlikely to comply with treatment. What is not so obvious, however, is that many physicians are unable to detect this type of noncompliance because their appointment systems are inadequate or because the patients do not take the step of making an appointment in the first place.

It follows, then, that an important method of detecting poor compliance is to watch the appointment book and day sheet. Although there is no guarantee that pa-

TABLE 11–2. DETECTING NONCOMPLIANCE

ASKING THE PATIENT

The easiest way to detect noncompliance is to ask the patient.

About 50% of noncompliant patients will admit to missing at least some medication.

If a patient admits to noncompliance, you can believe him or her.

Patients admitting to poor compliance are most responsive to attempts to improve compliance.

HOW TO ASK

Use "matter-of-fact," nonjudgmental, nonthreatening manner.

Use an introduction that allows a patient to "save face."

"Most people find it difficult to remember to take medicines. About how often do you forget yours?"

Source: Rakel RE. Textbook of Family Practice. 4th ed. Philadelphia, W.B. Saunders, 1990, with permission.

tients who keep appointments will comply with treatment, those who do not appear for follow-up have usually stopped taking their treatments as well. The importance of monitoring attendance cannot be overstressed: dropping out of care is one of the most frequent and most severe forms of noncompliance.

Response to Treatment

Provided that the treatment prescribed is known to be efficacious, failure of a patient to respond to treatment can be used as a readily available indicator of compliance levels. However, this method of assessing compliance is not infallible. For example, patients who appear to respond to treatment may do so because they were misdiagnosed or because their physicians' overprescribing is compensating for their poor compliance. Nevertheless, from the compliance perspective at least, there is less need to be concerned about patients who have reached the therapeutic goal. On the other hand, patients not showing a response to treatment will include patients who genuinely do not respond to therapy or who have been prescribed inadequate amounts and will also include a high proportion of poor compliers or noncompliers. Further detection methods are desirable positively to identify the latter.

Asking the Patient

Although it is not always reliable, asking the patient directly about compliance can be a very valuable and practical way of determining the pattern of medication consumption. When asked directly, about half of noncompliant patients will admit to missing at least some medication (Haynes, Taylor, et al). One can be assured that it is highly improbable that a *compliant* patient will admit to poor compliance, so patients admitting to missing medication have a very high likelihood of being poor compliers. The converse is not true, however, as even under optimal interview conditions about half of noncompliant patients will deny the fact. In addition, patients who admit to missing medication generally overestimate the amount of medication they do take. In one study, the average overestimate was in the region of 20%.

It must be emphasized that the method of questioning is of paramount importance. Asking in a threatening or belligerent manner, "*Of course, you are taking your pills, aren't you?*" will result in reflex affirmation. Approaching the patient with a face-saving, nonthreatening, nonjudgmental question will yield a higher proportion of accurate responses. For example: "*Most people find it difficult to remember to take medicines. Did you miss any of your pills during the last week?*" If the answer is affirmative, ask the patient to estimate the exact number of missed pills. Because of patients' tendency to overestimate compliance, it is important to take into account that admission of any noncompliance implies a compliance rate of less than 80%.

The methods of detecting low compliance described so far can be easily applied in any treatment setting and if applied with care will detect the majority of poor compliers. The following methods may be of help in detecting some of the remainder.

Counting Pills

As a method of providing a quantitative estimate of compliance over a period of time, pill counts can be relatively reliable so long as they are carried out in the patient's home with strict attention to bookkeeping (Haynes, Taylor, et al.). Unless the count can be carried out in such a manner that the patient is unaware of what is going on, it becomes a one-time-only procedure. Using pill counts in the office or clinic will result in a bias in the direction of overestimating compliance, in that many patients will consciously or unconsciously bring only *some* of their unused pills with them, giving the appearance that they have taken more medication than is actually the case, or they will "forget" to bring their pills or to come themselves.

Drug Levels

For some drugs, especially those with long serum half-lives resulting in relatively steady serum levels, the measurement of serum levels can be an extremely useful indication of compliance. The best examples are digoxin and phenytoin, for which plasma levels have been used successfully both to monitor compliance and to improve it through feedback to the patient. Other drugs commonly measured in this way are phenobarbitone and other anticonvulsants, theophylline, tricyclic antidepressants, lithium, and a variety of cardiac drugs. The caution is, however, that there is a great deal of individual variation in drug absorption, metabolism, and excretion. In addition, serum levels of drugs with short half-lives only indicate how recently a dose was taken and give no information on long-term compliance.

PREVENTION AND TREATMENT OF POOR COMPLIANCE

Misconceptions

Before discussing prevention and treatment, it is timely to reexamine some popular misconceptions about compliance.

The first misconception is that a good clinician can identify poor compliers. In fact, clinical judgment has a poor record of detecting compliance levels. *There is no stereotypical poor complier.* This is very important, because restricting prevention and treatment strategies to patients thought to be potentially poor compliers must result in neglect of a large number of patients who need attention, as well as unnecessary attention to some patients who do not require it.

Another popular and important misconception is that all that stops patients from being nearly perfect compliers is their ignorance of either the condition being treated or the treatment being used. While there is some

TABLE 11–3. KEYS TO SUCCESSFUL COMPLIANCE MANAGEMENT

DETECTION

Monitor attendance and achievement of the therapeutic goal.

Ask the patient.

PREVENTION

Make appointments convenient.

Simplify the regimen.

Give clear instructions, preferably written.

Make the patient an active participant

TREATMENT

Follow up nonattenders.

Increase attention and supervision.

Use cueing, feedback, and positive reinforcement.

Titrate frequency of visits to compliance need.

Involve spouse or other partner.

Maintain compliance interventions as long as compliance is desirable.

Source: Rakel RE. Textbook of Family Practice. 4th ed. Philadelphia, W.B. Saunders, 1990, with permission.

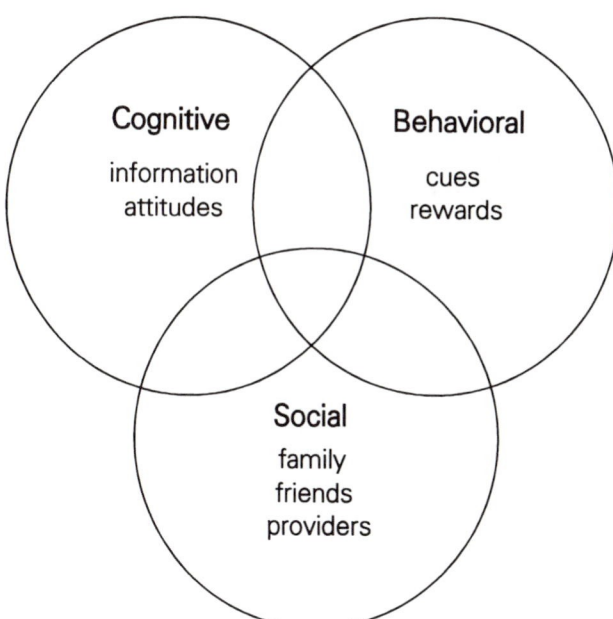

Figure 11–1. Factors influencing compliance.

evidence that written instructions help improve compliance for short-term regimens, even "mastery learning," in which patients were given detailed, step-by-step instruction on hypertension, had no beneficial effect on long-term compliance (Sackett et al.). The belief that it is possible to scare a patient into complying with treatment has also been dispelled (Leventhal et al.).

Although these popular beliefs have been discredited, the methods most commonly employed by physicians to improve compliance are predominantly those that have been found lacking. Methods that *have* been shown to be effective are not generally applied. Furthermore, changing the long-term behavior of physicians to manage compliance successfully cannot be done by simply informing or instructing them about efficacious interventions (Evans et al.; Haynes, Davis, et al.).

Figure 11–1 provides a framework for thinking about strategies for helping patients to comply. Success for long-term treatments generally requires adopting tactics from at least two of the areas in the figure. Thus, while addressing cognitive factors (providing the patient with clear information about the reason and administration of the treatment) is usually sufficient for a course of treatment that lasts 1 to 2 weeks, for longer treatments instruction must be supplemented by periodic reminders (cues) and reinforcement (rewards), and the patient's family may have to be recruited to help out. The details of the various approaches follow.

Prevention

The main thrust in the prevention of poor compliance is to remove barriers to compliance. Preventing patients from dropping out from care is of primary importance.

Longer waiting times are associated with higher "no-show" rates, so one aim is to keep patient waiting time to a minimum. Individual appointments at mutually convenient times help to achieve this goal. A system for follow-up, ensuring that patients leave the office with a *specific time* for a future appointment rather than with instructions to call for an appointment in, for example, 3 months, makes detection of those who do drop out much easier.

Simplifying the treatment regimen will remove another barrier to compliance. An essential element of this approach is to *eliminate unnecessary medications*. In addition, medications should be prescribed that need to be taken as few times daily as possible. The frequency of dosing with many drugs can be reduced below usually prescribed levels with no reduction in efficacy. For example, tricyclic antidepressants can be given as a single bedtime dose, thus reducing dosing frequency and timing side effects so that they occur mainly during sleep. A final strategy is to prescribe the least amount of medication necessary to achieve the therapeutic goal.

It has been shown that patients who feel that they are actively involved in their own care are better compliers than those who do not (Schulman). Studies have also shown that negotiating care with the patient rather than simply dictating or prescribing it results in better compliance (Eisenthal et al.; Tracy). Encouraging patients to take greater responsibility for their care by asking more questions of their physicians results in improved attendance (Roter). It follows that encouraging patients to participate in and take more responsibility for their own care is another strategy for preventing poor compliance, and it not only makes scientific sense but follows contemporary trends in physician–patient relationships.

Treatment

Dropping out of care constitutes a *compliance crisis.* Mail and telephone reminders to increase attendance, at least in the short term, can help prevent dropout. If the patient does fail to attend, it calls for prompt action by the receptionist or office nurse to reschedule nonattenders (Takala et al.). Personal contact of persistent nonattenders by the physician or the use of outreach services such as visiting nurses are other ways of "treating" nonattendance.

Low compliance is a chronic condition without a "one-shot" cure, so treatment of poor compliance must continue as long as the regimen of prescribed treatment. To make matters worse, none of the following has improved compliance when tested *alone:* special learning packages and pamphlets, special unit-dose "reminder" pill packaging, counseling about medication and compliance by a health educator or nurses, visits to patients' homes, provision of care at the worksite, self-monitoring of blood pressure, tangible rewards, and group discussions. Although these tactics have not worked alone, many have been part of more complex interventions that have been successful; whether they are essential parts of these complex interventions or just "along for the ride" is difficult to say.

Most successful compliance interventions have two features in common: *increased supervision* of, or attention to, the patient; and *intentional reinforcement,* reward, or encouragement of compliance (Haynes, Wang, et al.).

A variety of inducements to comply have been successful when combined with one another, including feedback of blood pressure response to hypertensive patients either by the provider or by the patient taking his or her own blood pressure, small tangible rewards for improved compliance and/or therapeutic response, medication tailored to daily schedules to decrease forgetting and inconvenience, encouragement of family support, stimulation of self-help through group support and discussion, negotiation of a brief written contract with the patient to improve health behavior, and calling back patients who miss appointments.

Many individuals other than physicians have taken an effective part in this process. Nurses, pharmacists, health educators, psychologists, and even individuals with no formal health training have played a key role in successful interventions.

In summary, the treatment of poor compliance involves many approaches. For short-term treatments, simple, clear instructions are sufficient. For longer-term treatments, there must be follow-up of nonattenders by telephone or mailed reminders. In addition, the practitioner must increase attention to, and supervision, of poor compliers and provide rewards or positive reinforcement for good compliance, such as simple praise and extending the time between appointments for those responding to treatment. Inui et al. have shown that most of these maneuvers can be incorporated with success into regular practice by simply focusing on compliance for a few moments during each encounter with the patient, emphasizing the importance of following the regimen, and tailoring medication to daily routines. This can be accomplished without necessarily prolonging the visit. And, most important, it is clear that all compliance interventions applied to noncompliers must be maintained as long as treatment is prescribed.

ETHICAL ISSUES

"Am I my brother's keeper?" (Genesis 4:9). This question highlights the dilemma in which most physicians find themselves when they are pressed to extend their compliance-improving strategies beyond the office visit. As with most questions of ethics, there is no easy answer.

The decision to apply tactics deliberately designed to change the compliance behavior of patients should meet the same types of ethical standards that apply to all therapeutic interventions (Levine). First, the diagnosis must be correct. Second, the therapy to be complied with must be of established efficacy. Third, neither the illness nor the proposed treatment should be trivial. Fourth, the patient must be an informed and willing partner in any attempt to alter his or her compliance. Finally, the method employed to improve compliance must also be of demonstrated effectiveness.

Having applied these standards and embarked upon a course of treatment, it makes no sense, ethically or otherwise, for the physician to abandon a patient at the first sign of poor compliance. Most physicians consider it *unethical* to withhold efficacious treatment from a patient with a serious physical disease. Why then should it be *ethical* to consider withholding treatment when the condition is *noncompliance?*

THE FUTURE

The advent of the personal computer has resulted in increasing use of microcomputers and microcomputer networks in physicians' offices. While initial applications have been for business and office management purposes, the computerization of health records affords a potential for monitoring patient compliance and assisting in the management of poor compliers.

Computerized appointment systems make it possible to provide patients with appointment times for long periods ahead and can be modified to flag nonattenders and produce automatic reminders. The ability to record age, sex, and diagnoses makes it possible to design a system that can improve *provider* compliance with screening and preventive maneuvers (Bypass et al.). Medication systems that store prescribing information can form the basis of a system that monitors whether patients are at least requesting prescription refills on time (Steiner et al.). The potential is great, but it will require both effort and expense by physicians or collaboration with pharmacists to make it work.

What of other advancements? The technology that brought us the efficacious treatments is also helping with compliance—drugs with long half-lives, long-acting parenteral preparations, conjunctival inserts, continuous transcutaneous absorption, insulin pumps, all are designed to make compliance easier, and more are on the drawing board.

CONCLUSION

In dealing with compliance we have consciously concentrated on medication, emphasizing long-term medications. This is not because we feel that noncompliance with short-term medications is inconsequential or that there is no problem of compliance with lifestyle or other behavioral changes. On the contrary, both of these areas are very important, and in fact noncompliance with lifestyle changes is a monster yet to be tamed.

The approaches to treatment we suggest are practical and well within the reach of practicing physicians. At last, after centuries of ineffectual ministrations, we have treatments that actually work; it behooves us, as providers of those treatments, to give them every opportunity to be effective.

The past decade, more than any other, has brought the therapist together with the patient, the family, and other members of the health care team in jointly working toward the full effectiveness of potent treatments. The rewards of this alliance are great—reduction of morbidity, disability, and preventable deaths.

REFERENCES

Becker MH. Sociobehavioral determinants of compliance. In Sackett DL, Haynes RB (eds.): Compliance with Therapeutic Regimens. Baltimore, Johns Hopkins University Press, 1976, pp. 40–49.

Best JA, Block M. Compliance in the control of cigarette smoking. In Haynes RB, Taylor DW, Sackett DL (eds.): Compliance in Health Care. Baltimore, Johns Hopkins University Press, 1979, pp. 202–222.

Bypass P, Hanlon PW, Hanlon LCS, et al. Microcomputer management of a vaccine trial. Comput Biol Med 1988; 18:179–193.

Closson R, Kikugawa C. Non-compliance varies with drug class. Hospitals 1975; 49:89.

Cody J, Robinson A. The effect of low-cost maintenance medication on the rehospitalization of schizophrenic outpatients. Am J Psych 1977; 134:73.

Eisenthal S, Emery R, Lazare A, et al. "Adherence" and the negotiated approach to patienthood. Arch Gen Psych 1979; 36:393.

Ettlinger PRA, Freeman GK. General practice compliance study: Is it worth being a personal doctor? Br Med J 1981; 282:1192.

Evans CE, Haynes RB, Birkett NJ, et al. Does a mailed continuing education program improve physician performance? Results of a randomized trial in antihypertensive care. JAMA 1984; 255:501–504.

Gilbert JR, Evans CE, Haynes RB, et al. Predicting compliance with a regimen of digoxin therapy in a family practice. Can Med Assoc J 1980; 123:119.

Glick BS: Dropout in an outpatient, double-blind drug study. Psychosomatics 1965; 6:44.

Haynes RB. Determinants of compliance: The disease and the mechanics of treatment. In Haynes RB, Taylor DW, Sackett DL (eds.): Compliance in Health Care. Baltimore, Johns Hopkins University Press, 1979, pp. 49–62.

Haynes RB, Davis DA, McKibbon A, et al. A critical appraisal of the efficacy of continuing medical education. JAMA 1984; 251:61–64.

Haynes RB, Sackett DL, Taylor DW. Practical management of low compliance with antihypertensive therapy: A guide for the busy practitioner. Clin Invest Med 1979; 1:175.

Haynes RB, Taylor DW, Sackett DL, et al. Can simple clinical measurements detect patient non-compliance? Hypertension 1980; 2:757.

Haynes RB, Wang E, Gomes MD. A critical review of interventions to improve compliance with prescribed medications. Patient Educ Counsel 1987; 10:155–166.

Inui T, Yourtee E, Williamson J. Improved outcomes in hypertension after physician tutorials. Ann Intern Med 1976, 84:646.

Leventhal H, Zimmerman R, Gutman M. Compliance: A self-regulation perspective. In Gentry D (ed.): Handbook of Behavioral Medicine. New York, Pergamon Press, 1984, pp. 369–434.

Levine RJ. Ethical considerations in the development and application of compliance strategies for the treatment of hypertension. In Haynes RB, Matteson ME, Engebretson TO, Jr. (eds.): Patient Compliance to Prescribed Antihypertensive Regimens. Washington, DC, U.S. Department of Health and Human Services, N.I.H. Publication No. 81-2102, 1980, pp. 229–246.

Rickels K, Boren R, Stuart HM. Controlled psychopharmacological research in general practice. J New Drugs 1964; 4:138.

Roter D. Patient participation in the patient-provider interaction: The effects of patient question asking on the quality of interaction, satisfaction and compliance. Health Educ Monogr 1977, 5:281.

Sackett DL, Haynes RB, Gibson ES, et al. Randomized clinical trial of strategies for improving medication compliance in primary hypertension. Lancet 1979; 1:1205.

Schulman B. Active patient orientation and outcomes in hypertensive treatment. Med Care 1979; 17:267.

Steiner JF, Koepsall TD, Fihn SD, et al. A general method of compliance assessment using centralized pharmacy records: Description and validation. Med Care 1988; 26(8):814–823.

Takala J, Niemela N, Rosti J, Sivers K. Improving compliance with therapeutic regimens in hypertensive patients in a community health center. Circulation 1979; 59:540.

Tracy J. Impact of intake procedures upon client attrition in a community mental health centre. J Consult Clin Psychol 1977; 45:192.

QUESTIONS

1. Which of the following patient factors affects compliance with medication?
   a. Gender
   b. Intelligence
   c. Economic status
   d. Disability
   e. Knowledge of long-term treatments

2. All of the following have a positive influence on compliance EXCEPT
   a. Degree of disability.
   b. Amount of supervision.
   c. Duration of treatment.
   d. Meeting patients' expectations.
   e. Patient satisfaction with care.

3. Which of the following has been shown to be ineffective in detecting poor compliance?
    a. Clinical judgment
    b. Asking the patient
    c. Monitoring response to treatment
    d. Counting pills
    e. Drug levels

4. All of the following maneuvers are useful in preventing poor compliance EXCEPT
    a. Making appointments convenient.
    b. Simplifying the regimen.
    c. Giving clear written instructions.
    d. Warning about the dangers of missing pills.
    e. Making the patient an active participant.

5. Which of the following is NOT effective in treating poor compliance?
    a. Following up nonattenders
    b. Increasing attention and supervision
    c. Using cueing, feedback, and positive reinforcement
    d. Involving a spouse or other partner
    e. In-depth education about the treatment

Answers appear on page 446.

DISEASE PREVENTION

R. MICHAEL MORSE and WARREN A. HEFFRON

ROLE OF THE FAMILY PHYSICIAN

The family physician has a special opportunity to be an effective force in disease prevention and health promotion. As the primary care provider for all ages in family units, the family physician has an inherent obligation to screen for a broad range of risk factors associated with preventable diseases and encourage appropriate preventive measures such as proper diet and exercise. To be most effective, many preventive activities are applicable to the entire family unit. These broader, family-wide, disease prevention and health promotion activities serve as the foundation for more age-specific recommendations and interventions for each individual family member.

While other medical/surgical problem areas may occasionally require subspecialty consultation, the family physician is the specialist to whom patients and other specialists look for provision of this broad range of health promotion and disease prevention activities.

Preventive activities are traditionally classified according to the phase of the disease process in which intervention occurs: tertiary (disease diagnosed and symptoms present), secondary (disease present and diagnosable, but no symptoms present), and primary (no diagnosable disease and no symptoms present).

The bulk of medical education focuses on the already ill patient (tertiary prevention); progressively less time is spent on secondary and primary prevention. This may lead medical students and physicians to provide evaluation and treatment primarily in "reaction" to patient symptoms, rather than in a "proactive" mode of care—that is, attempting to anticipate problems and prevent them.

Physicians may encounter a variety of obstacles to providing comprehensive preventive health services, including severe demands on the physician's time by patients already ill, lack of financial resources in the patient population, negative third party attitudes toward reimbursement for preventive care, and patients uninformed about the benefits of prevention.

EVALUATING PREVENTIVE ACTIVITIES

Not all diseases lend themselves well to the shift from medical intervention at the tertiary level to the secondary or primary level. Several parameters are used to determine the validity of such a shift for each disease and to determine the population group to whom the intervention should be applied. The general criteria are:

1. Is the disease worth screening for? Does it have a significant impact on the quality or quantity of life, and is it of sufficient prevalence in the population to justify screening?
2. Is sufficient information available to accurately identify, using risk factors and screening tests, the individual or groups likely to develop the disease? Or using diagnostic tests, is it possible to identify those likely already to have the disease at a presymptomatic stage?
3. Are the tests for the screening or early detection satisfactory in terms of accuracy, morbidity, cost, and acceptability to the patient and physician?
4. If it is possible to predict the disease or diagnose it prior to the onset of symptoms, is there a known intervention that will significantly alter the course of the disease?
5. Is the intervention or treatment satisfactory in terms of proven effectiveness, risk, morbidity, cost, and patient acceptability.

Table 12–1 is a mortality table for the United States. From it one can begin to understand the relative impact of various diseases on death rates. Also, the trend over 10 years for each disease is shown, allowing the reader to assess the degree of progress in prevention and treatment. In particular, the decreases in mortality from heart disease, stroke, accidents, liver disease, and perinatal diseases are highly encouraging and are due primarily to preventive measures. On the other hand, the slight increase in cancer deaths is worrisome, and the marked increases in chronic pulmonary disease, pneumonia, and influenza are very frustrating when one considers how preventable these deaths are.

TABLE 12–1. PERCENT OF TOTAL DEATHS AND PERCENT CHANGE FROM 1979 TO 1988 FOR FIFTEEN LEADING CAUSES OF DEATH: UNITED STATES, 1988

RANK ORDER	CAUSE OF DEATH	PERCENT OF TOTAL DEATHS	PERCENT CHANGE 1979 TO 1988
1	Diseases of the heart	35.3	−16.6
2	Malignant neoplasms[a]	22.4	1.5
3	Cerebrovascular disease	6.9	−28.6
4	Accidents and adverse effects	4.5	−18.4
	Motor vehicle	(2.3)	−15.1
	All others	(2.2)	−21.9
5	Chronic obstructive pulmonary disease[b]	3.8	32.9
6	Pneumonia and influenza	3.6	26.8
7	Diabetes mellitus	1.9	3.1
8	Suicide	1.4	−2.6
9	Chronic liver disease and cirrhosis	1.2	−25.0
10	Nephritis, nephrotic syndrome, and nephrosis	1.0	11.6
11	Atherosclerosis	1.0	−40.4
12	Homicide and legal intervention	1.0	−11.8
13	Septicemia	1.0	100.0
14	Perinatal diseases	0.8	−30.9
15	HIV infection	0.8	

Source: National Center for Health Statistics, 1990, with permission.
[a]Includes neoplasms of lymphatic and hematopoietic tissues.
[b]Includes other allied conditions.

INTERVENTIONS AND RECOMMENDATIONS. The 1989 recommendations of the U.S. Preventive Services Task Force will be referred to in this chapter. The student should recognize that these recommendations are for preventive activities for which there is a high level of proof of value. There are many additional tests and interventions that are used by many physicians as a result of recommendations by other highly respected medical authorities and organizations. The reasons for additions to the basic recommendations include expert opinion, a prolonged wait for a study that would prove effectiveness, and alternative interpretation of studies that have already been completed.

PREVENTION APPLIED TO SPECIFIC DISEASES

Atherosclerotic Diseases

Coronary Heart Disease

INCIDENCE. An adult male in the United States has a one in five likelihood of having a myocardial infarction by 60 years of age, twice that of females. The yearly national incidence of myocardial infarction is 1.5 million.

The yearly incidence of newly diagnosed coronary heart disease (CHD) is shown in Table 12–2. The majority of individuals with severe atherosclerosis of their coronary arteries do not have angina pectoris as a warning, but present with either an acute myocardial infarction or sudden death.

PREVALENCE. It is estimated that 5 million people alive today have symptomatic CHD.

By 20–24 years of age, about 44% of white males, 34% of black males, 11% of white females, and 43% of black females have raised lesions in their coronary arteries. By

self-report in a 1982 survey, 2.7%, or over six million Americans, have symptomatic CHD. A number of studies of angiographic and autopsy data estimate a prevalence of significant CHD (50% stenosis of at least one major vessel) in 4% to 4.5% of all asymptomatic adults. These autopsy studies show a range from 1.9% in 30- to 39-year-old men to 12.3% in men 60–69. Women in the same age groups ranged from 0.3% to 7.5%.

Although difficult, predicting the prevalence in *asymptomatic* adults is of importance to the physician if early aggressive intervention is to be targeted to the appropriate patients. These high-risk groups are identified by an analysis of the risk factors present for CHD.

COST/IMPACT ON SOCIETY. It is estimated that the cost of medical treatment and lost productivity for all cardiovascular disease in the United States in 1990 was $94.5 billion.

MORBIDITY/MORTALITY. CHD causes 28% of *all* deaths and 40% of deaths in the 35- to 64-year-old age group. Overall case fatality rate is 30% for the first and 50% for subsequent myocardial infarctions. Of those surviving, 13% of males and 40% of females will have a second infarct within 5 years. Ten-year survival for males is 50% and for females 30%. Two-thirds of myo-

TABLE 12–2. ANNUAL DIAGNOSIS OF NEW CORONARY HEART DISEASE

	MALE	FEMALE
Angina	420	370
Myocardial infarction	710	220
Sudden death	160	60
Total	1290	650

Incidence rates per 100,000 of new onset coronary heart disease by presenting signs and symptoms in U.S., ages 35–84. (From Framingham Study data: Kannel WB, Thom TJ, Hurst JW. Incidence, prevalence, and mortality of cardiovascular diseases. In Hurst JW (Ed.): The Heart, 6th ed. New York, McGraw-Hill, 1986, with permission.)

cardial infarction patients do not make a complete recovery, although 88% of those under age 65 are able to return to work.

IMPORTANT FACTS RELEVANT TO PREVENTION

1. Risk factor reduction will reduce the incidence of CHD, particularly when concentrated on blood cholesterol levels, hypertension, and cigarette smoking.

2. Changing the American diet to a low-saturated-fat, low-cholesterol diet will reduce the levels of serum cholesterol in the population.

3. No population in the world has been found with a combination of high total serum cholesterol levels and low CHD.

4. Regression of coronary lesions is possible with adequate treatment. Even a very low-fat diet combined with exercise and meditation, but without medication, has been shown to be effective.

Current national guidelines for determining CHD risk according to LDL cholesterol levels are listed in Table 12–3.

SCREENING TEST RECOMMANDATIONS

For the General Population

1. Measure cholesterol between 20 and 30 years of age and at least every 5 years thereafter. Earlier screening at 10–15 years of age should be considered for children with family history of CHD prior to 55 years of age. Physicians may wish to have the benefit of an LDL and HDL cholesterol to most accurately determine risk status. Certainly these tests, as well as triglycerides, should be done on all patients with elevated total cholesterol, a positive family history of CHD under 55 years of age, or other significant risk factors.

2. Measure blood pressure each office visit.

3. Update family history at least every 5 years.

4. Update smoking status:
   a) every 5 years in previous nonsmokers.
   b) yearly in previous smokers who have quit.
   c) every visit in current smokers.

5. Measure fasting blood sugar every 5 years. The presence of diabetes is a major risk factor.

6. Monitor activity levels at least every 5 years for every patient for the recommended 30 minutes of aerobic activity three times weekly.

7. Evaluate for obesity (greater than 20–30% over ideal body weight) yearly.

8. Monitor stress levels yearly (family, occupation).

PREVENTABLE ACTIVITIES RECOMMENDATIONS. All risk factors noted in Table 12–3 should be modified wherever possible.

Cholesterol Control. Physicians should prescribe a heart-healthy diet for *all* patients regardless of age or risk. It is particularly important that children learn healthy eating habits early in life. For patients less likely or able to follow the more extensive dietary instructions of the Step 1 diet as published by the American Heart Association (AHA), Table 12–4 gives very general guidelines that most patients can easily progressively implement.

All patients should be screened for risk status. The presence of other risk factors is used to determine the LDL intervention levels. Table 12–5 shows these recommendations for intervention with diet and medications.

Epidemiologic data show a significant CHD protective effect in populations consuming three or more servings of fish weekly. Also, a diet high in soluble fiber (oat bran products, legumes, and fruits) has been shown in some studies to reduce serum cholesterol, while nonso-

TABLE 12–3. IDENTIFYING RISK FOR CORONARY HEART DISEASE USING LDL CHOLESTEROL VALUES

HIGH-RISK GROUPS FOR CORONARY HEART DISEASE RELATED TO LDL CUTPOINTS
LDL cholesterol > 160 in any patient
or
LDL cholesterol > 130 in any patient with a history of CHD
or
LDL cholesterol > 130 in any patient with two or more of the following:
Prior history of CHD
Male sex
Family history of premature CHD (< 55 years of age)
Cigarette smoker (> 10 per day)
Hypertension
HDL cholesterol < 35
Diabetes mellitus
History of any occlusive vascular disease, peripheral or cerebrovascular
Severe obesity (more than 30% overweight)
Other risk factors to consider:
Elevated triglyceride levels
High-stress personality profile (probable)
Inactivity (probable)
Oral contraceptive use in smokers over 35

Source: National Cholesterol Education Program, with permission.

TABLE 12–4. SIMPLIFIED GUIDELINES TO HELP PATIENTS BEGIN LOWERING CHOLESTEROL AND FAT IN THEIR DIET

FOODS TO REDUCE OR ELIMINATE	RECOMMENDED SUBSTITUTIONS
Whole eggs	Egg whites (2 whites/whole egg) Egg substitute
Cheese	Whey cheeses Low-fat cottage cheese Low-fat (part-skim) cheeses Nondairy cheese
Whole milk	Low-fat or skim milk
Butter	Soft margarines Powdered butter flavoring
Ice cream Sherbets, sorbets	Nonfat "ice cream" and frozen yogurt Ice milks Vegetable oil-based frozen dessert Tofu-based "ice cream"
Fatty meats, hot dogs, luncheon sausage, bacon, poultry skin, internal organ meats	Lean varieties of red meats, meats less often and in smaller (3 oz.) portions Skinned chicken and turkey Fish Avoid frying Nonmeat meals Textured vegetable-based meat substitutes
Shellfish	Reduced portions if used Use lower-cholesterol varieties (crab, clams, scallops) Fish-based mock crab legs
Chocolate	Cocoa
Highly refined prepared foods High-fat prepared foods (bakery items, foods prepared with coconut, palm, palm kernel, or hydrogenated vegetable oils or animal fat or lard	Whole-grain varieties, fresh fruits and vegetables Homemade or prepared low-fat varieties using the unsaturated vegetable oils (soybean, canola or rapeseed, olive, corn or safflower, sesame, sunflower)

Source: Rakel RE. Textbook of Family Practice. 4th ed. Philadelphia, W.B. Saunders, 1990, with permission.

luble fiber (present primarily in wheat, vegetables, and fruits) has consistently shown no effect on cholesterol.

Other methods of altering risk secondary to hypercholesterolemia include weight control, exercise, and drug therapy.

Control of Hypertension.   Aggressive treatment of all patients with a systolic pressure greater than 140 or a diastolic pressure greater than 90 is essential. Risk is proportional to blood pressure even at diastolic levels between 80 and 90.

Prior to institution of drug therapy for hypertension, nonpharmacologic methods should be considered. These include salt restriction, weight reduction, biofeedback, and regular aerobic exercise.

Smoking Cessation.   Smoking may be the most correctable risk factor for CHD. Each physician should have a plan for assisting patients in smoking cessation which includes the following elements:

1. Patient recognition of smoking as a health problem.
2. A firm stance by the physician against smoking.
3. Encouraging a patient decision to stop.
4. Setting a target date for starting the program.
5. Multiple methodologies available, depending on patient needs and preferences: tapering, "cold turkey," substitution (e.g., nicotine gum or patch), counseling, hypnosis, support groups, buddy systems, and acupuncture.

TABLE 12–5. GUIDELINES FOR TREATMENT OF CHD RISK BASED ON LDL LEVELS (NATIONAL CHOLESTEROL EDUCATION PROGRAM, 1988)

RISK GROUP	INITIATE DIET	INITIATE MEDICATION*	GOAL LDL LEVEL
No CHD and < 2 risk factors	160 mg/dl	190 mg/dl	<160 mg/dl
Known CHD or ≥ 2 risk factors	130 mg/dl	160 mg/dl	<130 mg/dl

*Medication only begun if failure of Step 1 and 2 diets to achieve goal.

6. Structured long-term follow-up with maximal support and encouragement from physician and office staff.

Other Preventive Activities. It is recommended that physicians assist all patients to avoid risk factor development through encouragement of healthy lifestyles to prevent smoking, promote physical activity, cope effectively with stress, maintain ideal body weight, and provide periodic preventive health care.

DISCUSSION. The incidence of CHD in the United States has been decreasing significantly, as shown in Figure 12–1. Sixty percent of this decline is due to lifestyle changes, especially diet modification and smoking cessation. This encouraging information alone provides physicians sufficient reason to pursue further aggressive risk factor prevention and modification on a population-wide basis.

While total cholesterol measurement may be appropriate for mass public screening, use of LDL and HDL levels when determining risk for individual patients is more appropriate. These two values have a predictive power approximately six to ten times that of total cholesterol alone.

Triglycerides also can be very important in determining risk. In women, triglycerides predict risk as well as cholesterol except at very high cholesterol levels. In addition there is a very high-risk subpopulation with minimally elevated cholesterol and triglyceride who also have an HDL under 40.

Most authorities feel that use of the monounsaturated fats (olive oil, canola oil) should be emphasized in the total dietary fat allowance. This is based on epidemiologic studies and on the observation that these oils, when substituted for saturated fatty acids, reduce LDL cholesterol at least as much as the polyunsaturated fatty acids. Furthermore, they do not lower the HDL at the same time as do the polyunsaturated fats.

Recent data strongly suggest that sedentary lifestyle is a potent, independent risk factor that has a effect equal to the other major risk factors. It is likely that the national guidelines for risk assessment will eventually recognize sedentary lifestyle as a major risk.

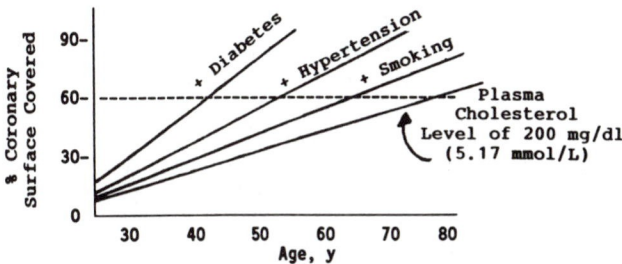

Figure 12–2. Relation of coronary atherosclerosis (percentage of surface of coronary arteries covered with lesions) vs. age as modified by addition of risk factors. In absence of other risk factors, patient with cholesterol level of 200 mg/dl (5.17 mmol/L) should reach critical stenosis at about age 70 years. Addition of smoking reduces age to 60 years, and addition of more risk factors (i.e., hypertension and diabetes mellitus) reduces age further. (*Source:* Grundy, SM. Cholesterol and coronary heart disease: A new era. JAMA 1986; 256:2848–2858, with permission.)

The issue of the effect of personality characteristics on CHD risk is poorly understood. Although type A personality has been traditionally implicated as a risk factor, studies are conflicting. There is general agreement that stress plays a significant role in CHD and that further study will reveal that specific identifiable characteristics such as suppressed hostility will increase risk.

Assessing total risk for individual patients may be complicated by the presence of more than one risk factor. A model for visualizing this process is shown in Figure 12–2. In this table one can better understand the effect of adding major risks to a baseline cholesterol of 200. However, it must be recognized that most major risk factors will vary in impact as their values change. Figure 12–3 shows this variable effect using increasing cholesterol values. Using the concepts in these two tables, a valuable paradigm is presented for cardiovascular risk assessment.

IMPACT ON FAMILY UNIT. The lifestyles that are important for prevention of CHD cannot be easily implemented by an individual without due consideration of the person's family and environment. The chances of abstinence from smoking are dimmed considerably

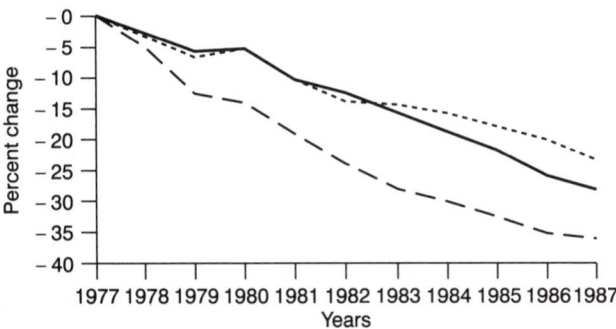

Figure 12–1. Cumulative percent decline in age-adjusted death rates for coronary heart disease, stroke, and total cardiovascular deaths, 1976 to 1987. Dotted line = coronary heart disease; dashed line = stroke; solid line = total cardiovascular deaths. (*Source:* American Heart Association. 1991 Heart and Stroke Facts, with permission.)

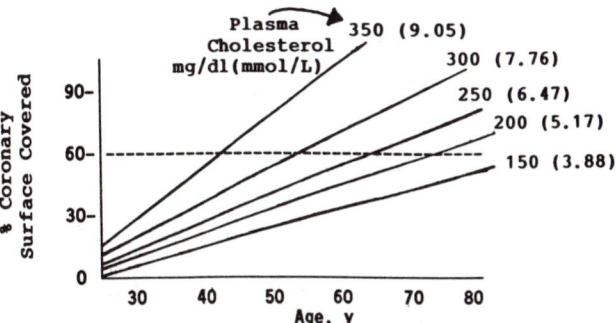

Figure 12–3. Relation of coronary atherosclerosis (percentage of surface arteries covered with raised lesions) vs. age at different levels of plasma cholesterol. At 60% of coronary surfaces covered with lesions, patients enter zone of markedly enhanced risk for clinical coronary heart disease. (*Source:* Grundy, SM. Cholesterol and coronary heart disease: A new era. JAMA 1986; 256:2848–2858, with permission.)

when there are other smokers in the home. Diet changes, especially, cannot be effectively implemented for only one individual in a family unit. Major changes in knowledge, attitudes, and habits in the entire family are often required so that the desirable foods can be purchased, properly prepared, and consumed with an agreed-upon common family goal of improved health. Anything less can lead to resentments, confusion, and outright rebellion.

When a family member needs dietary therapy, a family meeting at the beginning will enhance the chances of long-term success. This meeting can be used to educate the family about risk and diet, enlist the cooperation and support of all family members, and make plans for flexibility to meet everyone's needs. Fortunately, the AHA diets are nutritionally well balanced and can be recommended to all, regardless of risk status.

Helpful guidelines and educational materials are available from the AHA through local and state chapters. Several excellent cookbooks are also widely available. (Conner and Conner; Brody; Eshleman).

Cerebrovascular Disease

INCIDENCE. The incidence of stroke is 500,000 per year. The yearly incidence increases with age from 100/100,000 for ages 45–54 to 1800/100,000 at age 85. This translates into a 1 in 20 chance of having a stroke prior to age 70 for both males and females.

PREVALENCE. There are nearly 2 million living stroke victims in the United States. This, of course, does not include the millions of individuals with significant atherosclerotic cerebrovascular disease who are at an extremely high risk for stroke.

COST/IMPACT ON SOCIETY. The total yearly cost of stroke to society is estimated at $7.3 billion.

MORBIDITY/MORTALITY. Stroke is the third leading cause of death in the United States after CHD and cancer, resulting in a total of 149,200 deaths in 1987. Thirty percent of stroke victims die within 30 days and 43% within 6 months of the original event.

In addition to the high mortality, stroke carries a very high morbidity. Forty percent of stroke survivors require special services and 10% require total care.

IMPORTANT FACTS RELEVANT TO PREVENTION. The major risk factor for stroke is hypertension. The other risk factors for CHD are less predictive for stroke risk. However, the known presence of heart disease carries a high risk for emboli to the brain, causing an estimated 20% to 34% of cerebral infarcts. Diabetes mellitus, even if mild, carries a significant increased risk. This risk rises dramatically if both hypertension and diabetes are present.

Transient ischemic attacks (TIAs) confer a high risk of subsequent stroke. One out of five stroke victims has had at least one of the four major symptoms suggestive of TIA in the year prior: (1) temporary loss of vision (especially if in one eye), (2) unilateral numbness, (3) aphasia, and (4) focal weakness.

Patients with carotid bruits have a 2% incidence of stroke per year. Although aspirin, anticoagulants, and surgery are commonly prescribed, the current data are not sufficient to show that these treatments effectively reduce the risk of stroke in patients with asymptomatic carotid bruits. Such studies are in progress and will provide further guidance in the future.

Other risk factors for stroke include family history of stroke, cigarette smoking, oral contraceptive use, hyperlipidemia, and elevated hematocrit.

SCREENING TEST RECOMMENDATIONS. Elevated blood pressure, systolic *or* diastolic, is the single greatest risk factor for stroke and should be evaluated at each office visit. Other risk factors for atherosclerosis should be sought as previously recommended under coronary heart disease. Carotid bruits should be listened for every 5 years after age 40.

PREVENTIVE ACTIVITIES RECOMMENDATIONS. Prevention of stroke is aimed primarily at prevention and treatment of sustained, even mild, hypertension. Promotion of the healthy lifestyle habits discussed for CHD will be of likely, although unproven, benefit. Smokers, in particular, should be strongly advised to stop. Secondary prevention of completed stroke in patients with TIAs may include aspirin prophylaxis, anticoagulation, or carotid endarterectomy, depending on the clinical circumstances.

DISCUSSION. The most important reason to listen for carotid bruits is to document the existence of significant atherosclerosis and, therefore, alert the physician to the need to more aggressively modify risk factors. There is a risk, however, of initiating a process leading to angiography and endarterectomy, which carry substantial risk.

IMPACT ON FAMILY UNIT. The common results of stroke—physical disability, intellectual disability, depression—often cause a loss of independence. The family or friends are suddenly forced to help make parental-type decisions. Active participation in the rehabilitation and care of a stroke victim can create an enormous stress, financially and emotionally, on the family unit. Placement in a nursing home, however rational, will require a resolution of guilt within the family. The family physician plays a critical central role in the coordination of rehabilitation with the family and in helping the family to resolve conflicting feelings.

Substance Abuse: Alcoholism and Other Drug Dependency

INCIDENCE. Difficulties in clearly identifying the point in time at which an individual becomes an alcoholic make incidence rates very difficult to determine reliably.

PREVALENCE. Estimates of the prevalence of alcohol abuse or dependence range from 11 to 18 million Americans. In an ambulatory medical setting the prevalence of alcoholism is at least 10%. The rate for dependency on other drugs is about 2%. The rates of drug use and abuse in adolescents and young adults are particularly striking, as shown in Table 12–6.

COST/IMPACT ON SOCIETY. The estimated yearly cost of alcohol abuse in the United States is $115 billion in-

TABLE 12–6. PERCENTAGE ILLICIT USE OF DRUGS BY YOUTHS AND YOUNG ADULTS, 1982

	12–17 YEARS		18–25 YEARS	
	Ever Used	*Current Use*	*Ever Used*	*Current Use*
Alcohol	65	27	95	68
Cigarettes	50	15	77	40
Marijuana/hashish	27	12	64	27
Hallucinogens	5	1	21	2
Cocaine	7	2	28	7
Stimulants	7	3	18	5
Sedatives	6	1	19	3
Tranquilizers	5	1	15	2

Source: Adapted from Miller JD, et al. National Survey of Drug Abuse: Main Findings, 1982. Washington, D.C., U.S. Government Printing Office, 1983, with permission.

cluding $71 billion from lost employment and reduced productivity, and $15 billion in health care costs. The estimated 1983 total cost for illicit drug abuse was $60 billion.

MORBIDITY/MORTALITY. Patients with alcoholism have a 2.5-times-normal overall risk of mortality. An estimate for 1982 alcohol-related deaths was 138,027 or 7.6% of all deaths that year.

The morbidity for chemical dependency (alcohol and drug abuse) is substantial, ranging from the extremely high association with crime to cirrhosis, psychosis, depression, cardiomyopathy, peptic ulcer disease, overdose, cancer of directly exposed organs (lips, mouth, larynx, pharynx, esophagus, stomach, liver), pancreatitis, suicide, various infections (hepatitis, AIDS, endocarditis, pneumonia), fetal alcohol syndrome, and accidents of all types.

IMPORTANT FACTS RELEVANT TO PREVENTION. The most useful definition of chemical dependency is *the continued habitual use of a substance by a person despite resultant serious adverse effects on that person's life.*

Measures to increase enforcement of drinking and driving laws, to increase prices for alcoholic beverages, and to increase drinking age have been shown either to reduce alcohol consumption or to reduce the frequency of the legal consequences of drinking. Whether education will, in fact, reduce the rate of alcoholism is not known. Strong cultural biases (e.g., among Orthodox Jews) against drunkenness have a strong effect on the prevalence of dependency.

Children of alcoholics are at a three-times-greater risk of alcoholism, whether or not they are raised by their biologic parents.

While spontaneous recovery from alcoholism is reported in 4% to 26% of patients, treatment has been reported to result in a 70% recovery rate. One must remember that reports use a variety of definitions of "recovery." It is unrealistic, dangerous, and delusional for an alcoholic ever to attempt controlled drinking.

SCREENING TEST RECOMMENDATIONS. All patients over 12 years of age should be screened regularly for alcohol and substance abuse. A yearly frequency of screening will deliver a strong educational message to the patient.

Probably the single best screening is to ascertain through questioning if the patient has ever had a health, legal, or personal problem as a result of drinking alcohol. Two positives for the CAGE questions (Table 12–7) are also highly suggestive of alcohol abuse and require further investigation. The MAST (Michigan Alcohol Screening Test), as shown in Figure 12–4, can also be helpful in the diagnostic evaluation.

The presence or absence of alcoholism in first-degree relatives should be a part of the family history. All patients, including children, should be asked yearly if there are any problems within the family that involve alcohol.

PREVENTIVE ACTIVITIES RECOMMENDATIONS. Literature concerning the warning signs of alcoholism and sources of help should be freely available in every medical office. If the subject of chemical dependency is dealt with openly, there is an increased likelihood of seeking help through the family physician.

Patients with a family history of alcoholism should be counseled concerning their high-risk status and encouraged to become a member of Alanon or the Children of Alcoholics Foundation.

DISCUSSION. The same questions used for alcohol may be equally applicable to drug abuse.

Certain cues found in alcoholics and other drug-dependent patients will help lead to the correct diagnosis: problems with children, separation, divorce, job changes, depression, anxiety, hypertension, macrocytosis of red blood cells, low resistance to infections, recurrent accidents, any trouble with legal authorities (including driving while intoxicated), upper gastrointestinal complaints, and abnormal liver enzymes.

TABLE 12–7. CAGE SCREENING TEST FOR ALCOHOLISM (any two positives are highly suggestive)

CAGE QUESTIONS

C utting down?
A nnoyed by criticism of your drinking?
G uilty about your drinking?
E ye opener ever?

Source: Rakel RE. Textbook of Family Practice. 4th ed. Philadelphia, W.B. Saunders, 1990, with permission.

MICHIGAN ALCOHOLISM SCREENING TEST

QUESTION	YES	NO
Do you enjoy having a drink now and then?	0	_____
Do you feel you are a normal drinker? (By normal we mean you drink less than or as much as most other people and you have not gotten into any recurring trouble while drinking)	_____	2
Have you ever awakened the morning after some drinking the night before and found that you could not remember part of the evening?	2	_____
Does either of your parents, or any near relative, or your spouse, or any girlfriend or boyfriend ever worry or complain about your drinking?	1	_____
Can you stop drinking without a struggle after one or two drinks?	_____	2
Do you feel guilty about your drinking?	1	_____
Do friends or relatives think you are a normal drinker?	_____	2
Are you able to stop drinking when you want to?	_____	2
Have you ever attended a meeting of Alcoholics Anonymous? (AA)	5	_____
Have you gotten into physical fights when you have been drinking?	1	_____
Has your drinking ever created problems between you and either of your parents, or another relative, your spouse, or any girlfriend or boyfriend?	2	_____
Has any family member of yours ever gone to anyone for help about your drinking?	2	_____
Have you ever lost friends because of your drinking?	2	_____
Have you ever got into trouble at work or school because of your drinking?	2	_____
Have you ever lost a job because of drinking?	2	_____
Have you ever neglected your obligations, your school work, your family, or your job for 2 or more days in a row because you were drinking?	2	_____
Do you drink before noon fairly often?	1	_____
Have you ever been told you had liver trouble or cirrhosis?	2	_____
After heavy drinking have you ever had severe shaking, or heard voices or seen things that really weren't there?	2(5 DTs) _____	
Have you ever gone to anyone for help about your drinking?	5	_____
Have you ever been in a hospital because of drinking?	5	_____
Have you ever been a patient in a psychiatric hospital or a psychiatric ward of a general hospital where drinking was part of the problem that resulted in hospitalization?	2	_____
Have you ever been seen at a psychiatric or mental health clinic or gone to any doctor, social worker or clergy for help with any emotional problem, where drinking was a part of the problem?	2	_____
Have you ever been arrested for drunk driving, driving while intoxicated, or driving under the influence of alcoholic beverages or any other drug? If yes, how many times? _____	2 each _____	
Have you ever been arrested, or taken into custody even for a few hours, because of drunk behavior, whether due to alcohol or another drug? If yes, how many times? _____	2 each _____	

Figure 12–4. The Michigan Alcoholism Screening Test (MAST). Each response scores the number of points listed. A total of 0–3 points = probable normal drinker; 4 = borderline; 5–9 = 80% likelihood of dependence; 10 or more = 100% likelihood. (*Source:* Selzer, ML. Am J Psychiatr 1971; 127:1653, with permission.)

IMPACT ON FAMILY UNIT. The family is at the epicenter of the alcoholic earthquake. As the rumblings of the disease progress, so does pathology within the family. Most prominent is the role of the "co-alcoholic" or "enabler" who assumes the abnegated responsibilities of the alcoholic, covers for the alcoholic, and makes possible continued drinking. This person is often the major focus of the alcoholic's hostility. Treatment should include healing of the entire family.

Cancer

General Cancer Information

INCIDENCE. The number of estimated new U.S. cancer cases for 1988 (excluding carcinoma in situ and nonmelanotic skin cancers) was 985,000. The six most frequent cancers (excluding skin) are lung, colon-rectum, breast, prostate, urinary tract, and uterus. Thirty percent (75 million) of all Americans will eventually develop cancer.

PREVALENCE. There are over 5 million people alive today in the United States with a history of cancer. No data are available to indicate how many Americans have undiagnosed cancer at this time.

COST/IMPACT ON SOCIETY. The estimated U.S. total cost of medical care for cancer is over $10 billion a year. An additional $25 billion is lost in income.

MORBIDITY/MORTALITY. Cancer is second only to cardiovascular diseases as a cause of mortality in the United States and is responsible for over 22% of all deaths. The estimated mortality for 1988 is 494,000. The six leading causes of cancer death are lung, colon-rectum, breast, prostate, pancreas, and urinary system.

From 1930 to 1985 the U.S. mortality rate for cancer rose from 130 to 171 per 100,000. This rise has been primarily due to the continuing rise of mortality from cancer of the lung.

IMPORTANT FACTS RELEVANT TO PREVENTION. Thirty-five percent of all cancer deaths are thought to be related to diet (including obesity). Obese individuals have increased risk of colon, breast, and uterine cancers. High-fat diets are a risk factor for prostate, breast, and colon cancers. Foods rich in vitamin A (dark-green and deep-yellow vegetables and fruits) and vitamin C (citrus fruits, strawberries, and sweet peppers) and cruciferous vegetables (cabbage, broccoli, Brussels sprouts, and cauliflower) are all thought to have protective effects for various cancers. Salt-cured, smoked, and nitrite-cured foods increase the risk of upper GI cancers.

Smoking accounts for 30% of cancer deaths (primarily lung, urinary bladder, mouth, throat, and larynx), while alcohol is responsible for approximately 3% and occupational exposures for 5% of cancer mortality.

Therefore, diet, smoking, alcohol, and occupational exposures appear to account for over 73% of all cancer mortality. These are potentially preventable causes and are amenable to intervention by the family physician.

Early diagnosis and treatment (secondary prevention) is also of great benefit. Already 40% of newly diagnosed cancer victims have a 5-year survival. Of the 494,000 current yearly deaths, 174,000 might have been prevented by earlier diagnosis and treatment.

DISCUSSION. The prevention of cancer takes on a new urgency when one considers the likely dramatic increase due to the increasing number of elderly and success with decreasing mortality from other causes.

Lifestyle modification plus early diagnosis through screening could potentially reduce cancer mortality by 80% to 90%.

IMPACT ON FAMILY UNIT. For many of the cancers, a positive family history is a significant risk factor, opening the door for the physician to emphasize prevention and early detection for these families. It also may create a variety of behavioral problems within the family. Individual family members may experience hypochondriasis, depression, phobic disorders, generalized anxiety, and anger/hostility. These may be precipitated when issues of illness and death are being dealt with in the family.

Because of the great importance of lifestyle in the prevention of cancer, family health habits are the major source of successful cancer prevention. When one considers the fact that cancer will strike three out of four families, the value of generally applied preventive health measures within every family practice becomes evident.

Colorectal Cancer

INCIDENCE. Colorectal cancer has the second highest incidence of all cancers. The American Cancer Society estimated 147,000 new cases in 1988. The incidence of colorectal cancer begins to rise after 40, roughly doubling each decade. Ninety percent occur in the population over 50.

PREVALENCE. The exact prevalence in the population is not known. Most screening trials find 1–2 cancers and 80 polyps per 1000 screened patients.

MORBIDITY/MORTALITY. Mortality has been steady for almost 30 years at approximately 50% (62,000

TABLE 12–8. 5-YEAR SURVIVAL FOR COLORECTAL CANCER

SURGICAL PATHOLOGY	DUKES STAGE	% SURVIVAL*
In situ, mucosal invasion only	A	80–100
Muscularis invasion	B	60
Local nodes	C	22–43
Distant spread	D	1–4

*Range of reported survival in different studies.

deaths in 1988), despite the increasing vigilance of screening by physicians. This may be explained in part by shift of lesions from the rectum and sigmoid colon to the right colon where early detection by sigmoidoscopy is not possible.

The survival rate varies dramatically with the stage of the cancer, as shown in Table 12–8.

IMPORTANT FACTS RELEVANT TO PREVENTION. Colorectal cancer appears to arise almost exclusively from benign adenomatous polyps over a period of 5–10 years. However, only 20% to 30% of polyps are adenomas, and only 5% to 10% of adenomatous polyps become malignant. The appearance of adenomas occurs primarily between 40 and 45 years of age, with a significant increase in colorectal cancer in 5–10 years.

When compared with pathology found on colonoscopy, stool guaiac specimens (stool samples daily for three consecutive days) were 52% sensitive for carcinoma, 23% sensitive for polyps greater than 1.0 cm, and 4.4% sensitive for polyps less than 1.0 cm.

A major prospective study (uncontrolled) of over 20,000 patients followed for up to 25 years and screened periodically with only a 25-cm sigmoidoscope showed a 50% reduction of incidence of bowel cancers over that predicted.

Although there has been a progressive change toward polyps occurring higher in the large bowel, over 60% are still within reach of the 60-cm flexible sigmoidoscope.

Compared with the current 5-year survival rate of 55%, it is estimated that potentially 80% to 90% of all colon cancers could be prevented by screening stool for occult blood, sigmoidoscopy, and removal of adenomatous polyps found during further evaluation of positive screening tests.

Epidemiologically, 20% of colorectal cancers can be attributed to a dietary cause, especially lack of fiber. High-fat diets have also been implicated.

Risk factors for colorectal cancer are found in Table 12–9.

TABLE 12–9. RISK FACTORS FOR COLORECTAL CANCER

Age > 50
History of adenomas
Personal or family history of colorectal cancer or polyps
Ulcerative colitis
Crohn's disease affecting colon
Personal or family history of genital or breast cancer in females

Source: Rakel RE. Textbook of Family Practice. 4th ed. Philadelphia, W.B. Saunders, 1990, with permission.

SCREENING TEST RECOMMENDATIONS. Although these tests do not meet the criteria established by the Clinical Preventive Services Task Force, patients should be offered a rectal exam and a six-slide fecal occult blood test yearly after age 40, as well as flexible sigmoidoscopy every 3–5 years starting after age 40 and no later than age 50. (The American Cancer Society recommends two yearly exams starting at age 50 and every 3–5 years thereafter.)

PREVENTIVE ACTIVITIES RECOMMENDATIONS. Risk factor analysis should be performed at least by 40 years of age. Preventive activities include the surveillance described above, looking for presymptomatic carcinomas and lesions with malignant potential (adenomas). All patients, regardless of age, should be encouraged to eat a high-fiber, low-fat diet.

DISCUSSION. The ideal screening would be periodic colonoscopy on all high-risk persons. This is neither practical, cost-effective, nor acceptable to patients.

Knowing the 5- to 10-year natural history of progression from adenoma to cancer, one could reasonably decide to begin primary prevention at least this long prior to the age of 50 when the most dramatic increase in actual cancer incidence occurs.

IMPACT ON FAMILY UNIT. Since family history is a major risk factor, information obtained by the family physician should be used for family education concerning prevention.

Breast Cancer

INCIDENCE. In 1988 there were an estimated 135,000 new cases of invasive breast cancer and an additional 5000 carcinomas in situ. The lifetime incidence of breast cancer for females is now one in nine and appears to be slowly increasing. Twenty-eight percent of all new female cancers are breast cancers, compared with 16% for colorectal cancer, the next most common cancer in females.

PREVALENCE. Based on incidence and mortality statistics, the estimated number of patients with previously diagnosed breast cancer currently living is 432,000.

MORBIDITY/MORTALITY. The mortality rates for breast cancer from 1974 to 1985 were stable at 39,000 deaths per year. This accounts for 18% of all female cancer deaths, which is now second to the 20% of female cancer deaths caused by lung cancer. The 5-year survival rate for localized breast cancer is 90%, compared with 78% in the 1940s. In situ breast cancer has a cure rate approaching 100%. The survival rates at 5, 8, and 10 years were 88%, 83%, and 79% for breast cancers diagnosed through screening in the Breast Cancer Detection Demonstration Project.

IMPORTANT FACTS RELEVANT TO PREVENTION. The major accepted risk factors are listed in Table 12–10. Despite evaluation of risk factors, 75% of women with breast cancer have no risk factor other than their age. The risk rises progressively with age. A woman of 65–69 has over 200 times the risk of a 20- to 24-year-old and over four times the risk of a 35- to 39-year-old!

Breast self-examination alone has a sensitivity of 26%, compared to 45% for clinical breast examination and 71% for mammography, and 75% for a combination of mammography and clinical breast examination. Of significance, however, is the fact that in the Breast Cancer Detection Demonstration Project (BCDDP), 690 of the total 2675 breast cancers diagnosed were found by breast self-examination between screening visits. Nev-

TABLE 12–10. RISK FACTORS FOR BREAST CANCER

FACTOR	RELATIVE RISK
*Atypical hyperplasia and family history	11
*Family history premenopausal bilateral breast cancer	9
*Family history premenopausal breast cancer	3
Family history postmenopausal breast cancer	1.5
Family history bilateral breast cancer	5
*History previous personal breast cancer	5
Fibrocystic disease, proliferative type on biopsy	1.5–4
*Lobular carcinoma in situ	7.2
*Intraductal carcinoma in situ (risk >lobular CIS)	N/A
*Atypical lobular or ductal hyperplasia on biopsy	N/A
First pregnancy after 35	2–3
Nulliparous	3
Early menarche or late menopause	1.3–2.0
Increasing age	

Factors With Unclear Status
Alcohol intake
High-fat, low-fiber diet
Obesity
History of ovarian, endometrial, salivary cancers

*Factors for which there is a consensus to place a patient in a high-risk group needing special attention.
Modified from Love SM, Gelman RS, Silen W. Fibrocystic disease of the breasts—a non-disease? N Engl J Med 1985; No. 312(3):146, with permission.

ertheless, a definitive study showing a lowered mortality for those performing breast self-examination has not been done. Despite the lower sensitivity than mammography, clinical breast examination is thought to be useful. Up to 16% of cancers may be missed if no breast examination is included in screening. Half of these are minimal cancers and therefore highly curable.

The BCDDP was conducted over 5 years with 280,000 women ages 35–74 participating to evaluate a mass screening program for breast cancer. It did demonstrate that screening 40- to 50-year-old women was as effective in long-term survival rates as screening those over 50. However, the Health Insurance Plan of New York (HIP) study failed to show a statistically significant decrease in mortality for the under-50 age group, although there was a trend in that direction. The most important conclusion from the HIP study is that early detection of breast cancer does significantly decrease mortality.

A number of factors have been shown *not* to alter the risk of breast cancer. These include breast trauma, fibroadenomas, fibrocystic breast disease of the nonproliferative type, caffeine consumption, mastodynia with negative mammographic and clinical examination, breast feeding, and use of birth control pills or postmenopausal estrogen therapy.

SCREENING TEST RECOMMENDATIONS. Table 12–11 outlines the official guidelines of the U.S. Preventive Health Services Task Force, the American Academy of Family Physicians, and the American Cancer Society. These recommendations range from conservative to aggressive. Each physician must decide the level of preventive care to implement in practice. The Preventive Health Service Task Force guidelines represent the minimum level of preventive health care expected of primary care physicians.

PREVENTIVE ACTIVITIES RECOMMENDATIONS. Very little has been proven concerning the primary prevention of breast cancer. Diet may have a significant role. Pa-tients should be advised of the concern raised by the association of moderate alcohol ingestion, high-fat diets, and low-fiber diets with breast cancer. These dietary recommendations can be made on other grounds and are considered to be of general benefit. Therefore, physicians may wish to make these recommendations before a direct cause-and-effect relationship is firmly established.

Although of unproven benefit, breast self-examination is a logical, low-risk, no-cost activity. It should be taught to each female at the time of her first gynecologic examination and reviewed at each subsequent examination.

Every female should have an initial documented evaluation of risk factors for breast cancer at or before age 30. A long-term program for screening should be determined at that time.

Secondary prevention (early detection of disease prior to symptoms) is the focus of current major screening recommendations. All lesions of the breast should be promptly investigated. Any suspicious mass found on physician examination or mammography should be evaluated by needle aspiration, needle biopsy, or open excisional biopsy, depending on the clinical circumstances. A negative mammogram or negative clinical examination alone is never fully adequate to rule out cancer.

DISCUSSION. Environmental factors deserve more attention. The Japanese have a very low incidence of breast cancer. However, subsequent generations of Japanese immigrants to the United States have increasing incidence rates, eventually equalling the high U.S. levels. In addition, several recent studies have suggested a strong association between alcohol ingestion and breast cancer.

Certain factors (see Table 12–10) are considered adequate to place a female into the high-risk group. For instance, a mother and a sister with premenopausal bilateral breast cancer imparts a 30% lifetime risk.

TABLE 12–11. OFFICIAL RECOMMENDATIONS FOR BREAST CANCER SCREENING

Age	Test	AMERICAN ACADEMY OF FAMILY PHYSICIANS AND AMERICAN CANCER SOCIETY — Frequency	U.S. PREVENTIVE HEALTH SERVICE TASK FORCE — Frequency
20–34	BSE	Monthly	
	CBE	q3 years	
35–39	BSE	Monthly	
	CBE	q3 years	
	Mamm	Once	
40–49	BSE	Monthly	
	CBE	Yearly	Yearly
	Mamm	q1–2 years	
50–59	BSE	Monthly	
	CBE	Yearly	Yearly
	Mamm	Yearly	Yearly
60+	BSE	Monthly	
	CBE	Yearly	Yearly
	Mamm	Yearly	Yearly

BSE = breast self exam; CBE = clinical breast exam; Mamm = mammography.

A screening program that includes regular breast examination and mammography will miss very few breast cancers, but a large number of women will be falsely positive and will need to be evaluated with further diagnostic workup, such as needle aspiration, needle biopsy, or open biopsy.

The costs of mammographic screening remain a major concern. The 10-year cost of annual screening of only 25% of all women in the 40–49 age range would be $402 million. Even limiting mammography to those over 50 would result in a cost of $3.3 billion at the current average cost of $100 per examination. This is by far the most expensive preventive health care activity recommended.

The smaller the tumor when discovered, the better the prognosis. A review of several studies shows that nonpalpable mammographically detected cancers have a 13% to 20% incidence of metastatic spread, while those found by palpation have positive nodes 40% to 55% of the time. It has been calculated that the average time between the ability of mammography to first detect the cancer and the ability to palpate the mass is 2 years, which may be of some value in estimating the optimal interval for mammography.

IMPACT ON FAMILY UNIT. The fear of breast cancer can produce a great deal of anxiety. This fear is substantially heightened by a strong family history. As with other inherited predispositions to disease, the elements of guilt and resentment can have a profound effect on family functioning.

A major fear is associated with the patient's and husband's perceived loss of female identity. This can be allayed in part by a knowledgeable physician willing to discuss these issues openly and inform the patient and her husband of the variety of improved treatment alternatives now available. These include consideration of limited surgical procedures and radiation.

Once cancer has been diagnosed and a treatment plan decided upon, the family physician can play a critical role in preventing subsequent family dysfunction. The patient will need help in dealing with anger, helplessness, fear of recurrence, and the ill effects of treatments. Once cancer has been diagnosed, the emotional life of the family is changed forever. The family as a unit will require guidance and understanding.

Lung Cancer

INCIDENCE. Lung cancer now has the highest cancer incidence for both males and females in the United States. In 1988 the estimated number of new cases was 152,000.

MORBIDITY/MORTALITY. Lung cancer is the leading cause of cancer mortality for both males and females. The estimated number of deaths in 1988 was 139,000. Comparing the similarity of the incidence and mortality statistics, the grim nature of the prognosis is apparent, a 13% 5-year survival.

IMPORTANT FACTS RELEVANT TO PREVENTION. Except for the small minority of cases secondary to industrial exposure, the only known way to prevent lung cancer is not to smoke. Eighty-three percent of all lung cancers are directly attributable to smoking.

SCREENING TEST RECOMMENDATIONS. Although chest x-ray or sputum cytology may detect lung cancer at a presymptomatic stage, there is no study that shows a resultant improvement in the prognosis.

PREVENTIVE ACTIVITIES RECOMMENDATIONS. Patients at all ages should receive a strong health message from their physician concerning smoking: "It's addicting. Don't start. If you have started, stop." All preventive health checks should have an inquiry concerning smoking.

DISCUSSION. It is ironic that lung cancer has the highest incidence and mortality rate of all cancers, and yet is one of the most preventable. Physicians can continue to have a major impact on the risk of this disease through community and patient intervention and education. Excellent support materials are available from the American Academy of Family Physicians, the American Cancer Society, and the American Heart Association. Physician recommendation has a great potential impact on patients' decisions to stop smoking.

IMPACT ON FAMILY UNIT. A single smoker in a family can be a source of secondary smoke exposure for the rest of the family. Angina, respiratory symptoms, and increased risk of lung cancer can result in those exposed. Children from households with smokers have a higher school absence rate. Couples who smoke create a special problem for the physician who wishes to help. It is difficult to persuade one smoker to quit while the other continues, and it is equally problematic to bring two smokers to the point of wishing to stop at the same time. The withdrawal period is one of great stress and requires family education and support.

Carcinoma of the Cervix

INCIDENCE. The incidence of invasive cervical carcinoma is declining. There are now approximately 12,900 new cases of invasive cancer yearly. The incidence rises steadily through age 50 and then remains steady. Worldwide, cervical carcinoma is the most common malignancy in women, while in the United States it is seventh.

MORBIDITY/MORTALITY. The mortality for invasive carcinoma of the cervix is 7000 per year. The preinvasive cancer lesion of cervical intraepithelial neoplasia (CIN III or carcinoma in situ) has a 100% cure rate with proper treatment, while stage 1 disease has an 80% 5-year survival and stage 3, a 30% 5-year survival. Overall, the 5-year survival rate is 66%. The death rate has dropped 70% in the last 40 years. This is primarily a result of Papanicolaou smear screening programs detecting this disease at earlier stages when cure rates are higher.

IMPORTANT FACTS RELEVANT TO PREVENTION. Squamous cell carcinoma of the cervix occurs almost exclusively in women who have had coitus.

The mean time for progression from mild dysplasia (CIN I) to severe dysplasia/carcinoma in situ (CIN III) is 5.8 years, and the mean time for further progression to invasive carcinoma is an additional 10 years. The rate of progression for any one individual is unpredictable. CIN may regress spontaneously in 30% to 50% of cases. At least 30% of patients with CIN III will have progression to invasive carcinoma.

Major risk factors are early age for first intercourse, multiple sexual partners, herpes simplex virus infection, and history of condylomata (human papilloma virus or HPV) infection. Early sexual intercourse has an especially dramatic effect on risk. Females who have had coitus less than 1 year after menarche are 26 times more likely eventually to develop cervical carcinoma than the general population.

Fifteen to twenty percent of American women do not undergo regular Papanicolaou tests, and they account for the majority of cases of carcinoma of the cervix. A single Papanicolaou test is demonstrated to be 70% sensitive (30% of cases are missed).

SCREENING TEST RECOMMENDATIONS. All women should begin having Papanicolaou smears when sexual activity begins, but no later than age 18. The American Cancer Society recommends that each woman should have at least three negative annual Papanicolaou smears, at which time frequency may be reduced to as little as every 3 years at the discretion of the physician. Many physicians continue to advocate yearly screening. As yet, there appears to be no justification for screening high-risk groups more frequently. However, the 33% incidence of CIN in patients with HPV infections may represent a high-risk subgroup needing more frequent monitoring.

PREVENTIVE ACTIVITIES RECOMMENDATIONS. Risk status should be reevaluated at each preventive health visit, especially in groups who may have an increased likelihood of multiple sexual partners. Women should be advised of their risk status with emphasis on the importance of regular reevaluation. Although barrier contraception has only theoretical benefit, it can also be strongly recommended to help prevent sexually transmitted diseases.

DISCUSSION. There are other good reasons to see many women more often than every 3 years, such as monitoring use of birth control pills, dietary advice, contraceptive counseling, prepregnancy counseling, etc. It may be only a minority of women who will need to visit their physician less often than once yearly. Women have been educated for many years that the yearly Papanicolaou test is essential, but *not* that there are other important issues to be dealt with during these visits.

IMPACT ON FAMILY UNIT. Invasive cervical cancer occurring during the childbearing years will usually be treated surgically, ending chances of future pregnancy. This will have a profound effect on a single woman's approach to possible marriage and on a married couple's plans and relationship. The family physician's role only begins with referral for appropriate treatment. Preventive counseling is necessary in these situations. Women past the childbearing years may still suffer a loss of identity similar to, but not as intense as, the breast cancer victim.

Skin Cancer

INCIDENCE. There are 500,000 cases of skin cancer each year, of which 27,000 are malignant melanoma. This is over twice the incidence of cancer of any other organ system. The incidence continues to rise dramatically.

MORBIDITY/MORTALITY. Of the 7800 deaths each year, 5800 are from malignant melanoma.

IMPORTANT FACTS RELEVANT TO PREVENTION. The major risk factor for all skin cancer is exposure to ultraviolet (UV) light. Those who have had severe exposures as children and those with fair complexion are at particular risk. Occupational exposures to coal tar, pitch, arsenic, radium, and creosote all increase risk. Prior history of local treatment with ionizing radiation increases chances of localized skin cancers 25–30 years later.

SCREENING TEST RECOMMENDATIONS. During regular preventive health examinations, the skin should be thoroughly examined for suspicious lesions. All lesions suspicious for malignancy should be prophylactically excised and submitted for pathologic interpretation.

PREVENTIVE ACTIVITIES RECOMMENDATIONS. For primary prevention, all patients at risk should be counseled in measures for UV wave avoidance (sun or artificial tanning), protection with higher-number sunscreens (15 or greater), and use of protective clothing. Secondary prevention includes regular self-examination. This is a logical activity, especially for patients with already existing melanotic nevi.

The physician should also be alert to actinic keratoses and treat these as appropriate with 5-FU or retinoic acid topical application when generalized or with cryocautery when localized.

Endometrial Cancer

INCIDENCE. 47,000 cases per year.

MORBIDITY/MORTALITY. 10,000 per year.

IMPORTANT FACTS RELEVANT TO PREVENTION. Endometrial cancer is primarily a postmenopausal disease. The major etiologic factor appears to be unopposed estrogen, whether physiologic or iatrogenic. The most important early warning sign is abnormal vaginal bleeding. Risk factors are obesity, prolonged treatment with estrogen alone, age, and chronic anovulation. Hypertension and diabetes are associated with risk, probably because of the prevalence of obesity in these patients.

SCREENING TEST RECOMMENDATIONS. Abnormal endometrial cells are occasionally found on Papanicolaou smear, but this is not an adequate screen. *Any* endometrial cells found on a postmenopausal Papanicolaou smear should be considered abnormal.

All postmenopausal women with bleeding of any amount must have endometrial sampling performed.

PREVENTIVE ACTIVITIES RECOMMENDATIONS. Risk factors should be established at menopause and modified when possible. All women with an intact uterus who are treated with estrogen replacement therapy should be cycled also with a progestational agent.

Other Preventable Diseases

Osteoporosis

INCIDENCE. The incidence of fractures secondary to osteoporosis is 1 million per year. By extreme old age, one in every three women and one in every six men will have had a hip fracture, and one in three women over 65 will have vertebral fractures.

PREVALENCE. It is estimated that 15–20 million Americans have osteoporosis and are therefore at markedly increased risk for fractures.

COST/IMPACT ON SOCIETY. The direct and indirect cost of caring for patients suffering fractures secondary to osteoporosis is $6 billion each year.

MORBIDITY/MORTALITY. Between 12% and 20% of hip fractures lead to death, and 50% lead to significant disability.

IMPORTANT FACTS RELEVANT TO PREVENTION. Bone mass peaks in human beings at 20 to 30 years of age. Caucasian females have significantly lower peaks than males or darker-skinned females. In females after age 30, there is a 0.3% to 0.5% loss of bone mass yearly, which abruptly increases to 2% to 3% per year at menopause, and then, over the next 10 years, gradually returns to premenopausal rates. The rates of loss of trabecular bone and cortical bone are somewhat different. Trabecular bone loss (vertebra, distal radius) occurs earlier and in greater proportion during the menopausal years than cortical bone loss (long bones). The hip contains both types of bone. Men follow a similar sequence, but without the accelerated phase. The total loss of bone mass in males is about two-thirds that of females.

Prior to 30 years of age, the adequacy of calcium intake will affect the peak bone mass, and after 30 it will affect the rate of loss of bone mass. All women and men need 1.0 gm of elemental calcium daily to maintain a zero calcium balance. In postmenopausal women not prescribed estrogen replacement therapy, increasing this amount to 1.5 gm will not maintain zero calcium balance, will have no effect on trabecular bone, and will have minimal effect on cortical bone. There is an 80% prevalence of inadequate calcium intake among females.

Estrogen replacement therapy is the most effective method of preventing the accelerated phase of bone mass loss postmenopausally. Case control studies have shown significant decreases in postmenopausal fracture rates with estrogen replacement therapy. Discontinuation of estrogen results in a prompt return of accelerated bone loss. Other methods of maximizing peak mass and slowing bone mass loss include regular weight-bearing exercise. Actual gains in lumbar bone mass have been demonstrated in postmenopausal women placed on a weight-bearing exercise regimen. This effect was sustained as long as exercise was continued.

There are many primary risk factors for osteoporosis, plus multiple additional medical conditions that may make an individual at higher risk (Table 12–12). Contributing factors may be easily overlooked when an illness that may increase the risk of osteoporosis consumes

TABLE 12–12.   RISK FACTORS FOR OSTEOPOROSIS

Positive family history
Advancing age
Female
Caucasian or Asian
Early menopause (including surgical)
Underweight
Cigarette smoking
Calcium deficiency history
Hypogonadism (males)
Sedentary
Alcohol consumption
Subtotal gastrectomy
Hyperthyroidism
Hemiplegia
COPD
Glucocorticoid Rx
Anticonvulsant Rx

Source: Rakel RE. Textbook of Family Practice. 4th ed. Philadelphia, W.B. Saunders, 1990, with permission.

the focus of attention. A good example might be the elderly white female in otherwise good health who develops polymyalgia rheumatica. The attention required to make the diagnosis and treat with corticosteroids becomes the major focus. It is easy to forget that such a person, 2 years later, may be free of polymyalgia symptoms but debilitated by vertebral fractures.

Obesity, due to increased endogenous estrogen levels, and thiazide diuretics, due to decreased calcium excretion, have a protective effect.

SCREENING TEST RECOMMENDATIONS. There is no screening test that can be recommended. Specifically, densitometry has no place in routine preventive health care at this time.

PREVENTIVE ACTIVITIES RECOMMENDATIONS. All patients, especially females, should be educated regarding the recommended intake of 1000 mg of dietary calcium. Postmenopausal females not receiving postmenopausal estrogens should increase that amount to 1500 mg. Major nutritional sources of calcium are listed in Table 12–13. Recommendations for use of dairy products include the advice to use low-fat alternatives wherever possible as part of the overall prudent diet. Females of any age unable to meet minimal calcium needs through diet should be advised to use supplemental calcium.

TABLE 12–13.   NUTRITIONAL SOURCES OF CALCIUM

FOOD	SERVING SIZE	CALCIUM (mg)
Milk	1 cup	300
Cheese (low-fat)	1 oz	185
Yogurt (nonfat)	1 cup	450
Yogurt (whole milk)	1 cup	275
Cottage cheese (1%)	½ cup	70
Dark leafy greens	½ cup	150–180
Other vegetables	½ cup	30–100
Fruits	Average serving	<25

Source: Rakel RE. Textbook of Family Practice. 4th ed. Philadelphia, W.B. Saunders, 1990, with permission.

Risk status should be determined for all females, preferably at menarche, and reevaluated at the time of routine preventive health visits. Additional counseling concerning osteoporosis prevention should be given to those at higher risk.

Every female should be thoroughly evaluated at menopause for risk factors and possible estrogen replacement therapy. In general, most white females with any other risk factors are candidates unless there are specific contraindications. Therapy should be lifelong.

All patients should be counseled to maintain regular aerobic weight-bearing activity as part of the overall program for general preventive health care. Although 50–60 minutes of exercise three times weekly has been shown to increase bone mass, the minimum levels necessary have not been determined.

DISCUSSION. When prescribing estrogen replacement therapy, a daily dosage equivalent to 0.625 mg of conjugated estrogen has been documented as being effective; 0.3 mg may be equally effective. It is desirable to add progesterone for at least the last 10 days of each estrogen cycle, followed by 5–7 days without either hormone. Progesterone reduces or eliminates the increased risk of endometrial cancer associated with unopposed estrogen therapy. While estrogen replacement therapy appears to favorably affect the lipid profile, progesterone may partially negate this, and therefore it should be used in the lowest effective dose—the equivalent of 2.5 to 5.0 mg of medroxyprogesterone acetate.

IMPACT ON FAMILY UNIT. Family eating patterns will primarily determine the peak bone mass achieved. Therefore, counseling of women in the childbearing years should include recommendations for the entire family.

Elderly patients who are already at high risk create a dilemma for the family physician. Although several medications are being studied, there is little that is of proven value in not only replacing already lost bone mass, but also reducing fracture incidence. The process may be slowed with calcium, estrogens, and exercise. Exercise, in particular, places the osteoporotic patient at some increased risk for fractures. The resulting impact of severe fractures is sudden loss of independence. In an elderly family member, this has great impact in both emotional and financial terms. The resulting major decisions that must be made often reverse the parent–child roles.

Intimate knowledge of the elderly patient, his or her functional capacities, and the living situation place the family physician in a pivotal role in fracture prevention.

Sexually Transmitted Diseases

INCIDENCE. The peak incidence of sexually transmitted disease (STD) is in teenagers and young adults; teenagers alone account for 2.5 million cases. The reported incidence of gonorrhea is dropping from a peak in 1974 to current levels of 879,000 cases per year, with marked clustering in metropolitan areas. The true incidence may be twice the actual reported incidence. The estimated yearly incidence for chlamydia is an astounding 4.65 million cases. Each year, 120,000 infants are infected with chlamydia at birth. There are an estimated 724,000 new cases of herpes genitalis each year.

PREVALENCE. Because of the long duration of infection, the two most prevalent STDs are herpes simplex virus (HSV) and human papilloma virus (HPV). The cumulative prevalence of herpes simplex virus genitalis alone is 20 million cases at this time. Because of the asymptomatic nature of many chlamydia infections, it is estimated that the prevalence in the general population is 5%.

COST/IMPACT ON SOCIETY. For pelvic inflammatory disease (PID) alone, the costs per year are $2.6 billion.

MORBIDITY/MORTALITY. Over 200,000 women per year, one-fifth of those with PID, become involuntarily infertile, and 50% of all ectopic pregnancies are a result of PID. Twenty percent of females with one episode of PID will develop chronic pain.

IMPORTANT FACTS RELEVANT TO PREVENTION. All of the STDs have a high asymptomatic carrier rate, making prevention of transmission very difficult. Therefore, the single biggest risk factor is multiple sexual partners. Only abstinence, monogamy, or condoms will dramatically affect the risk.

SCREENING TEST RECOMMENDATIONS. No screening tests are recommended for the general population. High-risk groups should have a screening gonorrhea culture and direct fluorescent antibody test or enzyme-linked immunoassay for chlamydia performed at the time of routine pelvic examination. Persons with multiple sexual partners should be examined yearly.

PREVENTIVE ACTIVITIES RECOMMENDATIONS. Education should begin at least at, and preferably before, the beginning of sexual activity. All sexually active patients should be encouraged to seek medical evaluation for even apparently minor genital tract symptoms.

DISCUSSION. Physicians must maintain a high index of suspicion for all STDs, since there is a very high percentage of asymptomatic and minimally symptomatic patients. In high-risk populations, presumptive treatment for chlamydia, even with minimal signs or symptoms, is recommended by many experts. Treatment recommendations for gonorrhea now include coverage for chlamydia as well, for all patients.

IMPACT ON FAMILY UNIT. The incrimination that can result when a husband or wife is diagnosed with STD may lead to major family disruption. The physician will play the key role in interpreting the meaning of such an episode and bringing the couple to a mutual understanding. It is therefore critical that the physician know the natural course of the disease. For instance, 30% of women with gonorrhea may be asymptomatic carriers (in some populations the percentage for men may be almost this high), 70% of patients with genital herpes have no symptoms, and 70% of female lower genital tract infections with chlamydia are asymptomatic.

Human Immunodeficiency Virus Infection

INCIDENCE. The incidence of new cases of AIDS is rapidly increasing. In 1990 there were 43,339 new cases of AIDS reported (17.2 per 100,000). This is greater than one-fourth of the total number of cases since AIDS was first reported in 1981.

PREVALENCE. The Centers for Disease Control estimate that HIV infected 1.5 million Americans by 1987. Within 10 years of infection, 50% of individuals will develop AIDS and 40% will develop associated clinical illnesses. The prevalence of diagnosed cases of AIDS is estimated to be 365,000 cases in 1992.

COST/IMPACT ON SOCIETY. The cost of treatment alone is expected to go from $2.2 billion in 1988 to $13 billion in 1992.

MORBIDITY/MORTALITY. The case fatality rate is over 75% for persons with known AIDS for over 2 years.

IMPORTANT FACTS RELEVANT TO PREVENTION. The groups with the highest prevalence are hemophiliacs, homosexual males, intravenous drug users, individuals with multiple sexual partners, patients with multiple blood transfusions after 1977 and prior to blood screening in 1985, and babies born to infected mothers.

SCREENING TEST RECOMMENDATIONS. All patients should be screened for risk status. The frequency of screening will vary depending on the patient population cared for. Patients in high-risk groups should be strongly encouraged to be screened for HIV antibodies. One major reason for screening is to identify those individuals who are already infected so that intervention may be instituted to halt the further spread of the virus.

PREVENTIVE ACTIVITIES RECOMMENDATIONS. Education of patients is the number one priority for the individual family physician. At this time, the only real chance for meaningful intervention is to prevent exposure to HIV-infected individuals. Children and teenagers in particular must be helped to understand the reality of the risks of sexual contact (especially if unprotected with condoms) and intravenous drug use (especially using shared needles or syringes).

At-risk women in the childbearing years should be considered for yearly HIV antibody screening. Any of these women found to be HIV-positive should be strongly counseled against conception.

Within the office, the physician has a responsibility to employees and other patients to implement recommended measures to assure protection from inadvertent transmission.

DISCUSSION. In addition to individual action, there is a need for immediate, aggressive public health measures. These have been well outlined in the *Report of the Presidential Commission on the Human Immunodeficiency Virus Epidemic,* June 24, 1988. Major preventive recommendations in this report include: (1) institution of a confidential exposed partner notification system; (2) notification of all persons who received blood transfusions between 1977 and 1985 that they should be tested; (3) prevention and treatment of intravenous drug abuse as a top national priority; (4) prevention of drug and alcohol abuse (considered a facilitator for potential HIV exposure), especially through education of the nation's young people; (5) continual monitoring of blood supplies for safety; and (6) prevention of spread within health care facilities.

Secondary prevention will become increasingly important if methods to stop or retard disease progression in its presymptomatic stages become accessible and affordable.

IMPACT ON FAMILY UNIT. A special tragedy is the 35% potential for transmission of HIV from the mother to an unborn baby. Many of these infected babies are now left abandoned in the hospital.

Other Infectious Diseases and Immunizations

INCIDENCE. There are a number of infectious diseases that can be almost completely prevented by immunization. Many of these diseases have been public health scourges in the past and the source of great epidemics and even pandemics. These diseases include measles, mumps, rubella, hepatitis B, pneumococcal disease, influenza, pertussis, diphtheria, tetanus, poliomyelitis, and *Hemophilus influenzae* B disease. As can be seen from Table 12–14, the development of immunizations has cut this incidence a hundredfold or even a thousandfold in some cases.

Another group of preventable infectious diseases are those usually encountered by international travelers.

TABLE 12–14. U.S. CASES, DEATHS, AND VACCINATION RATES OF VACCINE-PREVENTABLE INFECTIOUS DISEASE

INFECTION	PREVACCINE CASES	LOW POSTVACCINE CASES	CURRENT CASES	TARGET GROUP VACCINATION RATE	YEARLY DEATHS
Measles	482,000	1497	18,200	85–95%	80–100 (est.)
Hepatitis B	N/A	Risen since vaccine in 1981	300,000	2–90%	250 (immediate) 5000 (sequelae)
Pneumococcal disease	N/A	N/A	N/A	10%	40,000
Influenza	N/A	N/A	N/A	20%	10–40,000
Pertussis	74,700	2820	4160	N/A	1
Diphtheria	9490	3	3	34–51%	1
Tetanus	601	48	53	16–59%	16
Paralytic polio	18,300	5	5	N/A	0
Hemophilus influenzae B disease	1 per 200 children prior to age 5	N/A	N/A	N/A	N/A
Rubella	3900	225	396	80–90%	0
Mumps	125,000	3020	5700	N/A	2

N/A: Not Available due to lack of reliable data.

The most common are malaria and travelers' diarrhea. The physician should provide information about mosquito avoidance, prophylactic medication, and food and water consumption.

COST/IMPACT ON SOCIETY. Although dollar values cannot be assigned for such a multiplicity of diseases, when the potential severe economic and health consequences of these diseases are compared with the marked efficacy of immunization, the cost-effectiveness is self-evident.

MORBIDITY/MORTALITY. In the past, these diseases had highly significant morbidity and mortality. Measles (rubeola) can cause death during the acute phase, while rubella can have a tremendous impact by causing congenital damage to the babies of mothers infected during pregnancy. Hepatitis has a low mortality rate of less than 1% during the acute episode, but up to 5% of victims may develop a chronic course with a need for extensive medical care that frequently ends in premature death.

Pertussis, diphtheria, tetanus, and *Hemophilus influenzae* B disease all had high incidence rates in the past, with an accompanying high death rate among the young. On the other hand, influenza and pneumococcal disease have had high incidence and mortality among the elderly. The latter two diseases still account for up to 80,000 deaths a year in the United States.

IMPORTANT FACTS RELEVANT TO PREVENTION

1. Immunization against these diseases will greatly decrease incidence, morbidity, and mortality.
2. Vaccines are available, relatively inexpensive, safe, and very cost-effective when compared to the costs associated with the morbidity and mortality of these diseases.

SCREENING TEST RECOMMENDATIONS

1. Each patient chart should contain a flow sheet recording the immunization status for each of these diseases, as well as rubella immune status for women in the childbearing years.
2. A quick review of the immune status should be made at each visit during the first 5 years of life and annually thereafter.

PREVENTIVE ACTIVITIES RECOMMENDATIONS

1. Each physician's office should be equipped to give needed immunizations when the screen reveals a need, or be prepared to refer to a facility that does. A sample schedule of recommended immunizations is found in Table 12–15.
2. All physicians should participate in community health education programs promoting public understanding of the need for appropriate immunizations.

DISCUSSION. Of all the activities carried out by physicians, the prevention of infectious diseases by immunization is the least expensive, takes the least effort, and is the most efficient. The control of the major infectious diseases has been a marked success for preventive medicine in the twentieth century.

Yet, despite the proven efficacy, there are major gaps in the full implementation of immunization. As can be seen in Table 12–14, measles has had a dramatic resurgence as a result of lax immunization practices. There are also major deficiencies in the levels of immunization for pneumococcal disease and influenza.

Health care workers in particular have an obligation to assure that they personally have an adequate immunization status for hepatitis B.

IMPACT ON THE FAMILY UNIT. A particular challenge for the family physician is the family that refuses to immunize its children for religious reasons or out of neglect. Other parents fear the potential side effects of vaccines (especially pertussis) and will rationalize that since most other children are immunized, the chances of their child's contracting the infection is near zero. Each physician should be aware of the relevant state laws and should have a strategy for dealing with these problems.

Moderate cost and occasional mild side effects such as fever, localized pain, or adenitis may cause some negative impact on the family. While a rare disastrous complication may occur, such as poliomyelitis in an unimmunized family member, these are so unusual that they are far outweighed by the benefits to the general popu-

TABLE 12–15. IMMUNIZATIONS: INDICATIONS AND SCHEDULES

IMMUNIZATION	0–15 YEARS OF AGE	16–64 YEARS	65 OR OLDER
DPT	2, 4, 6, 15 months and 4–6 years		
dT	15 years	Every 10 years	
OPV	2, 4, 6[a], 15 months and 4–6 years		
Measles	15 months and 4–6 years	College entrance[b]	
Mumps	15 months		
Rubella	15 months		
Hemophilus B[c]	2, 4, 12 months		
Influenza	Yearly if high risk	Yearly, high risk	Yearly
Pneumococcal		Once only when becomes high risk or at age 65	
Hepatitis B		Series of 3 when becomes high risk any age	

[a]Optional, except in endemic areas.
[b]If no previous booster. Other target groups if no previous booster are those leaving for foreign travel and health care workers.
[c]Conjugated vaccine: Schedule and number of injections may vary with vaccines from different manufacturers.

lation. The ultimate impact of a proper immunization program is healthier and more productive families with fewer congenital anomalies, fewer lost children, fewer paralyzed children and adults, and longer life spans for the elderly.

Accidents

INCIDENCE. The yearly number of accidents in the United States is over 60 million. The highest rate was found in the 18- to 24-year-old group.

COST/IMPACT ON SOCIETY. The estimated direct and indirect costs of injury in 1984 were nearly $97 million.

MORBIDITY/MORTALITY. There are over 95,000 deaths yearly from unintentional injuries. They are the fourth leading cause of death in the United States and the leading cause of death for those under 45. Almost half are secondary to automobile accidents. A distant second cause is falls, but these accidents are remarkable in that over 70% of them occur in the over 65 age group. The third most frequent cause of accidental death is drowning, followed by fire, poisoning, and unintentional firearm injuries.

IMPORTANT FACTS RELEVANT TO PREVENTION. Homes are the most common site of overall injury, while the automobile is the most common site for fatal injury. It is estimated that over half of all fatal automobile accidents involve a driver who has been drinking.

SCREENING TEST RECOMMENDATIONS. Screening for alcohol abuse is of top priority. Not only is it the major cause of traffic fatalities, it is also a major factor in all other types of traumatic accidents. Patients should be asked at the time of routine preventive health checks if they regularly use seat belts.

PREVENTIVE ACTIVITIES RECOMMENDATIONS. The guidelines for prevention listed under alcohol abuse and osteoporosis should be followed. Parents should be encouraged to assure that all children are taught to swim. Homes should be safety-proofed, especially when small children and the elderly live within the home. Use of seat belts and child restraint devices should be strongly encouraged. If available, air bags offer a significant additional degree of protection from automobile injury.

IMPACT ON FAMILY UNIT. In addition to the immediate trauma suffered, nonfatal accidents impact the individual and the family directly. An issue that must be confronted is the injured person's and the other family members' own mortality. Although some families will come closer at these times, others may distance as a defense mechanism.

Fatal accidents present a special problem. The loss is unexpected and often occurs in those who are otherwise young and healthy. The process of grieving may become particularly difficult or pathologic.

Glaucoma

PREVALENCE. The prevalence of increased intraocular pressure rises with age, from 5% at 40 years of age to 15% at 70–75 years of age. About 10% of those with increased pressure will have glaucoma.

IMPORTANT FACTS RELEVANT TO PREVENTION. The ultimate result of untreated glaucoma is blindness. The most common type of glaucoma, primary open angle, is asymptomatic until severe, often irreversible damage has occurred.

The three major criteria for diagnosis are elevated intraocular pressure, visual field defects, and optic disc pallor and cupping. In glaucoma, the cup's diameter is greater than 30% of that of the disc. The fundoscopic changes on direct ophthalmoscopy are best seen with the red filter.

Patients with upper normal intraocular pressure can have glaucoma and suffer from secondary blindness, while other patients can have elevated pressures without glaucoma. Both of these groups are exceptions to the usual course.

The risk factors for glaucoma are family history, black race, diabetes mellitus, and age.

SCREENING TEST RECOMMENDATIONS. The value of screening for elevated intraocular pressure with the Schiotz tonometer is controversial. If the family physician elects to use this method, patients should be screened starting at age 40 and every 5 years thereafter until age 60, at which time the screening interval should be reduced to 2–3 years. Fundoscopic evaluation by a well-trained physician at the time of tonometry will increase the sensitivity of screening.

PREVENTIVE ACTIVITIES RECOMMENDATIONS. There are no primary preventive measures available. Secondary prevention consists of educating patients of the need for regular evaluation for early detection and the warning signs of progressive glaucoma (e.g., blurring of vision and halos around lights).

DISCUSSION. Schiotz tonometry, although an accurate measure of intraocular pressure, has only a 66% sensitivity and a 91% specificity for glaucoma. Therefore, one-third of patients with glaucoma will have normal tonometry readings and will be missed. Also, 9% of those with elevated measurements will not have glaucoma. These facts make it imperative that high-risk patients have more extensive screening by an ophthalmologist, and that patients who are screened with tonometry only are advised that they are still at risk. The major value in screening is to detect those individuals with presymptomatic disease who would not ordinarily see an ophthalmologist. These individuals can then be referred for additional testing.

Diabetes Mellitus

Diabetes mellitus does not meet the criteria for mass screening, despite its high prevalence, high morbidity and mortality, long presymptomatic stage, and ease of diagnosis. Early diagnosis and treatment has not been shown to alter the prognosis. Nevertheless, screening has been advocated because the presence of diabetes is a major risk factor for coronary heart disease.

The only exception in which screening for diabetes provides clear direct benefit is during pregnancy.

TABLE 12–16. RELATIONSHIP BETWEEN COMMON PREVENTABLE DISEASES AND THE MOST COMMON RISK FACTORS

RISK FACTOR	DIET	HYPERLIPIDEMIA	OBESITY	HYPERTENSION	SMOKING	ALCOHOL	SEDENTARY LIFESTYLE	HEREDITY	STRESS AND DEPRESSION
Coronary heart disease	■	■	■	■	■		■	■	■
Stroke	■	■	■	■	■		■	■	■
Chemical dependence						■		■	■
Osteoporosis	■							■	
Accident/suicide						■		■	■
Sexually transmitted diseases and human immunodeficiency virus infection						■			
Lung cancer					■				
Breast cancer	■					■?		■	
Colon cancer	■								
Cervical cancer									
Endometrial cancer			■						

Source: Rakel RE. Textbook of Family Practice. 4th ed. Philadelphia, W.B. Saunders, 1990, with permission.

PREVENTIVE CARE FLOW SHEET
DEPARTMENT OF FAMILY MEDICINE
UNIVERSITY OF VIRGINIA

TEST	AGE IN YEARS									
	40	41	42	43	44	45	46	47	48	49
LIFESTYLE RISK ASSESSMENT	▬		▬		▬		▬		▬	
CHOLESTEROL HDL*	▬					▬				
STOOL GUIAC X3 RECTAL*	▬	▬	▬	▬	▬	▬	▬	▬	▬	▬
FLEXIBLE SIGMOIDOSCOPY*						▬				
Td	▬									
BREAST EXAM	▬	▬	▬	▬	▬	▬	▬	▬	▬	▬
MAMMOGRAM*	▬ ?		▬ ?		▬ ?		▬ ?		▬ ?	
PAP†	▬	▬ ?	▬ ?	▬	▬ ?	▬ ?	▬	▬ ?	▬ ?	▬

RISK FACTOR SUMMARY

Cardiovascular Risk
High LDL
Low HDL
+ Family History
Male
Tobacco
Hypertension
Diabetes Mellitus
Sedentary
Obesity
Stress
BCP > 35 y/o

Lung Cancer
Tobacco

Alcohol Abuse
Felt like Cutting down?
Annoyed by criticism?
Guilty about drinking?
Eye opener?
+ Family history
Problem in past related to alcohol?
   (legal, personal, health)

Suicide
Previous attempt
+ Family history
Depression

Glaucoma
+ Family history
Diabetes Mellitus
Black

Sexually Transmitted DIS/HIV
Blood transfusions (1978–85)
Multiple sexual partners
Bisexual/homosexual
Non-barrier contraception
Presence of or exposure to other STD
History of IV drug use

Osteoporosis
<1.0 gm. CA daily
Sedentary
+ Family history
Thin
White/oriental
Tobacco

Breast Cancer
+ Family history
Nulliparous
Primigravida at >35 y/o
Previous high risk biopsy

Cervical Cancer
History condylomata
History herpes
Multiple sexual partners
Early age first intercourse

Instructions for Use of Flow Sheet
Bars in boxes indicate appropriate age for test
Add a bar to a box if you plan to do the test at a
   different time or more often
Enter mo/yr in box when test completed
Write N/A if not applicable to patient
Write D/E in box if done elsewhere
Circle and date positive risk factors
To change a circled risk factor to negative write OK
   and date

*Controversial.
†May reduce to every 3 years after 3 normal Pap smears in low-risk groups.

Figure 12–5. Example of one of a set of flow sheets, each covering a decade.

Categories	Age Date	36	37	38	39	40	41	42	43	44	45	46	47	48	49	50
History and Physical Examination																
Blood pressure measured every year																
Dental examination every year																
Teach breast self-examination																
Menopause symptoms (present?)																
Contraceptive needs reviewed every year																
Laboratory Tests																
Baseline mammogram (under age 50)																
Cholesterol and high-density lipoprotein (baseline)																
Papanicolaou's smear (every 2 years—American Cancer Society; every 5 years Canada)																
Immunization																
Td (every 10 years)																
Counsel/Patient Education (Annually)																
Cigarette smoking																
Alcohol use																
Occupational hazards																
Skin cancer protection																
Seat belt use																
Exercise																
Life stages career/achievement family social stability																
Calcium supplementation																

Figure 12–6. Example of health screening flow sheet used in the department of family medicine, University of New Mexico.

LIFESTYLES FOR HEALTH

When one reviews the diseases discussed in this chapter, there is a strikingly common theme in their etiology and prevention: An individual's lifestyle is the major modifiable determinant of health.

Proper diet is of paramount importance to prevent the nation's number one killer, coronary heart disease; and it is estimated that 35% of cancers, the nation's number two killer, are secondary to diet. Fortunately, the specific dietary recommendations for prevention of one disease are also beneficial in general. Therefore, it is possible to make broad, prudent nutritional recommendations as a basis on which all physicians and patients can build: (1) total calories to achieve and maintain ideal body weight; (2) fat less than 30% of total calories; (3) saturated fat less than 10% of total calories; (4) cholesterol less than 300 mg per day; (5) carbohydrates 50% to 60% of total calories, emphasizing complex carbohydrates; (6) fiber, maximizing levels in diet, with emphasis on soluble fiber sources; (7) calcium, minimum of 1000 mg daily; and (8) sodium chloride, minimize to less than 3 gm of sodium (7.5 gm salt).

The importance of stress reduction and exercise in preventing disease is a subject of great interest. There is general agreement that they are of real importance. Recent studies have shown a significant protective effect for all-cause mortality for even modest levels of exercise.

Another common theme is the critical importance of avoiding toxins, especially the addictive substances nicotine and alcohol. Smoking accounts for 30% of all cancer deaths as well as being a major factor in coronary heart disease. Three hundred and twenty thousand deaths each year can be directly attributed to cigarette smoking. It is estimated that each pack of cigarettes sold results in a cost of $2.17 in medical care and lost productivity. Four percent of all male cancer deaths and 2% of all female cancer deaths are due to alcohol. Alcohol is a major contributor to morbidity and mortality from accidents of all kinds, liver disease, suicide, and homicide.

Table 12–16 shows the major diseases discussed and the number in which each of the above lifestyle issues is implicated.

DEVELOPING A PREVENTIVE HEALTH CARE FLOW SHEET

A simple and flexible flow sheet is essential for the continuity and comprehensiveness of preventive health care. Such a form can be effectively used as a tool for educating patients concerning their preventive health care needs. Patients at high risk for certain illnesses may need to have increased frequency of screening tests or special tests added. Also, recommendations for preventive activities will change as new information becomes available. An inflexible form will be of little use in 5–10 years.

An *informative* flow sheet will alert the physician to risk factors that have not been identified and proce- dures that have not been accomplished. Missing pieces of information should be obvious on even a cursory review of the form.

A deterrent to the use of any form or flow sheet is a need to duplicate data that are available elsewhere in the record. Therefore, the more data entry that is *unique* to the form, the more likely it is to be used.

Figures 12–5 and 12–6 show examples of flow sheets that family physicians have found useful.

GETTING STARTED

A comprehensive preventive health program is difficult to implement all at once in a busy physician's office. It often requires a new mind-set for physician and staff, a supporting set of educational materials and referral sources, and equipment. Adding new elements, one at a time, will obviate much of the potential threat posed by such a major undertaking. The office may decide to emphasize lipid screening or colorectal cancer screening at the beginning. Necessary staff and physician education, selection of appropriate educational materials, purchase of equipment, and implementation of the program can then take place in a longitudinal fashion at a comfortable pace. Once this is done to everyone's satisfaction, additional screening and preventive modules can be added, once again, one at a time.

The important thing is to begin.

BIBLIOGRAPHY AND SELECTED REFERENCES

American Heart Association. An Eating Plan for Healthy Americans. Dallas, American Heart Association.

American Heart Association. Dietary Treatment of Hypercholesterolemia—A Manual for Patients. Dallas, American Heart Association. 1988.

Brody J. Good Food Book. New York, W.W. Norton, 1985.

Castelli WP. Epidemiology of coronary heart disease: The Framingham Study. Am J Med, Feb. 27, 1984.

Conner WE, Conner SL. The New American Diet. New York, Simon and Schuster, 1986.

Eshleman R. The American Heart Association Cookbook. New York, NY. David McKay Co., 1984.

Hudson TW, et al. Clinical Preventive Medicine: Health Promotion and Disease Prevention. Boston, Little, Brown, 1988.

National Heart, Blood and Lung Institute. National Cholesterol Education Program. Bethesda, Md., National Institutes of Health, 1987.

Office of Disease Prevention and Health Promotion, U.S. Public Health Service. Disease Prevention/Health Promotion: The Facts. Palo Alto, Ca., Bull Publishing Company, 1988.

Riegelman RK and Povar GT. Putting Prevention into Practice. Boston, Little, Brown, 1988.

U.S. Preventive Services Task Force. Guide to Clinical Preventive Services. Baltimore, Williams and Wilkins, 1989.

QUESTIONS

1. Finding a small asymptomatic breast cancer on routine mammography is an example of
   a. Primary prevention.
   b. Secondary prevention.
   c. Tertiary prevention.
   d. Health promotion.

2. The major strategies for reducing cholesterol include (true or false)
   a. Exercising to maximum heart rate at least five times weekly.
   b. Reduction of dietary cholesterol.
   c. Supplements of omega-3 fatty acids.
   d. Reduction in dietary saturated fat.
   e. Meditation.

3. Documented major risk factors for coronary heart disease in the general population include (true or false)
   a. LDL cholesterol greater than 160.
   b. Type A personality
   c. Low HDL cholesterol

d. A family history of myocardial infarction under 55 years of age.

e. Cigarette smoking.

4. The marked reduction in the incidence of myocardial infarction in the past 10 years is primarily due to

a. Changes in methods of statistical analysis.

b. The "911" emergency system.

c. Lifestyle changes in the population.

d. Coronary bypass surgery.

e. Increasing premature cancer deaths.

5. In the general population, the greatest degree of proven benefit in reducing the incidence of stroke can be attained by

a. Dietary modification.

b. Regular aspirin therapy.

c. Carotid endarterectomy on all patients with carotid bruits.

d. Control of hypertension.

e. None of the above.

6. In the usual outpatient setting, the prevalence of alcoholism is generally measured at approximately

a. 10%.

b. 0.05%.

c. 3%.

d. 21%.

e. 1%.

7. Recommended strategies for dealing with alcoholism in the family practice outpatient setting include (true or false)

a. Including an instrument such as the CAGE questionnaire in preventive health risk screening.

b. Providing alcohol information sources in the office.

c. Documenting family history of alcoholism.

d. Encouraging abstinence for all patients.

e. Performing liver enzymes on all patients.

8. When considering a strategy for preventing colon cancer, which of the following are true?

a. There is no relationship in more recent epidemiologic studies between colon cancer and dietary fiber.

b. The majority of colon cancers are still within reach of the 60-cm flexible scope.

c. Colorectal cancer arises almost exclusively form benign polyps.

d. Family history has no effect on risk for colorectal cancer.

9. The major risks for cervical cancer include all of the following except

a. Infection with human papilloma virus.

b. Early onset of sexual intercourse.

c. Premature menopause.

d. Multiple sexual partners.

e. Severe dysplasia on Pap smear.

10. Which of the following are true about breast cancer?

a. About one in 20 females will eventually have breast cancer.

b. Since most females with breast cancer have known risk factors, screening programs can be focused just on this group.

c. Clinical breast exam is still important even if the mammography is negative.

d. There is a consensus among the national panels and organizations interested in breast cancer that screening should begin on all women at age 35.

e. A positive family history of breast cancer in a first-degree relative significantly increases the risk of a female patient.

11. Important strategies for the prevention of osteoporosis include (true or false)

a. 1000 mg of calcium daily for all females prior to menopause.

b. X-rays to determine bone density at menopause.

c. Consideration of postmenopausal estrogen therapy.

d. Postmenopausal progesterone therapy.

e. Regular swimming or other non-weight-bearing exercise after menopause.

12. You are asked to submit a list of screening tests and procedures for a local T.V. station to use in a health fair they are sponsoring. Criteria for tests to utilize would include (true or false)

a. Accuracy and reproductivity of the test.

b. A test which finds a disease after it is present.

c. A relatively inexpensive test.

d. Acceptability to the population.

e. A test for a rare disease with little morbidity.

13. Some tests you might recommend to the promoter of the health fair would include (true or false)

a. Baseline screening EKG.

b. Serum uric acid levels.

c. Serum cholesterol levels and lipid profile.

d. Blood pressure.

e. Smoking, drinking, and drug use questionnaire.

f. Mammograms for all women over 40.

14. Diseases for which you would plan screening activities would include (true or false)

a. Hypertension.

b. Down's syndrome.

c. Glaucoma.

d. Carcinoma of the lung.

e. Osteoporosis.

Match each of the following nutritional or medication recommendations with the clinical situations in questions 15 to 18:

 a. Decreased eggs, whole milk, butter, fatty meats, and shellfish; increased fiber.

 b. An ad lib "sensible" diet with sufficient calories to maintain an ideal weight.

 c. Initiate therapy with antilipidemia medication.

 d. A diet high in milk, yogurt, cottage cheese, green leafy vegetables, and fruits.

15. A 42-year-old man with a total cholesterol of 270 mg, LDL-C of 210 mg, and HDL-C of 30 mg who smokes two packs of cigarettes a day and whose father died of a myocardial infarction at age 50.

16. A 50-year-old woman with a total cholesterol of 160 mg, LDL-C of 100 mg, and FSH level of 89.

17. A 55-year-old woman, 6 years postmenopausal, whose grandfather had a "heart attack" at age 89 and who has a total cholesterol of 185 mg, LDL-C of 135 mg, and no other risk factors identified.

18. A 35-year-old man with an LDL-C of 125 and no other risk factors

19. The *single* drug most commonly used by young people in the United States is

 a. Marijuana.

 b. Cigarettes.

 c. Cocaine.

 d. Hashish.

 e. Alcohol.

20. The *two* most prevalent sexually transmitted diseases currently are

 a. AIDS.

 b. Chlamydia.

 c. Human papilloma virus.

 d. Syphilis.

 e. Gonorrhea.

 f. Herpes simplex.

Answers appear on page 447.

USING CONSULTANTS

ROBERT E. RAKEL

All physicians, regardless of their specialty, turn to other physicians at some time for advice. This process became formalized as physicians focused their training and limited their practice to a particular segment of medicine. The first specialty board, the American Board of Ophthalmology, was formed in 1917, and by 1989, there were 23 specialty boards and 51 subspecialty boards. The American Board of Family Practice established in 1969 was the twentieth primary specialty.

It is a common misconception of medical students that less information needs to be mastered in a narrow subspecialty than in family practice or other primary care disciplines. The fact is that the amount of information required to practice each of the 74 specialties and subspecialties is clearly defined and is about the same. What varies is the degree of breadth and depth in each.

In addition to being trained in a wide variety of clinical areas, family physicians are also trained to coordinate the care of seriously ill individuals who require a variety of consultants, orchestrating the skills of each to achieve optimum patient care and satisfaction (see Chapter 1). "Every patient should have a primary care physician who not only sees him for first-contact care, but who actively participates in his secondary and tertiary care by arranging and coordinating his consultant needs, by providing continuity, and by taking the patient back" (Stephens).

The appropriate use of the consultation process is an art that contributes to improved patient care when utilized properly by family physicians. Although there is a definite distinction between consultation and referral, the terms are often used interchangeably. Consultation is by definition the practice of one physician asking another for an opinion or assistance, whereas referral is the transfer of responsibility to another physician for the care of a specific problem. Referral usually involves one physician requesting the services of another for a particular purpose and for a limited time, such as referral to a surgeon for a cholecystectomy or to a cardiologist for coronary angiography. On the other hand, consultation is the process whereby one physician requests the opinion of a colleague regarding the diagnosis or management of a patient's problem. Regardless of this distinction, the physician initiating either process is spoken of as the referring physician, and the physician who is consulted or to whom the patient is referred is called the consultant.

In a study of patterns of consultation and referral, Geyman and associates found that 97% of the exchanges between family physicians and other specialists were referrals and only 3% were consultations. Fry notes with regret that consultation is no longer a deliberation between colleagues about diagnosis or proper treatment. He says, "We have come to view our specialist colleagues more as expert 'technicians' than as consultants." Although the system in the United Kingdom has been described as the specialist controlling the hospital and the general practitioner controlling the patient, this separation avoids much of the rivalry over patient care that occurs in the United States. Horder believes that "patients look to all of us for the same two things, technical competence and personal care. I believe that, at present, we have more cause to be concerned about the supply of personal care than technical competence."

WHEN TO REFER

It is wise to ask for a consultation whenever the patient or family expresses doubt or shows lack of confidence in the diagnosis or management. It is sometimes wise to obtain a second opinion for patients who have a life-threatening illness or a disease with a poor prognosis.

Consultation should also be considered when the family physician is dissatisfied with the patient's progress or is unsure of the diagnosis. One rarely gets in trouble asking for help with a difficult problem, but every experienced physician can remember at least one case in which a consultation should have been obtained. A consultation should be promptly initiated any time the patient or family requests or hints that they would like to have one. The physician must be alert to subtle clues of doubt indicating the desire for another opinion. If these clues are recognized and acted upon, confidence in the family physician increases. If not recognized, patient dissatisfaction leading to malpractice litigation may result. When doubt is recognized, the patient or family member should be encouraged to discuss this openly; consultation is then often unnecessary.

An early consultation is much less likely to damage patient confidence than a delayed one. The confident and secure physician who considers patient welfare to be of the utmost importance is not threatened and freely utilizes consultants at the appropriate, sometimes early, stage of a problem, before it has progressed to serious proportions that are more difficult to manage.

The patient's family is more apt to display doubt regarding the management of a case than is the patient. The physician who communicates easily with members of the family and is aware of their feelings will detect this insecurity earlier than the physician who is familiar only with the patient. The patient is less likely than other family members to express doubt regarding a diagnosis or method of management for fear of offending the physician. Whenever doubt is noted among the family members, the physician should suggest that the opinion of another physician be obtained.

RESPONSIBILITIES OF THE REFERRING PHYSICIAN

The consultation process involves approximately 12 decision points, beginning with the family physician's decision to refer and concluding with the family physician's providing feedback to the consultant regarding the eventual outcome (Table 13–1).

SELECTION OF THE CONSULTANT. The referring physician is responsible for the selection of the proper consultant for a particular patient. The family physician whose comprehensive training involves a broad range of disciplines has the insight needed to select the appropriate consultant for a specific problem. Care must be taken to select a consultant who has knowledge and skills appropriate to the patient's need, a personality compat-

ible with that of the patient, availability, competency maintained by frequent use of the required skills, and the ability to work well with the referring physician. Compatibility of personalities is an especially important factor to be considered, if at all possible, when selecting a consultant. A surgeon who alienates the patient, no matter how skilled, will be less effective than one who establishes good rapport and has the patient's confidence and cooperation.

Referrals to a psychiatrist sometimes pose special problems. Some patients resist such a referral and the family physician may also feel uncomfortable making the suggestion. However, the patient frequently welcomes psychiatric help and may be relieved by the recommendation. In a review of psychiatric problems encountered in hospitalized patients (Steinberg et al.), 50% of the patients for whom psychiatric consultation would have been helpful did not receive it because of physician resistance or failure to recognize the psychiatric problem. In those patients who later received psychiatric care, most of them accepted it well.

Patients are likely to benefit more from a psychiatric referral if they enter into the consultation with a positive frame of mind. Once the need for a psychiatric referral has been determined, the patient should be told the reason in an honest, straightforward manner. Questions about psychosocial problems should be incorporated into the history from the beginning of an illness, since they are a part of every problem, rather than being avoided until organic possibilities have been exhausted.

A perceptive family physician—through knowledge of the patient's personality, lifestyle, and previous reaction to similar situations—can best select the consultant and clinical setting to which the patient will respond positively.

ADEQUATE TRANSFER OF INFORMATION. The referring physician must be sure that the referral contract is clearly understood by the consultant. If the referring physician wants help with a diagnosis but does not say so, the consultant may assume that the request is for help with management, leading to dissatisfaction and unwarranted charges of "patient stealing." The referring physician should state the reason for the request and the action desired so that the consultant knows clearly whether the request is for an opinion only or also involves management.

The most common breakdowns of communication between referring and consulting physicians are the consultation request and the consultant's report. The referring physician must evaluate the problem adequately and transmit all necessary information to the consultant. Complete and accurate background information should avoid unnecessary duplication of diagnostic tests.

The process of information transfer varies with the nature of the problem. Some are straightforward, as for example a 67-year-old patient with an intertrochanteric fracture. If there are no medical problems and the patient is a good surgical risk, the transfer report can be brief. Other problems may require a complete summary of the office record, as in the referral of a 9-year-old pa-

TABLE 13–1. THE CONSULTATION PROCESS

1. The decision is made to refer.
2. Consideration is given to the patient's medical, emotional, cultural, and socioeconomic background.
3. Selection of the appropriate discipline (specialty field).
4. Selection of the appropriate physician in that field.
5. Preparation of both the patient and family for the consultation.
6. Preparation of the consultant.
7. The consultant provides feedback to the patient and family.
8. The consultant provides feedback to the family physician.
9. The family physician evaluates the appropriateness of the consultant's recommendations.
10. The family physician facilitates the patient and the family's acceptance of recommendations.
11. The family physician acts on the recommendations or selects another consultant in the same or a different field.
12. The family physician provides feedback to the consultant regarding eventual outcome.

Source: Modified from Barnett BL, Jr, Collins JJ, Jr. A new look at the consultation continuum. J Fam Pract. 1987; 5:665, with permission.

tient for recurring fever that lasts approximately 1 week every month despite negative laboratory studies.

The outpatient consultation or referral note should be in the mail within 24 hours or, better still, carried by the patient to the consultant, accompanied by a copy of the problem list and other pertinent items from the data base, including recent progress notes, laboratory reports, and x-ray films. The problem-oriented medical record is ideally suited to this, since it summarizes all major disorders affecting the individual and alerts the consultant to other past and potentially significant complications that should be considered in the management of the patient's current situation. An extensive referral note is not needed when adequate information is provided by the medical record.

PATIENT PREPARATION AND COMPLIANCE. Ten percent of all patients never keep the appointment with the consultant (Cummins et al.). Patient compliance may be improved if the patient feels more involved in the referral process. First, the referring physician should adequately inform the patient regarding the need for referral and ensure his or her understanding and cooperation. (The consent is particularly important if the patient is hospitalized, since almost half of the complaints to medical society grievance committees stem from patients receiving bills for hospital consultations that they had not authorized.) The informed patient understands what will occur and that the family physician will remain in charge or will resume responsibility at the conclusion of the referral. The understanding is important if the patient is to avoid feeling rejected or "sent away."

It is also likely that compliance will be increased if the patient is given some choice of consultants and control over the time of appointment. When the family physician recommends a consultation, the patient should be asked if a specific consultant is preferred. If not, then two or three qualified individuals should be suggested, with the positive features of each being identified. If the patient does not indicate a preference, then the family physician should make the final decision. Hines and Curry encourage the patient to review the referral form and accompanying materials when carrying them to the consultant. They feel this increases patient insight and cooperation, reducing "no shows" in the consultant's office.

Details about the appointment with the consultant may be difficult for the patient to remember, so providing a written note containing the consultant's name, address, and telephone number is helpful. It may also help to include directions to the consultant's office and to discuss with the patient what to expect during the visit, especially the amount of time it will take.

EVALUATION OF INFORMATION. It is the family physician's responsibility to continue to interact with the physician to whom the patient is referred and to lend assistance in the management of the case to the degree that is necessary for the best care of the patient. Even referrals that are for specific surgical procedures require that the family physician remain involved to manage concomitant medical problems, especially if they require cooperation from other family members. Carson found that only 7.8% of referrals were for the purpose of establishing a diagnosis. As in other studies, most referrals were for specific procedures, in this case to orthopedists, obstetricians, general surgeons, and dermatologists. Even when the consultation involves surgical or other technical skills, the family physician is responsible for ensuring that other aspects of the patient's medical background are not ignored and that the family is kept adequately informed.

Newly discovered information needs to be coordinated with that already recorded. When information is received from the consultant, the family physician must evaluate it within the context of the individual patient and the patient's family situation, work environment, expectations, and ability to comply. The family physician should also guide the consultant in the amount of information that should be given to the patient and family, being aware of how much information the family can tolerate and how it should be provided in order to enlist maximum support. Continued involvement of the family physician improves compliance with the treatment program and facilitates long-term rehabilitation.

FEEDBACK TO CONSULTANTS. It may be of value to keep a log of all referrals. Such a log, containing the patient's name, name of consultant, and date of referral, could then be checked when the report is returned to ensure that the patient actually sees the consultant and that a report is received. It would also help identify consultants who do not return information about patients. The log can be reviewed weekly and the consultant or patient contacted if no information is received after a specified time.

Family physicians should give feedback to the consultant regarding the outcome of an unusual case and not leave the consultant wondering whether the diagnosis was correct or the treatment successful. This is an especially appropriate courtesy if the consultant was prompt in reporting and in returning the patient. If the consultant has not provided information of value in managing the patient, then a second consultation should be seriously considered. Clarfield found that referring physicians felt that one-third of the time (31% of consultations) they had learned nothing of value from the referral. It is also important to let the consultant know if the consultation was inadequate. Experienced family physicians can help young consultants improve their "art of consultation" and should accept this as a responsibility, since consultants are rarely taught this skill during residency training. Bates believes that "nothing better expresses the ideal fraternity of medicine than an older family doctor helping a young specialist with professional relationships."

Suspecting that faulty consultation practices may be learned during residency training, McPhee and colleagues studied the communication between 27 general internists at a university medical center and their subspecialty colleagues who practiced in the same building in San Francisco. Even in this close academic setting where the referral rate was 9.4%, the referring physician did not receive a report 45% of the time. The poorest responding consultants were in ophthalmology (no response 69% of the time), obstetrics and gynecology (61%), orthopedics (57%), and dermatology (52%). A response was most likely to be received if the referring physician personally contacted the consultant.

RESPONSIBILITIES OF THE CONSULTANT

The consultant is expected to provide a prompt and concise report to the referring physician. The specific questions posed on the consultation request should be addressed and action limited to the amount of involvement requested. When the consultation involves a hospitalized patient, the consultant should see the patient promptly, provide an opinion and give therapeutic suggestions in a concise note on the consultation sheet, and, in general, not write orders unless there is this understanding with the referring physician.

The consultant has a responsibility to the patient and the referring physician to avoid unnecessary expense through duplication of studies recently obtained by the primary physician, unless there is good reason to doubt the results or there is sufficient need to repeat the test. Of course, the referring physician must have included the actual x-rays and adequate laboratory data as part of the referral document if such duplication is to be avoided. Adequate communication via the consultation request is essential, so that the consultant is made aware of the tests that already have been performed, the methods used, and the results obtained. The consultant's obligation is to build on this information, repeating procedures only when necessary to verify an abnormality or evaluate a change.

When a patient is referred for care, the consultant should remain in contact with the referring physician throughout the period of care and return the patient with a full written report when the problem is resolved or when no further involvement by the consultant is warranted.

A consultant should not refer patients to other consultants without the knowledge and consent of the primary physician, who should be coordinating or at least closely involved with this process.

The most common reason for discontinuing referrals to a particular consultant is failure to receive adequate reports or failure of the consultant to return the patient for continuing care. The latter occurs most frequently when the consultant also functions as a primary physician. The patient may "stay on" for continuing care if the consultant does not encourage his or her return to the referring physician. Even though a specific request was made for follow-up information, Cummins and associates received a report from the consultant only 62% of the time. Seventy-eight percent of consultants who were in private practice responded, but only 59% of those in university clinics did so. It was disappointing to note that the follow-up information was not better for patients who required continuing care by the family physician than for those with self-limiting problems. Even though one university stressed to its staff the importance of providing such follow-up information, the faculty did so only 75% of the time. It is distressing for the family physician who is responsible for continuing care of the patient to have the patient return after being hospitalized at a university center with no information having been sent regarding the treatment given or plans for follow-up. It is even more embarrassing to learn from a family member that a patient who was recently referred to a nearby medical center has died.

Curry and associates found that enclosing a return mailer with the consultation request (including a stamped, self-addressed envelope and a form specifically requesting feedback from the consultant) increased the percentage of consultant feedback from 39% to 60% and also increased the speed of the reply. These rates were significantly higher if the lack of reply from Veterans Administration Hospitals was excluded. Even with the higher response rate, it is unfortunate that 40% of the referrals resulted in no report to the referring physician.

Providing appropriate feedback to both patient and referring physician is a talent possessed by too few referral centers. The Mayo Clinic has an excellent reputation for providing good feedback to the referring physician. The Clinic also has a talent for maintaining or bolstering patients' respect for their family physician. Bates says, "The top notch consultant will render a report that informs without patronizing, educates without lecturing, directs without ordering and—sometimes most difficult of all—solves the problem without making the referring physician appear to be stupid. The real stars in this play are the consultants who discuss the differential diagnosis in such a way that they make a good case for the referring physician's previous diagnosis even when it was wrong."

The consultant's opinion should be weighed by the referring physician and the appropriate action taken, depending on the conclusions reached. The family physician may have already considered many of the recommendations the consultant makes but discarded them based on factors that may be unknown to the consultant.

Shortell and Anderson describe the rewards for both referring physician and consultant when their exchange is effective. For the referring physician, it is a positive and rewarding experience, knowing that the patient has received proper treatment. It will be a negative experience if the patient does not return or is disappointed with the consultant. The consultant will be flattered at being chosen as an expert and will enjoy receiving a well-prepared, cooperative patient. This could change to a negative feeling if the consultant receives an unpleasant, problem patient because the family physician does not want to be "bothered" any longer (i.e., the "dumping syndrome"), or if the consultant is called upon to treat patients without having been provided with adequate background information.

REFERRAL RATES

Rates of referral by family physicians in the United States and Canada average 2.7%, with a range of 1.0%

TABLE 13–2.   TYPES AND RATES OF REFERRAL FOR THE UNITED STATES

	CRUMP AND MASSENGILL	DOLEZAL ET AL.	GEYMAN ET AL.	GLENN ET AL.	MAYER	METCALFE AND SISCHY	MOSCOVICE ET AL.	RUANE	SCHMIDT	WHITE
Location	Alabama	South Dakota	California	Missouri	Minnesota	New York	Washington	Vermont	Massachusetts	Illinois
Year conducted	1977 to 1985	1977 to 1978	1974	1977 to 1979	1978	1973	1978	1978	1972 to 1973	1984
Length of study	9 years	1 year	2 months	3 years	1 year	1.5 months	3 months	7 months	1 year	2 months
Number of family physicians	161*	27*	8	>20†	3	4	6 and 1 surgeon	*++	1	17
Total number of patient visits during study period	177,838	15,609	6409 (office and hospital)	30,131	12,228	4604	6586	7220	5814 (office and hospital)	3975
Referral rate (per cent)	1.4	1	1.6	1.65	3.85	2.2	2.4	1.5	3	2.97

RANKING OF TOP FIVE SECIALTIES CONSULTED

Crump	Per Cent	Dolezal	Per Cent	Geyman	Per Cent	Metcalfe	Per Cent	Moscovice	Per Cent
ENT	13.4	Ortho.	17.9	Gen. Surg.	20.6	Gen. Surg.	25.5	Ortho.	21.2
Ortho.	13.3	OB-Gyn	17.3	Ortho.	15.8	OB-Gyn	10.8	Surg.	19.3
OB-Gyn	12.2	Gen. Surg.	15.4	OB-Gyn	11.9	Ortho.	9.8	ENT	10.6
Gen. Surg.	12.1	ENT	13.0	Ophthal.	11.1	ENT	9.8	Neurol.	7.5
Neurol.	8.0	Ophthal.	8.0	Urology	7.9	Urology	7.8	Gynecol.	5.0

				Mayer					
Ruane	Per Cent	Glenn	Per Cent	FEE-FOR-SERVICE	PER CENT	HMO	PER CENT	White	Per Cent
Gen. Surg.	22.0	Gen. Surg.	13.7	Gen. Surg.	17.3	Gen. Surg.	14.8	ENT	++
Ortho.	13.7	OB-Gyn	12.9	ENT	13.1	ENT	13.4	Surgery	++
ENT	12.7	ENT	11.9	Ortho.	12.5	Derm.	10.6	Neurol.	++
Univ. Hosp. Emerg. Dept.	10.8	Ortho.	10.5	OB-Gyn	10.7	OB-Gyn	9.5	OB-Gyn	++
		Ophthal.		Derm.					
Ophthal.	8.8		7.9		8.9	Ortho.	8.1	Ortho.	++
Derm.	6.9							Ophthal.	++

++Number not specified
*Residents and faculty.
†Residents, faculty, and nurse practitioners.

to 5.4%, as shown in Tables 13–2 and 13–3. Referral rates are greater for women than men and are highest in 15- to 44-year-old individuals. The National Ambulatory Medical Care Survey (1985) noted a 4.2% consultation rate in general and family practice.

The largest study of outpatient consultation rates by family physicians has been conducted by Crump and Massengill at the University of Alabama in Huntsville. This was a nine-year study involving 177,838 patient visits to 143 residents and 18 faculty members. The overall consultation rate was 1.4%; little year-to-year variation was noted (range 1.1–1.6%). Most of the referrals were to specialists in otolaryngology and orthopedics, followed by obstetrics and gynecology, general surgery, neurology, and urology.

In pediatrics and internal medicine, the two other primary care specialties, referral rates are somewhat higher. Internal medicine has a referral rate of 2.2% to 18.2%, and pediatrics has a range of 1.0% to 9.5% (Penchansky and Fox); however, the referral process in these specialties has not been studied in as much detail. It appears that this difference in rates can be explained by the less comprehensive nature of internists' and pediatricians' practices and their need for assistance in fields peripheral to areas of major emphasis in training. As noted in Table 13–2, most referrals are to a surgical specialty for a diagnostic procedure or specific therapy.

Ruane reviewed 108 consecutive referrals in a family practice and found a 1.5% referral rate. He noted, "The well trained family physician provides definitive care for the vast majority (in this study 98.4 percent) of patient encounters, contrary to the cherished beliefs of many medical school faculty." Twenty percent of the referrals were for the specific treatment of clear-cut problems (usually surgery). Sixty-four percent were for diagnostic tests not available to the primary care physician, such as allergy testing or arthrography. One family physician in his third year of practice found that less than one-half of 1% of patients were referred to a tertiary care center, and these were usually for the management of uncommon problems such as leukemia, sepsis, bone tumor, or cardiac bypass rather than for diagnosis (Schmidt).

Consultations in a rural practice have been documented according to the International Classification of Health Problems in Primary Care (Glenn et al., Table 13–2). By far, the most frequent problems requiring consultation involved the nervous system and sense organs. More than 86% of these problems were referred to specialists in neurology, ophthalmology, or otolaryngology. The second most common problems that needed referral were those associated with the genitourinary system, requiring consultation from a urologist or gynecologist. Data of this type may assist residency directors in emphasizing those areas during graduate training, although most referrals will continue to be for specific subspecialty procedures.

When referral rates for fee-for-service patients were compared with those for members of a health maintenance organization (HMO) in Minnesota (Mayer), the fee-for-service patients had a lower referral rate (3.19%) than the HMO patients (4.46%). Although the percentages of referral differed, the rank order of specialists that problems were referred to was remarkably similar and matched the specialists referred to most commonly in other studies (see Table 13–2).

What is not clear is whether a low rate of referral indicates that the physician is competent and requires assistance infrequently or whether that physician is incompetent and does not recognize problems that require referral. Other factors may play a role as well; the practice may consist mostly of healthy young adults, or consultants may not be available and referral may be difficult.

TABLE 13–3. TYPES AND RATES OF REFERRAL FOR CANADA

	Brock	Dixon	Hines and Curry
Location	Ontario (London)	Ontario (Rainy River)	Ontario (Toronto)
Year conducted	1975	1975	1975 to 1976
Length of study	1 month	1 year	1 year
Number of family physicians	39 (8 private practice; 31 residents and faculty)	1.7 (1 full time; 1 for 8 months)	3 Family Practice teaching units 9 full time faculty 17 part time faculty, residents and students
Total number of patient visits during study period	8616	6584 (estimated)	35,351
Referral rate (per cent)	5.4	3.3	5.3

Ranking of Top Five Specialties Consulted

	Per Cent		Per Cent		Per Cent
OB-Gyn	18.0	Gen. Surg.	35.9	Ophthal.	12.1
Gen. Surg.	13.0	Ortho.	16.6	OB-Gyn	10.9
Ophthal.	13.0	OB-Gyn	13.8	Gen. Surg.	10.2
Int. Med.	11.0	Int. Med.	12.4	ENT	9.2
ENT	8.0	ENT	6.0	Ortho.	8.3

SELF-REFERRAL BY PATIENTS

Patient self-referral plays a large role in the number of patients seen by physicians in consulting specialties in the United States. In 1971, 32% to 70% of patients seen by subspecialists in fields such as cardiology, gastroenterology, surgery, urology, and proctology were self-referred rather than being referred by a primary care physician (Shortell and Anderson). This figure is probably much greater today because of the dwindling number of primary care physicians in the United States.

SELF-REFERRAL BY PHYSICIANS

Physicians have come under considerable criticism when suspected of referring patients to colleagues or laboratories in which they have an interest or from which they derive some financial benefit as a result of the referral. Professional "kickbacks" in which the physician is paid for referring a patient have long been unethical. Receiving or paying a kickback for referring a Medicare patient is now a felony in the United States. Although few physicians would refer a patient to a poor quality physician or laboratory purely because of a financial kickback, it is also clear that "anyone's judgment can be subtly influenced by financial interests" (Stark). Any time a physician referral is thought to be in the physician's best interest rather than the patient's, the profession of medicine is at risk of losing its valued place in society. Physicians must avoid any referral that involves personal gain, since this practice runs the risk of influencing decisions and affecting patient care.

THE TEACHER-PUPIL RELATIONSHIP

The consultation process works best when two physicians work together as colleagues to solve a difficult patient problem. Since the process is usually a learning opportunity for the referring physician, it is easy for the consultant to assume the role of teacher and the referring physician the role of pupil. However, the process is not a superior–inferior or teacher–pupil relationship but rather two skilled physicians working together. The consultant has the responsibility to confirm the findings of the referring physician if no new information is detected. The consultant should not enter into a series of exotic tests merely because it is thought to be "expected" or because of fear that his or her prestige as a consultant will be jeopardized. The family physician may have requested another opinion primarily to confirm the diagnosis, perhaps wishing to obtain reassurance before telling the patient he or she has a permanent and incurable disease.

If the referring physician places the consultant in the role of "teacher," the consultant may feel obliged to make comments or recommendations that may not be necessary. The "pupil" likewise feels obliged to follow these recommendations. If the consultant's report is superficial, the referring physician is obliged to take only those actions that he or she feels are in the best interest of the patient. The family physician should accept full responsibility for interpreting and using the opinions of the consultant, in a manner similar to the evaluation of laboratory test results. The referring physician is as free to ignore the consultant's advice as to solicit it in the first place.

Balint feels that this teacher–pupil relationship interferes with patient care if the family physician is dissatisfied with the consultant's report but follows the advice solely out of respect for the consultant as the "expert." The consultant may have formed an opinion based on insufficient information or without total knowledge of the patient's emotional and medical background; or the opinion may have been generated, or even manufactured, as a result of having little additional information to offer. A good consultant will admit when he or she can think of nothing further that needs to be done and will not pursue unnecessary additional testing.

The consultation process is more successful when there is a personal interchange between two physicians rather than when communication is solely by letter. When the referring physician responds only to recommendations made in a report without the opportunity to discuss them with the consultant, inappropriate assumptions may be made. The more personal the interchange that occurs between the two physicians, the more effective will be the consultation.

COLLUSION OF ANONYMITY

A "collusion of anonymity" exists when neither the referring physician nor the consultant accepts responsibility for the patient (Balint). Inappropriate decisions regarding patient care can be made when neither physician accepts full responsibility. The problem is amplified when the family physician turns to a variety of consultants for advice, yielding to each, with no one person accepting ongoing responsibility for the patient. The consultation process is not a ritual of "passing the buck" but an integral part of the family physician's continuing responsibility for patient care. If the consultant does not provide meaningful or useful information, then additional consultations must be obtained until the problem is satisfactorily resolved. The term "primary physician" implies primary responsibility for the patient, not just physician of first contact.

THE FAMILY PHYSICIAN AS A CONSULTANT

It is unfortunate that too much responsibility for primary care is burdening many subspecialists. Referrals to family physicians are frequently made by physicians in the surgical disciplines for the care of families when psychosocial problems are prominent, for geriatric care, for the long-term management of a chronic illness, and for medical emergencies. Pediatricians frequently refer teenagers or young adults who have outgrown their practice.

In a survey of family physicians from five midwestern states, Amundson and Vogt found that 35% of the respondents received consultations and referrals from other generalist specialists and 28% received them from subspecialists. The most common reason for the referral was that the patient did not have a family physician, but the second most common reason, when the referring physician was another generalist, was for a procedure such as flexible sigmoidoscopy or vasectomy. One of the most common reasons for referral overall was for the family physician to serve as a coordinator of care.

The family physician can be a valuable consultant when comprehensive and continuing health care is in the patient's best interest or when there is a need for a physician skilled in coordinating the care of multiple specialists.

REFERENCES

Amundson LH, Vogt HB. The consultant family physician. J Am Brd Fam Pract 1989; 2(1):34–36.

Balint M. The Doctor, His Patient, and the Illness. London, Sir Isaac Pitman and Sons, 1964.

Barnett BL, Jr, Collins JJ, Jr. A new look at the consultation continuum. J Fam Pract 1977; 5:665.

Bates RC. The two sides of very successful consultation. Med Econ 1979; 56:172.

Carson ME. The referral process. Med J Aust 1982; 1:180.

Clarfield AM. A study of all referrals from a family practice unit. Can Fam Physician 1980; 26:527.

Crump WJ, Massengill P. Outpatient consultations from a family practice residency program: Nine years' experience. J Am Brd Fam Pract 1988; 1(3):164–166.

Cummins RO, Smith RW, Inui TS. Communication failure in primary care: Failure of consultants to provide follow-up information. JAMA 1980; 243:1650.

Curry RW, Jr., Crandall LA, Coggins WF. The referral process: A study of one method for improving communication between rural practitioners and consultants. J Fam Pract 1980; 10:287.

Dolezal JM, Amundson LH, Sinning NJ, et al. Pricare and ambulatory referrals. Continuing Education, January 1980, pp. 84–94.

Everett GE, Parsons TJ, Christensen AL. Educational influences on consultation rates of house staff physicians in a primary care clinic. J Med Educ 1984; 59:479–486.

Fry J. Hospital referrals: Must they go up? Changing patterns over 20 years. Lancet 1971; 2:148.

Geyman JP, Brown RC, Rivers K. Referrals in family practice: A comparative study by geographic region and practice setting. J Fam Pract 1976; 3:163.

Glenn JK, Hofmeister RW, Neikirk H, Wright H. Continuity of care in the referral process: An analysis of family physicians' expectations of consultants. J Fam Pract 1983; 16:329–334.

Hines RM, Curry OJ. The consultation process and physician satisfaction: Review of referral patterns in three urban family practice units. Can Med Assoc J 1978; 118:1065.

Horder JP. Physicians and family doctors: A new relationship. J R Coll Gen Pract 1977; 27:391.

Lawler FH. Referral rates of senior family practice residents in an ambulatory care clinic. J Med Educ 1987; 62:177–182.

Mayer TR. Family practice referral patterns in a health maintenance organization. J Fam Pract 1982; 14:315.

McPhee SJ, Lo B, Saika GY, Meltzer R. How good is communication between primary care physicians and subspecialty consultants? Arch Intern Med 1984; 144:1265–1268.

Metcalfe DH, Sischy D. Patterns of referral from family practice. NY State J Med 1973; 73:1690.

Moscovice I, Schwartz CW, Shortell SM. Referral patterns of family physicians in an underserved rural area. J Fam Pract 1979; 9:677.

National Center for Health Statistics. Unpublished data from 1985. National Ambulatory Medical Care Survey.

Nyma KC. Referral patterns in general practice. Aust Fam Phys 1973; 2:173.

Penchansky R, Fox D. Frequency of referral and patient characteristics in group practice. Medical Care 1970; 8:368.

Phelps LA, Renner JH. The development of a "Statement of policy regarding consultations." J Fam Pract 1977; 5:979.

Price PB, Loughmiller GC, Murray SL. Attributes of a good practicing physician. J Med Educ 1971; 46:229.

Ruane TJ. Consultation and referral in a Vermont family practice: A study of utilization, specialty distribution, and outcome. J Fam Pract 1979; 8:1037.

Saunders RC. Consultation-referral among physicians: Practice and process. J Fam Pract 1978; 6:123.

Schmidt DD. Referral patterns in an individual family practice. J Fam Pract 1977; 5:401.

Shortell SM, Anderson OW. The physician referral process: A theoretical perspective. Health Services Research, Spring 1971, p. 39.

Stark EH. Ethics in patient referrals. Acad Med 1989; March, pp. 146–147.

Steinberg H, Torem M, Saravey SM. An analysis of physician resistance to psychiatric consultations. Arch Gen Psych 1980; 37:1007.

Stephens GG. The Intellectual Basis of Family Practice. Tucson, Winter Publishing Company, 1982.

Tenney JB, White KL, Williamson JW. NAMC: background and methodology. Vital and Health Statistics, Series 2, No. 61, DHEW Publication (HRA) 74-1335, 1974.

White FZ. Referral patterns among family practitioners. Illinois Med J 1984; 166(1):31–33.

QUESTIONS

1. The first specialty board was the American Board of
   a. Family Practice.
   b. Internal Medicine.
   c. Pediatrics.
   d. Surgery.
   e. Ophthalmology.

2. The most common error in communication between referring physician and consultant is
   a. Consultation via the telephone.
   b. Talking to nurse instead of physician.
   c. Consultant report not sent.
   d. Inadequate information given consultant.

3. The most common reason for a family physician to no longer use a particular consultant is
   a. Lack of appropriate training of consultant.
   b. Personality of consultant.
   c. Limited hospital privileges of family physician.
   d. Failure to receive a report from consultant.
   e. Patient unhappiness with consultant.

4. The average rate of referral by family physicians in the United States is
   a. 3%.
   b. 10%.
   c. 15%.
   d. 25%.
   e. 50%.

5. Most referrals by family physicians are to
   a. Cardiology.
   b. Orthopedic surgery.
   c. Neurology.
   d. Ophthalmology.
   e. Urology.

Answers appear on page 447.

14

THE PROBLEM-ORIENTED MEDICAL RECORD

ROBERT E. RAKEL

A well-prepared medical record is among the most useful tools available to a family physician. When functioning effectively, it communicates the relevant facts regarding patient care to all health personnel involved and allows for the easy documentation and retrieval of information vital to the patient's ongoing care. The information should be organized in a systematic, logical, and consistent manner and should accurately reflect the patient's state of health. Orderly recording of data is vital to efficient care, and although the information should be simplified as much as possible, it must likewise be both complete and accurate. Family medicine involves the care of patients over a prolonged period of time. Acute illnesses cannot be treated as totally isolated events but must be viewed in the total perspective of a person's or a family's long-term care. A pregnant woman, for example, may have a slightly elevated blood pressure, which should be compared with readings prior to and following pregnancy to assess its true importance. (Similarly, her smoking habits, alcohol intake, caffeine intake, weight, and other physiologic and psychologic functions should be noted and followed.)

An office record system will maintain its usefulness and efficiency over time only if it is individually designed to match the objectives and the personality of the physician using it. The chart should be developed and organized based upon the individual physician's preferences and needs. Some will enjoy using flow sheets frequently; others will be turned off by them. Some will prefer, and will be able to maintain, an adequate medication list; others may find it impossible to keep such a list current. The ideal record must also be kept simple and must not handicap or confine the busy physician's productivity by requiring unnecessary paper work. The lengthy, illegible, and poorly organized office record of the past has developed into a logical, well-structured account that lends itself to quick and easy retrieval of information and ready assessment of the patient's present health care needs and potential health hazards. It also assists the physician in predicting the patient's potential future state of health by identifying significant risk factors.

THE PROBLEM-ORIENTED, OR PATIENT-ORIENTED, MEDICAL RECORD (POMR)

The stimulus for change in record-keeping came in 1969, when Weed developed the problem-oriented medical record (POMR). Although this innovative concept was originally applied to the hospital record, its principles have served as the nucleus for major changes in outpatient records as well. The "pure" form proposed by Weed has required some modification to be adapted to family practice, but its basic concepts serve as an excellent foundation for an efficient office medical record. The POMR has also been called the "patient-oriented medical record," since it helps to avoid depersonalization and emphasizes individuality of the patient by listing the specific problems unique to that person. Hence, the patient is not just another person with gallbladder disease but an individual with a unique combination of associated problems that identify him or her as different from other patients with gallbladder disease.

The POMR achieves its maximum potential in the hands of a family physician. It works especially well in the continuing care of patients with chronic illness and in complex cases involving multiple problems. Since these are areas in which family physicians are especially effective, it is no wonder that they are the greatest promoters of the POMR. Now that many patients who suffer from previously fatal illnesses are surviving, the family physician is involved in the continuing care of ever increasing numbers of the chronically ill. Management of patients with these chronic illnesses requires a dynamic record that accurately reflects at all times the patient's present and past medical problems and assists the physician in remaining aware of other potential problems that can become significant at any time.

IMPROVED COMMUNICATION

As our society becomes more mobile and medical technology becomes increasingly complex, we need a well-organized medical record system that permits easy communication and transfer of information among health professionals, both within the same office and at separate sites. No longer can the record be a document understood only by the physician who places data in it. It must permit other physicians, as well as an increasing number of other health personnel, who also depend on the record, to readily assess the patient's condition, understand the plan of management, and recognize all elements important to the patient's ongoing care. As long as the record is able to communicate information in this manner, it will serve as an effective tool for all members of the health care team.

The maintenance of a complete and well-organized medical record over a prolonged period of time contributes to high-quality care by permitting attention to be focused on preventive measures. Increased emphasis is being placed on the assessment of the quality of care, and outpatient records need to be organized in a manner that permits review, just as hospital records are reviewed. Terminology is also being influenced by third-party payers. The physician and other health professionals, such as the dentist, nurse, and therapist, are now called providers, and the office visit is an encounter. It is hoped that in family practice an encounter will remain a friendly interaction between physician and patient, rather than follow Webster's definition of "a meeting of adversaries or hostile persons to engage in conflict." It is no wonder that many physicians bristle at the use of this term to refer to their relationships with patients.

Improved patient care must remain the primary objective of any newly structured record system. As Murnaghan stated: "Data collection and information systems cannot be justified if they subvert the process of patient care and fail to benefit the patient and provider either directly or indirectly. The growth of public, as opposed to private, responsibility for personal health services means that more and more data requirements will be placed upon the providers of care." Data collection must not be allowed to become threatening to either the patient or the physician but must be an obvious asset to the care and management of all problems related to patients.

PATIENT ACCESS TO MEDICAL RECORDS

Use of the computer in medical record keeping has focused more attention on confidentiality of the medical record. Access to medical records for management purposes is being given to more and more non-health professionals who are neither sensitive to patients' concerns about confidentiality nor bound by strong ethical or professional codes of conduct regarding the use of such information. A fine balance between confidentiality and access will have to be struck.

The Federal Privacy Act of 1974 (Public Law 93–579) establishes the patient's right to obtain the medical record in federal institutions. A number of states also have statutes as well as precedent court decisions permitting direct access of patients to their medical records. Usually, physicians own the pieces of paper the medical record consists of, but the patient has the right to access the information contained in the record. For example, the Medical Practice Act of Texas states, "A physician shall furnish copies of medical records requested, or a summary or narrative of the records, pursuant to written consent for release of the information."

Controversy still exists about the effect this will have on clinical care. Although there is no proof that sharing the record with the patient improves the quality of care, there is general agreement that it improves patient understanding and compliance. Dr. H. I. Schade, a family physician in Los Gatos, California, allows patients to keep their own complete medical record, and he maintains only a brief office record in note form. Patients thus have the record available if they are seen in an emergency room or by a consultant or when moving to a new area. He believes that making the records available to the patients not only enables them to develop a keen understanding of their medical problems and treatment but actually discourages rather than encourages malpractice suits (Schade).

One survey of patients (Michael and Bordley) found that 80% felt they should be permitted to see their medical record, but they were not convinced that possessing a copy was as important as reading it. Regardless of local law, the best policy is to allow patients to examine and copy their records upon request unless there is a valid medical reason for refusing to do so. Tufo and colleagues gave patients copies of their medical records in an attempt "to provide a clear statement of problems and plans to emphasize self-help and patient responsibility." They feel that the patient's audit of the record provides feedback concerning the accuracy of the information and the level of patient understanding.

Fischbach and associates promote the involvement of the patient; in developing their problem list and progress notes, they state, "The attitude that 'what you don't know won't hurt you' is proving unrealistic; it is what patients do not know, but vaguely suspect, that causes them corrosive worry."

Sharing the medical record with the patient certainly has its place and can be of value, yet discretion is called for since it can also be harmful. For example, some elderly patients may become depressed or confused by seeing a problem list containing 10 to 12 items and multiple medications. Patients with emotional problems may have difficulty understanding or coping with the content of progress notes.

INFORMATION RETRIEVAL

The medical record is rapidly becoming less the private property and sole responsibility of the physician and more the joint responsibility and common property of the physician, other health providers, and the patient. Information in the medical record should be highly visible, clear, and concise so that it can be retrieved easily to allow for effective and efficient use of time by the physician and other health professionals.

The use of facsimile (fax) transmission greatly facilitates the transfer of medical information, including the electrocardiogram. In many ways, fax transmission is superior to telephone voice communication, express mail, and electronic mail. It can be especially useful in emergency care.

TRANSFER OF INFORMATION

It is important that the family physician incorporate the patient's entire medical background into the record so that the total comprehensive picture is constantly available to the physician and other health personnel who need it. Valuable medical information is often scattered in a variety of locations and thus becomes relatively inaccessible or unavailable when needed.

When new patients are seen, a strong effort should be made to acquire all medical information from other physicians, government services, hospitals, and other health agencies previously involved in the patient's care. A great deal of unnecessary effort and expense results when each physician, in turn, must establish full medical data for every patient, since a variety of diagnostic tests and therapeutic trials must be needlessly repeated. When the transferred record is in the form of the POMR or some similarly concise system, putting it to use is a simple matter.

A well-organized record system, such as the POMR, also allows the referring family physician to communicate the patient's total health status more effectively to consulting physicians by submitting the problem list with the consultation request. This prevents the specialist from merely "treating his own disease" and ensures awareness of all of the patient's medical, social, and psychiatric problems, as well as the problems for which the consultation is being requested. When a cardiologist is asked to consult about a seriously ill patient in the coronary care unit, the problem list clearly illustrates other problems to be considered and managed and makes the need for continuing involvement by the family physician readily apparent. Subspecialists are prevented from concentrating on a single part to the detriment of the whole patient.

LEGIBILITY

Legibility is necessary if any data, no matter how systematically organized, are to be retrieved and collated in a rapid, accurate, and useful manner that will permit the quick review of a patient's total health status. The well-known illegibility of physicians' handwriting is an understandable product of conditioning during many years of rapid note taking. This handicap, the greatest barrier to effective communication and good records, is now being removed as a rapidly increasing number of physicians turn to dictating their records and using secretarial services for transcription to obtain clearly typed progress notes. This improved legibility is an obvious advantage in group practices, in which more than one physician and several nurses or other health professionals are likely to depend upon the same chart. The POMR, because of its structure, lends itself well to dictation with a minimum of confusion.

ORGANIZATION OF A RECORD SYSTEM

Filing

A record-keeping system, no matter how well organized, is of little value if the medical record cannot be found. Much time can be saved by using an efficient filing system.

Alphabetic Filing Systems

This is a popular method of record storage, especially for small practices. Records are filed alphabetically according to surname. Because of the similarity of many names, however, misfiling is common. Strong ethnic backgrounds in a community may lead to heavy concentrations of similar names. Family filing is also difficult with the alphabetic system, particularly when there are different surnames in the family.

Color coding of alphabetical filing systems limits misfiling and eases retrieval. Each letter has a distinctive color. Colored labels representing the first two letters of the patient's last name are fixed to the tab on each file. Misfiling is common however, when there are many charts filed under common family names such as Smith, Jones, and Young.

Numeric Systems

Terminal digit filing appears to be the more efficient system for family practice. Fewer charts are misfiled using this system, and it allows for a more rapid and accurate placement and retrieval of records. The only significant disadvantage is the need to maintain an alphabetic and numeric cross-reference index.

Color Coding

Color-coded terminal digit filing largely eliminates the possibility of misfiling or at least limits it to a narrow area. Ten colors are used, one for each of the 10 Arabic numerals 0 (zero) to 9, as opposed to the large number of colors needed in alphabetic systems. This permits ready recognition of visually distinct categories, especially when open shelving is used. Records are arranged according to the last two digits. Each number is keyed to a color on the record jacket edge. The two colors representing the two digits are easily recognized if the record is misfiled. Records with the same two terminal digits are then arranged in sequence according to the numbers preceding the two terminal digits. Thus, chart 00–00–13 will be followed by 00–01–13, 00–02–13, and so on.

Open Shelving

Color-coded terminal digit filing works best with open-shelf filing, although it can be adapted to drawer files as well. Shelves are better than drawers, however, since they can be stacked higher and it is easier for more than one person to have access to them at a time.

Inactive Records

Purging of inactive records avoids burdening the record system with unused charts. To keep the unnecessary volume to a minimum, records of patients who have not been seen for 2 or 3 years should be considered inactive and removed from the active file. This weeding out can be a relatively simple process. A color-coded tab or mark corresponding to the year can be added to the margin of each chart. Each year the color is changed when a member of the family is seen so that the color represents the most recent year in which the patient or family was seen. If yellow was the color 3 years ago, it is an easy task to pull all charts with yellow tabs. For the system to work, however, the receptionist or nurse must check this tab each time the chart is pulled to make sure the color corresponds to the current year.

Family Charts

The physician's care of families is facilitated by a record system that focuses on the family. Family folders are filed under the name of the head of the household or the person responsible for the account. With the numeric filing system, there is only one possible shelf location for the family folder regardless of the variety of surnames involved. Even if surnames vary within a family because of children from previous marriages or because the wife's parents live with the family, each individual is identified by a one- or two-digit modifier within the family number.

The family folder usually consists of an outer file jacket containing selected family information as well as the individual charts of each family member. The first item in the family folder is the *family registration form* containing family demographic data that are usually obtained at the first office visit. It maintains a prominent location in the chart because it is a ready source of reference for the names and ages of all family members and includes occupational and insurance information. The purpose of the family chart is to provide the physician with as much information as possible relating to factors involving the entire family that could have an impact on the health of any individual member. It is important for the physician to note when the problems involving one family member influence the health of another.

It is also useful to have a corner or prominent area in the chart to record events that are important occurrences in the patient's life so that these can be recalled and mentioned during subsequent visits. Reference to or questions about events such as the birth of a grandchild, move into a new home, or trip abroad will be appreciated by the patient.

FAMILY MEMBER VISIT REGISTER. Family stress may become evident by a clustering of problems in many family members. The *family member visit register* can assist the family physician in identifying these problems early. Widmer et al. have shown that early signs of depression include an increased number of visits by all family members and frequent complaints of pain, anxiety, and functional problems by the patient and other family members for up to a year before the depression becomes obvious.

Patterns heralding serious diseases of this nature can be identified earlier if the family physician maintains an overview of the interpersonal dynamics within a family.

The family member visit register (Fig. 14–1) is placed in a prominent area of the family folder and records the dates, names, and major reasons for visits by all family members. A glance at this form shows whether other recent problems prominent within the family have a bearing on the present complaint. It may also serve as a reminder to the physician to ask about the progress of another family member who was recently ill. In this way the physician can assess the degree of recovery or the likelihood of a continuing disability and can be constantly prepared to deal with family problems in addition to serving as the personal physician for individual family members.

Chart Organization

The organization of material within the chart will vary with the type of chart selected, but in all cases the material should be organized in a consistent and predefined manner. If a folder is used, the problem list is usually the top sheet on the left, with the family registration record beneath it. The top sheet on the right contains the most recent progress notes, with previous progress notes beneath it, followed by the data base, electrocardiograms, and correspondence. If possible, each of these sections should be divided by tabs or by some other method to allow easy identification, perhaps by using different colors for each section. A more economical method than purchasing chart dividers is to cut away the edge of progress note pages to make the underlying data base accessible.

Using the POMR

Weed describes four basic elements as the nucleus of the POMR: the data base, problem list, initial plan, and progress notes. Although his initial plan applies primarily to the complete workup of a new office patient or the admission workup of a hospitalized patient, most physicians prefer to incorporate it into ongoing patient care as a feature of the progress note (Fig. 14–2). The logical approach to record-keeping, then, calls first for the establishment of a data base, after which a problem list is developed, initial plans are identified, and the patient's progress is monitored with continual updating of the data base and problem list.

Problem List

Although the problem list is developed largely from information accumulated in the data base, it is the most important single ingredient of the POMR. A problem is anything that requires diagnosis or management or that

FAMILY MEMBER VISIT REGISTER

NAME _DALY_

NUMBER _50-00-03_

Given Name	LLOYD	DAWN	PEGGY	KEVIN	MICHELLE	MRS. VAN	
Date of Birth	3/18/39	5/12/41	11/29/60	8/20/64	5/5/71	4/20/02	
DATE	PROBLEM	PROBLEM	PROBLEM	PROBLEM	PROBLEM	PROBLEM	PROBLEM
3/17/75	ulcer						
4/3/75		Headache			well child exam	BP check	
4/7/75				sore throat			
5/12/75			school prob.				
5/30/75	Alcoholism						
7/8/75		Fatigue					
7/23/75		Depression					
8/19/75				Cough			
9/4/75	Ulcer check						
9/22/75						BP check	
10/1/75					Otitis media		
10/10/75					FU - OM		
11/12/75			Drug Prob.				
12/6/75		Depression					
1/17/76				Laceration			
2/10/76		Marital Prob.					

Figure 14–1. Family member visit register, University of Iowa. (From Rakel RE. Textbook of Family Practice. 4th ed. Philadelphia, W. B. Saunders Company, 1990, p. 1701, with permission.)

interferes with quality of life as perceived by the patient. It can be either a firm diagnosis, a physical symptom, or a social or economic problem. It is any physiologic, pathologic, psychologic, or social item of concern to either the patient or the physician.

The problem list serves as a comprehensive overview of the patient's present and past state of health. It indicates whether the problems are active or have occurred in the past but are at present inactive. The problem list is a reminder of what has occurred so that the physician

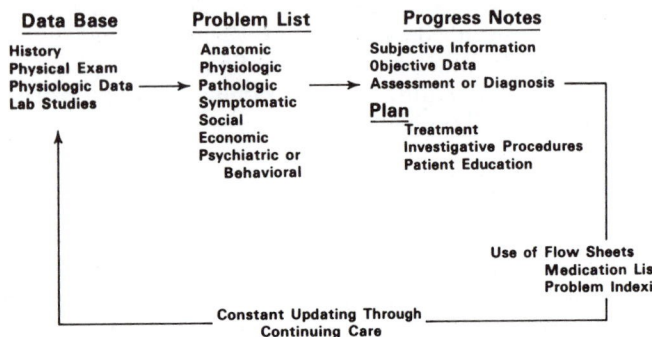

Figure 14–2. Basic elements of the problem-oriented medical record. (From Rakel RE. Textbook of Family Practice. 4th ed. Philadelphia , W. B. Saunders Company, 1990, p. 1703, with permission.)

can be helped to remember that the patient had a cholecystectomy or hysterectomy and thus does not continue to ask about the function of these organs while obtaining a history.

Problems can be any of the following:
1. Anatomic (hernia)
2. Physiologic (jaundice of unknown etiology)
3. A sign (hepatomegaly)
4. A symptom (dyspnea, fatigue)
5. Economic (financial difficulty)
6. Social (marital discord, spouse alcoholic)
7. Psychiatric (depression)
8. Physical handicap (paralysis, amputation)
9. Specific diagnosis (acute rheumatic fever)
10. Abnormal laboratory test (elevated blood urea nitrogen, elevated sedimentation rate)
11. Risk factor (family history of diabetes mellitus or cancer)

Each problem is numbered, and when possible the progress notes are keyed by number to the appropriate problem on the list, thereby reflecting its present state of resolution.

The types of illness seen by a family physician are often more appropriately described as symptoms or undifferentiated problems than as diseases. *Disease* implies a full understanding of the pathology and etiology of the illness, whereas many of the illnesses encountered by the family physician involve a varying degree of insight into the underlying etiology and a varying severity of the illness, which occasionally resolves while still in the undifferentiated state.

The problem list is a dynamic picture of the patient's health problems and is continually changed by updating, as new problems are added or old problems are carried to a greater degree of resolution. It should contain all of the patient's continuing problems and should have a prominent position in the record, so as to constantly remind the physician to care for the whole patient and not to limit attention to the current problem. One value of the problem list is that it continually "stares back at you" and prevents the physician from focusing on too limited an area to the exclusion of the patient's total health picture. With such a format, it is possible to rapidly orient oneself to the most important current problem without forgetting the others.

All problems can be kept in proper perspective. One physician on call for another can rapidly grasp the essential nature of a case by scanning the problem list and thereby can make a more rational decision regarding the acute presenting problem. To do this, however, the problems should be *printed* for ease of reading and rapid scanning.

The basic concept of the POMR is that the problem is the functional unit. All activities relating to the care of the patient, including progress notes, history, physical findings, and therapy, refer to the specific problem for which treatment was initiated. The constant surveillance of the patient's state of health by the physician and allied health personnel and their efforts toward establishing effective health maintenance require constant monitoring of health hazards and risk factors. These risk factors should be identified on the problem list and should serve constantly to alert all health personnel to their presence.

It has been appropriately said that the main value of the POMR is not its structure but its honesty. The POMR demands that all problems be described straightforwardly and at their present stage of development and resolution, no matter how elementary the terms used to describe them may be. It insists that physicians list only what they *know* to be present, not what they *think* to be present. The principle to be followed is "record what is known, not what is supposed." The POMR discourages guesswork and insists on an accurate listing of actual problems and observed facts. As Weed has said, "The problem list should not contain diagnostic guesses; it should simply state the problems at a level of refinement consistent with the physician's understanding, running the gamut from the precise diagnosis to the isolated, unexplained finding."

The POMR does not demand excessive compulsiveness but does require that all significant factors be displayed so that they cannot be ignored. Abnormal data should be placed on the problem list and accounted for. The logic behind clinical decisions will be apparent in the POMR, and caution should be taken to avoid drawing conclusions prematurely.

Design of the Problem List

The problem list can be structured in a variety of ways. Physicians should select those components considered most desirable and arrange them in the manner most appropriate to their practice. Most practices design their own problem list, but a large variety of formats are available commercially. The University of Iowa problem list (see Fig. 14–3) has separate columns for coding, problem number, problem, date of onset of problem, date problem recorded, and comments. Another format is that used at Baylor College of Medicine listing acute and chronic problems on the same page (Fig. 14–4).

ACUTE, SELF-LIMITED PROBLEMS. Some programs use a separate problem list for acute, self-limited problems, since only chronic problems should be placed on the master problem list. These temporary problems can be listed separately, as shown in Figure 14–4, or on a separate page entirely. The frequency of recurrence is indicated by dates of occurrence. In this manner, recurring acute problems, such as otitis media or acute bronchitis, which can be threatening to the patient's future health, can be identified and transferred to the major problem list.

An alternative method for identifying acute problems is to list them as "Problem No. 2," as in Figure 14–3. When this method is used, all acute, self-limited problems are labeled Problem No. 2 in the progress notes, with the name of the problem also listed next to the heading of No. 2. In a similar manner, the label "Problem No. 1" is permanently assigned to health mainte-

PATIENT PROBLEM LIST

FAMILY # 50-13-62

NAME *Wanda Smith*

DATE OF BIRTH *8-25-21*

HOSPITAL # *70-59438*

Code	No.	Problem	Date Onset	Date Recorded	Comments:
	1	Health Maintenance			
	2	Acute Episode			
	3.	*Hypertension*	*1970*	*1/14/82*	
	4.	*Degenerative Joint Disease*	*1976*	*1/14/82*	
	5.	*S/P Hysterectomy*	*1976*		*Fibroid*
	6.	*Depression*	*1980*		
	7.	*Rt. Carotid Bruit, Asymptomatic*	*1981*		

ALLERGIES:

Code	RISK FACTORS	Date	Comments:
	Strong Family History of Diabetes		
	Carcinoma of Breast in Mother		

IMMUNIZATIONS	DATE	DATE	DATE	DATE	DATE	IMMUNIZATIONS	DATE	DATE	DATE
DTP						Influenza			
TOPV						Pneumovax	*1/14/82*		
Indicate one: DT, Td, Tet Tox									
Tuberculin Test									
MMR									

3/82

Figure 14–3. Problem list, University of Iowa. (From Rakel RE. Textbook of Family Practice. 4th ed. Philadelphia, W. B. Saunders Company, 1990, p. 1704, with permission.)

nance activities and stresses the emphasis on preventive measures in family practice.

Many physicians believe that temporary problems can be handled in the progress notes only and need not be identified on the problem list. This simplifies the record system but runs the risk of failing to recognize recurring acute problems that deserve greater visibility and continuous monitoring. Most acute and temporary problems that are encountered, however, are self-limiting and usually do not recur with a frequency that requires their being placed on the master problem list.

COMPONENTS OF THE PROBLEM LIST. Legibility is an important component of the problem list. Problems should be either typed or printed in large letters to support the major function of the list: that the problems be visible at a glance.

A variety of methods can be used to illustrate the active or inactive status of each problem. Those problems

that have been resolved but may have an impact upon the patient's future health must be retained on the problem list for continued visibility. A resolved problem can be transferred to a separate inactive column, or it can be identified by indicating the date of resolution under "comments" or in a separate column. It can also be identified by drawing a line or arrow through the problem.

When a higher level of understanding or sophistication is reached for any active problem or combination of problems, these should be changed to a single, new problem. This resolution to a higher level can be indicated by listing the date of resolution of the earlier problem and adding the newer problem at the bottom of the list. Another method is to draw an arrow from the previous problem to the newer designation while maintaining the same problem number and position on the problem list, space permitting. If a comment column is used,

MR-1-11/88

BAYLOR FAMILY PRACTICE CENTER
PROBLEM LIST
Please Print

Name _Smith, Sandra_   Date of Birth _7-13-32_

NO.	DATE	CHRONIC PROBLEMS AND RISK FACTORS	COMMENTS
1.	2/86	HEALTH MAINTENANCE	
2.	2/86	Hypertension	
3.	2/86	FH Colon CA	
4.	7/89	CA Breast	℞ Mastectomy - 2 pos. nodes
5.	9/89	Depression	
		ALLERGIES	PCN

	DATE	ACUTE PROBLEMS	RECURRENCES										
	3/20/86	Bronchitis											
	5/30/87	Low back pain											
	6/21/87	Contact dermatitis											
	6/88	Vaginitis											
	3/89	UTI											

Figure 14–4. Problem list, Baylor College of Medicine, Houston, Texas. (From Rakel RE. Textbook of Family Practice. 4th ed. Philadelphia, W. B. Saunders Company, 1990, with permission.)

the reason for this change can be noted. Otherwise, future information can be identified by placing over the arrow the date of the office visit at which information leading to the increased resolution was obtained. An example of such a change in problem status is the listing of "dyspnea on exertion" and "peripheral edema" as sep-arate problems that are then resolved to "congestive heart failure," once the presence of renal disease has been ruled out. Another example would be the change of the problem of "pain, right knee" to "degenerative joint disease" when x-ray exams identify the specific cause.

FAMILY PROBLEM LIST. Family problem lists are a method of depicting the problems of each family member on the same page, along with problems that involve the entire family unit. Many family physicians prefer to include this information as part of the family genogram instead of using a family problem list.

Whatever the method of organization, this comprehensive, visible, and concise overview of problems enables the physician to provide family-oriented care while keeping the ongoing problems of individual members in proper perspective. The only real disadvantage of a family problem list is the limited amount of space available and, thus, the limited amount of information that can be documented. If a family problem list is used, it should be prominently displayed in the family folder and should be the only place that master problems are listed. This should force the physician to look at the family as a whole. Unfortunately, there is some risk that the physician may focus on the individual's record to the exclusion of information in the family folder.

The family problem list emphasizes the fact that no one in the family can have a problem without affecting other members in some manner; in fact, the problems of greatest importance are those that by their very nature affect each family member (Grace et al.). The family problem list gives the physician an awareness of the entire family's health problems. It serves as a reminder of the problems of other members who are not being seen but may need attention or follow-up.

Data Base

The data base is the first step toward developing the problem list. It is the platform upon which the structure of the POMR depends for stability. The data base consists of the history (chief complaint, present illness, past history, family history, social history, and review of systems), physical examination, physiologic data, and baseline laboratory studies. The data base on each patient varies depending upon age, sex, and race.

The data base serves as the groundwork for each patient's future care and should include those tests that are effective screening procedures for significant disease or are likely to be good reference points for future problems; for example, elevations of blood pressure can have a significant long-term detrimental effect, and a mild elevation may go undetected if an earlier baseline determination is not available for comparison. The data base should concentrate on the problem that cannot afford to be missed and should include those tests that are of greatest value in detecting these problems. Active debate will continue regarding the need for various routine tests; the issue of which test is the most reliable indicator of potentially significant disease will be settled only by further research. Tests to be emphasized in the data base are those that detect disease at its earliest, presymptomatic phase so that the normal course of the disease can be interrupted and its impact minimized.

A complete data base is so essential to the success of the POMR that many physicians place "incomplete data base" as "Problem No. 1" on the list, where it remains until all required data have been obtained. A commitment should be made to obtain all of the data within a given period of time. If a complete history and physical examination cannot be obtained at one visit, information can still be collected bit by bit during a series of visits over a period of time. The visibility of an incomplete data base as Problem No. 1 serves as a constant reminder to continue accumulating the data, regardless of the nature of the episodic visit.

History

A variety of new methods for obtaining the medical history have been developed to save the physician time and still allow for an in-depth accumulation of valuable historical information. These health history questionnaires are available as printed forms for the patient to complete, either in the office waiting room or at home prior to the visit. A questionnaire can be either self-designed or purchased commercially.

When a complete history is being obtained, it is important to have available the records from the patient's previous physicians because the patient may have an unrealistic impression of the pathologic findings present, and accurate assessment of past problems is possible only by reviewing the actual records or a summary from the physicians involved. This information should become a permanent part of the data base and should serve as a reference point for all present and future difficulties in the same areas.

Physical Examination and Physiologic Data

One advantage of using a printed physical examination sheet is the ability to easily identify information that has been obtained in part but has yet to be completed. A highly structured "check-off" format is sometimes used. This makes it possible to set a goal for completeness and to know when that goal has been reached or what remains to be done. With a nonstructured, open-ended format, it is difficult to tell how much remains incomplete.

Some practices insist upon a comprehensive data base for all new patients and will not accept patients for treatment beyond the second visit for an episodic illness until the standard comprehensive examination is completed. Following the completion of this examination, the patient is sent a summary of the findings, including a problem list and the plans for following each problem. The patient is asked to review the material for accuracy and to keep it for a permanent record.

Laboratory Data

A valuable time-saving practice is to transfer all laboratory report slips to a standard laboratory data sheet. This method avoids the bulk and confusion that a mass of laboratory slips in a variety of colors and sizes contributes to the medical record. Fears that mistakes can be made when transferring the data have been shown to be mostly unfounded, and the significant amount of time saved in retrieving and comparing a sequence of laboratory information arranged side by side chronologically is well worth the time and effort involved. This ability to follow the variations of single or multiple tests over time on a single page is of significant benefit in maintaining an accurate overview of the patient's laboratory data, especially when compared with the system of "shingling" laboratory slips that requires a variety of slips to be found and lifted if one is to follow a sequence of tests such as serum potassium, glucose, or cholesterol.

Standard computer printouts of laboratory tests performed outside the office are popular and are reported in a variety of formats. Some of these can be designed to allow placement in the chart so that chronologic documentation of single tests is possible.

It is also useful to document chronologically the dates and results of Papanicolaou smears, electrocardiograms, x-ray exams, and other selected items. The actual report forms (if they contain a more detailed description of an abnormality) can be filed to the rear of the chart. Once complete information is transferred to the appropriate section of the data base form, the slip can be discarded.

The data base should also identify all allergies and should include a summary of all immunizations, hospitalizations, and consultations. In this manner, the physician can note at a glance whether a patient has any allergies, has ever been hospitalized, or has ever required consultation by other physicians. Organizing data in this manner may take slightly longer, but the time saved in retrieval more than compensates for the effort. The chronologic order of information in both the progress notes and the laboratory data is particularly useful in family practice because changes over time and frequency of involvement can be visualized and coordinated. When there is an abnormal laboratory or physiologic finding that cannot be explained by a problem already on the problem list, it is included as a new problem and maintains that visibility until it is resolved by further diagnosis or treatment.

Progress Notes

Well-organized and logically structured progress notes in combination with the problem list are the secret of the POMR's effectiveness in promoting continuing patient care. Progress notes are divided into four main components: subjective information, objective data, assessment, and plan (Fig. 14–5). These components correspond to the history, physical examination, diagnosis, and treatment sections of the traditional record. The acronym SOAP is used to describe the POMR format of a progress note and is a more descriptive and more easily pronounced term than would be the acronym HPEDT. An essential feature of any useful record is the organization of major components of the progress notes, placing the most important features in a consistent and readily identifiable position. The historical or subjective data should consistently occupy one specific position and the plan of management, or therapeutic data, an-

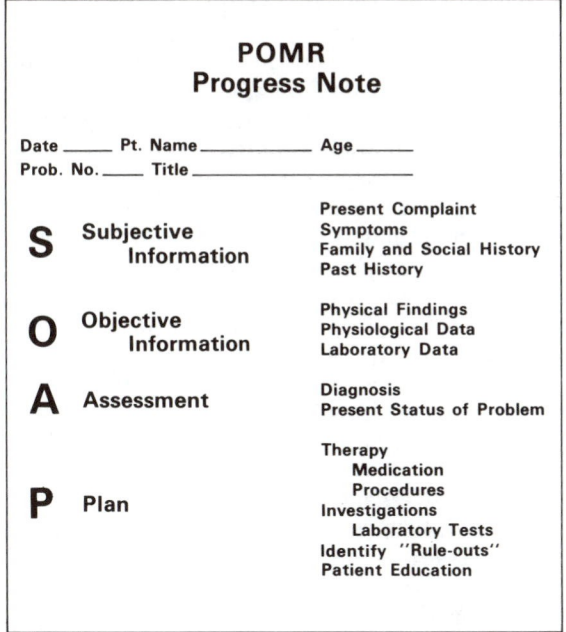

Figure 14–5. Major components of the POMR progress note. (From Rakel RE. Textbook of Family Practice. 4th ed. Philadelphia, W. B. Saunders Company, 1990, p. 1712, with permission.)

other. The actual location is insignificant, as long as each maintains a separate, easily located, and readily visible identity.

Every problem need not be described in a progress note at each visit. Comments need be made regarding only those problems that are pertinent to that visit and for which some change of status or new information is noted. Likewise, every item or component of the progress note need not be commented upon at each visit. If there is no change in status or no new information available, that section, whether it be the subjective, objective, assessment, or plan, should be omitted or a dash inserted to indicate "no need for comment." Meaningless terms such as "doing well" or "status quo" are of little value and should be avoided.

SUBJECTIVE INFORMATION. This includes the history of the problem and all descriptive information perceived as important by the patient, including symptoms and feelings. This is an interpretation of the problem from the patient's point of view.

OBJECTIVE DATA. This term refers to those items noted on examination by the physician or allied health personnel. These data include all measurements and factual information obtained by independent observers, and they represent the facts undistorted by bias. Information within this section should also be arranged consistently in the same order, e.g., data concerning blood pressure, temperature, pulse, and respiration.

ASSESSMENT. This refers to either the diagnosis or a description of the problem at its present stage of resolution. Guesswork is not permitted, and only the degree of resolution that can be supported by data is described.

Problem-solving techniques are a fundamental component of traditional medical education. Problem recognition, however, is too often modified by a haste to play the academic game of one-upmanship and to establish a diagnosis rapidly and with the least amount of data. The POMR lays bare any attempt to shortcut the establishment of a sound diagnosis based on the logical acquisition of adequate data. This does not mean, however, that a differential diagnosis is to be avoided, since all "rule-outs" and potential causes for the problem should be reflected accurately in the record so that the problem can be pursued to a definite conclusion. This conclusion may be either the complete disappearance of the sign or symptoms without a final diagnosis ever being reached or the combining of a variety of symptoms and signs into a definite diagnosis.

PLAN. This refers to the diagnostic and therapeutic modalities used in the management of the problem. This section should include all present medications, laboratory tests, procedures (such as exercise or inhalation therapy), further diagnostic plans (such as x-ray studies), patient education (such as informative literature and diet instruction), counseling methods, and the use of consultants. The entire plan (or treatment) section is the most important portion of the progress notes and should be prominently located so that it can be easily found, since future evaluation requires the comparison of outcome with previous treatment plans to determine whether the results obtained match previous expectations. In this manner, the success or failure of earlier plans can be measured. If the progress note is handwritten, the use of a green or red pen will make this section stand out and be easily identified.

A well-thought-out plan helps to maintain continuity of care and allows the physician to communicate to an associate the plans for the patient's management. Three major subdivisions constitute the execution of the plan:

1. *Diagnostic studies* should contain the "rule-outs" and the tests to be used in this process of differential diagnosis; for example, to rule out peptic ulcer, obtain an upper gastrointestinal tract series, stool guaiac determination, and so forth. Under the heading of diagnostic studies would also be included the laboratory tests to be done at the next visit. The nurse or laboratory technician will then be alerted to obtain these prior to the physician's involvement. The diagnostic studies category means that more information is needed, and it lists the tests to be conducted to assist in the future evaluation of a problem.

2. *Therapeutic measures* include medications and other treatment modalities.

3. *Patient education* consists of the factors necessary for patient understanding and compliance. This, too, is often a neglected area and therefore warrants visibility by including it as a regular item in the progress notes. The patient education section is of greatest importance for patients with chronic problems, since treatment of one form or another will be a constant feature throughout their lives. The patient should know what to expect from treatment, what side effects are possible, and how a specific medication might react with other drugs or foods. Unexpected events should be avoided as much as possible so that maximum compliance will be maintained. The patient also needs adequate insight into the

problem to know when to seek help without further delay. When patient instruction is given, such as the distribution of an American Heart Association booklet on hypertension or information about the hazards of smoking, it should be documented in the record so that other health personnel who share responsibility for continuing education of the patient will remain informed.

Hospital Discharge Summaries

These summaries should also be organized in the POMR format, with each problem being identified and numbered and the pertinent information "SOAPed." This record (the discharge summary) is then incorporated into the office record to assist in the continuing care of the patient during future office visits.

AVOIDING LEGAL PITFALLS

Juries have a tendency to believe that if an event is not recorded it never occurred, so a complete and accurate medical record is the physician's best defense in a malpractice suit. Often there is a 2- or 3-year delay before a case reaches court and recall from memory will be difficult. Therefore, an accurate and legible record is essential.

Every page of the medical record should bear the patient's name. Progress notes should be signed, dated, arranged chronologically, and if not typed then written in ink, never pencil.

Derogatory, trivial, or loose comments about patients or colleagues should not be recorded; they could prove embarrassing if publicized during a legal review. Similarly, vague and ambiguous statements, such as "the patient is feeling better," should be avoided.

Altering a Record

Adding or changing a statement is no problem if done correctly and if no suit is pending. However, altering the record after a suit has been filed is the kiss of death. This is considered tampering and arouses suspicions that are difficult to dispel. If it is necessary to change an entry in the chart because of an error, the inaccurate material should be crossed out with a single line so that the words remain legible. The change should be initialed and the date and time noted in the margin with a note explaining why the change was made.

Documenting Phone Calls

It is wise to document every telephone call received in the office. Requests for prescription refills should be documented in the medical record as should any call involving medical advice or treatment.

Words to Avoid

Medical records are not privileged and confidential; the information belongs to the patient. Maligning or deprecatory remarks are certainly inappropriate. Words that should be avoided are "simple," "routine," and "uncomplicated," since they suggest a guarantee or predict a good outcome. If the patient is described as uncooperative, the reasons should be documented. Similarly, if patients refuse certain diagnostic tests or procedures this should be documented along with the reason for recommending the test. The fact that the patient was informed of the need for the test is also important. A suit has never been successfully brought because the physician gave the patient too much information.

FLOW SHEETS

Flow sheets are a useful adjunct to any medical record system, particularly when the POMR is used in conjunction with continuing patient care and the management of chronic illnesses. It is sometimes difficult to review the course of a single problem over time using progress notes because a great deal of page turning is required to pick out that problem on successive visits. Placing the prolonged course of a single problem, or even selected multiple problems, on one flow sheet greatly facilitates comprehension and management. Flow sheets are also useful in any clinical situation requiring the monitoring of multiple laboratory and therapeutic data over a long period of time. They present an overview of the illness, compressing events over time onto one page, and allow the physician to identify current values as well as observe trends in the course of a disease. Flow sheets permit speedy retrieval of data and facilitate the ongoing analysis of the stage of chronic illness by indicating changing trends in response to therapy.

Once the parameters to be monitored have been identified, the flow sheet serves as a constant reminder to review these items and acts as an early warning system for potential problems by indicating variations from the previous pattern or baseline. Such sheets allow for a large amount of physiologic and management data to be accumulated in a compact area and observed at a glance.

The flow sheet permits ready comparison of all determinations of a single test. It also permits physiologic and laboratory data to be monitored on the same time scale as therapeutic management. When material is categorized in this manner, physicians tend to write more concise and clearer notes, including fewer irrelevant details.

The time required to enter data on a flow sheet is much less than the time that is lost in sorting out disorganized information in the traditional record. A partially used flow sheet, however, can be more inefficient than none at all, since the physician is then required to search back and forth among the flow sheet, progress notes, and data base for the complete information.

The flow sheet can be a simple piece of graph paper, a self-designed form (Fig. 14–6), or a preprinted form. In each instance, the left-hand column should contain the elements considered essential to the ongoing management of the problems being followed. Just as the data base must be individually designed for each practice, the flow sheet must be suited to the preferences of the physician and must be designed to measure those items considered most important in the management of the illnesses for which it is used.

Items to be monitored on a flow sheet usually include:

1. Frequency of symptoms
2. Physiologic data, such as weight, edema, and blood pressure
3. Laboratory data, such as fasting blood glucose levels, urine cultures, and serum cholesterol levels
4. Medications
5. Nondrug therapy, such as diet and physical therapy
6. Patient compliance
7. Patient education

Flow sheets serve as memory aids and guard against the possibility of important aspects of a patient's continuing care being overlooked by the physician. For example, when monitoring the course of a diabetic patient, the physician may forget to regularly check the fundi or peripheral pulses for potential vascular change. Listing these as areas to be evaluated at prescribed intervals, along with other specifics, will serve as a reminder to all office personnel. The data-gathering activities of allied health personnel can easily be incorporated into the structure of the flow sheet by identifying those parameters to be measured at the next visit prior to the physician's examination. The flow sheet should monitor problems at intervals that will reflect the degree of stability of the illness; the more acute and unstable the problem, the more frequently measurements will be required. Items should be monitored often enough to ensure good care without undue expense. In an intensive care unit, the intervals between items are minutes or hours, whereas in the outpatient setting, they are days, weeks, or months.

The chart format of a flow sheet also minimizes problems caused by illegible handwriting. Effective use of flow sheets may obviate the need for progress notes when repeated visits relate only to the ongoing management of the chronic illnesses followed on the flow sheet. When progress notes are necessary, "see flow sheet" will frequently suffice in lieu of entries in the objective and plan categories.

MEDICATION LISTS

Almost from the beginning, medication lists have been a component of the problem-oriented medical record as it is used in family practice. Chronic medications are frequently documented on a separate page or below the problem list. It is difficult, however, to keep these lists current, for as soon as omissions occur, the list becomes more trouble than it is worth since it must be checked against the progress notes for accuracy. A variety of other methods are in use, the most accurate involving a direct copy of all prescriptions written. Figure 14–7 is an illustration of the medication list used at the University of Iowa, where pressure-sensitive paper, upon which the prescription is placed when written, is

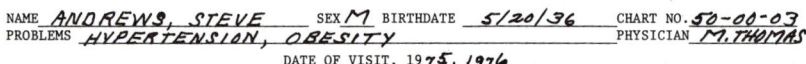
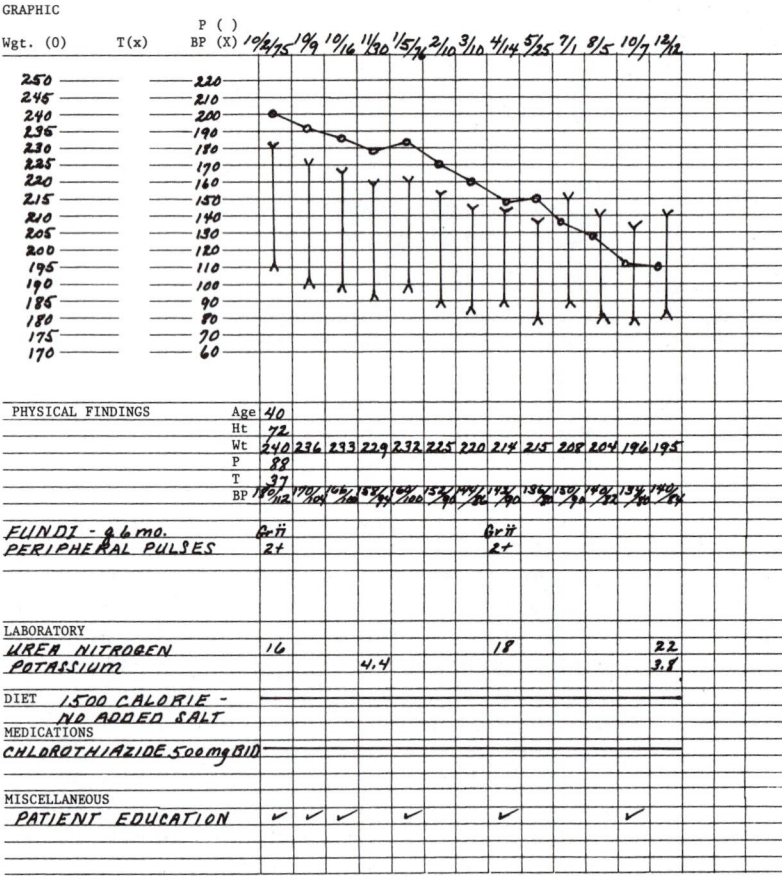

Figure 14–6. Flow sheet for a patient with hypertension and obesity. University of Iowa, Family Practice Center. (From Rakel RE: Principles of Family Medicine. Philadelphia, W. B. Saunders Co., 1977, with permission.)

used. Although redundancy occurs, the usefulness of this list lies in its accuracy. Problems arise only if prescriptions are written without being placed over the appropriate area on this sheet.

One way to avoid this problem is to use a medication list such as that developed in the Department of Family Medicine at Baylor College of Medicine. Prescriptions are fixed along the left side of the page by a perforation. An actual copy of the medication prescribed is left on the underlying pressure-sensitive sheet. No loose prescription pads are used, so this almost ensures an accurate record of all medications prescribed, plus their strength, quantity, instructions, and number of refills. Space is also allotted for recording the date and reason for discontinuing a drug.

STANDARD GENOGRAM STRUCTURE

The family genogram is a tool used by physicians to summarize on one page a large amount of information relating to the family. It includes a family's hereditary background and the risk this places on current members, along with other major medical, social, and interactional influences. The genogram is also referred to as the family pedigree, family tree, or genealogic chart.

The genogram should indicate those conditions in the family that have hereditary significance, but it can also be used to depict problems of a less well-defined hereditary nature that appear to have a high incidence in a family. Even if these problems are not purely genetic, they may be related to social or environmental factors or to family traits or habits that predispose future family members to the likelihood of that problem developing. The genogram can also demonstrate problems of unknown etiology that are common in a family. Regardless of the cause of the problem, demonstrating its trend throughout succeeding generations of a family is valuable, because it gives offspring some idea of whether they might develop the condition. Thus, charting the incidence of cancer, heart disease, or asthma in a family alerts the individual patient to factors that should be watched for closely.

Jones, Robert
Name

DRUG ALLERGIES Penicillin

| | 7-13-32 | 50-16-32 | |
| Date of Birth | Chart No. | Date |

Date	Prescription	Strng.	Quant.	Sig.	# Re-fills	Problem	Subsequent Refill Information
5/4/82	Hydrochlorothiazide	50mg	100	ī twice daily to lower blood pressure	0		7/1/82 #100
5/4/82	Tetracycline	250mg	40	ī four times daily until gone	0		
9/14/82	Theodur	200mg	120	īī tabs P.O. b.i.d.	4		
9/14/82	Hydrochlorothiazide	50mg	120	ī tab P.O. b.i.d	2		
10/19/82	Tetracycline	250mg	40	ī tab qid	0		

Figure 14–7. Medication list, University of Iowa, Family Practice Center. (From Rakel RE. Textbook of Family Practice. 4th ed. Philadelphia, W. B. Saunders Company, 1990, p. 1717, with permission.)

Family History

Family background and family influences are not merely incidental items to be considered briefly during the care of an individual; they are essential to the continuing and comprehensive care of that individual and family. The family history has long been a major component of the medical record, since information concerning family background is a potential source of valu-able diagnostic information. Too often, however, family data are treated superficially when the physician asks questions regarding the frequency of hereditary or transmissible problems within the family. This ritualistic inquiry is often no more than a recitation by the physician of diseases, such as tuberculosis and diabetes, for which a yes or no answer is requested and that yields data of only limited usefulness. The astute diagnostician delves into the patient's background more thoroughly,

Figure 14–8. Basic genogram containing family names, first names, and ages or birthdates. (From Rakel, RE. Textbook of Family Practice. 4th ed. Philadelphia, W. B. Saunders Company, 1990, with permission.)

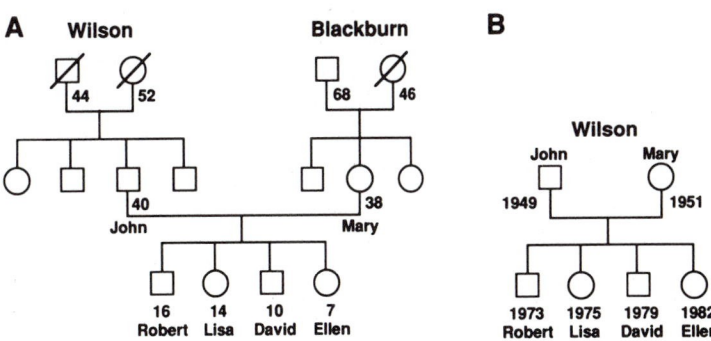

attempting to uncover subtle trends or relationships between significant past events and the present problem. The family physician usually accumulates a complete family history over a period of time, gradually adding items to the picture during a series of patient visits. In this way the patient, by asking other family members for additional data and clarification, is able to add more information at subsequent visits. Families usually enjoy developing a family genogram and cooperate in constructing one that not only reflects their lineage but also remains a dynamic picture that can be of medical value to future generations.

One example of an important hereditary influence is inborn errors of metabolism. Although these are rare and normally occur at a rate of only one in every 10,000 births, the carriers of these diseases experience a rate of one per every 100 births or less. The probability of one carrier's marrying another is sufficiently high to cause concern, and since many of these disorders can be prevented or managed if diagnosed early, the identification of these affected individuals, or carriers, assumes greater importance. Over a thousand genetic abnormalities caused by single mutant genes in humans have been identified.

Basic Design of the Genogram

The purpose of the family genogram is to develop a realistic overview of the family's background and potential health problems. The techniques and symbols used should be those that physicians consider most meaningful in their practice and with which they feel most comfortable. Because the objective is to provide this information at a glance, the chart should be kept simple and brief. The more complicated the symbols and the more cluttered the design, the more time and effort it takes to construct the chart and to retrieve the information. Symbols requiring the least possible amount of explanation should be selected to represent specific problems.

The standard family genogram chart consists of three or more generations, representing all members of both spouses' families. The generations can be identified by roman numerals. The first-born members of each generation are the farthest to the left, with siblings following to the right in order of birth. A single generation is represented on the same line, and symbols should all be the same size. In generation I, it is traditional to place the husband's symbol on the left. The children of that

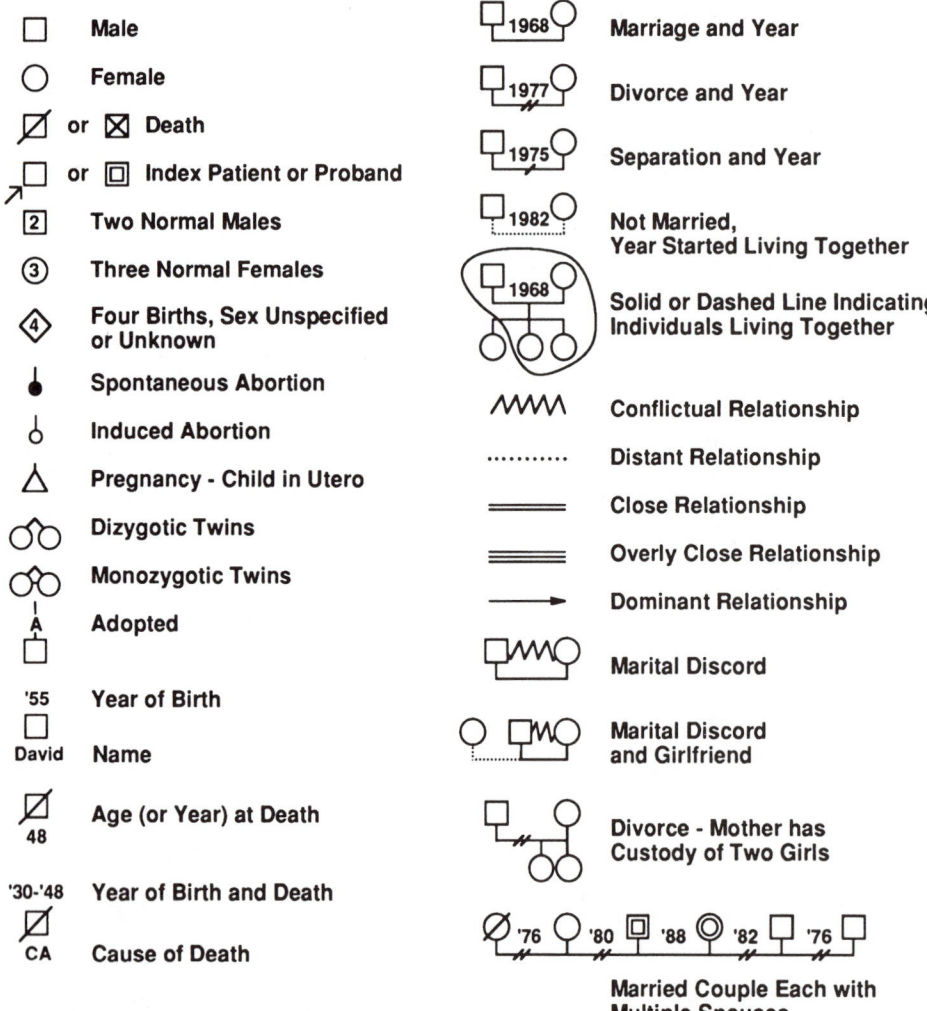

Figure 14–9. Standard genogram symbols. (From Rakel RE. Textbook of Family Practice. 4th ed. Philadelphia, W. B. Saunders Company, 1990, p. 1725, with permission.)

marriage are indicated on the next generation line. In later generations, the first pregnancy (or first-born child) is placed to the left. The family name is placed above each major family unit, and the given names are placed below each symbol. An indication of either the patient's age or birthdate with each symbol is also useful. When ages are shown, it is important to indicate the date on which the chart was developed so that these ages can be adjusted over time. The other method is to show the dates of birth, as in Figure 14–8.

There is often one member of the family who is of greater medical significance because of a chronic disease or an overwhelming problem. If such an individual is the major reason for developing a genogram, this person is called the *index person* (similar to the *proband*) and is identified by an arrow, double square, or double circle (Fig. 14–9).

The components of a genogram include the following:

1. Three or more generations
2. The names of all family members
3. Age or year of birth of all family members
4. Any deaths, including age at or date of death and cause
5. Significant diseases or problems of family members
6. Indication of members living together in the same household
7. Dates of marriages and divorces
8. A listing of first-born of each family to the left, with siblings listed sequentially to the right
9. A key depicting all symbols used
10. Symbols selected for simplicity and maximum visibility.

Familiarity with the standard symbols (Fig. 14–9) allows for more rapid retrieval of information. These standard symbols should be used whenever possible, but variations can easily be developed to provide more accurate or useful information.

Standard symbols that maintain simplicity and avoid competition can be used with most family genograms, since only a few conditions normally require representation. When a variety of problems are represented in one genogram, the selection of symbols should be made with special care to assure that they are noncompetitive. Cluttered symbols are more difficult to interpret and may defeat the chart's primary purpose. Additional notations on selected individuals regarding their occupation, level of education, general state of health, or other medical problems can usually be listed beneath the symbol or beneath the chart to give a more complete picture of that individual.

When family members assist in constructing a genogram, they may gain additional insight into risks inherent in the family system and an increased awareness of the importance of some problems. For example, if repeated suicides occur, increased attention can be given to recognizing the early signs of depression.

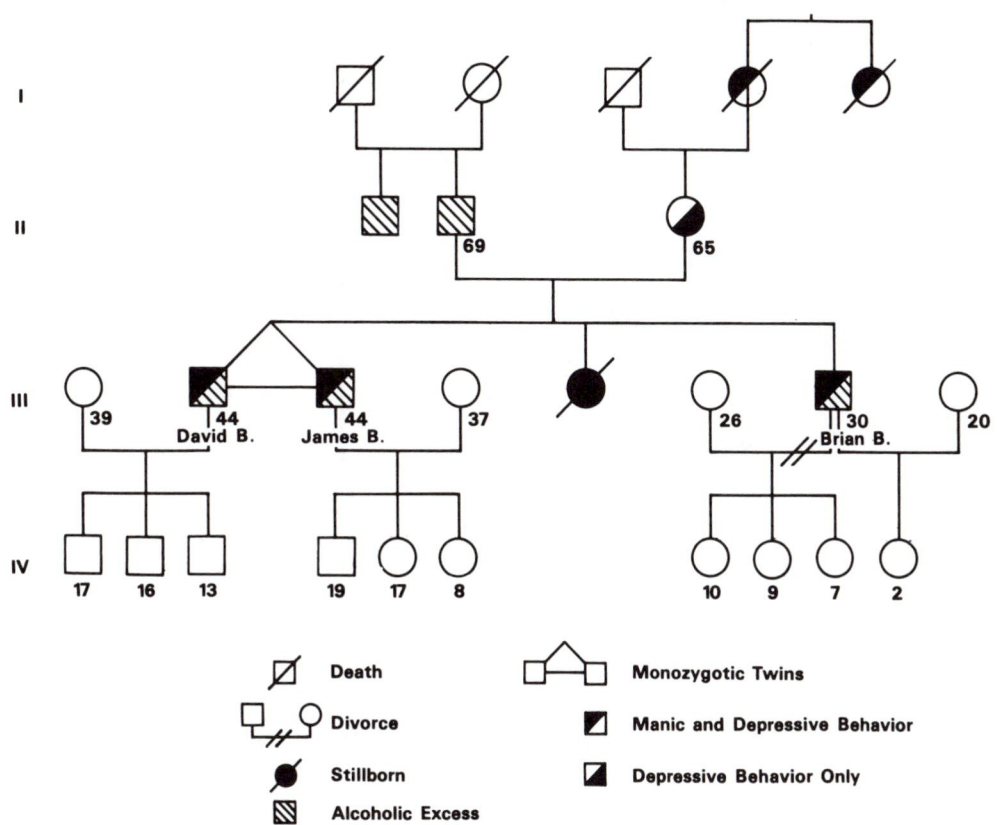

Figure 14–10. Family genogram with bipolar affective disorder. (From Rakel, RE: Principles of Family Medicine. Philadelphia, W. B. Saunders Company, 1977, with permisssion.)

It may be useful to highlight critical medical information on the genogram, using a yellow highlighter or colored pen. In this way, significant problems can be immediately recognized by anyone working with the family. This technique may be useful in educating family members about the importance of these items. For example, if cancer or heart disease is highlighted, the family can be told about the particular risk of continuing cigarette smoking.

The genogram shown in Figure 14–10 was developed by a family practice resident investigating the frequency of manic depression in a family and its relationship to alcoholism (Geron). An apparent X-linked inheritance was noted. Of medical significance to the family is the fact that the affected individuals in generation III first developed symptoms at ages 22 and 32. The predictive significance for generation IV is obvious. Prompt recognition and treatment of symptoms will be possible when the problems first occur rather than later, after significant hardship has been experienced, as is so often the case.

Functional Charting

An additional dimension can be added to the genogram by including the functional components shown in Figure 14–9. In this way, the social and interpersonal influences that operate within a family can be shown in addition to hereditary influences. Such a picture, which includes evidence of the emotional relationships between individuals living together, gives a more dynamic image of the family and allows for greater insight into patterns of behavior. This visualization of family roles and interpersonal relationships allows one to judge the totality of the family unit—its strengths and weaknesses, its degree of solidarity, and its ability to withstand future stressful situations.

A clinical example is shown in Figure 14–11. Kathryn is a 2-year-old child who is seen 2 days after her second birthday complaining that her stomach burns. Functional abdominal pain may be one of the biopsychosocial hypotheses to be considered. The genogram in Figure 14–11 may be useful in testing this hypothesis. The genogram is read as follows:

Family Structure: Single-parent family with one child at home

Family Demographics: High school–educated parents, mother employed; status consistent with that of other family members

Family Life Events: Divorce of patient's parents 1 year prior to visit; patient's birthday 2 days prior to visit

Family Problems: Patient's father has emotional and work problems; this also appears to be a pattern among his siblings

INTERPRETATION. From an individual and family life cycle perspective, the patient may not be progressing

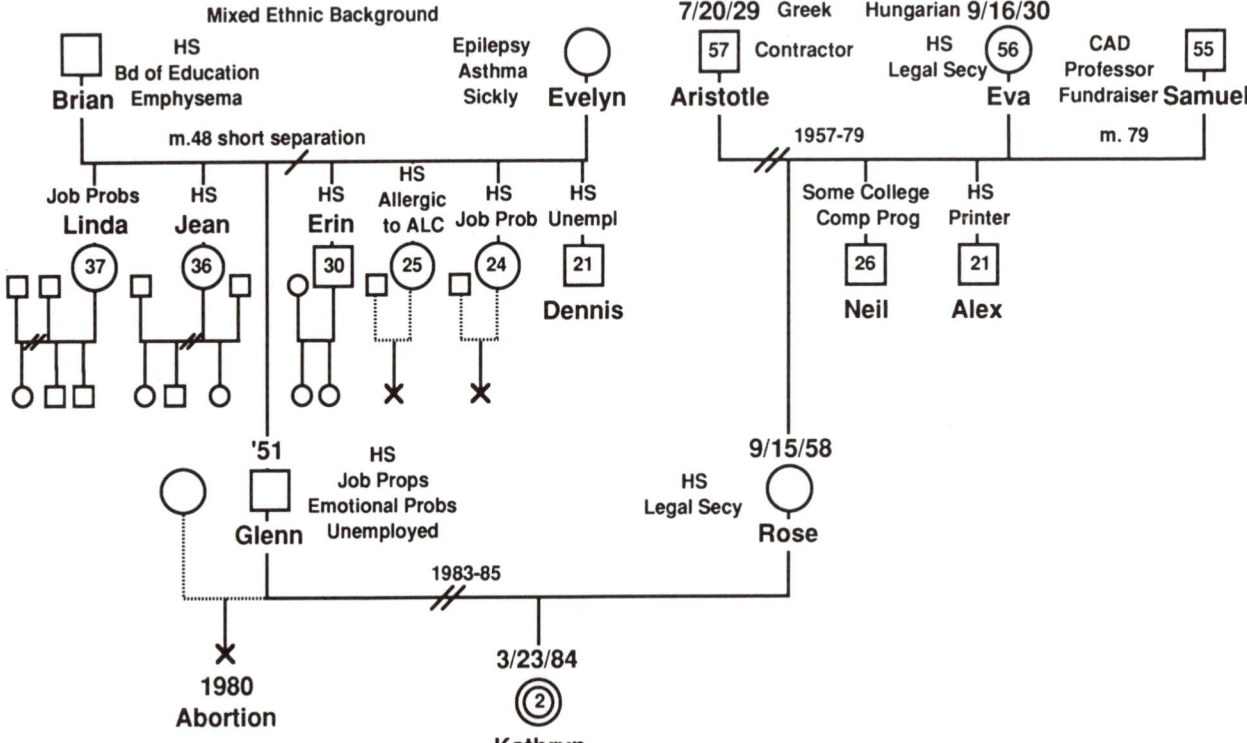

Figure 14–11.   Case Example: Kathryn. (From Rakel, RE: Textbook of Family Practice, 4th ed. Philadelphia, W. B. Saunders Company, 1990, with permisssion.)

adequately in her development because of the absence of her father. Normal family development has been disrupted by the divorce, and, depending upon the father's visitation privileges, the patient may be having inadequate contact with a male parental figure. From a stress–social support perspective, the divorce of the parents within the last year is a major life event, as is the child's second birthday 2 days before the visit. The impact of these events on the child may need to be explored further. In addition, there are the daily problems of attending day care while the mother works and the fact that only a single parent is home during evenings and weekends.

The interpretation of this genogram suggests that there is the necessary and sufficient information to support a functional abdominal pain hypothesis. A standard biomedical evaluation is of course indicated to evaluate that clinical hypothesis, and more focused family information may need to be gathered further to test the psychosocial hypothesis. The genogram reading and interpretation provide a guide to help the clinician efficiently gather the most relevant additional family data.

REFERENCES

Bjorn JC, Cross HD. Problem Oriented Practice. Chicago, Modern Hospital Press, 1970.

Fischbach RL, Sionelo-Bayog A, Needle A, Delbanco TL. The patient and practitioner as co-authors of the medical record. Patient Counseling and Health Education, First Quarter 1980, pp. 1–5.

Geron M. Genetics of Bipolar Affective Disorder and Its Application in Family Practice. Iowa City, University of Iowa, June 26, 1976.

Grace NT, Neal EM, Wellock CE, Pile DD. The family-oriented medical record. J Fam Pract 1977; 4:91–98.

Michael M, Bordley C. Do patients want access to their medical records? Med Care 1982; 20:432–435.

Murnaghan JG. Ambulatory medical care data. Review of the conference proceedings. Report of a conference on ambulatory care records, Chicago, April 1972. Med Care 1973; 11(Suppl):13.

Schade HI. Office Policies Statement of the Schade Medical Clinic, Los Gatos, California, 1980.

Texas Revised Civil Statues Annotated art 4495b, sec 5.08(b) (West Supp 1987).

Tufo HM, Bouchard RE, Rubin AS, Twitchell JC, Van Buren HC, Bedard L. Problem-oriented approach to practice: II. Development of the system through audit and implication. JAMA 1977; 238:502–505.

Weed LL. Medical Records, Medical Education and Patient Care. Chicago, Case Western Reserve University Press, 1971.

Widmer RB, Cadoret RJ, North CS. Depression in family practice: Some effects on spouses and children. J Fam Pract 1980; 10:45.

QUESTIONS

1. The most important component of the Problem Oriented Medical Record is the
   a. Data base.
   b. Problem list.
   c. Progress notes.
   d. Flow chart.
   e. Filing system.

2. Which of the following are components of the data base?
   a. Physical examination
   b. Laboratory results
   c. Family history
   d. Past medical history
   e. Present illness

3. SOAP stands for
   a. Systemic, Objective, Assessment, Plan.
   b. Symptoms, Objections, Arrangements, Proposals.
   c. Subjective, Objective, Assessment, Plan.
   d. History, Physical Findings, Diagnosis, Treatment.
   e. Symptoms, Findings, Assessment, Plan of Therapy.

4. Flow sheets include which of the following?
   a. Laboratory results
   b. Physiologic data
   c. Selected medications
   d. Problem list
   e. Consultant reports

5. Which of the following are standard components of a genogram?
   a. Three or more generations
   b. Deaths
   c. Names of family members
   d. Divorces
   e. Significant diseases

6. A genogram using functional symbols
   a. Emphasizes problems of parents.
   b. Focuses on the most ill family member.
   c. Shows interpersonal relationships.
   d. Depicts strong relationships.
   e. Shows discord.

Answers appear on page 447.

15

ECONOMICS OF MEDICAL PRACTICE

E. LEE TAYLOR

The highest use of capital is not to make more money, but to make money do more for the betterment of life.

HENRY FORD

Economics is the science of the production and distribution of goods and services. Medical economics is that part of the national economy that focuses on the production and distribution of health care goods and services. It is imperative that family physicians in this modern, complex, and rapidly changing medical economics system have an understanding of the basic national economic system and the role that medical economics plays within the system. Without that understanding, it would be difficult for any physician to maintain a practice that meets the growing demand for delivery of high-quality health care services in the most cost-effective manner.

THE LAW OF ECONOMICS: SUPPLY AND DEMAND

One basic law of economics—the law of supply and demand—states that *when demand for a product or service is high, price will rise, and when the demand for a product or service decreases, the price will fall, provided all external forces remain stable.* The external forces that affect supply and demand in the health care system are numerous. The effects each force may have on the supply or demand side of the economic scale would require volumes to explain. One can see from Figure 15–1 that it is an almost impossible task to perfectly balance the economic elements of medical care. Many of these forces may affect either side of the scale—supply or demand for health care service.

A perspective of the present-day medical economy can be gained by a review of its historical development. Knowledge of the rapid changes in our health care system will provide some understanding of the many external forces that have produced the present medical economic environment.

THE EVOLUTION OF MODERN MEDICAL ECONOMICS

Before 1940, there was little interest in medical economics, especially by the federal government. Most people, except the indigent, paid their own medical bills. The indigents were cared for by physicians who agreed to provide services for the poor in exchange for hospital privileges. A small number of group health insurance plans existed, but relatively few people belonged or subscribed to them. Medical care, in comparison with other costs, was not considered to be expensive. The government financed only 20% of the total national health care costs at that time. Today, the government's share of health care has more than doubled to over 40% of total national health care expenditures. Many events have led to today's large expenditures for health care; most have occurred since 1940.

THE MOVE TO SPECIALIZATION

World War II brought about rapid changes in the health care system. During this time, antibiotics, anesthesia, and many medical and surgical techniques were developed and improved at a rapid pace. Before the war, most physicians were general practitioners. Fewer than 25% of physicians in the United States were in specialty training. Most physicians leaving the military after the war went back to specialty training because of increased technology and the new G.I. Bill of Rights, which provided educational stipends for veterans. The stipends supplemented these physicians' residency incomes and made additional training affordable. The federal government also started programs that subsidized medical schools and hospitals with large amounts of research funds. Consequently, the age of specialization was inevitable. By the 1950s, almost 20,000 physicians were in specialty training (Campion). In 1990 only 8.3% of the 85,330 residents in training were in family

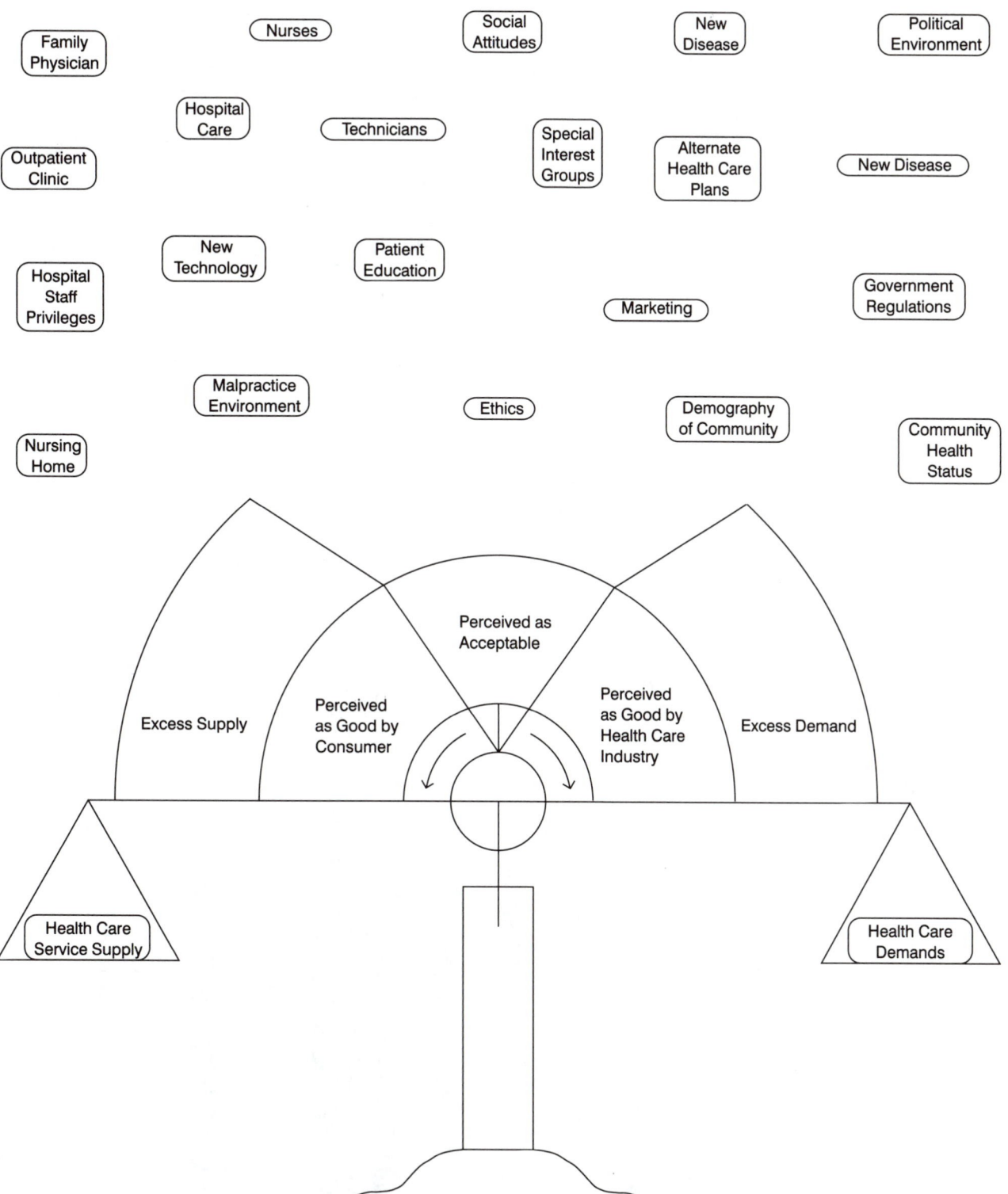

Figure 15–1. Health care economic scale and additional economic weights. (From Taylor, EL. Economics of family practice in Rakel RE (ed): Textbook of Family Practice, 4th ed. Philadelphia, W. B. Saunders Co., 1990, p. 1741, with permisssion.)

practice programs (Rowley et al.). By 1946 the general practitioners were feeling a drastic reduction in both their numbers and their influence. Within the medical profession, some were losing hospital privileges because specialized hospital staffs were often requiring board certification or residency training rather than granting privileges on the basis of proven capability (Council on Long Range Planning and Development). As a result, the American Academy of General Practice was formed in 1947.

PHYSICIAN SHORTAGE

As specialization continued, the shortage of primary care physicians (general practitioners, general internists, and general pediatricians) grew worse. The lack of primary care physicians, especially family physicians, and a general shortage and geographic maldistribution of physicians became a concern of the profession, the public, and the federal government. In 1948 the Ewing Report from the Federal Security Agency and a bill introduced by Senator Claude D. Pepper (D., Fla.) proposed a 5-year program of support for medical schools to address the predicted shortage of 42,000 physicians by 1960. The amount of federal funds to subsidize medical schools for research, training, and construction grew rapidly, and increasing specialization continued (Campion).

The 1950s saw the concern about a physician shortage continuing, and a series of reports led to the passage of the Health Professions Education Assistance Act of 1963. This act was intended to increase enrollment in medical and other allied health science schools. It provided loans to students and funds for renovating and constructing new facilities. Around the early to middle 1960s, the perception was that more economic stimulus was needed to increase the number of health care workers. Federal legislation to fund operational support for schools was provided contingent on each school's increasing its enrollment (Council on Medical Education). This funding stimulated the increase in the number of medical schools from 85 in 1957 to 127 by 1982. The number of medical school graduates more than doubled, from 7264 in 1963, at the time the legislation was passed, to 15,667 by 1981. The number has remained relatively stable over the past nine years (Fig. 15–2).

PRIMARY CARE DEVELOPMENT

Until the 1960s very few efforts were made to control specialization. Even when efforts were made, there were no limits or restrictions. The 1960s produced several reports indicating the need for primary care physicians. The Ad Hoc Committee on Education for Family Practice (The Willard Report) recommended that family practice be designated a specialty and that board certification be provided (Council on Medical Education). By 1969 The American Board of Family Practice was established; family practice became the twentieth specialty and formal residency programs began. In 1971 the American Academy of General Practice changed its name to the American Academy of Family Physicians.

In 1975 the Coordinating Council on Medical Education reported that the percentage of primary care

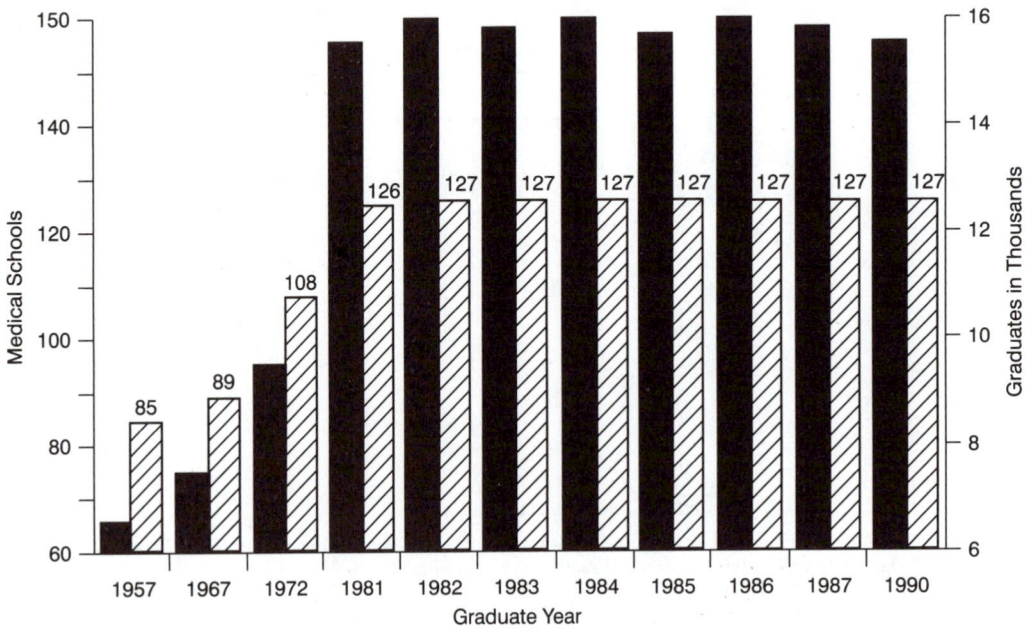

Figure 15–2. Medical school growth and graduates, 1957–1990. Solid black bars represent the total number of graduates in thousands, and dashed black bars represent the number of medical schools for a given year. (From Jonas HS, Etzel SI, Banznasky B. Graduate medical education in the United States. JAMA 1990; 264:801–809; Crowley AE, Etzel SI, Shaw HA. Graduate medical education in the United States. JAMA 1987; 258:1031–1040; Campion FD. The AMA and U.S. Health Policy Since 1940. Chicago, Chicago Press, 1974, with permission.)

physicians (general practitioners, general internists, and general pediatricians) had decreased from 43% of all physicians in 1965 to 34% in 1972. Congress had attempted to stimulate interest in the family practice specialty with the Family Practice of Medicine Act in October 1970. At that time, the American Boards of Internal Medicine and Pediatrics were advised to make primary care careers in their specialties more attractive (Council on Medical Education).

PUBLIC DEMAND AND EXPECTATIONS

Before 1940 medical care was not considered an important issue because medicine was frequently considered somewhat ineffective and not too expensive. During and after the war, with the advent of antibiotics, new surgical procedures, and the therapeutic success of medicine, medical care became a desired and demanded service of our society. The new demand for medical services created the rapid spread of health insurance. The number of people covered by health insurance grew from a very few in 1950, to 72.3% of the population in the 1960s, and to 86.4% of the population by the 1970s. With the enactment of Medicare for the elderly and Medicaid for the indigent in 1965, a significant additional demand was placed upon the profession for medical care and health care services. Many of the health care services being purchased were no longer personal, out-of-pocket expenses paid for by the individual consumer. Not only did the number of patients per physicians increase, but the number of visits per patient increased also. Physician visits per patient per year increased from three in 1940 to five in 1984 (Campion).

Society's greater expectations from medical care also produced a malpractice crisis. The number of claims increased from 2.9 per 100 physicians before 1976 to 6.2 per 100 physicians by 1981. The size of awards to patients also increased, as did the premiums for professional liability insurance, at a rate of 14% annually after 1976 (Campion).

EVOLUTION OF HOSPITAL AND SERVICES CARE

Many factors contributed to the growth of hospitals. Some of these were increased medical technology, new surgical procedures, federal grants for research, the Hill-Burton Act of 1946, private health insurance, and specialty training for physicians. As public demand for the quality of care being provided in hospitals rose, annual admissions increased from 13.6 million in 1940 to 36.2 million in 1980. Outpatient visits to hospitals increased by 44% between 1970 and 1979 (Campion).

As accessibility of health care grew, so did cost. This was logical, but it was the degree of growth in expense that caused concern. In 1970 the Nixon administration recognized that the Medicare hospital program would cost $2.7 billion more than anticipated 5 years earlier. At this time the focus of the federal government began

to shift from the previous concern for access to health care to cost containment. As the cost of hospital care increased, many programs were instituted by the federal government to review hospital utilization and to limit the number of hospital days and services provided during an admission (Campion).

The prospective payment system was enacted in 1983, a system of hospital reimbursement based on over 400 Diagnosis-Related Groups (DRGs). Under DRGs, hospitals are reimbursed at a fixed rate for diagnosis and treatment of the DRG, regardless of the length of stay or service provided. The prospective payment system has encouraged hospitals to provide only required services and to reduce the length of stay in the hospital.

As of 1986 the average length of stay in hospitals had decreased and was at a 16-year low for patients under 65 years of age and at a 5-year low for patients 65 years of age and older. These shorter lengths of stay are due to the prospective payment system implemented by the federal government in 1983 and the response of the health care profession to pressure from private businesses and health care insurance companies to reduce health care costs (Arnett and Freeland).

UNDERSTANDING GENERAL ECONOMICS

As evidenced by the historical events since 1940, we have seen the effects of technology, public attitudes, demand for services, politics, and the massive federal economic stimulus that has brought us to today's complex system of medical economics.

To gain an understanding of today's medical economic environment, it is necessary to understand how the national economy is measured and evaluated. This will give physicians a better understanding of why there is so much private, public, and political interest in health care costs. Some important terms often used in describing the medical economic environment are described below.

GROSS NATIONAL PRODUCT

The gross national product (GNP) is the total market value of final goods and services produced by a national economy over a specific period of time. This is usually reported on an annual basis and is frequently used to measure the standard of living and the rate of economic growth. The rate of growth of a specific product or service is expressed as a percentage of the total GNP. National health care expenditures were 11.6% of the United States GNP in 1989.

CONSUMER PRICE INDEX

The consumer price index (CPI) is the measurement of the average change in the price for goods and services that are bought for everyday living. This includes the costs for physicians, dentists, drugs, and other health

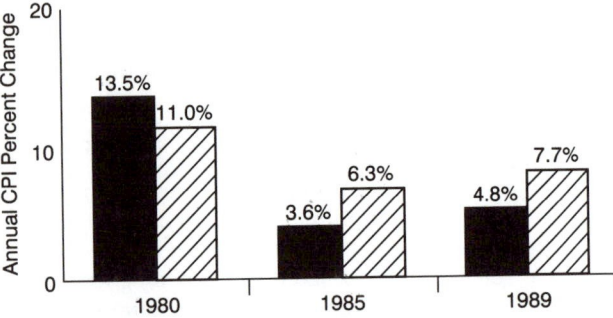

Figure 15–3. Average consumer price index—urban (CPI-U), 1980–1989. Medical care versus all goods and services. Solid black bars represent percent change in all goods and services, and bars with diagonals represent percent change in medical care. (From Bureau of Labor Statistics, U.S. Labor Dept., with permission.)

care. The CPI is usually published each month and averaged over a period of one year. The CPI measures the changes in the price of goods and services from a reference date, at which time the index base was equal to 100 (The World Almanac). The reference year is selected by the federal government.

An increase of 300 in the CPI would mean that there was a 200% increase in the price of a product or service since the reference date. The average percentages of increases and decreases are referred to in the medical economic reports published by the government and presented to the public by the media. The average CPI for medical care compared with all other goods and services from 1982 to 1989 can be seen in Figure 15–3.

NATIONAL HEALTH CARE ECONOMICS TODAY

The national annual health care expenditures have grown from $40 billion in 1940 to over $600 billion in 1989. Our health care bill is now 11.6% of the GNP, and we now spend $2354 per person on annual health care. Table 15–1 demonstrates the trends in health care expenses in our national economy.

There have been significant changes in shifting the cost from private households to business and government. In 1960 individual out-of-pocket expenses were 49%. In 1989 the out-of-pocket expenses dropped to 21%. However, the cost to private business has in-

creased from 27% to 37%, and the government cost has increased from 24% to 42% (Figure 15–4). This transfer of cost to business and government is strongly affecting their ability to grow and compete in the marketplace.

GROSS NATIONAL PRODUCT MEASUREMENT OF HEALTH CARE COSTS

National health expenditures have increased for the last 50 years as a percentage of the GNP. In the 1970s the GNP increased at a rate of 2% to 6% a year while health care expenses grew at a rate of 12.7%. In 1980 and 1981 the growth of national health care expenses was 15%, whereas the GNP grew at an annual rate of only 8.3%. In 1989 health care spending increased 11.1%, and the GNP grew only 6.7% (HHS News).

The highest health care expenditures on a national basis are for hospital care and physician services. Before 1965 and the enactment of Medicare and Medicaid programs, national expenditures for hospital care were $13.9 billion. This had increased to $176.6 billion by 1986. By 1986 physician service payments, which account for approximately 20% of the national health care dollar, had increased to 10 times the total 1965 charges (Reuter). One should note, however, that the percentage of the health care dollar that was spent for physician services ranged from 18% to 20% of total health care expenditures over a 25-year period (Table 15–2).

It is important to remember that after passage of the Medicare and Medicaid legislation in 1965, financial access to health care was provided for many who previously had had no health care coverage. Hospital admission rates increased 25%, surgical procedures increased 40%, and the number of hospital days per person over 65 years of age rose 50%. Since the group of these aged 65 or older accounts for 10% to 12% of the population and needs more medical care than the younger segment of our society, it is not surprising that they account for over one-fourth of the total medical expenditures (Campion). It was during this time of Medicaid and Medicare implementation, as discussed previously, that the number of medical school graduates was doubled in an attempt to meet the demand for services.

CONSUMER PRICE INDEX MEASUREMENTS OF HEALTH CARE COSTS

Medical care prices have grown rapidly, as shown by the CPI. Inflation in the medical economic area is about twice the rate of inflation in the general economy (Reuter).

As an example of CPI measurement, Figure 15–3 compares the average CPI for all medical care with the average total CPI for all goods and services from 1982 through 1989. The costs for medical services and total medical care have shown significant increases above the average CPI for all other goods and services.

TABLE 15–1. TRENDS IN HEALTH CARE EXPENSE GROWTH

ITEM	1960	1980	1989
Total expenditures	$27.1 billion	$249.1 billion	$604.1 billion
U.S. population	190.1 million	235.2 million	256.6 million
Per capita expense	$143	$1050	$2354
Percent of GNP	5.3%	9.1%	11.6%

Source: HCFA, Office of the Actuary: Office of National Cost Estimates, with permission.

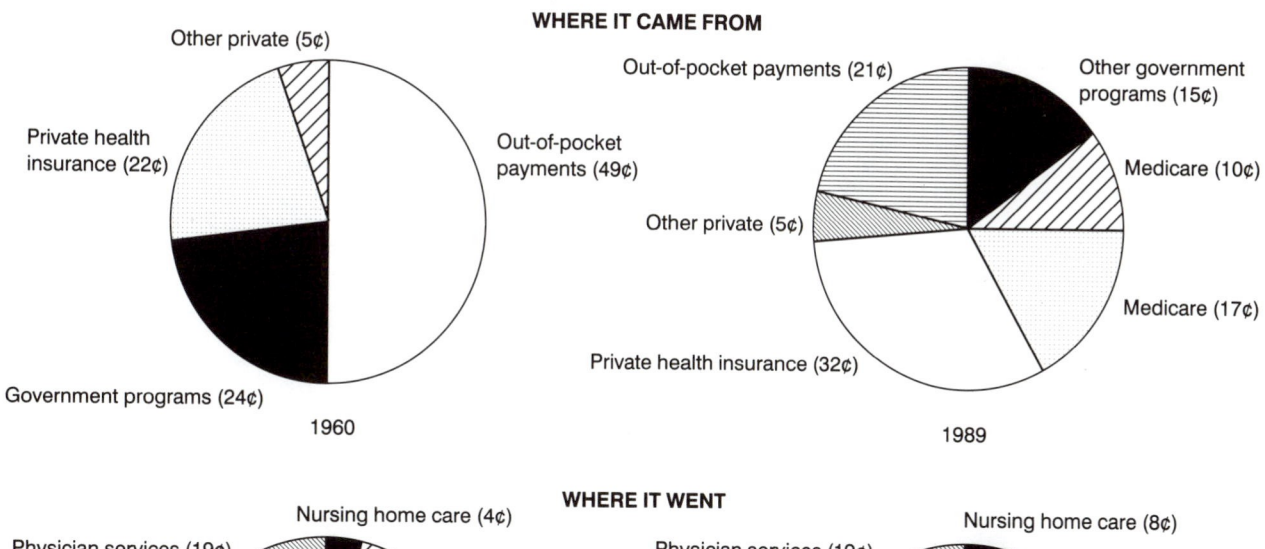

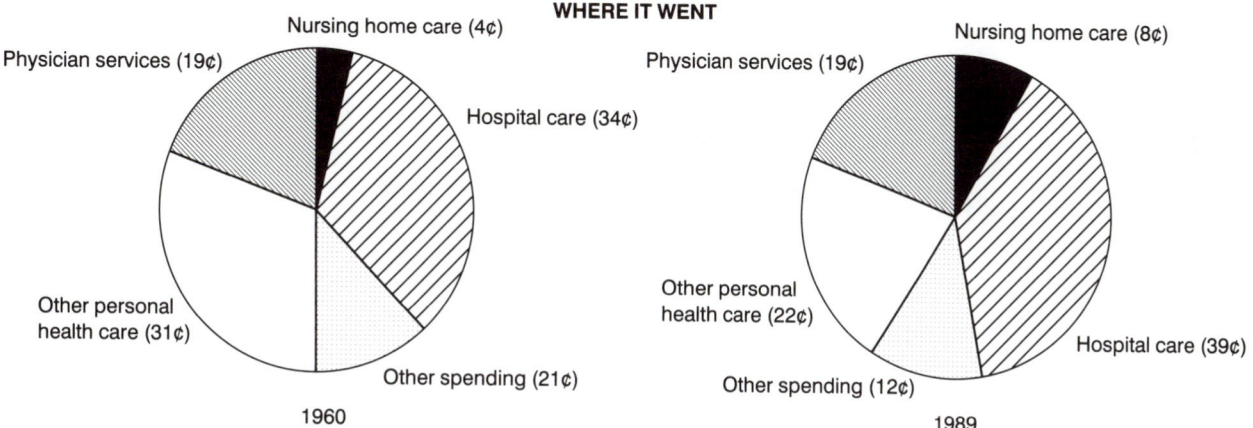

Figure 15–4. The nation's health care dollar, 1960–1989: Where it came from—where it went. (From Health Care Financing Administration, Office of the Actuary: Data from the Office of National Cost Estimates; HCFA Review 1990; 11(4):3, with permission.)

TABLE 15–2. PARTIAL LIST OF U.S. HEALTH EXPENSES (BILLIONS OF DOLLARS)

TYPE OF EXPENSE	1965 (%)	1980 (%)	1989 (%)
Total cost	$41.6	$237.9	$604.1
Hospital care	8.5 (20.3)	101.6 (41.0)	232.8 (38.5)
Physicians' service	2.1 (20.3)	46.8 (18.9)	117.6 (19.5)

Source: HCFA, Office of the Actuary: Office of National Cost Estimates, with permission.

ATTITUDES OF SOCIETY

To gain some perspective on our society's attitudes, one needs also to observe the personal spending habits of our society on goods and services outside the health care economy (Figure 15–5). As one can see, eating out and recreation are significant parts of American lifestyles.

PHYSICIAN SUPPLY AND DEMAND

Although a physician shortage was predicted in the 1950s and every economic effort was made to correct that undersupply, the nation faced a new issue in 1978: Would there be too many physicians in 1990 if the present rate of production continued? To address that issue, the Graduate Medical Education National Advisory Committee was established by the Department of Health and Human Services. After two years of study, the committee reported in 1980 that there would be an oversupply of 75,000 physicians by 1990 if the present rate of graduation from medical schools continued. As a result of this report, Congress decreased and eliminated much of the funding to medical schools that had begun in 1963 (Council on Medical Education).

In July 1988 a new council was appointed to advise Congress on federal policies regarding physician supply and demand for services. The Council on Graduate Medical Education (COGME) reported the following (Residency Assistance Program Newsletter):

There is an undersupply of family physicians.
There is a geographic maldistribution of physicians, with few physicians in many rural and inner-city areas.
There is an adequate supply of pediatricians.
There may be an impending undersupply of general internists.
More minorities should be represented in medicine.

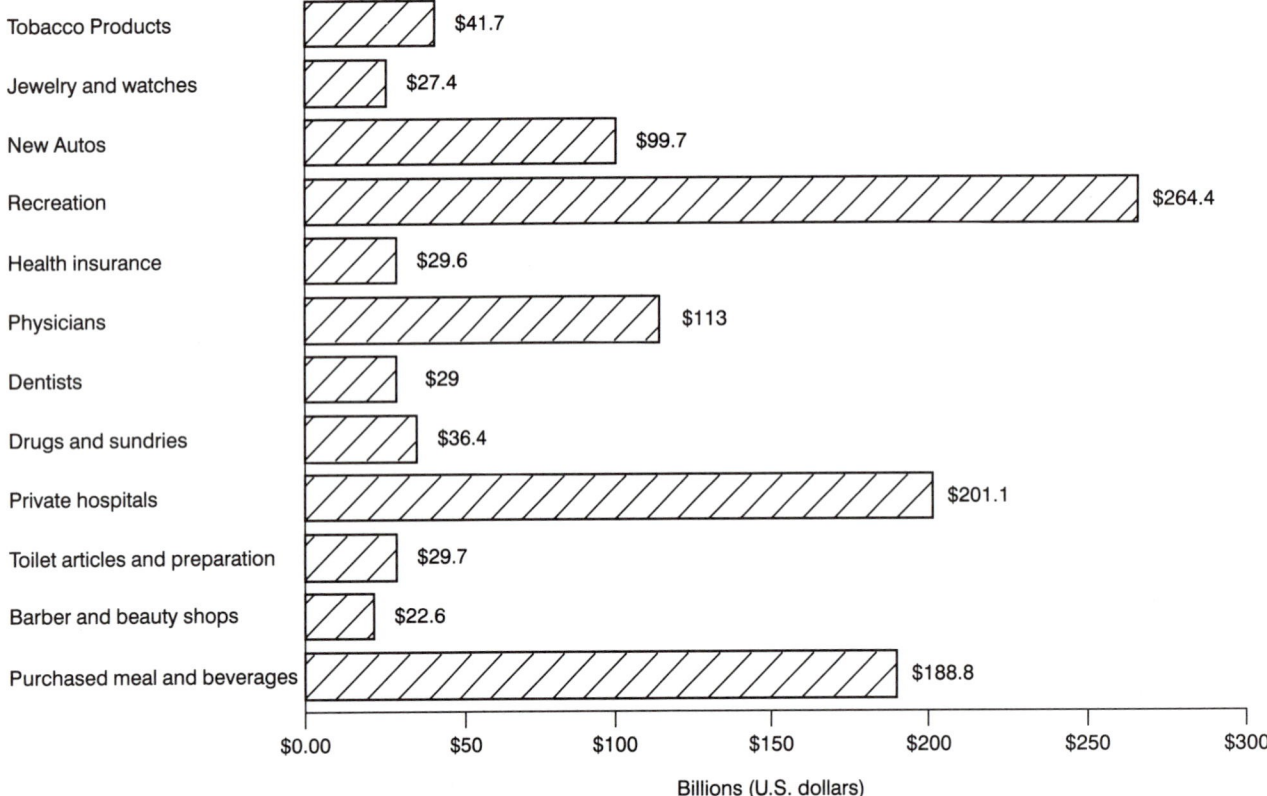

Figure 15–5. Personal consumption expenditures in the United States. (From the World Almanac and Book of Facts, 1988, p. 113; Bureau of Economic Analysis, U.S. Commerce Dept., with permission.)

The present health care financing system decreases the attractiveness of certain disciplines to students and presents incentives that tend to produce a concentration of physicians in what may be oversupplied specialties.

By 1988 it appeared that the physician supply of medical school graduates was remaining stable or decreasing slightly.

Future changes in reimbursement policy may play a greater role in increasing the number of primary care physicians, including family physicians. There have been discrimination patterns in the reimbursement system in the following ways:

Physicians in rural areas have not been reimbursed at the same rate as those in urban areas. This includes reimbursements from Medicare.
Primary care physicians, including family physicians in some cases, have received lower reimbursement than other specialists or subspecialists for performing the same procedures.

In an attempt to correct reimbursement inequities, The Harvard Resource Based Relative Value Scale study, directed by William S. Hsiao, was submitted to the Health Care Financing Administration (HCFA) for review in 1988. The reimbursement design, if accepted by Congress, will compensate more for cognitive skills and reduce the rate for some procedural and surgical treatments. The Health Care Financing Administration will also submit its own recommendations to Congress. It is expected that primary care physicians will receive more equitable reimbursements for their service. A long, drawn-out debate is expected, with the largest opposition coming from the surgical and internal medicine subspecialists because of the possibility of a reduction in some of their fees. This reimbursement plan may be implemented by 1992.

FAMILY PRACTICE PHYSICIAN SUPPLY AND DEMAND

In 1975 family physicians accounted for 13.8% of the total physician population. As of 1989 they accounted for about 11.9% of the total (Council on Long Range Planning and Development). Part of this decreased percentage is a result of the increased number of graduates from medical schools and the overall increase in physicians.

Although composing only 11.9% of the physician population, family physicians manage 30.5% of the more than 636 million office-based outpatient visits per year in the United States. Internists manage 11.6% and pediatricians 11.4% (Council on Long Range Planning and Development). Representing only 11.9% of the physician supply, this country's family physicians see approximately one-third of the nation's total office visits.

The 1985 demographic analysis of family practice office visits compared with visits to other physicians can be seen in Table 15–3. It should be noted that about 20% of office visits to family physicians were made by patients

65 years of age or older. Visits to family physicians accounted for 30% of the total geriatric office visits to all physicians. With the rapidly growing geriatric population now at 12% of the United States population, this is economically significant since all patients over 65 years of age are covered under the Medicare program. The increasing aging population will continue to place an increasing demand on the specialty of family practice as well as on the entire health care system.

DISTRIBUTION OF FAMILY PHYSICIANS

The geographic distribution of family practice graduates of 1990 can be seen in Table 15–4. Of the 1990 family practice graduates, 42.3% practice in geographic areas with a population less than 25,000 and 26.3% practice in areas more than 25 miles from a large city (AAFP).

This geographic trend is more common for family physicians than for the other primary care specialists. From 1970 to 1983 the overall physician supply increased in metropolitan and in rural areas, but the percentage slightly decreased in rural areas (Mead and Seidman). Although the Graduate Medical Education National Advisory Committee in its 1980 report predicted physician oversupply in many specialty areas (including pediatrics, obstetrics and gynecology, and certain internal medicine subspecialties), the trend toward specialization has continued. The recent Report of the Council on Graduate Medical Education has confirmed this trend which is creating the undersupply of family physicians. From 1970 to 1983 internal medicine showed an increase of physicians of 95.6%; pediatrics, 80.6%; obstetrics and gynecology, 55.3%; surgical spe-

cialists, 51.3%; and family practice, 10.7% (Mead and Seidman).

The 1990 annual report of the American Board of Medical Specialties indicates that 61.4% of those completing internal medicine residencies subspecialize and do not enter primary care. About 9.9% of the obstetrics and gynecology residents and 15.6% of pediatricians also subspecialize. This means that most internal medicine residents and significant numbers of the other specialists do not enter primary care and must remain in larger metropolitan areas in and around large hospitals or medical centers in order to be provided with the consultations and high-technology equipment necessary to practice their subspecialties. In fact, only 8% of internists, including subspecialists, and 9.5% of pediatricians practice in nonmetropolitan areas (Barnett and Midtling).

FAMILY PRACTICE INCOME

There are many factors that affect an individual's income. The economics of the community and the nation, the number of years one is in practice, the practice type, and, of course, the time and dedication one places in patient care and practice management all have an impact on personal economics.

Table 15–5 compares the median incomes and expenses of the primary care specialties with 1989 receipts. This information is provided by an ongoing survey that is conducted periodically by the journal, *Medical Economics*. This survey is representative of specialty, geographic area, and age of physician. Overall, there are some general trends that can be seen from the *Medical Economics* continuing survey.

TABLE 15–3.   NUMBER AND PERCENT DISTRIBUTION OF OFFICE VISITS BY SEX AND AGE OF PATIENT AND BY FAMILY PHYSICIANS IN THE UNITED STATES FOR 1985

SEX AND AGE OF PATIENT	ALL PHYSICIANS		FAMILY PRACTICE		OTHER PHYSICIANS	
	Number of Visits in Thousands	Percent Distribution	Number of Visits in Thousands	Percent Distribution	Number of Visits in Thousands	Percent Distribution
TOTAL	636,386	100.0	193,995	100.0	442,391	100.0
FEMALE						
Total female	387,480	60.9	117,685	60.7	269,795	61.0
Under 15 years	58,175	9.1	14,699	7.6	43,475	9.8
15–24 years	48,883	7.7	16,679	8.6	32,204	7.3
25–44 years	118,557	18.6	35,797	18.5	82,760	18.7
45–64 years	82,331	12.9	26,915	13.9	55,416	12.5
65 years and older	79,535	12.5	23,595	12.2	55,940	12.6
MALE						
Total male	248,906	39.1	79,310	39.3	172,593	39.0
Under 15 years	60,594	9.5	14,960	7.7	45,633	10.3
15–24 years	25,081	3.9	9,672	5.0	15,408	3.5
25–44 years	57,167	9.0	20,251	10.4	36,978	8.3
45–64 years	55,060	8.7	17,081	8.8	37,978	8.6
65 years and older	51,004	8.0	14,346	7.4	36,657	8.3

Excludes physicians in anesthesiology, pathology, and radiology.
Source: United States Department of Health and Human Services, Public Health Service, National Center for Health Statistics, National Ambulatory Medical Care Survey: Unpublished Data, and Facts About Family Practice. Kansas City, Mo., American Academy of Family Physicians, p. 23, with permission.

TABLE 15–4. DISTRIBUTION OF 1990 GRADUATING FAMILY PRACTICE RESIDENTS BY COMMUNITY SIZE

CHARACTER AND POPULATION OF COMMUNITY	NUMBER OF REPORTING GRADS	PERCENTAGE OF TOTAL REPORTING GRADS	CUMULATIVE TOTAL OF REPORTING GRADS
Rural area or town (less than 2500) not within 25 miles of large city	86	5.4%	5.4%
Rural area or town (less than 2500) within 25 miles of large city	53	3.3%	8.7%
Small town (2500–25,000) not within 25 miles of large city	279	17.6%	26.3%
Small town (2500–25,000) within 25 miles of large city	254	16.0%	42.3%
Small city (25,000–100,000)	266	16.7%	59.0%
Suburb of small metropolitan area	55	3.7%	62.7%
Small metropolitan area (100,000–500,000)	192	12.1%	74.8%
Suburb of large metropolitan area	212	13.4%	88.2%
Large metropolitan area (500,000 or more)	155	9.8%	98.0%
Inner city/low-income area (500,000 or more)	32	2.0%	100.0%
	1584	100.0%	

Source: American Academy of Family Physicians, 1991, with permission.

One trend is that all physicians' incomes tend to peak when physicians are between 45 and 54 years of age and reach their highest levels when physicians have been in practice between 10 and 20 years. In addition the survey shows that 48% of the family physicians surveyed had net annual practice earnings of $100,000 or more after expenses and before taxes.

ALTERNATIVE HEALTH CARE PLANS

The alternative health care plans, such as Health Maintenance Organizations (HMOs) and Preferred Provider Organizations (PPOs), are heavily recruiting family physicians because of their broad base of expertise in providing health care to all ages and both sexes. It is imperative that family physicians understand these health care systems very thoroughly in order to avoid economic pitfalls.

Health Maintenance Organizations

HMOs experienced rapid growth as a result of the federal law enacted in 1973 to provide federal grants to private HMOs. This law was a result of pressure from private industry to cut health care costs. As of 1985,

TABLE 15–5. PRIMARY CARE SPECIALTIES MEDIAN INCOMES: GROSS AND NET (1989)

SPECIALTY	PRACTICE GROSS*	PRACTICE NET†	PRACTICE EXPENSES
Internists	$216,990	$110,500	$ 94,260
Pediatricians	$209,130	$101,800	$ 94,720
FPs	$211,540	$ 97,340	$106,750
All MDs	$248,070	$132,550	$ 98,740

*Gross represents physicians' individual shares of 1989 gross receipts from practice before professional expenses and income taxes.
†For unincorporated physicians, net is 1989 individual income from practice minus tax-deductible professional expenses, before income taxes; for incorporated physicians, it is total compensation from practice (salary, bonuses, and retirement set-asides) before income taxes.
All figures are medians for 1989.
Source: Medical Economics Continuing Survey of M.D.s in private practice. Medical Economics, Sept. 3, 1990, with permission.

over 21 million Americans were enrolled in prepaid plans such as HMOs. This number is expected to increase to approximately 50% of the population by the year 2000 (Aluise).

HMOs have several unique characteristics that differ from traditional health insurance. A fixed number of patients enroll in a plan with a physician or group practice. A contract is entered into to provide comprehensive health care services to patients enrolled in the plan. The physician receives a fixed amount of money to provide specifically defined care and services. This fixed payment per enrollee is received regardless of use by the enrollee. Some patients use more than the allocation; some use less. Few patients use none of this allocation.

The physician is at risk financially and can experience an economic loss if costs for excessive visits, health services, or serious illnesses exceed the fixed allocations per patient or enrollee. The process of providing care to an HMO community must be monitored very closely, and the family physician must be very careful to assess the amount of administrative time that the HMO places upon his or her present practice and office staff. In addition to financial and administrative burdens, the family physician must be aware of the possibility of being placed in an adversarial relationship with a patient when he or she denies a patient's requests for laboratory and x-ray procedures or consultation services that may be unnecessary but that the patient perceives as otherwise. As a so-called gatekeeper in this system, the family physician may often find that he or she is in another adversarial role with consultants regarding the number of visits or health care services the consultant perceives as necessary (Aluise).

Preferred Provider Organizations

The PPOs combine the philosophy of fee for service with an HMO type of health care plan. PPOs operate within a system that comprises a panel of health care providers and includes physicians, hospitals, diagnostic centers, and other entities to form a contractual team concept. A fee schedule for each service is negotiated and agreed upon before the service is provided. Patients are given a choice of services within that health care system. The fee schedule is usually 10% to 20% less than the area's prevailing charges. In PPOs cost-effective health care is encouraged through incentives for patients to use more outpatient services such as surgery, home health care, and rehabilitation services. They may also require preadmission certification and second opinions. PPOs closely monitor costs and productivity patterns of the physicians and other providers of health care services. Some malpractice policies may not cover a physician while participating in a PPO contract (Aluise).

As of July 1986, 650 plans enrolling 24 million people were in business. Membership growth has been over 25% annually. Many concerns have been expressed regarding the possible conflict of prepaid arrangements and the potential for lowering the quality of care and placing the patient at risk by limiting services. Consequently, physicians must continue to maintain high ethical standards and be patients' advocates. Third-party payers can be held liable if they are considered to have unreasonable cost-containment provisions that may adversely influence medical decisions (Cook and Rodnick).

FUTURE DIRECTIONS

The present medical economy has evolved at a rapid pace, primarily since 1940. The influence upon the medical economic environment has come from numerous sources: the government, the public, special-interest groups, professional societies, and the explosion of scientific knowledge and technology. The federal government has played a significant role in the advancement of health care access and quality of care in this country; however, it must also accept and share the responsibility for the increased costs that have been created by social medical programs. Although political leaders are focusing upon the cost-effective side of health care costs in the face of a large national budget deficit, they will find it difficult to place any of the burden on private citizens. Health care is now viewed as a basic right and not an economic commodity, as other goods and services are considered to be.

The federal government must address several issues. Physician supply and reimbursement policies affect medical students' selections of specialties and often influence physicians to choose geographic locations other than underserved rural or urban areas. Little has been done in most medical schools to provide adequate or realistic incentives for students to enter family practice or to practice in rural areas. The number of students who have chosen family practice as a specialty has fallen far below the level that had been expected. The national goal had been for 50% of all graduates to enter primary care specialties, with half of that number entering family practice (Rakel and Pisacano). The number of students entering family practice each year has ranged from 10% to 15% and has never reached that goal. Overall, rural and inner-city areas have had little gain in overall physician supply, although more than 40% of family practice graduates go to these areas.

The federal government, medical schools, and state legislatures must provide visible and positive encouragement as well as economic stimulus in order to increase student interest in family practice. Family physicians as well as all other physicians must practice good management and understand the political and economic facets of health care delivery.

In 1978, Rogers recognized problems which remain more than a decade later:

Academic medical center faculties do a poor job of preparing physicians for a generalist role.
Family physicians and general internists in rural areas receive less remuneration than specialists who practice fewer hours in major hospitals. This needs to be corrected.
Physicians do not have a sufficient understanding of the financial aspects of health care.
A geographic maldistribution of physicians creates problems of access to health care for many patients.

Health care is not being adequately delivered on an ambulatory basis.

Efforts to correct the situation have been slow because of the misdirection of medical education, economic stimuli, and political attitudes within our medical schools and the medical profession. Family physicians will determine their destiny by their participation in and response to these challenges, but appropriate stimuli from medical schools and the political and professional environment will be mandatory to reach any type of medical economic balance in our society. The prominent leaders in medical education must sincerely and visibly support and encourage medical students to enter family practice as a specialty and our political leadership must correct inequities in reimbursement and discover innovative incentives that encourage more students to choose underserved geographical areas where there is inadequate access to health care.

REFERENCES

Aluise JJ. Essentials of Family Medicine. Baltimore, Williams and Wilkins, 1988.

American Academy of Family Physicians (AAFP) Directors Newsletter. Kansas City, Mo., 10:14, 1988.

American Academy of Family Physicians (AAFP) Residency Assistance Program Newsletter. Kansas City, Mo., 2:2–3, 1988.

American Board of Medical Specialties Annual Report and Reference Handbook. Evanston, Ill., American Board of Medical Specialties, 1990.

Arnett R, Freeland M, McKusick D, et al. National health expenditures: 1986–2000. Health Care Financing Review, Health Care Financ Admin 1987; 8:1.

Barnett PG, Midtling JE. Public policy and the supply of primary care physicians. JAMA 1989; 262:2864–2868.

Campion FD. The AMA and U.S. Health Policy Since 1940. Chicago, Chicago Press, 1984.

Cook JV, Rodnick JE. Evaluating HMO/IPA contracts for family physicians: One group's exposures. J Fam Pract 1988; 26:325.

Coordinating Council on Medical Education, 1975

Council on Long Range Planning and Development, American Medical Association: The future of family practice. JAMA 1988; 260:1271.

Council on Medical Education: Future Directions for Medical Education. Chicago, American Medical Association, 1982.

Crowley AE, Etzel SI, Shaw HA. Graduate medical education in the United States. JAMA 1987; 258:1031–1040.

HHS News. U.S. Department of Health and Human Services 1990; 12:20.

Jonas HS, Etzel SI. Undergraduate medical education. JAMA 1988; 260:1067.

Jonas HS, Etzel SI, Barznasky B. Graduate medical education in the United States. JAMA 1990; 264:801–809.

Mead D, Seidman B. National Physician Trends from 1970–1983. Chicago, AMA, Department of Data Release Services, 1986.

Rakel RE. Textbook of Family Practice. 3rd ed. Philadelphia, W. B. Saunders, 1984, p. 17.

Rakel RE. Textbook of Family Practice, 4th ed. Philadelphia, W.B. Saunders, 1984, p. 1751.

Reuter JA. Health Care Expenditures and Prices. Major Issues System Brief. The Library of Congress, Washington, D.C., Congressional Research Service, 1988; pp. 1–12.

Rogers DE. American Medicine Challenge for the 1980s. Cambridge, Mass., Ballinger Publishing Co., 1978; pp. 77–86.

Rowley BD, Baldwin DC, McGuire MD, et al. Graduate medical education in the United States. JAMA 1990; 264:822–832.

The World Almanac and Book of Facts 1988. New York, Newspaper Enterprise Association, 1988.

QUESTIONS

Matching Questions

Match each of the following amounts and percentages with the items in 1 through 10.

   a. Over $600 billion
   b. 11.6%
   c. $264.4 billion
   d. $27.1 billion
   e. $41.7 billion
   f. 3%
   g. 30.5%
   h. fewer than 25%
   i. 11.9%
   j. 39%
   k. 19%
   l. $41.6 billion

1. Annual consumer spending on tobacco products
2. Annual consumer spending on recreation
3. Cost of National Health Care, 1989
4. Cost of National Health Care, 1960
5. Percent of physicians in specialty or subspecialty training in 1940
6. Percent of health care dollar spent for physician service
7. Percent of all office visits seen by family physicians
8. Percent of physicians in the United States who are in family or general practice
9. Percent of national health care dollar paid to hospitals
10. Annual consumer Health Care Bill percent of Gross National Product

Match each of the following phrases in a–f with the statement or phrase in items 11–17.

   a. The Willard Report
   b. Medicare and Medicaid
   c. Created a decrease in hospital length of stay
   d. Total market value of final goods and services produced by a national economy
   e. Measurement of the average charge in the price for goods and services bought for everyday living
   f. Pays physician a fixed amount of money for each enrollee in the plan
   g. Operates within a system of health care which

contracts for health care services from many health care providers

h. Economic measurement of military health care spending

11. HMO
12. Government health insurance for the elderly and indigent passed in 1965
13. Recommended that family practice become a specialty
14. PPO
15. Diagnosis Related Groups (DRGs)
16. Gross National Product (GNP)
17. Consumer Price Index (CPI)

True or False Questions

18. Each statement listed in a–f should be identified as a true or false statement.
    a. The U.S. population over 65 years of age is decreasing as a percentage of the national population.
    b. The two highest health care costs are for hospital and physician services.
    c. Diagnosis Related Groups (DRGs) were designed to increase hospital length of stay.
    d. The government share of national personal health care expenses is increasing.
    e. Business has experienced a decrease in the amount of the health care bill that they pay.
    f. Private individuals are paying more out-of-pocket expenses as a percentage than they did in 1960.

19. Some malpractice policies may not cover physicians who participate in
    a. DRGs.
    b. Medicare or Medicaid.
    c. PPO.
    d. Workmans Compensation.

20. Identify as true or false each statement in a–d that has had an impact upon health care cost.
    a. DRGs
    b. Malpractice cost
    c. Overspecialization
    d. Medicare and Medicaid

Answers appear on page 447.

16

RESEARCH IN FAMILY MEDICINE

RICHARD L. HOLLOWAY and JOHN C. ROGERS

FAMILY MEDICINE: A RESEARCH DISCIPLINE

You may have read the title of this chapter as "Research in Family Medicine?" because you may not have known before that family medicine has a research agenda, or you may have wondered why family physicians would even want to do research. After all, most students, including those entering family practice, have little or no experience with or interest in research. Most students want to become practicing physicians and appreciate the importance of research in clinical medicine, but do not want to be directly involved in the process. This is often particularly so because the research that students learn most about during the preclinical years of medical school is bench-type laboratory research. Basic science lecturers who go on about the details or significance of their own research tend to further disinterest students, who, in general, endure the preclinical years of medical school to finally get to what they really want to do, namely clinical medicine. Yet more and more family physicians are doing research, and you may come to understand the specialty of family practice better by learning about the research conducted by practicing family physicians and medical school faculty.

Research creates new knowledge, and that is its fundamental purpose. Individuals have many personal reasons for getting involved in research, but medical specialties or academic disciplines conduct research in order to develop a knowledge base. This new and evolving knowledge helps define the discipline and advance the practice of the specialty. Some see family practice as an amalgamation of other clinical specialties such as internal medicine, pediatrics, obstetrics and gynecology, psychiatry, dermatology, orthopedics, otolaryngology, ophthalmology, and general surgery. From this perspective, research in family practice seems unnecessary, since new knowledge provided by researchers in the other specialties should be sufficient for the practicing family physician. Family practice researchers take a different point of view and assert that the knowledge produced by these other specialties contributes to family practice but is not sufficient to help family physicians meet the challenges they confront in primary care. The body of knowledge that provides the scientific basis for the specialty of family practice includes, but also goes beyond, the knowledge produced by researchers in other medical specialties. In academic terms, this scientific foundation is referred to as the discipline of family medicine.

Research in family medicine does, of course, deal with many diseases or health conditions studied by other fields, but family medicine investigators may ask different types of research questions, study different types of populations, and use different types of research methods. For example, a great deal of the biomedical research funded by the National Institutes of Health is directed at explicating the mechanisms of disease such as the pathophysiology or the ultimate cause at the molecular biology level. This research is intended to provide new treatments and perhaps "cures." This basic science research and the clinical research conducted by other fields are asking what could be done or what should be done to treat biological diseases. Some family medicine investigators ask these questions, but others ask how biomedical treatments affect patients' functioning, how organization and financing of the health system affects access to and quality of care, how psychosocial factors are related to illness and functioning, how human values and the meaning of illness are involved in clinical care, how patients and physicians make medical decisions, and how prevention can become a routine part of medical care. These questions extend beyond what is wrong biomedically and how to fix it technologically to all of the factors that interact when one human being with health concerns goes to another for care.

Besides asking different questions, family medicine investigators may study different populations than investigators in other fields. For example, many of the patients studied in academic health centers have been selected through a filtering process of referral and consultation and may have more severe or unusual forms of a particular disease than do all individuals with the same condition in the general population. Family medicine researchers typically focus on patients seen in primary care settings or even people in the community who do not come through doctors' doors. In addition, family medicine researchers may study not only patients but also doctors and patients as they interact together, or patients in their families. These different questions and different populations obviously may require research methods other than those using biomedical technology, such as questionnaires and videotapes.

There are five U.S. family medicine journals that publish peer-reviewed research papers which are then included in *Index Medicus*. These journals record the original work of the field: *Journal of Family Practice, Family Medicine, Family Practice Research Journal, Archives of Family Medcine* and *Journal of the American Board of Family Practice*. Other countries (Japan, Israel, Australia, Great Britain, the Netherlands) have national family/general practice journals, and in 1984 the World Or-

ganization of National Colleges, Academies, and Academic Associations of General Practitioners/Family Physicians (WONCA) started its official journal *Family Practice—An International Journal*. Fifteen years of papers published in the *Journal of Family Practice* reveal the subjects of interest to these authors and the types of scholarship they produce. Figures 16–1 and 16–2 present general categories of the content and types of papers. For a more specific view of what family medicine investigators are now doing, simply visit the faculty, department, or medical library near you.

Now you know that family medicine has its own scientific literature which may be very different from that of other disciplines. The next goal is for you to learn how to be an intelligent consumer of family medicine research and clinical research in general. Toward that end, the rest of this chapter will introduce you to some general concepts about the research process. By under-

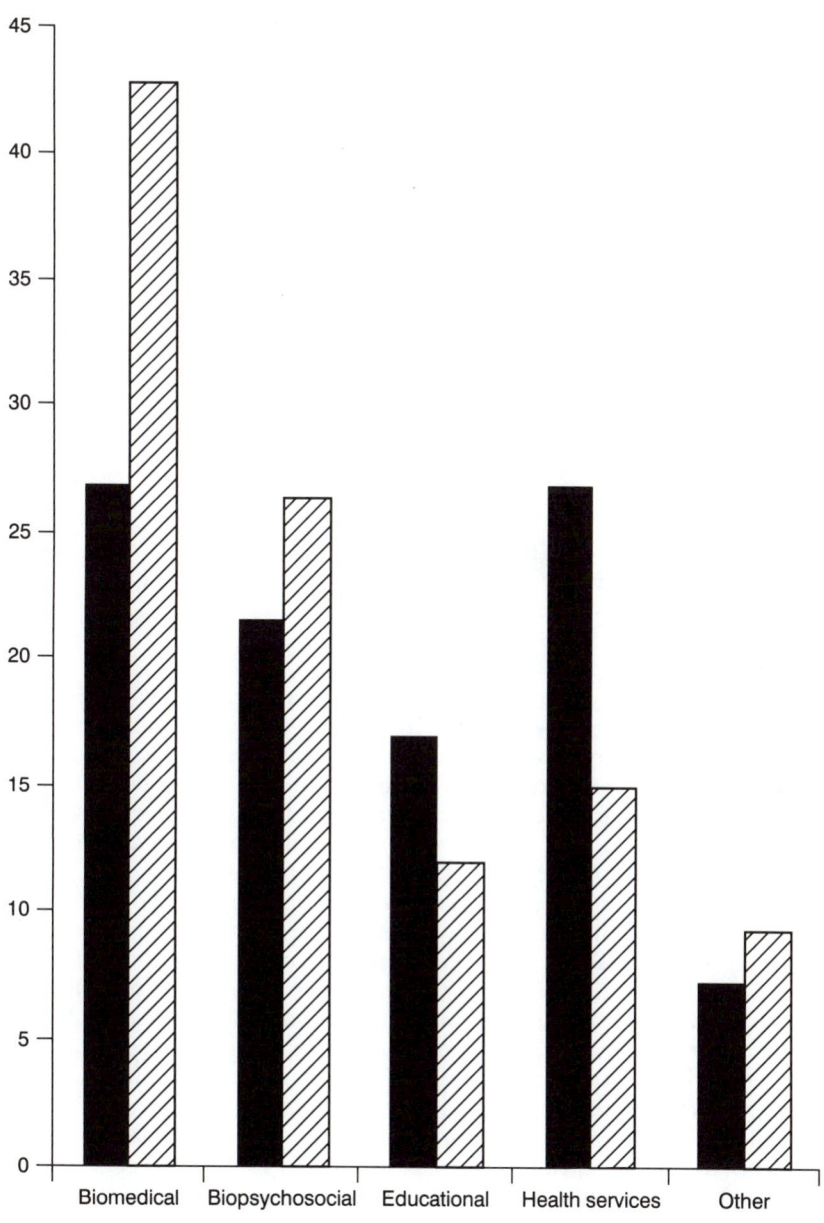

Figure 16–1. Overall percentage of all papers published in the Journal of Family Practice by major content area. The period 1974–1983 is represented by the black bars, and the period 1984–1986 is represented by the bars with diagonals. (From Geyman JP and Berg AO. The Journal of Family Practice 1974–1988: Window to an evolving academic discipline. J Fam Prac 1989; 28(3) 301–304, with permission.)

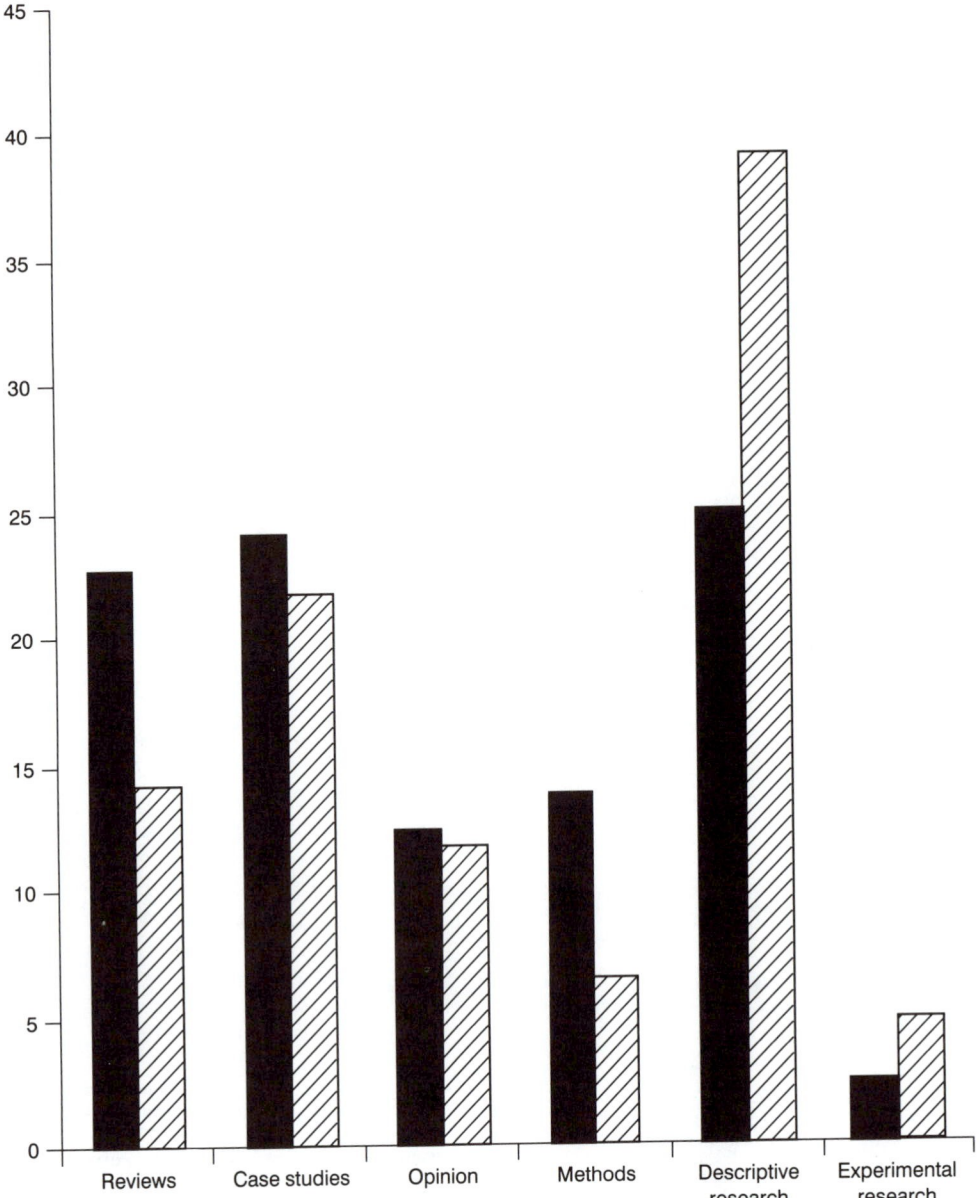

Figure 16–2. Overall percentage of all papers published in the Journal of Family Practice by type. The period 1974–1983 is represented by the black bars, and the period 1984–1988 is represented by the bars with diagonals. (From Geyman JP and Berg AO. The Journal of Family Practice 1974–1988: Window to an evolving academic discipline. J Fam Prac 1989; 28(3) 301–304, with permission.)

standing various research activities and issues, you should better understand any academic discipline and the growing knowledge base that provides its scientific foundation.

GETTING TO KNOW THE FIELD: THE LITERATURE SEARCH

Drawing from an established body of knowledge can enrich the researcher's understanding of the study area. The literature search can determine if a particular study has already been done, but its usefulness does not end there. Chances are the study has been done before but perhaps not in just the same way or with a different emphasis or context. A review of the literature can give important support to the choice of topic as well as ensure the study adds to what has already been done before.

SECONDARY SOURCES. Investigators begin reviewing the literature by conducting a general reading program in the area of interest. Typically, this involves a review of secondary sources, usually textbooks or review articles, in which authors present the works of others rather than their own research. The goal is to get an overview that provides clues to definitions, historical data, classic studies, and perhaps a bibliography or list of references. In addition, a secondary review can give information about key researchers and important centers or institutions where the seminal work has been conducted. However, a secondary review is only a beginning and has significant limitations. In secondary sources, authors present the work of others and incorporate their own biases into the literature chosen for review. Furthermore, the information rarely is as current as that found in primary sources. Secondary sources can generate and help determine the scope and usefulness of various works. References in secondary sources should be used to develop a starting point from which to begin a more specific literature search.

PRIMARY SOURCES. Primary literature sources are usually journal articles, although they can be book chapters, technical reports, dissertations, or government documents. Primary sources contain the author's report on his or her original work. Once an area of interest has been identified, researchers concentrate more and more on a narrow band of primary sources, which usually are not part of a general reading program because they tend to be quite specific. Concentrating on a particular area helps to identify primary sources that focus on a particular aspect of the research.

The human element is crucial when reviewing the literature. One of the joys of the research process is the development of colleagues. People who research a given area usually are accessible and delighted to talk with others interested in that particular area. Researchers need not be intimidated by the thought of calling a world-renowned expert to discuss a particular research area. People who have spent a long time researching an area have valuable insights and advice on how to proceed.

RESEARCH QUESTIONS

In the process of identifying and declaring an area of interest, a number of potential research questions come to mind. Many will be dismissed as the literature leads to greater familiarity with the field. New questions are stimulated and others are refined as the reading reveals what questions have been asked and how they have been addressed. Through the iterative process of reading and questioning, the researcher's questions become more specific and the procedures necessary for addressing the questions become more apparent.

A persistent issue in family medicine research has been the link between the clinical and research worlds. A barrier to understanding the research process has arisen from the assumption that research questions and findings must have immediate clinical applicability to be useful in family medicine. Because the purpose of research is to build a knowledge base, that assumption simply is not true. Clinical applicability usually follows the research process after a period of time. Sometimes research questions and their associated findings never result in clinical applicability. Clinical practice has a natural independence from the research process, a point that needs underscoring. To be sure, research questions are expected to be useful at some level in clinical reasoning and practice. But to limit research only to questions with immediate applicability to clinical practice is to restrict the researcher's creativity unduly and may undermine the ultimate utility of the research and development process.

A researcher begins by asking a question driven by the "core of doubt" and suggested by the existing research, then sets out purposefully and systematically to answer that research question. The researcher does not try to prove a point, support a set of beliefs, or find reasons for a specific predetermined course of action. Instead, the researcher tests a range of plausible hypotheses about factors that may or may not be related to a particular outcome. Often, research is best done in teams because team members can share differing perspectives on hypothesized connections.

RESEARCH THINKING

Physicians are socialized throughout medical school, residency training, and practice to the types of thinking expected within clinical medicine. Unstated presumptions and rules govern how to gather and evaluate evidence, how to develop diagnostic formulations from incomplete and conflicting information, how to test clinical hypotheses, and how to choose among therapeutic options. This type of thinking is not formalized, usually occurs unconsciously, and continues after the clinical encounters are over, such as during lunch, dinner, recreation, and social events. Researchers' thinking differs in some respects, but experienced investigators' thinking also may become subconscious, occurring at all times (even in dreams) and evolving through an extended socialization process.

Although various authors disagree about the nature of research reasoning, a point of consensus is that the purpose of research is to build knowledge. The researcher uses a combination of methods aimed at building a fundamental understanding of a phenomenon. Researchers use data collection and deduction to develop answers to their questions. Deduction comes in the formulation of a question and the development of logical reasoning around the topic. The process requires nothing but the researcher's brain and can occur at any time of the day or night, irrespective of allotted research time.

Research questions arise, in part, from some theoretical understanding of a phenomenon. Whether this theoretical understanding has been formalized into a structured body of work or merely exists as a common understanding among clinicians, theories produce questions through the logic of deductive reasoning. Questions also may evolve through inductive reasoning such as from a well-established line of empirical research that has suggested future study. Every physician has seen the last paragraph of a research article suggesting that because of the observed findings, future investigators should examine questions X, Y, and Z. Research questions arising from theoretical understanding and induction are part of the process Thomas Kuhn characterized as "normal science."

HYPOTHETICAL REASONING

To aid in the formulation of sound research questions, researchers have developed a reasoning process that begins with the assumption that an experimental group does not differ from a control group (the way the things are done typically under normal circumstances).

This reasoning, called the "null hypothesis," presupposes that the results will be the same for the experimental and the control group. Although this may seem peculiar, it is understandable that the researcher would begin with a conservative assumption supporting the way "things are" rather than with a subversive assumption favoring the experimental intervention.

The task of the researcher then is to see whether or not the experimental intervention produces a result that differs from the normal condition. This assumption, which underlies the entire research process, is critical to understanding research methodology. Understanding statistical significance, biases in research design, selection biases, sampling, and other forms of research reasoning is rooted in the fundamental principle of assuming no difference between the experimental and normal conditions.

The researcher begins by asking what is the probability that results favoring the experimental intervention would have occurred by chance? The answer comes in the form of a probability statement, such as "The probability that the positive results occurred by chance is less than 5% ($P < 0.05$)."

Answers to research questions rely on a delicate linkage between the conceptual understanding of a question and the testing of that question under normal conditions. If positive results of an experimental intervention are sufficiently improbable by chance alone, the researcher concludes the research hypothesis is tenable. Notice that we use the term "tenable" rather than true. If we err on the side of caution, it is because the research process has a level of credibility that may carry an overrated force of truth.

THE RESEARCH TEAM

With few exceptions, clinicians work on a one-to-one basis with patients. Other members of the health care team are called in to increase the efficiency of the physician and to perform services the physician does not provide. The family physician feels a sense of responsibility to the patient and assumes the role of case manager and primary provider. In a research project, the principal investigator assumes a similar role. The principal investigator drives the project. Also, the principal investigator energizes the process through the "core of doubt," dictates the specific techniques necessary for his or her questions, and determines what co-workers (co-investigators) or consultants are needed due to his or her limitations. Other members of the team (research assistants, programmers, and secretaries) carry out tasks that increase the efficiency of the investigators, whereas co-investigators and consultants lend expertise the principal investigator does not personally possess. Colleagues who are not directly involved in a project become invaluable critics and supporters as the principal investigator strives to be at the cutting edge of research in the area, refines questions and designs, revises grants and manuscripts, and advances his or her thinking. The more people who know about and have discussed a project, the stronger is the foundation of the project. But with few exceptions, research cannot be completed successfully by a committee but only by a principal investigator who has the motivation to complete a project. Guided by this leadership, the other players in the process conduct their roles and perform their tasks.

RESEARCH TECHNIQUES

The research process requires some general techniques and some highly specialized techniques. Through reading, a researcher becomes familiar with the design, measurement, and analytic procedures frequently employed in the field. Specialization is inevitable if a researcher wants to develop a program of research and contribute substantially to a body of knowledge. Resisting this aspect of research socialization is futile; accepting it as a natural part of the research role is extremely rewarding and beneficial.

A few general research techniques provide a necessary foundation for specialization. They include (1) developing hypotheses, (2) selecting subjects, and (3) assessing internal validity.

Developing Hypotheses

Once a question has been developed, a researcher probably has some expectation of the results. Since any expectation may bias the results, a researcher can impose many controls to reduce the amount of bias inherent in the research process. Research expectations are called "hypotheses," since they are speculations about the relationship among the variables within the question.

DEFINING VARIABLES. Simply stated, a "variable" is anything that varies. Variables are implicit in the research question itself and give it meaning. For example, "Is patient compliance enhanced by patient education?" represents a question that has been researched and discussed frequently in family medicine. Within that question, two variables emerge: patient compliance and patient education. One need not look beyond the research question to find the variables of interest. Certainly, other variables might emerge that have an impact on the outcome of the question, but the first step is to look at the question itself and to determine the central variables of interest to the researcher. Additional variables will come later, including confounding variables that interfere with the researcher's ability to draw conclusions about the relationships among the basic variables of a study.

With a question like the one involving patient compliance and patient education, a researcher might hypothesize that systematic patient education would improve compliance. This hypothetical relationship suggests that the use of patient education in a prescribed number of patient encounters will produce greater levels of compliance than would be seen with no patient education. This is just one interpretation of how the question might be investigated.

OPERATIONAL DEFINITIONS. For each variable of compliance and patient education, the researcher has a conceptual understanding. At this point the researcher is still working on the level of abstract thinking, and the understanding of compliance and patient education need not come from any source other than experience. The next step in defining variables produces a level of information that most researchers do not have readily available. To measure a variable such as compliance or patient education, the researcher needs to develop specific definitions. These definitions, called "operational definitions," provide an understanding of the operations the researcher will use to define each variable. Compliance might be defined as a specific formula or outcome measurement, such as blood tests, self-reports, urine samples, or pill counts.

Patient education might be defined in terms of a specific activity within parameters defined by the researcher. In this example, patient education is the independent variable because the researcher can manipulate the variable as a purposeful intervention. Independent variables are manipulated to have an effect on an outcome (or dependent variable), in this case compliance.

After operationally defining variables, the researcher develops working hypotheses, which suggest how variables might relate to one another. At this point, the hypotheses become more specific. For example, in a study of patient education and compliance, the researcher might hypothesize that compliance will be enhanced by a systematic application of patient education, as predicted by a specific set of findings in previous literature. After refining the research question with well-defined variables that can be manipulated (independent) or measured as an outcome (dependent), the researcher invokes the null hypothesis to help remove bias from the study.

Selecting a Representative Sample

Researchers frequently ask statistical consultants what sample size is needed to ensure the validity of results. The answer is twofold, but perhaps it is simpler than one might imagine. The basic principles of subject selection are sample size and sample representativeness, each of which warrants significant independent attention.

The first and perhaps most important job of the researcher is to determine the representativeness of the sample. Under ideal circumstances, subjects should be selected randomly from a defined population and randomly assigned to treatment or control conditions under controlled circumstances. Though conditions are rarely ideal, the sample always should be selected in a purposeful, systematic manner that should provide a truly representative group of individuals from a defined population. Before considering sample size, the researcher must ensure that each member of the sample is as representative as possible of a defined population. A population is a theoretically infinite set of individuals with some shared characteristics. These characteristics may be as few or as numerous as is reasonable for the purposes of research. For example, a study often focuses on a population of individuals who have a particular disease. The researcher begins by defining the characteristics of the disease, then seeks to sample individuals who have those characteristics.

Sample size becomes a consideration only after the population has been defined. Numerous guidelines and texts give excellent direction for selecting research samples. Each formula for calculating sample size considers at least some of the following elements:

1. The relative homogeneity or heterogeneity of the individuals within the population. The more individuals differ, the larger the sample size needed.
2. The number of planned comparisons the researcher will make. The more planned comparisons, the larger the sample size.
3. Meaningful differences. As a general rule, larger sample sizes allow detection of smaller differences. From a practical standpoint, however, a researcher must ask whether or not a difference is worth detecting. A blood pressure drop of a single point, for example, may not be clinically useful, even though it could be statistically "significant" in a very large study. The researcher must anticipate a useful or meaningful change in scores and choose the sample size accordingly.

Other aspects of choosing a sample size include practical considerations such as resources available and the kind of precision the researcher wishes to have with regard to results. A consulting statistician can calculate a precise sample size that is tailored to the research question.

Assessing Internal Validity

The purpose of research design is to control for unintended influences that might interfere with the understanding of the relationship between the independent and dependent variables. As a result, the design must cover a range of potential unintended influences. These unintended influences have a number of different names, but they commonly are called "threats to internal validity." A study's internal validity may be defined by its freedom from unintended influences. Therefore, the more a study can control threats, the more likely it will be able to support conclusions about the relationship between the independent and dependent variables.

A refined organization of threats to internal validity was introduced by Campbell and Stanley. Since the introduction of their terminology, threats to internal validity have been discussed at length, and authors differ on the specific interpretation of different kinds of threats to internal validity. For the purposes of this discussion, we have categorized threats to internal validity into four basic areas:

1. *Time and history.* Effects due to historical events or the maturation of subjects.
2. *Experimentation and observation.* Effects resulting from the performance of the experiment itself.

3. *Selection.* Biases due to assignment or attrition of subjects.

4. *Regression to the mean.* An effect due to the selection of subjects from extreme groups.

TIME AND HISTORY. A caption underneath a picture of a particularly disheveled W. C. Fields states, "Things happened." Things happen during the performance of a research project, too, and a good design controls for the impact of unintended historical events. Two major sources account for the majority of time and history effects. "History" refers to events that occur outside the study but that have an impact on the outcome of the study. For example, a dissertation student at the University of Minnesota was interested in studying the effects of Tylenol marketing on the drug-consuming public. He scheduled his study for 1982. His timing was particularly poor since that was the year that a number of cases of "Tylenol tampering" were reported in Chicago. Could these effects have been avoided? Perhaps, but only if one were to select a particularly insulated sample that was protected from any knowledge of the events surrounding the tampering incidents.

Maturation can exert an effect as subjects grow older during a study. Sometimes effects occur only because subjects age, not because they grow smarter, learn patient education materials better, or respond better to treatment. "Tincture of time" is a common clinical term for the self-resolution of an illness. Maturation also can be effectively controlled by the use of a control group. At the very least, a control group can reveal the effect maturation has on subjects, as compared with the effect of an intervention.

EXPERIMENTATION AND OBSERVATION. The numerous effects of experimentation and observation have inspired texts, articles, journals, books, pamphlets, and probably a few leaflets. Some of the most prominent effects follow.

Repeated measurement occurs when the investigator uses a number of measurements over a period of time to observe profiles within patients. This is particularly evident in studies of issues such as blood pressure, task performance, knowledge tests, and psychological questionnaires. Subjects may respond differently at the beginning of the study than later as they become used to the measurement. The researcher must determine then how much of the variation is due to true observed differences as opposed to how much of the variation involves acclimation to the measurement.

Experimental effects parade under a number of fairly colorful names, such as the Hawthorne effect, the halo effect, the John Henry effect, and others. Each of these effects refers to subjects' responses to the process of being studied. The Hawthorne effect, for instance, refers to a subject's response to the novelty of participating in an experiment. (This effect is so named because of its association with an electrical company's Hawthorne plant, where a study of worker productivity was conducted in the early twentieth century.) The halo effect reflects the tendency of raters, observers, or any measurement tool to generalize across a number of categories when the effect in only a single category is known. This type of effect can be observed in clinical ratings, educational studies, and a number of other ratings-based experiments.

The John Henry effect is named for its association with the legendary John Henry of the nineteenth century, who beat the steam-powered railroad spike-driving machine in a contest. John Henry was the control group in this experiment, and he beat out the experimental group (the steam-powered machine). This happens in real experiments, too. If the control group learns of its status, the members attempt to outperform the experimental group. This has been observed in a number of community trials involving health promotion and emphasizes the need to protect the control group from knowledge of the experimental materials.

Observer bias may occur in any kind of study that uses observers as a primary source of measurement. The best way to overcome this bias is to train observers carefully and make sure they are not tempted to rely on their own internal criteria for measurement but use the criteria set by the study.

A final effect of experimentation and observation, which demands much more discussion than is possible here, is that of recall biases (selective recall). Many studies, particularly those using retrospective methodologies such as case-control studies, require subjects to recall something about their past behaviors. Although this may seem like a simple task, everyone has a tendency to recall some things better than others. When asked to recall particulars of health or specific exposures, many people have difficulty because of bias by their current state of health. Many studies involve people who are seriously ill. They tend to recall vividly some parts of their behavior and suppress others. It is only human nature to do so. Case-control studies are particularly vulnerable to this type of bias. The best case-control studies are those that control recall bias as thoroughly as possible. They employ highly structured questionnaires, present questions in several different ways to check the validity of responses, and make use of trained raters and observers who consistently follow a rigorous course.

Having collected data, a rigorous investigator calculates the reliability of any questionnaires used and determines the reliability of the observers who conducted the interviews. The researcher can then be assured that data were collected in a consistent and correct fashion.

SELECTION. Selection effects arise any time subjects have not been randomly selected and then assigned randomly to experimental and control conditions. Any time nonrandom methods are used, individuals may be assigned to experimental conditions in a way that might bias the sample. This bias may become evident through unbalanced responses to questions, one study group containing people who have more of a certain characteristic, or in more healthy people being contained in one group than another. Randomization is the only way to control completely for such unintended influences, but as a secondary measure, investigators often measure as many important characteristics as possible as to account for potential differences. The problem with such a strategy is the impossibility of measuring all characteristics of interest. However, given a selective list of important characteristics, an investigator may support the case that bias has been reduced.

One of the primary sources of control in an experiment is the control group. An ideal control group would consist of members who are identical in every respect to the experimental group but who have not received the experimental treatment or intervention. A control group typically is selected at the same time as the experimental group by random selection from a defined population. Only through randomization can the experimenter be relatively sure that any extraneous characteristics have been equally distributed between groups.

Other forms of control include crossover designs, in which members of the control and experimental groups literally cross from one to the other after a period of time. This assures the experimenter that nothing inherent to the control or experimental groups might have caused some differences. Double-blind studies control for the effect of the expectations of the experimenter on the study. In double-blind studies, a physician who does not know the identity of experimental and control groups administers treatments to reduce the potential for bias.

Attrition is particularly problematic in long-term investigations, such as cohort studies. Attrition is also a factor in questionnaire-based studies that depend upon high response rates for accurate results. The only universal rule of thumb is to make sure that as many people as possible from the beginning of the study are represented in the sample at the end of the study. Many investigators who conduct long-term studies have employed relatively elaborate strategies to keep people in their studies to ensure the validity of their results. For example, investigators conducting a hypertension reduction program in Minnesota sought advice from clinical psychologists to determine why individuals were leaving the study and to devise strategies to keep them in. Any time a study subject is lost to follow-up, a potentially important piece of information is lost.

REGRESSION TO THE MEAN. The final threat to internal validity is regression to the mean, a peculiar phenomenon that occurs when subjects have been selected on the basis of extreme scores of one form or another. When individuals have been selected because of an extreme characteristic (high blood pressure, for example), the categorization of "extremeness" is a relatively arbitrary one. If everyone with a diastolic pressure of greater than 100, for example, was categorized as high, one might argue that 100 is an inappropriate figure just because it is arbitrary. Ninety-nine might be better, or 101; the point is that the choice is arbitrary and thus is subject to error. The cutoff point depends on precision measurement to classify individuals as above or below 100. Individuals who are erroneously classified for whatever reason are not "true members" of the extreme group. Statistically, the more one diverges from the average score, the more likely it is that an error will occur from the measurement to the "true" score.

Extreme scores have a natural tendency to rebound slightly on repeated measurement. This is not due to any inaccuracy on the part of the investigator or anything else. It is merely a statistical phenomenon reflecting the fact that the more extreme a score, the less likely it is that the true score is that extreme. In studies that depend on extreme scores, erroneously classified individuals sometimes may have true scores that are somewhat lower or higher. This may interfere with interpretation of a study treatment intended to raise or lower scores, since the investigator may not know whether a change in those scores reflects treatment efficacy or a statistical phenomenon. A control group provides a good remedy for this kind of problem, as does careful attention to the statistical significance assigned to the study.

As clearly indicated, research designs have plenty of potential for error. Words like "bias" and "control" have loaded meanings in their everyday usage and can scare even the most hardy clinician away from research. Honest research depends upon the researcher's disclosing as much information as possible so other people might replicate the study and determine whether or not the results fit their own setting and circumstances. Eliminating bias and controlling for unintended influences are challenges in every study.

DESCRIPTION OF STUDY TYPES USED IN FAMILY MEDICINE

A recent analysis of a sample of the family medicine literature revealed that four study types were used most often among researchers in this field. We will, therefore, concentrate on these four types and discuss them from the point of view of the critical features that students encounter as they confront each design or study type. Table 16–1 summarizes the four designs and their critical features. The four designs are the clinical trial (experimental), the cohort or prospective (longitudinal) study, the case-control study, and the cross-sectional study. We will discuss each of these types and their design features in terms of the activities associated with each critical phase of the research: the participation of the researcher, the selection of subjects, the composition of study groups, the timing of various observations, and the temporal relationship among variables.

Clinical Trial (An Experimental Study)

The researcher conducting a clinical trial is an active manipulator of conditions who tests for hypothesized outcomes. The defining features of such a trial are that it is a well-controlled, unbiased intervention on a randomly selected and assigned group of subjects. The purpose of a clinical trial is to establish a causal relationship between this intervention and the hypothesized outcome. An experiment conducted in this way is the only type of research that can claim to establish a cause-and-effect relationship since it controls for the greatest number of threats to internal validity (as discussed above). In other words, a clinical trial is capable of isolating the ef-

TABLE 16–1. FEATURES OF ANALYTIC STUDY TYPES COMMONLY USED IN FAMILY MEDICINE

DESIGN FEATURES	CLINICAL TRIAL (EXPERIMENTAL STUDY)	COHORT STUDY	CASE-CONTROL STUDY	CROSS-SECTIONAL STUDY
Participation of researcher	Conducts intervention	Observes naturally occurring events over time	Retrospectively determines presence or absence of risk factors	Records coexistence of variable
Bases of selection of subjects	Random selection	Population without outcome and with and without risk factor	Population with and without disease (outcome)	Convenience sample
How study groups composed	Random assignment to intervention and control groups	Two groups defined by presence or absence of risk factor	Two groups defined by presence or absence of outcome	Single group for which association among variables sought
Timing of observation	Subjects assessed before and after intervention or control procedure	Subjects assessed repeatedly during course of study	Subjects assessed for outcome at beginning of study then questioned for risk factors	Data obtained on all variables concurrently
Temporal relationship among variables	Intervention precedes outcome	Risk factor precedes outcome	Presence of risk factors presumed to exist before outcome	No temporal relationship assumed—variables exist at same point in time

fect of an intervention on a group of subjects by eliminating most other sources of competing explanations for the results.

While few clinical trials have been conducted in family medicine research, it is becoming an increasingly popular choice among those researchers who wish to describe the impact of an intervention on various types of patients. Many such interventions are drugs; however, the intervention may consist of a patient education strategy, a procedure, or other nondrug intervention. An example of a clinical trial is the AMA Physicians' Health Study investigation of the impact of aspirin on the reduction of cardiovascular disease. Physician subjects were assigned randomly to either a treatment (aspirin) group or a placebo control group and asked to participate in the trial for a period of years. Various measures were taken before and after the trial, including previous cardiac history and cardiovascular illness (stroke and myocardial infarction). The outcomes of greatest interest to the researchers were cardiovascular events. Data showed that there was a significant reduction in cardiovascular events in the aspirin group.

So the experimental study derives its strength from several important sources of control: before/after measurement, the random assignment of subjects to experimental and control groups,[1] and the elimination of competing sources of influence over the results by carefully controlling the intervention (sometimes using a placebo, an intervention which is identical to all aspects of the true intervention with the exception of the main variable of interest). The experimental study, finally, offers the assurance that the intervention or independent variable has preceded the outcome in time. Thus, it is the most powerful design available.

Cohort Study (Prospective)

The *cohort study* is a kind of prospective study, named because it follows a group (cohort) of individuals over time. Approximately 8% of studies conducted in family medicine use this methodology. Its relative rarity may be due to the fact that it is a difficult type of study to conduct and takes a great deal of time and effort (not to mention money!) to reach fruition. But the benefits of such a study are enormous.

The Framingham Heart Studies are responsible for much of what we know about the risk factors in cardiovascular disease. These studies have followed a sample of the population of Framingham, Massachusetts, since about 1950 to study the effect of risk factors for cardiovascular disease. These cohort studies identified approximately 5000 patients at risk who were "free of coronary heart disease" and measured important hypothesized risk factors which could be correlated to the outcomes associated with coronary artery disease. The study was initially planned to last about 20 years but has continued, unabated, to the point of this writing. In

addition, several "spin-off" studies have been conducted.

These studies have had enormous impact because they are conducted "in the real world," involve relatively large numbers of subjects, and assure that the risk factors precede the outcome in time (as you will soon see, cross-sectional and case-control studies cannot make this claim). So, despite the incredible amount of time, energy, and money they consume, cohort studies can be immeasurably useful. As you may already have guessed, you will not see them very often—they take a while to come to fruition for publishable results. But when they do, their impact is impressive.

Case-Control Studies (Retrospective)

A clever researcher has referred to the case-control study as a "trohoc" study (cohort spelled backwards) because a case-control study seeks to replicate the approach of a cohort study, but by *beginning at the end*. This relatively peculiar strategy has enormous benefits for the researcher, not the least of which is a reduction of the lengthy wait for the development of disease the cohort researcher must endure. Those using case-control methods begin with patients with a diagnosed disease and also find an appropriate number of nondiseased individuals who are like the diseased in all other characteristics. The researcher then conducts a kind of detective search for antecedent conditions that may have caused the disease. This search usually takes the form of questions asked of the patient or his/her family.

For example, researchers who were investigating the association between Reye's syndrome and aspirin usage first identified children who had the disease and others who did not have it, and then questioned their parents about a multitude of potential causative hypotheses, including factors unrelated to the treatment of the antecedent viral illness (asbestos, drinking water, etc.). From 72 potential exposure hypotheses, only aspirin was shown to be dramatically related to the development of the syndrome. Children who were treated with aspirin were nearly twice as likely to develop Reye's syndrome than those who were not. These results were combined from two studies done in Michigan; it was noted by the authors that while Reye's can develop without aspirin consumption, it is much more likely when aspirin is given.

The way in which the above results were discussed reveals some of the limitations of the case-control approach. We cannot talk about causation, only of association between the purported cause and the disease or the odds of disease in those with the purported cause when compared to those without the purported cause. This so-called relative risk or odds ratio is a mathematical expression of the increased likelihood of contracting the disease when one has the identified risk factor. For example, the relative risk of contracting Reye's syndrome based on the study reported here is about 1.54 (study results combined), meaning that a child who takes aspirin is a little more than 1½ times as likely to contract Reye's than one who does not. This information can be

---

[1] Ideally these subjects have also been randomly selected from a population, although this is frequently more difficult to accomplish.

clinically, as well as academically, useful because it provides some guidance for decisions.

Cross-Sectional Studies

By far, the most prevalent type of study in family medicine is the cross-sectional approach, sometimes referred to as a correlational approach. Perhaps the main reason for the choice of this type of study is its convenience. Most cross-sectional studies are conducted on existing databases. A researcher who conducts this type of study identifies variables of interest and determines the strength of their correlation in a given population. By correlation, we mean the mathematical degree of association between two variables, usually expressed as a correlation coefficient (to be discussed below). Sometimes these studies are conducted as a collection of new data; usually they are conducted as an analysis of existing data or a "convenience sample" (such as hospital records, medical charts, census, or disease report data). When they are conducted from newly collected data, it is often the result of some form of questionnaire.

The results of a cross-sectional study usually appear as a correlation coefficient that varies between -1 and $+1$. A perfect one-to-one association between variables would be a $+1$. A perfect negative relationship (as one variable increases, the other decreases) would be a -1.

Zero or near-zero correlations indicate that there is no systematic association between variables. A strong association between variables means that they share some important characteristics, but it in no way implies causation. The reason for this is primarily that data are collected at the same point in time, and the researcher cannot be assured that either variable preceded the other. Also, there are simply too many other variables that cannot be controlled for and may influence the final result.

Most cross-sectional studies will make suggestions for future research. This is wise, because cross-sectional studies are admittedly limited in their power to predict relationships between variables. When many data have been collected for a variety of purposes, there is always a possibility that relationships may be found in error. Thus, more well-controlled follow-up studies are usually advised to clarify the relationships between these variables.

The family medicine literature is not yet 20 years old, but it is dynamic with recent changes in both the subjects and types of studies. As family medicine builds its scientific foundations, it strives to define itself as an academic discipline and to provide new knowledge for practitioners of the clinical specialty. Whether future researchers or not, students need to know about the various processes of research to intelligently read and interpret original works. This chapter has provided an introduction to the most basic research processes.

REFERENCES

Berg AO, Gordon MJ, Cherkin DC. Practice Based Research in Family Medicine. Kansas City, Mo., American Academy of Family Physicians, 1986.

Campbell DT, Stanley JC. Experimental and Quasi-experimental Designs for Research. Chicago, Rand McNally, 1963.

Feinstein AR. Clinical Biostatistics. St. Louis, C. V. Mosby, 1977.

Friedman GL. Primer of Epidemiology. New York, McGraw-Hill, 1980.

Fromm BS, Snyder VL. Research design and statistical procedures used in the Journal of Family Practice. J Fam Pract 1986; 23:6.

Gehlbach SH. Interpreting The Medical Literature: A Clinician's Guide. Lexington, Mass., D. C. Heath, 1982.

Geyman JP (Ed.): Special Issue on Research in Family Practice. J Fam Pract 1978; 7:1.

Kerlinger FN. Foundations of Behavioral Research. New York, Holt, Rinehart & Winston, 1973.

Krathwohl DR. How to Prepare a Research Proposal. Syracuse, N.Y., Syracuse University Bookstore, 1966.

Kuhn T. The Structure of Scientific Revolutions. Chicago, University of Chicago Press, 1964.

Leaverton PE. A Review of Biostatistics: A Program for Self-Instruction. Boston, Little, Brown, 1986.

Lilienfeld AM, Lilienfeld DE. Foundations of Epidemiology. 2nd ed. New York, Oxford University Press, 1980.

Marks RG. Designing a Research Project and Analyzing Research Data: The Basics of Biomedical Research Methodology. Belmont, Ca., Wadsworth, 1982.

Marsland DW, Wood M, Mayo F. Content of Family Practice. In Geyman, JP (Ed.): A Statewide Study in Virginia with Its Clinical, Educational, and Research Implications. New York, Appleton-Century-Crofts, 1976.

Physicians' Health Study Research Group. Preliminary Report: Findings from the aspirin component of the ongoing Physicians' Health Study. N Engl J Med 1988; 318:2.

Riegelman RK. Studying a Study and Testing a Test: How to Read the Medical Literature. Boston, Little, Brown, 1981.

Sackett DL, Haynes RB, Tugwell P. Clinical Epidemiology: A Basic Science for Clinical Medicine. Boston, Little, Brown, 1985.

QUESTIONS

1. Which of the following designs is capable of supporting inferences about causation?
   a. Cross-sectional
   b. Case-control
   c. Experimental
   d. Cohort

2. Which of the following is a purpose of a research design?
   a. To identify a research area
   b. To control for unintended influences
   c. To measure outcomes
   d. To measure independent variables

3. What is a "threat" to internal validity?
   a. An unintended influence interfering with inferences
   b. A challenge to the integrity of the researcher
   c. A mistake in the reporting of research results
   d. An offense committed against a research subject

4. What is the purpose of a null hypothesis?
   a. An expectation of significant results
   b. A prediction of significant results
   c. An expectation of no difference
   d. An expectation of negative results

5. Which of the following is true regarding sample representativeness?
   a. The larger the sample, the more representative of a population it is.
   b. Small samples are unrepresentative of a population.
   c. Sample representativeness may be assured by a 25% sample.
   d. Sample representativeness is considered independently of sample size.

6. Why is selection bias a potential threat to internal validity?
   a. Some people select the wrong answers.
   b. Some people select the wrong study.
   c. Some studies do not randomly assign subjects.
   d. Some studies do not randomly select variables.

7. What is the purpose of a control group?
   a. It controls access to the study.
   b. It controls measurements of subjects.
   c. It controls the flow of information to the researcher.
   d. It controls for unintended influences on subjects.

8. What is the meaning of a zero correlation?
   a. There is no systematic relationship between variables.
   b. As one variable increases, another decreases.
   c. As one variable decreases, another increases.
   d. There are insufficient data for interpretation.

9. Why was the case-control approach developed?
   a. To replicate cohort approaches with more power.
   b. To replicate experimental studies with fewer subjects.
   c. To replicate cohort approaches with more efficiency.
   d. To replicate experimental studies with less time.

10. Which of the following is a limitation of secondary literature sources?
    a. They are more detailed than primary sources.
    b. They are biased by the author's summary.
    c. They are difficult to find in most libraries.
    d. They contain erroneous information.

Answers appear on page 447.

17

HOW TO READ MEDICAL JOURNALS

JOHN W. McCALL and LARRY CULPEPPER

There are only a handful of ways to do a study properly, but one thousand ways to do it wrong.

McMASTER UNIVERSITY

PROBLEM OF KEEPING UP

The publication of medical journals can be traced to the early 1600s, and a look at their evolutionary growth reflects the history of both medical science and practice (Booth). The number of scientific journals has increased an estimated fourfold over the last decade, with the medical sciences representing the most explosive field. The total number of medical journal publications increased seven and one-half times (Bowker). Today there are well over 20,000 biomedical journals (McMaster University); new articles appear at a rate of at least one every 26 seconds (Krogh). Therefore, even a speed reader, reading 24 hours a day, could not keep up with all the medical literature. "If practitioners were to attempt to keep up with the literature by reading two articles per day, in one year they would fall fifty-five centuries behind. Put another way, if physicians were to read everything of possible biomedical relevance, they would need to read 5500 articles per day" (Haynes et al.). Given this information, why should one even attempt to keep up—is it necessary?

FIRST PRINCIPLE: UNDERSTAND WHY IT IS IMPORTANT TO KEEP UP WITH THE MEDICAL LITERATURE

Several studies have documented journal reading to be the most important continuing education activity in terms of physician preference, frequency with which it is used, amount of time devoted to it, and frequency with which it leads to changes in practice (Gehlbach, Geyman, Haynes et al.). "The use of medical journals consistently ranks above the use of other sources of literature such as newsletters, textbooks, and monographs, as well as above the use of other means of continuing education such as personal contact with colleagues, making of clinical rounds, continuing education courses, and contact with pharmaceutical representatives" (Haynes et al.).

Reasons for keeping up with the medical journal literature in clinical practice include: (1) to stay current with medical trends and maintain competence; (2) to seek solutions to specific patient care problems; and (3) to nourish a personal sense of curiosity and interest about medical conditions. Regular journal reading will yield insights into the clinical course and prognosis of human illness, new diagnostic procedures, new treatments, and dangerous drug interactions and side effects (Gehlbach, Haynes et al., McMaster University). The ultimate application of keeping up is to make rational decisions about changing one's practice of medicine. Good reading habits and skills should contribute to the appropriate and timely adoption of new knowledge into practice.

Before one can read competently, minimal skills and a basic strategy on "how to read" must be developed. Even the most dedicated readers will receive few benefits for their efforts if they lack the ability to separate the valuable contributions from trivial or misleading articles. Many physicians lack the skills, or, if they have the skills, they may have low confidence in their ability to read critically (Alguire et al., Geyman). "How should family physicians respond to the contemporary plethora of epidemiological data, recommendations, and warnings?" (Stephens). These skills are seldom taught formally during medical school or residency training (Alguire et al., Krogh, Riegelman). Almost 60% of all graduating medical students responding to the 1989 Association of American Medical Colleges questionnaire reported that the time devoted to the teaching of literature analysis skills was inadequate. A result of regular reading is the development of competence and confidence in distinguishing new findings that are reliable and valid from those that are not and deciding when new information should lead to a change in clinical practice.

SECOND PRINCIPLE: DETERMINE WHAT TO READ

Once the need is recognized and the commitment is made, the next step is to decide "what to read." For this step, it is important to have a working knowledge of the types of journals and types of articles in those journals.

TABLE 17–1. A GRAMMAR FOR INTERPRETING THE MEDICAL LITERATURE

FIRST PRINCIPLE Understand why it is important to keep up with the medical literature.

SECOND PRINCIPLE Determine what to read.

THIRD PRINCIPLE Determine whether to read an article.

Rule One Look at the title to determine general interest.

Rule Two Verify the article's relevance by reading the summary or abstract.

Rule Three Scan the article to determine technical complexity.

FOURTH PRINCIPLE Determine how to read medical journals.

Rule One Understand the general concepts.
Step 1: Know the standard article format for most clinical studies.
Step 2: Be skeptical.
Step 3: Don't judge an article by the journal in which it is published.
Step 4: There is more to an article than the abstract.
Step 5: Recognize there is no such thing as a perfect study.
Step 6: Judge the author's treatment of contradictory studies.
Step 7: Recognize that validity and reliability are crucial.

Rule Two Determine what is being studied.
Step 1: Determine the study questions or hypothesis.
Step 2: Identify the specific study variables under study.
Step 3: Determine how the variables are defined and measured.

Rule Three Determine who is being studied.
Step 1: Determine the characteristics of the study subjects.
Step 2: Determine how subjects were selected.
Step 3: Determine if the sample size is adequate.

Rule Four Determine the type of study and assess validity.

Rule Five Determine how the data have been statistically analyzed.
Step 1: Recognize the fundamental importance of good descriptive statistics.
Step 2: Determine the types of inferential statistics used.

Rule Six Understand that statistical tests do not by themselves determine causation.

Rule Seven Decide whether the results and recommendations warrant any change in your clinical practice.

Journals, like people, have unique personalities reflecting their mission or special focus. Two methods for classifying journals are by topic, i.e., general purpose to highly specialized, and by the type of articles most often published, i.e., original research, review, established protocols for treating patients, etc. Under the first method, there are three categories: (1) general, e.g., *New England Journal of Medicine, JAMA,* or *Lancet;* (2) medical specialty, e.g., *Journal of Family Practice, Annals of Internal Medicine,* or *Pediatrics;* and (3) subspecialties, e.g., *Circulation* or *Archives of Dermatology.* In addition to the *Journal of Family Practice,* major family medicine journals include the *American Family Physician,* the *Journal of the American Board of Family Practice,* and *Family Medicine* (a joint publication of the Society of Teachers of Family Medicine and the North American Primary Care Research Group). International journals of note include *Family Practice: An International Journal* and the *Journal of the Royal College of General Practice.*

The typical family physician should read at least six to eight journals. These journals should represent a mix from the two methods weighted toward the patient composition of the physician's practice. A physician's list of regularly read journals should fit his or her reading style and provide a mix of original research and review articles. In addition, Reinharth advocates that the physician select some journals and articles outside of his or her specialty and include some basic science articles.

Regarding the mix of original articles versus review articles or other nonoriginal contributions, Haynes and colleagues strongly condemn reading any article that is not original and peer-reviewed. However, Patrick describes this approach for the family physician as narrowminded. Our view is that the mixture of reading material should reflect the purpose for reading. Physicians often encounter a patient with an unusual disease or combination of diseases about which they need specific information. For this purpose, scanning a textbook, followed by reading a quality review article, is an excellent initial approach. This process may be followed by scanning articles from "how to" journals such as *Patient Care* to identify practical insights. Finally, scanning original research articles will identify recent advances. In contrast, reading to keep up generally should include a few good review articles as they appear and scanning reports of original research.

Good clinical review articles often include enough basic science background to allow physicians who regularly read them to stay current. We recommend that the family physician limit reading basic science articles, unless he or she simply finds pleasure in such reading. Original articles regarding new drugs should be limited primarily to clinical trials and postmarketing (FDA release) reports. Studies investigating drugs that are close to being licensed by the FDA for general use are referred to as Phase III studies. Of very limited interest for clinical application are reports of animal studies (Phase I) or preliminary human trials (Phase II). Parts II and III of the articles by Haynes and colleagues provide further information about deciding which journals to read.

THIRD PRINCIPLE: DETERMINE WHETHER OR NOT TO READ AN ARTICLE

Once one decides on a general game plan of what to read, the next step is to determine the rules related to whether to read a particular article. Gehlbach describes this process as learning how to "taste" an article; it also has been described as separating the "wheat from the chaff" (McMaster University).

Rule One: Look at the Title to Determine General Interest

The reader should have a vested interest in the article to be read. Look at the title. If the article is not interesting or appears not to be relevant to the reader's practice, move on.

Rule Two: Verify the Article's Relevance by Reading the Summary or Abstract

"At issue here is not whether the article's results are true, but whether the results, if true, are useful" (McMaster University). The question to ask is whether the new clinical information would be of practical use for the reader, given his or her particular practice setting and patients. Would the differences lead to different results?

Rule Three: Scan the Article to Determine Technical Complexity

If the technical complexity of the article far exceeds the ability of the reader to comprehend it, the effort would be inefficient and frustrating.

FOURTH PRINCIPLE: DETERMINE HOW TO READ MEDICAL JOURNALS

This section is the heart of this chapter. The emphasis in this section is on how to read a clinical research study to determine whether the results are believable and applicable to the reader's practice.

Rule One: Understand the General Concepts

Step 1: Know the Standard Article Format for Most Clinical Studies

This format usually consists of the abstract or summary; the introduction (definition of the problem and review of the literature); the methods (design of the study, description of the sample, data-collecting procedures, any treatment administered and data analysis); the results (of data analysis); the discussion (of results and study limitations, relationship of results to previous studies); the summary and/or conclusions; and the bibliography. A quick scanning of the abstract, introduction, and conclusions usually will let the reader identify whether articles with interesting titles are truly of interest. If so, more time can be spent on the results, discussion, and methods sections.

Step 2: Be Skeptical

The reader should be skeptical of all articles. One should not accept a study's results and conclusions as "truths" unless one understands the general techniques of critical reading and has reviewed the study and understood its limitations. These techniques involve the ability to understand the format of an article, analyze the process by which the study was done, recognize the limitations of the work, and critique the results and interpretation. The critical reader should ask the following seven questions (Crocker): What is the purpose of the study? How does this research relate to the current body of knowledge in the professional discipline? What measures are used? Do the sample size and sampling procedures permit results to be generalized to a larger population? What is the design of the study and what are its inherent limitations? What is the outcome of the data analysis? What (if any) are the implications for practice?

Step 3: Do Not Judge an Article by the Journal in Which It Is Published

A naive view is that one does not have to worry about the credibility (validity and reliability) of an article if it appears in a peer-reviewed journal, particularly a prestigious one. Although some journals do have more rigorous standards than others, to use this factor to judge the merits of a particular article is dangerous. "The review and editorial policies of even the best and most highly respected journals provide incomplete protection from error" (McMaster University).

It also is dangerous to judge the validity of an article by its packaging; the right jargon and inclusion of complicated tables generated by sophisticated computer statistical packages do not ensure quality. An outstanding parody on this line of thinking is the article "The Teething Virus" (Bennett and Brudno). The tragic side to this humorous article, according to the authors, is that they get requests for additional copies from physicians who think it is legitimate. Only after a critical review can the physician derive valid and useful conclusions from an article and appropriately apply its findings to practice (Cuddy et al.).

Step 4: There Is More to an Article Than the Abstract

The good abstract is informative and should be able to stand apart from the article, but it cannot be the sole basis for a critical opinion of the study's validity (Cuddy et al.). A complete abstract should include information that identifies the study purpose, research design, methods, results, conclusions, and recommendations. Sometimes the author's abstract of the article contains more wish than reality and presents a distorted view of the work that follows (Gehlbach).

Step 5: Recognize That There Is No Such Thing as a Perfect Study

At the opposite extreme, there are those who are overly critical of everything published and only consider the weaknesses of a study. To operate at this extreme is a folly equal to overlooking all weaknesses of an article. There is a big difference between the ideal study design (as in any blueprint) and the final product. The critical questions are, (1) Do the strengths outweigh the weaknesses? and (2) Is there something in the study that adds new knowledge that improves patient care? (Elenbaas et al.). Every research publication is likely to have a flaw; occasionally, some flaws invalidate the entire study (Cuddy et al.). However, even when an overt investigator bias or a design flaw is in evidence, it is incorrect to reject the author's conclusion immediately or substitute the opposite. "The only conclusion that a reader should make from a poorly designed study is that no conclusion can be made" (Elenbaas et al.).

As discussed later, different study designs are particularly susceptible to different problems. An informed reader should be aware of these when evaluating an article. When a design flaw or other bias is identified, the reader should consider whether it is likely to make the findings more or less extreme than those actually reported. Often, a study design problem may be such that a perfect study would have found an even more extreme finding than that reported. In such cases, the existence of the finding can be accepted from the flawed study even though the estimate of the strength of a reported finding might be subject to question.

Step 6: Judge the Author's Treatment of Contradictory Studies

It is the responsibility of the investigator to include both sides of an issue in his or her literature review, usually presented in the introduction. A literature review should relate the current study to previous studies and show how this study will attempt to answer questions not resolved by these studies (Crocker). An important indicator of author bias is the treatment of contradictory studies. The critical reader should assess whether the author has emphasized only particular previous results that favor his or her objective and ignored those that disagree with or discount his or her findings. A related serious error that occasionally is committed is that an author will select a previously published study and draw conclusions regarding efficacy by comparing its results with the results of the current study (Elenbaas et al.).

Step 7: Recognize That Validity and Reliability Are Crucial

The core issues for how to read the medical journal literature are summarized in two words: *validity* and *reliability*. Reliability is the degree of consistency between repeated measures of the same thing: if I repeated the study, would I get the same data? Validity is the degree to which a study achieves the aim for which it was designed: does it represent the truth? Is it unbiased? Is it applicable to practice? Will the patients we see and treat respond in the same way as those described in the study? Does the paper really support its claims (Crocker, Gehlbach)? Of the two concepts, validity is the most important but the most difficult to assess and the more subjective of the two (although the two are not mutually exclusive). A study's findings may be very reliable yet invalid.

There are two types of validity: internal and external. Internal validity usually refers to the ability of the study design to measure what it was intended to measure within the confines of the study. External validity is more commonly referred to by physicians as "generalizability." Generalizability has to do with whether conclusions can be applied to settings different from that used for the study, including the reader's practice (Gehlbach). "The reader should be wary of statements of invalid extrapolation to clinical situations that were not within the study scope" (Elenbaas et al.). Different types of studies are prone to different internal validity problems. These will be discussed after we have identified the various types of studies. Generalizability is discussed further under Rule Three.

Rule Two: Determine What Is Being Studied

Rules two through four represent the "what," "who," and "how" of reading the medical journal literature.

Step 1: Determine the Study Questions or Hypothesis

What is the subject of the investigation? Is it hypertension, pregnancy outcome, patient compliance, or treatment efficacy? More specifically, what is at issue, e.g., the relationship between, the effect of, or the cause of? In short, what is the hypothesis? The research question or hypothesis is usually in the introduction as part of the statement of the problem, although it is usually implied rather than formally stated. A hypothesis is a statement of the predicted outcome of the study design, and results are compared to it.

Step 2: Identify the Specific Variables under Study

These can usually be identified in the abstract, introduction, or methods section. Variables are so named because they may "vary" according to the circumstances surrounding them at any given time. Descriptive studies report information about variables of interest and the relationships among them.

In analytic studies there are two types of variables: independent variables and dependent variables (e.g., smoking and cancer, monosaturated fats and cholesterol, family well-being and diabetic control). The *independent variables* can be described simply as the variables under study, which are presumed to influence the dependent variable. A *dependent variable* is exactly that. It is defined as being dependent on other variables for its outcome, shape, or existence. Therefore, a study that has a title such as "The effect of passive smoking on lung cancer mortality rates of nonsmoking female airline attendants" is saying that passive smoking has been identified as the independent variable and lung cancer mortality as the dependent variable.

A special group of independent variables are referred to as *confounding* variables. Confounding variables are associated with the independent variables of interest in the study and also are independent risk factors for the disease of interest (the outcome). Differences in outcomes between groups in a study actually may be due to the confounding variable rather than to the independent variable under study. For example, if various occupations are being investigated for risk of lung cancer, and it also is known that smoking varies between occupations, unless the frequency of smoking in the various groups is taken into account in the analysis, associations between the occupational risk of interest and lung cancer will not be valid. Confounding variables are particularly important to analytic studies that seek to draw cause-and-effect conclusions. While authors might not specifically label variables as confounders, the readers should look for whether other risk factors known to affect the outcomes in question in the study have been taken into consideration, particularly if they also are likely to be related to the potential cause under study.

Step 3: Determine How the Variables are Defined and Measured

These elements are referred to as *operational definitions*. The specific definitions and measures greatly influence the results and are directly related to the issue of validity considered later. For example, how does the investigator actually define and measure passive smoking, family well-being, diabetic control, or monosaturated fats? In many articles, the variable definitions and measures are not reported and the reader is asked to assume that they were adequate, valid, and reliable. Sometimes they are reported in fine print or as footnotes to save space. Find them and do not assume that print size is related to level of importance.

Rule Three: Determine Who Is Being Studied

Rule Three is critical when it comes to making a decision about the applicability of study findings to your clinical practice. A study's methods and procedures may be very reliable, but the results may still not be applicable to patients in a different practice. The characteristics of the sample have a great deal to do with this question of external validity or generalizability—the appropriateness of applying the findings from a study setting to a specific practice. In determining who is being studied, several steps must be followed (Cuddy et al.).

Step 1: Determine the Characteristics of the Study Subjects

This factor includes such characteristics as the subjects' age, sex, occupation, education, and medical condition. What were the "inclusion and exclusion criteria"? Investigators will sometimes restrict their study to a very homogeneous group of subjects. For example, studies of aspirin in the prevention of cardiac or stroke events might be restricted to white males age 45–65. One view is that such restriction limits the application of the study findings. However, it greatly reduces the likelihood of erroneous conclusions due to age, sex, or race differences between intervention and control groups. Thus, a reader is left with greater confidence in the validity of the study but also with the sometimes difficult problem of deciding the biological plausibility of applying the results to individuals who were not represented in the study.

For family physicians, the generalizability of studies conducted on hospitalized patients and patients from subspecialty referral practices, clinics, and emergency rooms is often questionable. Such studies may involve patients who are different enough from those of family physicians that the results of a similar study done with the family physician's practice would be different. These differences may be of a demographic nature (age, race, sex, education, inner city–rural, married–single parent, etc.). They may be subtle; duration and severity of illness, time differences in diagnostic assessment, compliance, practice staffing, and physician continuity are a few such areas of difference that might affect the results of a study. For example, in studies investigating treatment of urinary tract infections, few women at initial presentation in private practice had antibody-coated bacteria in their urine (which possibly indicates duration and severity of infection), while such was commonly found in hospital clinic patients and in a majority of emergency room patients.

Step 2: Determine How Subjects Were Selected

This information goes beyond simple inclusion and exclusion criteria (Crocker, Cuddy et al., McMaster University). This question actually refers to the type of sample—random (or probability) sample versus a nonrandom (or availability) sample. It is the method used to obtain a "representative" sample, i.e., a sample that is typical of the entire population from which the sample was drawn. Most clinical studies are based on "availability" samples, i.e., all subjects (up to a certain number) that meet the inclusion and exclusion criteria.

A false assumption is to equate "randomized" with a "random sample" (Crocker). A randomized study often uses an availability sample and assigns the patient or subject to one group or another based on the principle of "randomness," i.e., giving each subject equal chance of being put in one group or another. A true random sample gives an equal chance of being in the study to every subject meeting inclusion criteria in the population. Theoretically, a nonrandom or availability sample could be just as representative of some population as a random sample if the investigator knows all the important characteristics of the population to be studied and carefully selects subjects based on them. However, most investigators are not willing to make such an assumption (nor should the reader) and opt for a random sample whenever feasible.

Step 3: Determine Whether or Not the Sample Size Is Adequate

Sample size is a very important question, since it directly affects statistical significance and, therefore, error type (see Rule Five). Unfortunately, the answer to this question is usually much more elusive than we like to think and often is more art than science. Mathematical formulas for determining sample size do exist, but they are highly dependent on the validity of specific information used in the calculations about the condition in the population to be studied. Consequently, the number produced by a sample size formula is no more reliable than the assumptions used. Accurate data for such use often are not available. In reality, the critical reader cannot do much more than determine whether or not the sample size appears reasonable within the context of the practical limitations of the study, i.e., time, resources, complexity of the exclusion and inclusion criteria, and rarity of the disease or variables under study. One advantage of studies that report results using confidence intervals is that the breadth of such intervals provides a good indication of sample size adequacy (see Rule Five).

Rule Four: Determine the Type of Study and Assess Validity

With the general concepts covered, it is time to construct a specific framework for dissecting journal articles that report clinical or epidemiologic findings. To start, determine the type of study from the title, abstract, or introduction. This imposes a logical structure to the article, guides the reader in assessing critical issues, and narrows the possible conclusions. For example, one would approach a descriptive article (e.g., prevalence or cross-sectional study) differently than an analytic study (e.g., case-control or cohort study).

We recommend that the inexperienced reader not memorize a complicated taxonomy of research designs. In fact, some types of studies are sometimes referred to in different ways, e.g., cross-sectional or prevalence, retrospective or case-control, prospective or cohort study. Very often, a study may be a combination of two or more classical types. A quick test of the reader's level of ability to comprehend types of studies may be found in the response to the question "Does a clear mental image emerge when one reads the following: a multicenter, prospective, randomized, double-blind, crossover clinical trial?" Until a reader gains confidence with his or her own classification system and own set of definitions, we recommend that a practical approach is to keep one or more glossaries of terms close by. A glossary of terms can be found in most epidemiologic textbooks or textbooks on clinical research methods.

In a very broad sense, there are only two types of studies: *descriptive* and *analytic*. Types of descriptive studies include case reports and series, correlational studies, and cross-sectional (also termed prevalence) studies. Case reports and their expansion into case series are the most basic types of studies and often serve to alert the medical community of new medical phenomena. In cross-sectional studies, all information is gathered at the same time from participants available at that time. Because of this they are sometimes called prevalence surveys.

CROSS-SECTIONAL STUDIES. This type of study has two major problems. First, since it takes a snapshot at one point in time, the relative contribution of frequency of occurrence, severity of a disease, and effectiveness of any treatment cannot be separated. For example, a frequent but rapid fatal disease will be under-represented in the study population, while an infrequent but chronic disease will be over-represented. Second, since information about both diseases and their potential causes is collected at the same time, it may be very difficult to decide whether the potential cause really preceded the disease.

CORRELATIONAL STUDIES. This type of study uses information on the entire population rather than individuals. The major limitation of such studies is the inability to link data at the individual level. For instance, the frequency of cigarette smoking in various countries has been correlated with the frequency of cardiac deaths. It is assumed that smokers are the ones dying more frequently of cardiac disease. A related concern is the lack of ability to control for the effects of confounding variables. For instance, diet actually may lead to cardiac deaths rather than cigarette smoking, with diet varying across countries in a pattern related to cigarette smoking.

A major disadvantage of all *descriptive* study types is that no cause-and-effect relationship can be established. The advantages, however, are that they can be done simply and economically and are useful for identifying potential relationships for investigation using analytic study designs. For example, case reports provided the first evidence of the existence of AIDS. These were followed by cross-sectional studies that began to identify how prevalent the condition was and the characteristics of patients affected. This information could not prove cause-and-effect relationships but provided an informed basis for design of case-control and cohort studies of hypotheses regarding blood, sexual, and other transmission vectors.

In *analytic* studies, the investigator exercises direct or indirect control over the variables of interest so that cause-and-effect conclusions can be drawn from comparisons between groups of subjects. Variables of interest may be exposures to potential causes of disease (e.g., smoking), preventive measures, diagnostic tests, treatments, or other medically related events. These types of studies often involve observations that span a significant period of time. Analytic studies may be divided into "intervention studies," including clinical trials and quasi-experimental designs, and observational studies," including case-control and cohort studies. Each of these designs has particular advantages and is prone to specific validity problems. These elements are discussed in more detail in sections that follow.

INTERVENTION STUDIES. In these studies, the investigator intervenes to control the treatment, diagnostic test, preventive measure, or exposure (potential cause of a disease) under investigation. The outcomes of interest are subsequently measured, and the experience of those individuals receiving the intervention is compared to that of those who did not. Sometimes the comparison is between two or more "active" agents, between an active agent and a placebo, or between an active agent and a control group in which no intervention is made. At times ethical considerations preclude use of a control group, and a study will be between the currently accepted treatment and an experimental treatment. The comparison group may be the same patients as those receiving the intervention with measurements taken at an earlier point in time (self controls), or a different group of patients who were measured at the same time or at an earlier time (the latter are often referred to as "historical" controls) may be used.

The key questions for assessing the validity of an intervention study include: How comparable were the intervention and comparison populations? What was done with information about patients who either did not agree to take part in the study or left the study (including those who died) before final outcome measurements were obtained? How comparable were the effects of being in the study for the two groups other than the specific intervention under investigation? How adequate were the measurements in measuring the changes of interest? Was compliance measured, and how was information about patients who were not compliant managed?

With regard to the first and second questions, the double-blind randomized clinical trial is the gold standard. In this design, subjects are enrolled and informed consent obtained prior to their being randomly assigned to receive the intervention under investigation or a placebo (or alternative treatment). For large samples, this design, if properly carried out, makes the likelihood very high that the control and intervention groups will be similar in all characteristics other than the intervention. Most other intervention designs also seek to obtain groups that are equal with regard to all characteristics other than the intervention under study. In articles reporting such studies, the first table should be a presentation of the characteristics of the control and intervention groups. Did the investigator's randomization or other selection process really result in equal comparison and intervention groups? If not, how likely are the differences to have affected the results? Were differences in socioeconomic factors or geographic location likely to lead to different outcomes? Were the morbidity of the two groups and the severity of illness equivalent? For studies using historical controls, were other changes in medical care or society during the intervening time likely to alter the outcome?

In addition, the reader must determine the difference between the beginning sample and the sample the investigator finally used. The reader must determine the characteristics of the patients who withdrew from the study or were lost to follow-up. For studies in which this is an issue, a second table in the article should contrast the baseline characteristics of those who completed the study with those who withdrew before completion and any differences between the comparison and intervention groups. This information may be used to evaluate the likely affects of those dropping out on the reported study outcome. In most situations, the most valid approach to analyzing data is to leave dropouts in the group to which they were originally randomized. Were the dropout rate and the reasons for dropping out similar in the two groups? Did dropouts actually represent an adverse outcome such as death? Did patients with the most severe disease or ones with a specific comorbidity leave the intervention group more frequently? Did subjects drop out due to side effects or poor compliance (possibly indicating side effects)? When more than 10% to 20% of subjects drop out of a study, the validity of the results becomes increasingly tenuous. Similarly, measurement of compliance is crucial to knowing whether the intervention group actually received the intervention. This is particularly important in studies with negative results.

Investigators routinely present t-tests or other tests that judge the statistical significance of differences in groups or between groups and those lost to follow-up. However, such tests are of little value in deciding the larger questions of the effects of group differences or of loss to follow-up on the study results. This is a matter of judgment. If certain outcomes primarily occurred in certain groups of patients or in those lost to follow-up, would the conclusions be different?

The nature and adequacy of the measurement tools used must be understood to know what an intervention has actually achieved. For such instruments, whether they have undergone a standardization and validation process is important. In assessing measurement tools, the reader should ask not only whether the measurement instrument was appropriate to the change of interest but also whether it adequately reflected changes in the range of interest. Functional assessment tools may be used as an example. While several can adequately measure the functional status of patients, their maximum discriminating ability is among patients who have significant existing disability (e.g., cane- or wheelchair-dependent) as opposed to those with less severe disability.

Traditionally, the best measures have been considered to be those reflecting direct biological information, such as blood pressure, weight, or morbidity outcomes (new heart attacks, deaths, etc.). Symptom reports and other questionnaire data are thought to be "softer" and more subject to differing interpretations by respondents. In this area, one dilemma of interest to family physicians is that while "hard" biological data may be the most important in deciding whether an intervention works, "soft" quality-of-life information, only obtainable through questionnaires, may be important in deciding the overall value of the new intervention.

COHORT STUDIES. Cohort studies are used primarily to investigate the effects of being exposed to some condition on the subsequent development of an outcome (usually a disease). Cohort studies are particularly suited to the study of possible causes, including rare causes, of common diseases. They must be very large and, consequently, costly and inefficient, if the outcome occurs infrequently or requires a long follow-up interval. These studies also can help determine time relationships between being exposed and the development of the outcome.

In cohort studies, two or more groups are set up with subjects allocated based on exposure status. These studies generally are done prospectively, that is, the groups are constructed at a time when all subjects are free of the outcome (usually a disease). The groups should be similar on all characteristics known to be related to the outcomes of interest. One group is the exposed group; the other group is the unexposed comparison group. The groups are then followed for an interval of time, and the rates of developing the outcome for the exposed and unexposed groups are compared. Two issues are critical to the validity of the results from cohort studies.

First, the exposed and unexposed groups must indeed be similar in all other characteristics related to the outcome(s), except for the exposure of interest. For some cohort studies, particularly those focusing on occupational exposure, data from the general population often are used since the general population is rarely exposed. However, such studies may be subject to a "healthy worker" bias, since the general population comparison group may include individuals with chronic illness and lifestyle habits that prevent them from working.

Crucial to the validity of the study is that whatever procedures are used to identify outcomes must be applied equally to both exposed and unexposed individuals. To ensure that the groups being compared are similar with respect to characteristics that might affect the disease outcome, except for the determinant understudy, it is important to check that the information obtained from the two groups is adequate and of comparable quality. Thus, for example, the validity of a study should be questioned if the cause of death for the comparison group was determined from death certificates and, for the exposed group, from hospital records. The adequacy and nature of measurement tools, as discussed for intervention studies, are equally important for cohort studies.

A second major problem in cohort studies is the information on subjects lost to follow-up. If the number of patients lost to follow-up is related to the exposures of interest or to the outcomes, the validity of the results will be in jeopardy. Concerns regarding those patients lost to follow-up discussed for intervention studies apply to cohort studies as well.

CASE-CONTROL STUDIES. Although cohort studies are particularly useful for investigating the possible effects of exposures, case-control studies are used for identifying one or more causes of a single disease, particularly a rare disease. Since both the exposure and the development of the disease have occurred at the time of the study, they can be conducted far more rapidly and less expensively than cohort studies, which require a follow-up period. Thus, case-control studies are of great value in studying rare diseases and particularly those with long latent periods. However, they are not very useful in investigating rare exposures, unless study groups can be identified for which the exposure is not uncommon (such as special occupational groups).

In case-control studies, subjects are identified by whether they have the disease (cases) or do not have the disease (controls). Cases are usually identified from an available population, such as patients attending a practice or admitted to a set of hospitals. In reading a case-control report, one should look for a very specific set of criteria by which patients were judged to have the disease. Whenever possible, patients should be individuals identified at the time of diagnosis (incident cases) rather than all those existing at a point in time (prevalent cases). Otherwise, the prevalent cases will reflect determinants not only of the development of the disease but of disease chronicity.

The selection of the control group is the most critical issue in designing a valid case-control study. In general, controls should be individuals who, if they had developed the disease, would have been counted as cases in the study. Thus, controls represent nondiseased members of the larger theoretical population of which the cases represent all the diseased individuals. If cases and controls have been adequately selected, differences in exposure rates in the two groups may be considered to be associated with the frequency of developing the disease. (Such association does not necessarily imply a cause-and-effect relationship.) The control group in most studies should not be the general population, for the same reasons as in cohort studies.

As with previously discussed study designs, the sources of information should give comparable quality information for both cases and controls. Probing for exposure information may be different in different settings, e.g., smoking or drug abuse history may be probed in greater detail at the time of hospitalization than at the time of initial office workup. If office records are used to obtain the information on controls, office records also should be used to obtain information on cases. Otherwise, the results may represent differences in how the information was obtained rather than in true patient status.

Case-control studies have the potential of developing more problems than clinical trials or cohort studies. Sometimes in ways that are not immediately obvious, the selection of cases or controls depends on the exposure being investigated. This factor will invalidate a case-control study. For example, in a recent study of the relationship of pancreatic cancer to caffeine intake, controls were selected from the practices of gastroenterologists who were the physicians for the cases. However, patients seeing gastroenterologists for reasons other than pancreatic cancer are likely to have been instructed in the past or to have decreased their coffee intake spontaneously. In this particular example, the finding of an increased rate of caffeine intake among those with pancreatic cancer was invalid. A second major problem for case-control studies is the role of recall on the part of study subjects giving information. Individuals with the disease are likely to ponder potential causes and recall exposures that have been forgotten by the nondiseased controls.

RETROSPECTIVE AND PROSPECTIVE STUDIES. The reader will frequently encounter these two terms, which refer to the temporal sequencing of study events rather than the basic design. A retrospective study is one in which all the events have occurred (both exposure and outcome) prior to data collection. Retrospective studies are usually studies in which subjects are examined for some common factor in their history, and are often descriptive in design. Case-control studies are also retrospective. Prospective studies are those in which subjects are followed from identification of the characteristic of interest to the time of outcome, e.g., disease. In many instances, a prospective approach will be used simply to observe the effects of a treatment or other event over time. Most intervention studies and cohort studies are conducted prospectively.

Rule Five: Determine How the Data Have Been Statistically Analyzed

The overall objective of the statistical analyses reported in an article is to reduce the data into simple groupings with numerical values that can be interpreted in unbiased ways. In reality, this part of the article may leave many readers confused. Consequently, many readers skim data analysis information. This makes the reader almost totally dependent on the investigator to make judgments about the appropriateness of the analyses and limits the reader in making an informed decision about changing clinical practice based on the results. The following steps may be helpful in evaluating the statistical sections of articles. A number of journal articles have discussed statistical interpretation in more depth (Elenbaas et al., LeFevre, Sheehan).

Step 1: Recognize the Fundamental Importance of Good Descriptive Statistics

The reader may not understand all the nuances of statistics, but all readers should be able to make some judgment about the results and recommendations based on good frequency tables, e.g., numbers, percentages, means, etc. A good article, even one constrained by space, should have good descriptive statistics as a foundation to the results section.

Step 2: Determine the Types of Inferential Statistics Used

There are three basic types of inferential statistics: (1) tests of statistical significance, (2) tests of association or strength, and (3) tests or techniques that have predictive capability.

TESTS OF STATISTICAL SIGNIFICANCE. Frequently used tests of significance are the chi-square test and the t-test. Analyses of variance or covariance are basically t-tests for assessing the difference in means for more than two groups. They also allow for statistically taking into account the effects of other variables including potential confounding variables. Test of significance are reported in terms of the P value. Most studies that use inferential statistical techniques begin with a test of significance to determine the P value. The P value is the probability that a finding involving grouped data could have occurred by chance. Simply interpreted, $P < .05$ means that there is at least a 95% probability that the finding did not occur by chance alone and a less than 5% probability that the finding occurred by chance.

Conclusions using P values are subject to error in two directions. The error of deciding that a finding is not due to chance alone, when in fact it is, is known as an "alpha" or "type I" error. On the other hand, concluding that the finding is due to chance, when in fact it is not, is a "beta" or "type II" error. A small sample greatly increases the chance of making a beta or type II error. Although there is nothing magical about a $P < .05$, this has become a benchmark for statistical significance. However, the reader should always keep the concepts of statistical error (alpha and beta) in mind in making his or her own interpretation. If the results are "negative" (P value $> .05$), then a report of the "power" of an analysis is useful. It is the chance that a type II error did not occur.

TESTS OF ASSOCIATION. A test of association, such as a *relative risk ratio* (*RR*) or *odds ratio* (*OR*), is a test of the strength of the relationship between two or more variables or outcomes. The relative risk is the ratio of the likelihood of an event occurring in one group in comparison to its occurring in a second group (often called the "comparison" or "reference" group). For example, a value of 1 indicates an equal chance, a value of 1.3 indicates a 30% increase in likelihood of the event occurring, a value of 2 indicates a doubling in likelihood, and a value of 0.7 indicates a 30% decrease in likelihood. *Confidence intervals* are often reported for relative risk (*RR*) measures or other statistics. They indicate the range within which the true value is likely to be at a given level of certainty. For example, $RR = 1.5$ (90% C.I. 1.3–1.8) indicates that the best estimate is a 50% increase in risk of the event occurring with a 90% chance that the true value lies between a 30% and 80% increase in risk. Larger samples give narrower confidence intervals, indicating more precision in the result obtained. Relative risks give information about the magnitude of the findings as well as the certainty of the estimate. They are related to P values, in that if $P < .05$, the 95% confidence interval will not include 1.0. If the P value exactly equals .05, one extreme of the 95% confidence interval would be 1.0 (e.g., 95% C.I. 1.0–1.8).

An R value or *correlation coefficient* is another statistic indicating association between variables. It has a range of -1 to $+1$. If there is no linear relationship between two variables, the value of the coefficient is 0. If there is a perfect positive linear relationship, the value is $+1$, and if there is a perfect negative linear relationship the value is -1. However, two variables can have a correlation coefficient close to zero and still have a strong nonlinear relationship (Norusis). A correlation coefficient measures the strength of the relationship but relays no information about statistical significance, nor can causation or prediction be assumed (Crocker, Elenbaas, McMaster University).

TESTS OF PREDICTION. Common statistical techniques employed for this purpose include some types of analysis of variance and covariance, multiple regression, and logistic regression. These last two elements often report results in terms of relative risks adjusted for the effects of other variables.

Determining the appropriateness of a test or set of tests is often difficult and requires a level of expertise that is beyond the scope of this chapter. There are a number of assumptions that must be considered in determining statistical test appropriateness, such as sample size, level of measurement of the data, type of sample distribution or shape (normal or otherwise), power, and so forth. If the reader is concerned about the appropriateness of a test, it may be necessary to consult an introductory statistics textbook.

Rule Six: Understand That Statistical Tests Do Not Determine Causation by Themselves

A cause-and-effect relationship can never be established by a statistical test alone. Statistical significance only indicates that the association between two variables is not likely to be due to chance alone. For example, a comparison of mortality and morbidity between hospitals and steel mills would find a stronger association or correlation between hospitals and mortality and morbidity than for steel mills. However, this does not mean that hospitals are a major cause of mortality. In addition, if one was interested in studying the cause of fires, one would find a very high correlation between fires and fire trucks; however, it would be foolish to assume that fire trucks cause fires.

The decision to consider a relationship to be one of cause and effect requires consideration of several issues other than statistical results. First, one must determine whether the design of the research reported was of an analytic nature (i.e., case-control, cohort, or intervention design) and whether the results can be considered valid based on issues already discussed. Descriptive studies cannot prove a cause-and-effect relationship.

Additional criteria that can help in assessing an article on a cause-and-effect relationship include information about the temporal sequence of events reported, the strength of the association reported, the presence of a dose-response relationship, the biological credibility of the proposed association, and the consistency of the findings with other published work. The first three of these issues can be evaluated using information presented in the article. An absolute criterion for a cause-and-effect relationship is that the cause preceded the effect. This is easily confirmed in clinical trials and cohort studies. However, it is a critical issue to confirm in assessing a case-control report. The greater the magnitude of the observed association, the less likelihood that it is due to factors not considered by the investigators, including undiscovered causes. Similarly, the presence of a dose-response relationship can be considered some-

what supportive of a cause-and-effect relationship if other criteria are met. However, by itself it is a weak criterion, since such a dose-response relationship may be due to the influence of extraneous variables. The lack of a dose-response relationship may simply indicate the existence of an all-or-nothing type of phenomenon.

If the study is judged to be indicative of a cause-and-effect relationship based upon the above criteria, further support for the relationship might be inferred from the investigator's reporting of other supportive articles in the review of the literature (introductory and discussion sections). Further support can be derived from general knowledge about the logical plausibility of the relationship. This is not an absolute requirement, since cause-and-effect associations often are identified years prior to development of an understanding of the specific biological pathways involved. Once again, this can be judged, in part, based on the author's discussion and introductory sections.

Rule Seven: Decide Whether or Not the Results and Recommendations Warrant Any Change in Clinical Practice

A considerable percentage of the medical literature provides support for the use of new diagnostic studies, medications, history-taking methods, and patient education efforts about causes of disease. Over time, many initial reports are brought into question or disproven by subsequent studies. For example, it is not uncommon for drugs to be removed from the market within one or two years of release due to newly discovered side effects. Two-thirds of the studies appearing in medical journals have been judged to contain some unwarranted conclusions (Sheehan). Therefore, it is important for the physician to be aware of the pitfalls discussed in this chapter—when to reject, when to take a wait-and-see attitude, or when to make actual changes in clinical practice. The clinician-reader needs to develop an approach for deciding when to put new findings into practice.

We propose the following steps for the physician to take in making such decisions. First, articles that report completely new causes of disease or first-time reports of the effectiveness of a diagnostic test or treatment should be viewed as preliminary only. The readers should identify whether the results, if supported in the future, would be applicable to his or her practice. If so, the reader can keep an eye out for further supportive literature. Another practical reason to develop an understanding of major new reports is that if they also are reported by the news media, patients may question the physician about the findings.

If other articles subsequently report the same findings, the reader may seriously consider incorporating the findings into practice. The validity of such articles must first be verified by critical reading: "Before accepting the conclusions of such studies, clinicians should be satisfied that the improved patient outcomes following therapy are so great that they cannot be explained by one or more biases in the assembly of the study patients or in the assessment or interpretation of their responses to therapy" (McMaster University).

As a second step, the opinion of clinical experts should be obtained prior to clinical application. Editorials accompanying articles may serve this purpose. In addition, the physician may want to discuss them with the specialty consultants he regularly uses. Consultants will frequently have additional information available to them from subspecialty meetings and discussions with university-based investigators. Generally, one should not consider using a new medication or procedure prior to its use by the local consultants. Because of the increased frequency with which subspecialty consultants see patients with diseases in their area, they are likely to be more aware of practical issues and potential complications in the treatment of these patients. For a new medication, once the conditions mentioned earlier have been satisfied, the physician may decide to begin its use in his or her practice. To start, we recommend use with particularly reliable patients who are likely to recognize and report side effects early. As the physician gains ex-

perience, it is reasonable to use new clinical tools that have demonstrated advantage on a routine basis.

A final activity in keeping up with the literature is keeping up with changes in medical literature itself: "In the next decade, I believe academics and publishers will have to increase their efforts to make medical publications more relevant and to keep practitioners up-to-date. The general medical journal will have to change. Though it will still be the first to report important results, it will become less a multispecialty showcase, less an archive for curiosities, and more a forum for critical analysis and rapid exchange of comment. Its ultimate task will be to firmly integrate new results into the existing body of knowledge. This means the journals will have to link academics, medical educators, professional writers, and learned societies more closely—a big job but medical journals will have to respond to the increasingly complex challenge of keeping up" (Morgan). However, the responsibility and the challenge to keep up and to do so correctly will remain primarily with the physician.

REFERENCES

Alguire PC, Massa MD, Lienhart KW, Henry RC. A package workshop for teaching critical reading of the medical literature. Med Teacher 1988; 10:85–90.

Association of American Medical Colleges. Graduation questionnaire results: The University of Tennessee College of Medicine. Washington, D. C., AAMC, 1989.

Bennett HJ, Brudno DS. The teething virus. Pediatr Infect Dis 1986; 5:399–401.

Booth CC. The origin and growth of medical journals. Ann Intern Med 1990; 113:398–402.

Bowker RR. Ulrich's News: Serials trends: Scientific publishing boom. R.R. Bowker's International Serials Database 1988; 1:2.

Crocker LM. Linking research to practice: Suggestions for reading a research article. Am J Occup Ther 1977; 31:34–39.

Cuddy PG, Elenbaas RM, Elenbaas JK. Evaluating the medical literature part I: Abstract, introduction, methods. Ann Emerg Med 1983; 12:549–555.

Elenbaas JK, Cuddy PG, Elenbaas RM. Evaluating the medical literature part III: Results and discussion. Ann Emerg Med 1983; 12:679–686.

Elenbaas RM, Elenbaas JK, Cuddy PG. Evaluating the medical literature part II: Statistical analysis. Ann Emerg Med. 1983; 12:610–620.

Gehlbach SH. Interpreting the Medical Literature: Practical Epidemiology for Clinicians. 2nd ed. New York, Macmillan, 1988.

Geyman JP. Critical reading habits and the maturation of family medicine. J Fam Pract 1987; 25:115.

Haynes RB, et al. How to keep up with the medical literature: I—Why try to keep up and how to get started. Ann Intern Med 1986; 105:149–153.

Haynes RB, et al. How to keep up with the medical literature: II—

Deciding which journals to read regularly. Ann Intern Med 1986; 105:309–312.

Haynes RB, et al. How to keep up with the medical literature: III—Expanding the number of journals you read regularly. Ann Intern Med 1986; 105:474–478.

Krogh CL. A checklist system for critical review of medical literature. Med Educ 1985; 19:392–395.

LeFevre ML. Statistical analysis in family medicine research. Fam Med 1988; 20:359–363.

McMaster University. How to read clinical journals: I—Why to read them and how to start reading them critically. Can Med Assoc J 1981; 124:555–558.

McMaster University. How to read clinical journals: III—To learn the clinical course and prognosis of disease. Can Med Assoc J 1981; 124:869–872.

McMaster University. How to read clinical journals: V—To distinguish useful from useless or even harmful therapy. Can Med Assoc J 1981; 124:1156–1162.

Morgan P. Are physicians learning from what they read in journals? Can Med Assoc J 1985; 133:263.

Norusis, MJ. The SPSS Guide to Data Analysis. Chicago, SPSS, 1986.

Patrick JK. Controlling the medical magazine monster. J Ark Med Soc 1988; 84:480–482.

Reinharth D. Keeping up with the medical literature. Ann Intern Med 1986; 105:807–808.

Riegelman RK. Studying a Study and Testing a Test: How to Read the Medical Literature. Boston, Little, Brown, 1981.

Sheehan TJ. The medical literature: Let the reader beware. Arch Intern Med 1980; 140:472–474.

Stephens GG. Epidemiological abuse. J Am Bd Fam Pract 1990; 3:305–308.

QUESTIONS

1. Sound advice for reading the medical literature would include (true or false)
   a. Limiting clinical reading to only original and peer-reviewed articles.
   b. Judging the credibility of an article based on the journal's level of prestige in the medical community.
   c. Seeking solutions to specific patient-care problems.
   d. Recognizing that there are no perfect studies.

e. Limiting the number of basic science articles on preliminary human trials.

2. Research rarely includes the entire population in the study. Important points to remember about sampling are (true or false)

a. A randomized sample and a random sample are slightly different terms, but they mean the same thing.

b. Theoretically, a nonrandom or available sample could be just as representative of a population as a random sample, if the investigator knows all the important characteristics of the population to be studied and carefully selects subjects based on those characteristics.

c. Sample size directly affects statistical significance and, therefore, error type.

d. When one doesn't know anything about the demographic characteristics of the population to be studied, simple mathematical formulae can easily be applied to determine the sample size needed for a study.

3. External validity is more commonly known by physicians as "generalizability," which refers to

a. The general application of the results to the clinical setting.

b. The general significance of the research question.

c. The general reliability of the methods.

d. Whether or not the general conclusions can be applied to a setting different from that used in the study.

4. "Confounding" variables are best described as those which

a. Are associated with the independent variables of interest in the study and independent risk factors for the disease of interest.

b. Add confusion to the conclusions.

c. Are considered in a study design but which are found to be without foundation.

5. A prevalence survey, which gathers all information at the same time from participants available at that time, is also known as a

a. Cohort study.

b. Case-control study.

c. Cross-sectional study.

d. Intervention study.

6. A double-blind randomized clinical trial is best described as

a. A cohort study.

b. A case-control study.

c. A cross-sectional study.

d. An intervention study.

7. The investigation of possible causes, including rare causes, of common diseases, as well as determining time relationships between being exposed and the development of the outcome, should be conducted in a(n)

a. Cohort study.

b. Case-control study.

c. Cross-sectional study.

d. Intervention study.

8. The appropriate use of statistics adds strong support to the credibility of an article. The inappropriate use can be very deceptive and lead to false conclusions. Judge the following statements:

a. A correlation coefficient measures the strength of the relationship but relays no information about statistical significance, nor can causation or prediction be assumed.

b. When a journal limits the length of an article, descriptive statistical information should be dropped in favor of inferential statistics.

c. There are a number of assumptions that must be considered in determining statistical tests of appropriateness, such as sample size, level of measurement of the data, type of sample distribution or shape, and power.

d. Statistical significance and clinical significance are the same.

9. Some types of analysis of variance and covariance, multiple regression, and logistic regression are best described as tests of

a. Statistical significance.

b. Association.

c. Prediction.

d. Noninference.

10. One should decide whether or not the results and recommendations warrant any clinical change in clinical practice according to the following criteria (true or false):

a. Articles that report completely new causes of disease or first-time reports of the effectiveness of a diagnostic test or treatment should be viewed as preliminary only.

b. If other articles subsequently report the same findings, the reader may seriously consider incorporating the findings into practice.

c. The opinion of clinical experts should be obtained prior to clinical application.

d. In prescribing a new medication, use only the most reliable patients.

Answers appear on page 448.

PROBLEM SOLVING IN FAMILY MEDICINE

JOHN C. ROGERS and WENDY S. BIGGS

A major shift occurred in medical education approximately two decades ago, when medical educators began to place more emphasis on the teaching and assessment of problem-solving skills. New curricula were developed in some medical schools in North America to initiate problem-based learning, such as those at McMaster and Harvard (New Pathway). The ideas quickly spread to other medical schools, such as Bowman-Gray and Southern Illinois University. The new programs asserted that clinical skills consist of a set of reasoning strategies that are easily learned and enable students to solve any problem successfully, even novel, complex problems. However, research showed that the correlation between problem-solving performances in different clinical domains, such as nephrology and gastroenterology, was low. Elstein and colleagues called this "content specificity," implying that specific biomedical knowledge along with a set of generic problem-solving skills was necessary for expert problem-solving. Thus, although problem-solving performance is highly dependent on the solver's knowledge base relevant to a specific problem, teaching basic problem-solving steps does provide a foundation for clinical reasoning (Schmidt et al.).

Expert reasoning is characterized by knowledge structures known as "illness scripts." "Illness scripts" are created in memory from "book learning" and actual patients or cases and contain prototypic descriptions of how clinical features are interrelated in various diseases. Early clinical medical students have few firsthand experiences on which to draw, and thus, their prototypes are sparse, resulting in reasoning that is predominantly convoluted, based on the pathophysiology learned in the classroom. Later in medical training, case presentations become more concise, since more experienced students possess refined scenarios and concepts with which to categorize the illnesses (Schmidt et al.).

Second-year introduction to clinical medicine courses have typically presented students with one model for approaching clinical problems, that is, the complete history and physical. This is the standard assessment performed when a patient enters the hospital. It consists of the chief complaint, statement of the reliability of the patient as a historian, history of the present illness, past medical history, social history, family history, review of systems, complete multisystem physical examination, and laboratory data followed by an impression and initial plans. This map for doctor–patient encounters is followed very rigorously on internal medicine rotations where typically three to five patients per week receive a "complete workup" by the student. This general map is also followed on pediatrics, and in an abbreviated form on surgery and obstetrics/gynecology where a single problem is more typically the focus of the admission. When students enter the ambulatory arena, they quickly realize that the complete history and physical is an inappropriate map for these brief doctor–patient encounters. Although daily hospital visits are similar in that they are problem-focused, they, too, are an inappropriate map for ambulatory visits. Some of the distinctions between the daily rounds and ambulatory visits include:

1. Reasonably well defined problem versus often undifferentiated problems
2. Total physician control versus a large degree of patient control
3. Rapid access to laboratory and consultation services versus low access
4. Patient availability for reevaluation versus patient unavailability after completion of the encounter
5. Predominantly curative medicine versus often supportive and preventive medicine

In addition to these contrasts, the ambulatory experiences provide students with two other challenges: the types of problems confronted and the stages of the diseases. First, outpatient medicine includes numerous conditions that are either not seen or ignored during hospital admissions and that receive little attention in most medical curricula. Most medical students are trained in university medical centers, and, as noted in

Chapter 2, these centers admit a very small fraction of patients seen in primary care. Hence, students are not exposed to numerous illnesses which present to primary care doctors, and are unprepared to evaluate them. Second, the stages of diseases and appropriate therapeutic interventions differ considerably between hospital and ambulatory settings. For example, the Coronary Care Unit routines for unstable angina and "rule-out MI" bear little resemblance to the office management of stable exertional angina. Similarly, the treatment for diabetic ketoacidosis or the care of an acute COPD exacerbation differ greatly from therapy for the patient with non-insulin-dependent diabetes or the patient who smokes and has early signs of obstructive lung disease on pulmonary function tests. These two factors affect the illness scripts students have for problems seen in primary care.

There are three additional factors which further complicate the business of student training in generalist ambulatory care settings. First, since in family practice there is no filtering or focusing of patients or problems by age or organ system as in the other specialties, students must be prepared to confront a broad range of problems (see Tables 2–3 and 2–4 in Chapter 2). The top 30 diagnoses seen by office-based family physicians constitute only about two-thirds of all problems seen in the outpatient setting; furthermore, only three problems (general medicine examination, acute upper respiratory tract infection, and hypertension) are each seen in more than 5% of the visits (Rosenblatt et al.). In other words, the next patient to be seen could be any age and may present with any of more than 100 problems involving virtually any organ system and any pathophysiologic process. Family physicians also see a wide variety of clinical conditions in the hospital setting: The 50 most common hospital diagnoses by office-based family physicians constitute only 60% of the total list of problems treated by family physicians in the hospital (Rosenblatt et al.).

The second complicating factor is the amount of time dedicated to each of these ambulatory visits. The mean time per encounter for the 25 most frequent diagnoses ranges between 9 and 17 minutes, with the bulk of the mean times between 10 and 14 minutes (Rosenblatt et al.). Not only must the primary care physician deal with an extremely wide variety of problems, but he or she must do so within a relatively short time.

The third complicating factor differentiating ambulatory care from hospital care is the availability of the patient, especially for certain tests. In a hospital, the patient is virtually always "in the house" when the test is ordered, when it is done, and when the result is known. In the ambulatory setting, however, the patient is usually present in the doctor's office when the test is ordered, virtually always gone when the test is done, especially if it is done in an outside laboratory or radiologist's office, and only sometimes present when the result is known. These contrasts between the hospital and ambulatory settings underscore the need for an organized, disciplined approach to the ambulatory visit which cannot be taught in the hospital setting.

One way to view the ambulatory encounter consists of defining five major tasks for the clinician:

1. Construct a problem list.
2. Assess the patient's expectations.
3. Establish a therapeutic relationship.
4. Negotiate a management plan.
5. Learn from the encounter.

Each of these tasks consists of several steps (Table 18–1). A student should strive to complete each step, no matter how briefly, in order to master the components of the complete ambulatory encounter.

TASK 1: CONSTRUCT A PROBLEM LIST

The primary task is to construct a problem list (see Chapter 14). Most clinicians do this without consciously realizing it. Students, however, may need more guidance, because a problem list may include more than the patient's biomedical disease. Dr. I. R. McWhinney describes the difficulty in constructing problem lists:

1. The patient often presents more than one problem at the same visit.

2. The problems are often not presented in order of priority. The most serious problem may be left until last or not even mentioned at all.

3. The most sensitive problems may be expressed in indirect or metaphorical language.

4. The problem is not necessarily the same as the disease.

5. Much of the information presented by the patient

TABLE 18–1.   ENCOUNTER CHECKLIST

Task 1: Construct a Problem List
Acquire information
Generate biopsychosocial hypotheses
Interpret information
Evaluate hypotheses

Task 2: Assess the Patient's Expectations
Solicit patient's goals
Solicit patient's requests
Elicit patient's explanatory model
Elicit patient's prototypical experiences

Task 3: Negotiate a Management Plan
Develop a decision tree with options and outcomes
Determine likelihood of outcomes
Obtain patient's evaluations of outcomes
Select course of action

Task 4: Develop a Therapeutic Relationship
Gather contextual information
Solicit patient's cognitive appraisal
Elicit patient's emotional response
Elicit patient's coping response
Demonstrate unconditional regard

Task 5: Learn from the Encounter
Identify own problem-solving method
Identify standard operating procedures, rules, or protocols
Identify doctor–patient relationship model
Declare intentions for behavior change

is "noise," that is, it is not useful in solving the patient's present problems (Rakel).

Thus, a problem list may include a somatic complaint, an abnormal physical examination or laboratory finding for which an exact biomedical diagnosis has not been established, an emotional problem or significant social event that affects the patient's general health, or disease prevention and health promotion, in addition to any established biomedical and/or psychiatric diagnoses.

The four steps required to construct a problem list are rather obvious:

1. Acquire information.
2. Generate biopsychosocial hypotheses.
3. Interpret information.
4. Evaluate hypotheses.

Research findings for these steps are summarized in Table 18–3 (Elstein et al.). Much of the information gathered during the patient visit for assessing a patient's expectations (task 2) and developing a therapeutic relationship (task 3) is useful for diagnosing or defining the patient's problem. The nonverbal cues, the body language and facial expressions of the patient, as well as data from physician's direct inquiries, that is, the history, physical examination, and laboratory testing, are useful for diagnosing and defining the patient's problems. Sources of information other than the patient, such as the clinical setting, the medical record, other health professionals, and the patient's family, are also important for reliable and valid problem definition.

A major error in information gathering is failure to recognize a relevant or critical cue. Medical students are taught to be extremely thorough early in their training. As they gain more experience, the relevant or critical cues become more evident and the history and physical become more concise. The interview technique is important in obtaining as much information as possible. Open-ended questions allow the patient to tell his or her story and what is personally most important. Patients report the greatest satisfaction when doctors use open-ended questions and listen more (see Chapter 10). Then the interviewer can focus on the details that seem most relevant by asking the patient to elaborate. Asking "yes-no" questions may be most expedient, but they are often leading and disguise the patient's true problem. These questions should be saved for last to get information not covered well or to clarify points. By carefully directing the patient's discourse, a physician can obtain all the information needed and promote a good doctor–patient relationship simultaneously.

HOW TO DEVELOP A DIFFERENTIAL DIAGNOSIS

The generation of biopsychosocial hypotheses that can explain a patient's constellation of symptoms is one of the most critical steps in problem definition, and a source of continuing challenge to neophytes as well as experienced clinicians. A systematic approach initially aids in generating a differential list of diagnoses or hypotheses—the hypothesis matrix. In developing the matrix, one localizes the patient's problem and then considers the organ systems that could be involved, such as musculoskeletal, central nervous system, cardiovascular, lymphatics, pulmonary, gastrointestinal, or skin and connective tissue. Then, one considers the basic pathophysiologic processes responsible for somatic symptoms and diseases. Most medical students learn a mnemonic for this process such as KITTEN.

K (C)	-Congenital
I	-Infectious
T	-Toxic or metabolic
T	-Traumatic
E (I)	-Inflammatory
N	-Neoplastic

The mnemonic is by no means totally inclusive. Other processes to consider are degenerative, demyelinating, mechanical, immunologic, psychogenic, and idiopathic. Using these categories allows construction of a hypothesis matrix, for example, in a patient presenting with chest pain. The clinician first directs evaluation to general organ systems by asking system-specific questions, such as, for the cardiovascular system: anterior chest pain, palpitations, or dyspnea on exertion. This eliminates some organ systems from consideration when there are no relevant symptoms and focuses on the systems with positive findings. Next, possible pathophysiological processes are considered, such as inflammatory versus infectious, and the matrix is filled in with specific diagnoses, for example, pericarditis versus myocarditis. A matrix for a patient presenting with chest pain could look like the one in Table 18–2.

The hypothesis matrix can be used in a hierarchical manner. When the evaluation leads to a specific diagnosis, such as infectious pericarditis, there are further levels of differentiation to consider. The etiology of infection may be fungal, parasitic, bacterial, or viral. Similarly, if signs and symptoms point to bacterial pericarditis, it may be from *Staphylococcus aureus*, *Streptococcus pneumoniae*, or *Haemophilus influenzae*. Progressing

TABLE 18–2. HYPOTHESIS MATRIX FOR CHEST PAIN

PATHOPHYSIOLOGIC PROCESS	ORGAN SYSTEM		
	Cardiovascular	*Pulmonary*	*Gastrointestinal*
Mechanical	Myocardial infarction or dissecting aneurysm	Embolism	Achalasia
Inflammatory	Pericarditis	Pleuritis	Ulcer
Infectious	Endocarditis or myocarditis	Pneumonia	Gastroenteritis

from general to increasingly specific levels in a hypothesis matrix can be an efficient and effective strategy for thinking comprehensively about diagnostic possibilities in a manageable way without unnecessary detail.

Recognizing the major errors in generating diagnostic hypotheses is discussed in Table 18–3. Some errors are typical as students develop into experienced clinicians. On new rotations, common problems include failure to generate any hypotheses or the profuse generation of hypotheses, where every finding seems to suggest another disease. Increasing familiarity with problems seen in a specialty may overcome the first errors; however, the problem of failing to generate the correct diagnosis as a hypothesis or failure to generate a replacement hypotheses may still exist. The error of recurrent generation of hypotheses, which is thinking of the same disease in all the right and wrong places, may occur if an important diagnosis was missed in the past. Knowing what kinds of errors are common may not prevent them entirely, but may limit their frequency. One strategy is to stick to the hypothesis matrix and always state three to four hypotheses at any point in the encounter. This is useful on clinical rotations when cases are presented to residents and attendings. Quickly rattling off three or four possible diagnoses shows that the student is thinking!

Factors leading to the generation of hypotheses are extremely important (Table 18–4), and deliberate attention to them is critical to prevent serious omissions and harm to patients, and to preclude unfortunate commissions which may lead to unnecessary expense and also possible harm to patients.

TABLE 18–4. HYPOTHESES FORMATION

FEATURES OF HYPOTHESES
1. *Multiple systems.* Typically more than one organ system and more than one pathophysiologic process included in differential diagnosis.
2. *Hierarchical organization.* Starts general and becomes more specific.
3. *Competing formulations.* Diagnosis A versus diagnosis B. One condition *or* another, such as myocardial infarction versus pulmonary embolism.
4. *Functional relationship.* Diagnosis D secondary to diagnosis E. One diagnosis *and* another, such as transient ischemic attacks secondary to chronic atrial fibrillation with atrial thrombus.

FACTORS LEADING TO GENERATION OF HYPOTHESES
1. *Probability.* What is the likelihood of a condition's being the explanation?
2. *Treatability.* What could be wrong that can be treated and that if not diagnosed could harm the patient?
3. *Severity.* What could be the most serious condition that if missed could harm the patient?
4. *Salience.* How is this case just like the one seen recently?
5. *Novelty.* Is this an interesting or rare case, a "zebra"?

Source: Elstein AS, Shulman LC, Sprafka SA (Eds.): Medical Problem-Solving: An Analysis of Clinical Reasoning. Cambridge, Harvard University Press, 1978, with permission.

TABLE 18–3. STEPS IN CONSTRUCTING PROBLEM LISTS

I. *Acquire Information*
1. All relevant cues are not usually obtained; students are expected to be thorough, but "real" doctors are not.
2. Thoroughness is weakly associated with diagnostic accuracy; thus experienced clinicians can cut corners.
3. Efficiency is not related to diagnostic accuracy.

Major Error: Failure to acquire a relevant cue.

II. *Generate Biopsychosocial Hypotheses*
1. Hypotheses are generated early in encounter. Four to five hypotheses are considered within first 5 minutes after obtaining only three to five relevant cues.
2. Number of hypotheses is a function of the capacity of the short-term memory.
3. Number of hypotheses is fairly constant throughout encounter as diagnostic hunches from general to more specific are generated.

Major Errors
Failure to generate hypotheses: "Cannot think of a thing" (common for beginners).
Failure to generate correct formulation as hypothesis: "You cannot diagnosis it if you do not think of it."
Failure to generate competing hypotheses: "Can only think of one thing."
Failure to generate replacement hypotheses: "Premature closure."
Recurrent generation of hypotheses: Have favorite diseases and always look for them, even in the wrong places.
Profuse generation of hypotheses: Think of many possibilities but cannot focus them (common for beginners).

III. *Interpret Information*
1. Clinicians use a three-point scale: for (+), noncontributory (0), and against (−).
2. Overemphasize "for" information: Tend to look for information that supports various diagnoses and to pay little attention to findings that go against hunches in the differential diagnosis.
3. Accuracy of cue interpretation related to diagnostic accuracy: Must know what findings are associated with what diseases in order to make the correct diagnosis.

Major Errors
Clinicians ignore unreliability of cue—do not consider whether the cue may be wrong.
Often do not interpret available cues—gather information but do not use it in decisions even though it is relevant.
Often make interpretive errors:
   Overinterpretation: Saying "for" or "against" when really "noncontributory"
   Underinterpretation: Saying "noncontributory" when really "for" or "against"
   Misinterpretation: Saying "for" when really "against," or vice versa

Source: Elstein AS, Shulman LC, Sprafka SA (Eds.): Medical Problem-Solving: An Analysis of Chemical Reasoning. Cambridge, Harvard University Press, 1978, with permission.

The first factor to consider is "probability" what are the most likely (most common) explanations for the patient's problems? Uncommon and rare conditions are indeed rare in primary care where there is no filtering by referral to a medical center. The old truism applies: The uncommon manifestations of common diseases are more common than the common manifestations of uncommon disease, or as some people say, "When you hear hooves, think of horses, not zebras."

The next two factors to consider are "treatability" and "severity." A rank order of possibilities with the most likely at the top often has the severe treatable conditions at the bottom. In other words, the most common problems are not terribly dangerous on an acute basis, and the dangerous ones are seen infrequently. One of the intellectual challenges of primary care is to differentiate between common problems and the uncommon or rare condition that is severe and treatable, because to miss it could do irreparable harm to the patient. Severe diseases that are untreatable are important but not urgent, since the course of the disease cannot be altered and the passing of time until the next visit has no deleterious health implications. On the other hand, it is not acceptable to let a patient leave the office without first considering the severe, treatable conditions. The physician must be certain enough that the patient will be safe until the next visit. The degree of certainty required depends upon the patient's and the physician's tolerance of ambiguity and uncertainty as well as the expense and difficulty of definitively testing for the hypothetical conditions. One cannot afford to completely test for and rule out every possibility, but thorough knowledge of history and physical findings characteristic of the serious conditions can usually test the hypotheses to a sufficient degree of certainty.

The last two factors in Table 18–4—"salience" and "novelty"—may play a role in the generation of diagnostic hypotheses, but are not strongly recommended. Salience or "I recently had a patient with Q that presented this same way"—is very often invoked by clinicians, but commonly leads to errors. Typically, this factor brings to mind unusual or rare conditions that the clinician places high on his or her own priority list, often because the condition was missed previously and the patient had a bad outcome. This leads to more extensive, expensive, and possibly more invasive testing than would be indicated by a more objective estimate of the likelihood the patient has Q. Novelty is thinking of the esoteric diseases to have intellectual fun and to make patients "interesting cases." This strategy is a useful teaching and learning exercise and is often stimulating, but

can lead to excesses if the "zebra" is put near the front of the herd of horses.

Once the information has been gathered and hypotheses generated, the information must be interpreted with regard to the clinical hypotheses (Table 18–1). Knowledge about health conditions and associated symptoms, physical findings, and laboratory abnormalities is used to decide whether the presence or absence of a specific piece of information supports or refutes a particular hypothesis. A matrix helps organize the cues obtained during the patient interview (Table 18–5). Using the diagnoses from the diagnostic hypotheses matrix, one can synthesize information to systematically rule in or eliminate diagnoses by mentally placing +, 0, or − in each column according to data obtained during the patient encounter.

Various strategies exist to evaluate hypotheses and trim a bulky matrix of differential diagnoses to a working diagnosis. First, one can rule out possibilities if the patient has several absent findings or negative cues. Second, patients may give positive cues that help rule in a condition. Especially helpful is the "pathognomonic" cue, one that is consistent with the condition and whose presence helps rule in the condition. Of course, ruling in those hypotheses that best account for the positive and negative findings depends upon biomedical knowledge and clinical experience, so that narrowing down the matrix becomes more rapid with time. The only evidence that this process occurs in the physician's or the student's mind is the statement "I think the problem is _____."

The rule-out strategy is used a great deal in primary care, especially for the severe treatable conditions that are uncommon. To effectively rule out these diseases, clinicians look for the absence of findings that are frequently seen in patients with the conditions. Such findings are "exquisitively sensitive" in that they have a high true positive and a low false negative rate. The absence of such a sensitive finding is strong evidence against the possibility that the patient has the disease. This strategy is also used for more common conditions, since it can efficiently trim a rather long, comprehensive list of hypotheses. Telling patients what they "don't have" reassures them, even if what they "do have" is not known.

When applying the rule-in strategy, clinicians look for the presence of findings that are "extremely specific," that is, they have a low false positive and a high true negative rate. Such findings seldom appear in the absence of the disease, so their presence is strong evidence in support of the disease. Pathognomonic findings are usually 100% specific by definition. This strategy is used to

TABLE 18–5. INTERPRETING INFORMATION TO EVALUATE HYPOTHESES

CUES	Pneumonia	Pulmonary Embolism	Dissecting Aneurysm	Pericarditis
Risk Factors				
Pain syndrome				
Associated signs and symptoms				
Laboratory results				

confirm a diagnosis after the other leading contenders are eliminated by the rule-out strategy.

Unfortunately, many historical and physical findings (symptoms and signs), and even laboratory tests, are not "exquisitively sensitive" or "extremely specific," but they may be all the information available. How are the true and false positive rates balanced if the finding is present or the test result abnormal? Likewise, if the finding is absent or the test normal, how are the true and false negative rates balanced? An approach for combining these factors is important, since few patients have the classic manifestations of diseases described in textbooks. Even in textbook descriptions, qualifiers, such as "very often," "usually," "sometimes," and "rarely," are used to indicate variability in the sensitivity or specificity of clinical data. These words are obviously too vague to combine in a way to give precision to the interpretation of data and evaluation of hypotheses.

Likelihood ratios can be used to quantify and interpret data in clinical practice (Griner et al., Sackett et al.). For positive or abnormal results, calculate the ratio of the true positive rate and the false positive rate (TPR/FPR). For negative or normal results, calculate the ratio of the false negative rate and the true negative rate (FNR/TNR). These likelihood ratios indicate the degree to which the odds or likelihood of a disease is affected by the presence (positive likelihood ratio) or the absence (negative likelihood ratio) of a particular finding. The odds of a disease are changed as the physician acquires each additional piece of data. Except for unusual exceptions, the prior odds of a possible diagnosis are decreased when the physician learns the patient does not have a sign or symptom or an abnormal test (negative likelihood ratio), and the prior odds are increased when the physician learns the patient does have the sign or symptom or abnormal test (positive likelihood ratio).

This is the same logic as the rule-out and rule-in strategies, but made more explicit and precise. When an "exquisitely sensitive" finding is absent, the negative likelihood ratio is expected to be quite small due to the very low false negative rate, that is, FNR/TNR is small so the prior odds of the disease are decreased substantially. Similarly, when an "extremely specific" finding is present, such as a pathognomonic finding, the positive likelihood ratio is expected to be quite large due to the very small false positive rate, that is, TPR/FPR is large so the prior odds are increased substantially.

The ratios extend this logic, however, by simultaneously considering a finding's sensitivity and its specificity. If a test were both "exquisitely sensitive" and "extremely specific," the negative likelihood ratio would be very, very small due to the low false negative rate and the high true negative rate (FNR/TNR). The positive likelihood ratio would be very, very large due to the high true positive rate and the low false positive rate (TPR/FPR). Findings with various combinations of levels of sensitivity and specificity will produce likelihood ratios of varying magnitudes, and hence, information of varying usefulness to the task of evaluating diagnostic hypotheses such that most are ruled out and a working diagnosis is selected or ruled in.

An example illustrates these ideas. A common problem in ambulatory care is the selection and interpretation of laboratory tests for patients with sore throat. Table 18–6 displays several options, including various streptococcus culture media, rapid strep tests, and EBV-mononucleosis tests. First, by comparing these tests, how the sensitivity affects the likelihood ratios when the specificities of the tests are equal (standard versus selec-

TABLE 18–6. SELECTING TESTS FOR PATIENTS WITH SORE THROATS

Blood Agar Cultures for Streptococcus

	STANDARD	SELECTIVE	DETECKTA-KIT
Sensitivity	.92	.85	.97
Specificity	1.00	1.00	.98
LR+	∞	∞	48.5
LR−	.08	.15	.03
Time	12–24 hours, perhaps 36–48 hours		

Rapid Strep Tests

	DIRECTIGEN	STREP-ID	STREP-A-FLUOR
Sensitivity	.88	.72	.44
Specificity	.92	.98	.78
LR+	11.0	36.0	2.0
LR−	.13	.29	.72
Time (minutes)	65	10	15

Gram Stain of Erythematous Area or Exudate for Strep*

Sensitivity	.73
Specificity	.96
LR+	18.25
LR−	.28
Time (minutes)	5

Tests for Epstein-Barr Virus–Mononucleosis

WBC Differential >50% lymphocytes, usually atypical lymphocytes		Rapid Slide Test (Positive Monospot equivalent to heterophil >1:224)	
WEEK 1	**PEAK**	**WEEK 1**	**PEAK**
Sensitivity .82	.90	.85	.96
Specificity .98	.98	.98	.98
LR+[a] 41.0	45.0	42.5	48.0
LR−[b] .18	.10	.15	.04

Heterophil ≥ 1:224

		EBV antibody >1:10
	WEEK 1	**PEAK**	**PEAK**
Sensitivity	.85	.97	.99
Specificity	.99	.99	1.00
LR+†	85.0	97.0	∞
LR−‡	.15	.03	.01

*Positive = spherical gram-positive cocci, singly or in pairs, in association with disrupted PMNs (neutrophils).
†LR+ Positive likelihood ratio.
‡LR− Negative likelihood ratio.

tive culture medias; WBC differential versus rapid slide test) becomes evident. Similarly, how the specificity affects the likelihood ratios when the sensitivities are the same (selective culture media versus rapid slide test at one week or heterophil at one week; Deteckta-kit media versus heterophil at peak) is apparent. Second, by comparing the ratios for the alternative tests, one can choose the preferred test based on how positive and negative results for the various tests affect the odds of strep throat or mononucleosis. Third, one may decide to use a sequential testing strategy, such as a strep culture after a negative rapid strep test, because the rapid strep test's negative likelihood ratio does not decrease the odds of strep enough to rule it out. Finally, once a clinician routinely chooses a test, he or she can remember how much the results of the test increase or decrease the odds of the disease, that is, how much information is obtained in exchange for the effort, time, and expense of the test(s).

Clinicians do not go through this type of analysis every time they order a test, interpret clinical findings, or evaluate hypotheses. However, the knowledge of likelihood ratios and this type of analysis can be used to develop decision rules or standard operating procedures that are routinely applied in common clinical situations. The analysis can also help the physician decipher difficult or puzzling cases. Table 18–7 reviews some general rules physicians use for evaluating hypotheses.

Experienced clinicians typically arrive at a diagnosis without being explicitly aware of having performed the four steps required to construct a problem list during the clinical encounter. They are much like the tennis pro who concentrates on the strategy of the game and has little or no conscious awareness of the movements required for placing the serve or the forehand passing shot to take advantage of the opponent's weakness. A student is like a beginning tennis player who must learn the component parts of a forehand swing and practice them repeatedly alone, as well as with an instructor pres-

TABLE 18–7. HYPOTHESIS EVALUATION

DECISION RULES: METHODS TO TRIM DIFFERENTIAL DIAGNOSIS

1. *Pathognomonic.* Use a "diagnostic finding" to rule in or rule out a diagnosis by depending on presence or absence of a particular finding.

2. *Reject: Most Negatives.* Rule out those possibilities with several "against" findings. Either patient does not have features common in condition (absent, therefore "against") or patient has features that are inconsistent with the condition (present, therefore "against"). Very often used as a strategy.

3. *Select: Most Positives.* Rule in those possibilities with the most "for" findings, ignoring any "against" findings. Not a very good strategy, since unable to explain the "against" findings.

4. *Pattern.* Rule in those diagnoses that best account for the "for" findings, even considering the "against" findings—is the pattern of findings consistent with the condition? Probably most commonly used strategy.

Source: Elstein AS, Shulman LC, Sprafka SA (Eds.): Medical Problem-Solving: An Analysis of Clinical Reasoning. Cambridge, Harvard University Press, 1978, with permission.

ent. These four steps—acquiring information, generating hypotheses, interpreting information, and evaluating hypotheses—are the components of the task of constructing a problem list, and each must be deliberately practiced many times over for the student to become a competent clinician.

TASK 2: ASSESS THE PATIENT'S EXPECTATIONS

Assessing patients' expectations can determine the need for and guide patient education. In addition, the process of learning patients' understanding or perceptions can be used in future encounters to negotiate the treatment plans with the patients and thus enhance compliance. As noted in Table 18–1, there are four key concepts involved in this task: patients' goals, patients' requests, patients' explanatory model, and patients' prototypic experiences.

Patients' goals are the ends that they wish to achieve with regard to health, functional ability, or symptoms. Typically, this is not made explicit during the encounter and often cannot be easily articulated by patients, or even by physicians for that matter. Sometimes patients clearly state that they need to be well by such and such date because of some important event, such as a wedding or vacation or graduation. Others simply want to be rid of the symptoms because they are uncomfortable. Others want to be reassured because they are alarmed or concerned about bodily sensations. Still others wish to be able to perform certain levels of function for their job or personal satisfaction. Finally, others may want to live long enough to see some critical personal event, at which time their lives can be complete. Attempting to identify as explicitly as possible a patient's goals can help form a strong alliance between the doctor and the patient, particularly if both can agree on a unified commitment to the achievement of the stated goal.

As they go through medical training, physicians learn to work toward implicit goals of curing disease, relieving symptoms, and discovering causes of signs and symptoms. If at all possible, the primary goal is to cure disease. Usually clinicians accept relieving symptoms until the cure removes the symptoms or the disease resolves itself, or in the case of chronic incurable diseases, function is maintained. The driving force for physicians, however, is finding an explanation for symptoms and signs, for it provides the basis for providing cures and symptomatic relief.

These goals work well in most clinical encounters. Patients visit doctors wanting to be "fixed," returning to their normal state of health as soon as possible. If patients cannot be cured, usually they are satisfied with symptomatic relief until the condition resolves itself. When neither cure nor relief of symptoms is possible, knowing the cause of their troubles and explaining how, maybe why, they are ill, satisfies most patients. Sometimes, however, these goals lead to problems in the doctor–patient relationship. Physicians may become so preoccupied with curing disease that they feel powerless when cure is impossible and caring and palliation are all they can offer. Physicians may not appreciate how important caring is to patients, perhaps more important than curing, and that patients certainly see caring as "doing something" (see also Chapter 7, "Care of the Dying Patient").

Another major problem occurs when physicians are unable to find reasons for patients' symptoms or to relieve them. The search for the cause of the symptoms may escalate to more and more tests and more and more doctor visits: an expensive and potentially risky search that repeatedly finds "nothing wrong." For these patients, reassurances based on negative test results are often interpreted as, "The doctor said it was all in my head." In addition, if an explanation is not found, attempts to control the symptoms may repeatedly fail. Here attempts to achieve the implicit goals lead to frustration and a "stuck" feeling for both doctors and patients. One effective strategy is the opposite of the physician's usual "take charge" approach to clinical problems: "Don't just do something, stand there!" By altering the goal of explaining symptoms to one of maintaining function despite persistent symptoms and no identifiable cause, the destructive spiral may be broken. After abandoning the fundamental goal, the physician can tell the patient that a cause will probably never be found and the symptoms probably will never be resolved or even controlled, and that together the patient and the physician must focus on getting on with life (functional abilities) in the face of persistent, unexplainable problems. The patient may stay and strive to become optimally functional, or may never return to the practice. Either way, the physician has not contributed to additional unwarranted testing or treatments, has minimized personal frustration from repeatedly thwarted goals, and may have weakened the patient's fixation on an unattainable goal. This strategy is useful whenever somatization is present and the patient's resistance to psychosocial exploration, much less psychogenic explanation for symptoms, is very high. Making patients' and physicians' goals explicit allows them to be validated, negotiated, or changed as needed to achieve the best outcome for both parties.

Patients' requests are their notions of the means needed to achieve their goals (Like and Zyzanski). Patients often want medical information about their problems, such as what it is called, what causes it, how long it is going to last, and what tests may be needed. At other times, patients want emotional assistance and are not seeking physical examination or laboratory testing. Very often in ambulatory care, patients simply want the physician to listen while they share their own perspective about the problems. Other patients want advice about general health matters such as diet and exercise. Finally, patients often want some biomedical treatment for their physical discomfort such as medications or surgery. Patients sometimes are very explicit about what they expect the doctor to do, but often this is only indirectly mentioned during the visit. By explicitly determining a patient's request for the visit, the clinician can address this issue and negotiate directly with the patient if there

seems to be disagreement between the physician's recommended means of achieving the goal and the patient's desired means. This, of course, presumes that both parties are working toward the same goal.

Typically, one source of patients' requests is their explanatory model. The concept of explanatory model comes from the anthropological literature and refers to the theory about the disease (Kleinman). There are a number of available models about the causes of diseases, their prognosis, and appropriate treatments, such as the western biomedical model taught in allopathic and osteopathic schools of medicine, the chiropractic theory, and numerous others not typically taught in U.S. medical schools, such as those followed by lay healers. In any community there may be specific cultural theories, which may follow the biomedical model but with misunderstandings, distortions, and unsubstantiated speculations. Nevertheless, the beliefs that patients hold often drive their requests and strongly influence what they expect of physicians and what they are willing to do for themselves in order to achieve their goals.

Another determinant of patients' requests is their prototypic experiences. There are three main sources of these experiences: personal experience with a problem, experience of a family member or friend, or reading or hearing about the issue through media such as magazines and television (Like and Steiner). Sometimes these sources of information, particularly significant family members or friends, have much more influence in patients' lives than do physicians. If strong experiences in these areas have led to a request that is contrary to the physician's recommendations, then the doctor's plans for the patient may not produce the desired result unless this conflict and its source are addressed directly.

The task then is to gather information related to each of these four concepts before attempting patient education or negotiating the management plan. This inquiry may reveal that there are no conflicts, no critical gaps in the patient's understanding, and no need for a long-winded discussion by the physician. Alternatively, the doctor and patient may discover areas where brief, focused education and dialogue could be very effective and satisfactory for both parties. This inquiry may even reveal major gaps or conflicts that perhaps could be resolved after serious negotiation or that may lead to the decision that the doctor and patient could not have a successful working relationship. This approach to clinical encounters is sometimes described as "patient-centered care" in contrast to the focus on diagnostic reasoning or "doctor-centered care" covered in Task 1.

TASK 3: DEVELOP A THERAPEUTIC RELATIONSHIP

To be a healer and help solve patients' problems, the physician must foster a relationship of mutual trust and respect. In primary care, where a patient may be seen for many years, there are many opportunities to establish a workable therapeutic relationship. However, when the doctor and patient do not have a long-standing interaction, a therapeutic relationship must be developed in a brief period of time.

Although a physician's nonverbal cues to the patient may be a major determinant in establishing an effective relationship, the direct inquiries he or she makes will foster the desired relationship. The four areas in which the physician can inquire include:

1. Contextual information about family, work, and sociocultural environments
2. Information about patients' cognitive appraisal of their context
3. Information on patients' emotional response to their context
4. Information on the patients' efforts at coping with their context, appraisal, and emotional response (Table 18–1) (Stuart and Lieberman)

Gathering contextual information indicates to the patient that the physician is not interested simply in a diseased organ system or pathophysiologic process, but is concerned about the person who is experiencing the illness. In addition to listening carefully and maintaining eye contact, asking a patient about work, family life, and social world demonstrates the physician's regard for the patient as a person. This conversation also allows the doctor and patient to have a human connection on a basis other than the reporting of physical complaints and the prescribing of biomedical treatments.

By gathering information about the patient's cognitive appraisal, emotional response, and coping efforts, the physician reinforces the view that the patient's physical complaints cannot be considered in isolation from the rest of the patient's life. This acknowledgment of the interaction of the patient's emotional life and physical well-being also contributes to the development of a personal bond between doctor and patient which is necessary for an optimal healing relationship. Asking people questions about who is at home, what type of work they do, if they have a confidant or tangible social support or physical help, and what they think about what is going on in their lives is relatively easy to do. Treading on emotional ground and asking people how they feel about their lives, however, takes more courage. Peoples' responses are unpredictable. The possibility of "opening Pandora's box" usually intimidates students, residents, and many practicing physicians, who feel they do not have enough skill to deal with strong emotions, especially negative ones. People usually do not expect the physician to solve these problems. Instead, most are very grateful that their physician has taken the time to ask and listen. Most importantly, verbally and nonverbally expressing empathy manifests the unconditional regard necessary in any therapeutic relationship (Stuart and Lieberman).

Asking how someone is coping with a situation or feelings is more straightforward and less difficult than asking about feelings. Coping mechanisms can be categorized into three types: (1) attempt to change the problematic situation, (2) change the way an unchangeable situation is thought about, and (3) decrease the stress from situations that cannot be changed or

thought about differently. By challenging a patient's restricted range of coping mechanisms and outlining alternatives he or she may not have considered, the physician may expand the patient's repertoire of coping mechanisms. Patients also may gain specific coping skills through assertiveness training (type 1), cognitive restructuring (type 2), or stress management, specifically meditation, progressive relaxation, self-hypnosis, biofeedback, or exercise (type 3). Asking questions about the patient's context, cognitive appraisal, emotional responses, and coping skills goes beyond the biomedical model and may develop a therapeutic relationship that will intervene in patients' lives in a meaningful manner.

TASK 4: NEGOTIATE A MANAGEMENT PLAN

Being a master diagnostician is often viewed as one of the higher levels of achievement in the medical art. Each week, the case study in the *New England Journal of Medicine* provides a challenge for those who aspire to become proficient diagnosticians and illustrates how some of the best physicians perform the art. By observing their dialogue and reflecting upon our own approach, we note how people may take different paths to arrive at a diagnosis. We also note how the process of diagnosing may be similar among practitioners, and finally, whether the selected hypothesis is the "correct diagnosis."

When it comes to management and discharge plans, however, the variability among practitioners is often even more dramatic than that observed for the diagnostic process. There may be a "treatment of choice" or a series of "appropriate" treatments of which one may be "preferred." Even when the choice is limited to two or three different treatments, the process by which one course of action is selected is often unclear to the accomplished physician and even more obscure to the student.

Although it is not fully understood how experienced clinicians make management decisions, there are steps that at least help structure and define the decisions that must be made (Weinstein et al.). The first is to develop a decision tree that includes the therapeutic options and the outcomes that can result from each option. This structure outlines the treatment alternatives from which the physician and patient can choose, as well as the potential outcomes or consequences, both minor and major, of each selection, as in Figure 18–1A. This step may be more difficult than it sounds; thus, just as patients may unconsciously restrict their range of coping responses, the clinician may unduly restrict the number of management options under consideration. Early in physicians' training this may be due to lack of knowledge, but later it may occur because time pressure promotes automatic and unconscious judgment of options that eliminates many from consideration even before they are mentioned to the patient. Always listing at least three treatment options prevents closed thinking about alternative choices.

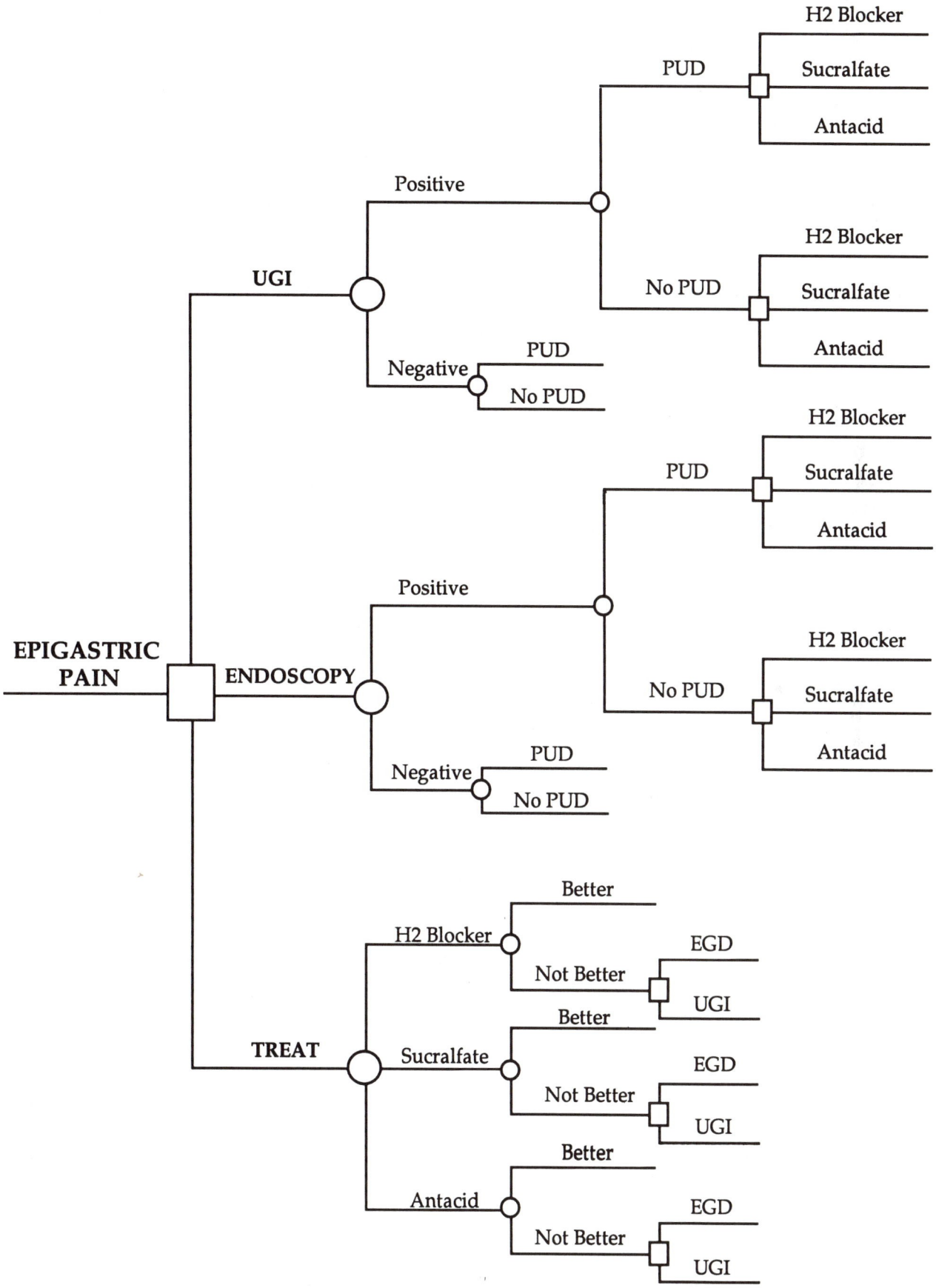

Figure 18–1A. Outline of a decision tree. Each branch would end with specific outcomes. PUD = peptic ulcer disease; UGI = barium x-ray of upper gastrointestinal tract; EGD = endoscopy of esophagus, stomach, or duodenum.

Often, it is important to ask patients if they have any ideas, particularly if they know a lot about their disease or have had the problem previously. Stating several options to patients does not take much time and involves the patients in their own care. Sometimes by drawing the decision tree as in Figure 18–1A, both the physician and the patient can visualize and openly discuss the various options.

Just as three or more options are considered, three or more outcomes should be pondered (Figure 18–1B). A clinician should know what the desired outcome is, what serious, even life-threatening complications can occur, and what minor side effects patients may experience. Patients will want to know about all three in order to make an informed choice. Patients also may wish to know the likelihood of each of the outcomes.

The next step is to obtain the patient's preference with regard to the outcomes and the treatment alternatives. There are formal ways of assessing a patient's preferences, such as category rating, time tradeoff, and standard gamble (Weinstein et al.). However, physicians usually use these formal methods in informal ways without they or the patients realizing it.

The study that quantified the amount of stress (adjustment) associated with life events or changes (Holmes and Rahe) used the category rating technique. The death of a spouse was considered to be the most stressful and was given an arbitrary score of 500 points. People then gave points to other life events, such as marriage and divorce, childbirth or child leaving home, new mortgage, loss of a job, and so forth. Similarly, scales of 0 to 10 or 0 to 100, with 10 or 100 being the most stressful or undesirable outcome, are used to get information from patients on levels of pain or other symptoms. This also may be done for the various outcomes that could occur after different treatments. This strategy helps rank order the outcomes by desirability as well as providing data on relative weights of the patient's preferences.

In time tradeoff, people state how many years of a completely healthy life they would exchange for 10 years in a state of health described by one of the outcomes of the decision tree, considering disability, limited activities, pain, and so forth (Weinstein et al.). This method provides values for the various health states that could occur as a result of the treatment, and helps physician and patient better understand the magnitude of the difference in value those alternative outcomes hold for the patient.

For the standard gamble, patients choose between staying in a particular state of health or taking a gamble with two possible outcomes. The best outcome is usually perfect health, and the worst is immediate death (Llewellyn-Thomas et al.). By varying the likelihood of the best and worst outcomes (always equaling 100%, since these are the only two possibilities) the value of the particular state of health is determined by when the patient stops taking the gamble but prefers to stay in the described state of health. Physicians often use a variation of the standard gamble when talking with patients about treatment options. Physician and patient both recognize that each treatment is a gamble of sorts, with potentially good and bad results. Usually physicians present the facts as they know them based on the likelihoods of the good and not-so-good outcomes and ask patients if they want to take the gamble.

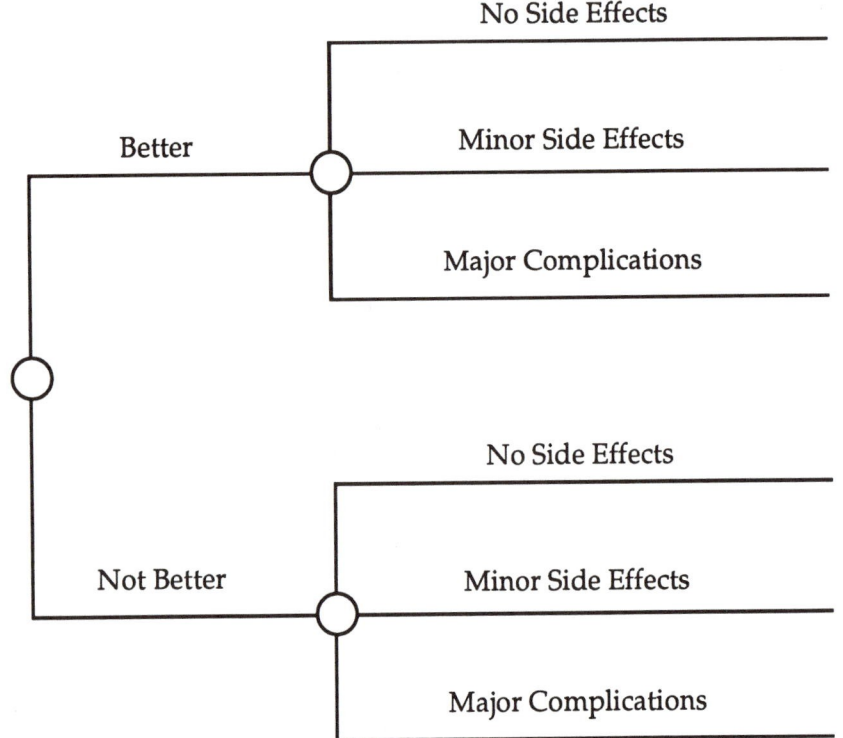

Figure 18–1B. Decision tree. General outcomes.

Unfortunately, in category-rating, time tradeoff, or standard gamble, clinicians may subtly, even nonverbally, reveal their biases. They typically "accentuate the positive and eliminate the negative" when discussing options, even when the options are statistically equivalent. If the options are put in positive terms, patients will tend to accept treatment. For example, if treatment is presented as having a 90% chance of no serious complications instead of as a 10% risk of serious complications, patients will tend to accept the treatment. However, to inform truly rather than convince patients, the physician must give a balanced message using parallel phrases: 10% chance of major complications or 90% chance of no complications. Then, when a patient selects an option, it is not skewed by the style of presentation, and it more accurately represents his or her values.

You may not go through these processes explicitly during every encounter, since you will not have time, and patients vary in their desire for direct involvement in medical decisions that affect them. On the other hand, you may do it informally and quite quickly in your head once you have command of the components of the methods. If, at a minimum, you share your thoughts with patients about three options and their major results, patients will be very grateful. They will know why you are recommending tests or treatments, will feel more involved, and will be more likely to comply with your suggestions or directions. Also, it takes a burden off you, since your patients now own and are more responsible for their health and the medical decisions that affect their health. This strategy permits real negotiation between you and your patients about your advice and what they choose to do about the problems they bring to you. By simply providing the patient with the likelihoods and getting an idea of the patient's preference through one of the three techniques discussed, you can usually quickly choose a course of action that is based on the best medical knowledge and the patient's values.

TASK 5: LEARN FROM THE ENCOUNTER

Learning from a patient encounter is a principal way physicians continue their education on a day-to-day basis. Reflecting on the encounter can help the physician determine ways in which the relationship with a particular patient and the management of that patient's problems can be improved as the care continues. Physicians can also develop a fuller understanding of the patient's problems in more general terms so that the care of other patients is improved.

There are four key components to learning from the encounter:

1. Identify the problem-solving method used or errors in the process committed during the encounter.
2. Identify the type of doctor-patient relationship.
3. Identify decision policies, rules, or protocols used during the encounter or at least applicable to the clinical problems involved in the visit.

4. Declare an intention for behavioral change.

Reviewing the processes by which a diagnosis was made and the management plan implemented can identify biases or pitfalls that may become habitual and lead to misdiagnosis or inappropriate management decisions. For example, there are specific errors that can occur at each of the four steps of the diagnostic process as outlined previously (Table 18–3). In addition, the heuristics or rules of thumb used to make judgments can often lead to biases, as described by Kahneman, Slovic, and Tversky in their classic book *Judgment Under Uncertainty: Heuristics and Biases* (1982). There are also a series of decision-making styles that have been described by Barrows (Table 18–8). These errors in problem solving cannot be completely avoided, but by reflecting upon encounters and noting when errors occur, clinicians may make these errors less frequently and may avoid the self-deception that all is well with their decision making.

One simple way of characterizing the type of doctor-patient relationship involves three different models: active-passive, guidance-cooperation, and mutual participation (Szasz and Hollender). In the active-passive relationship, the physician is presumed to know what is best for the patient in all ways, and the patient is presumed to be unable or unwilling to make independent decisions and assume responsibility for the consequences of those decisions. In this model, the physician is often seen as paternalistic or maternalistic by being very protective and directive of the patient. The patient in this model is passive and overtly or covertly says, "Tell me what to do, Doc."

The mutual participation model is more common as patients become very knowledgeable about their bodies, factors contributing to illness and health, and the risks

TABLE 18–8. PROBLEM-SOLVING STYLES

Eureka	Pathognomonic or powerful piece of information brings to mind one obvious diagnosis.
Buckshot	Disorganized interview and inordinately large number of diagnostic possibilities.
Basket	Every conceivable question and nearly every organ system before any diagnostic possibilities considered
Single Diagnosis at One Time	One diagnostic possibility ruled in or ruled out; if the diagnosis is ruled out, another diagnostic possibility is considered.
Cookie Cutter	Preset diagnoses for patients with certain demographic characteristics and presenting complaints force the patient to fit.
Disease of the Week	Same diagnostic possibilities and same interview and examination for each patient.
Cookbook	Rigidly follows an algorithm outlining appropriate interview and examination for specific presenting complaints or problems.
Stepwise	Several appropriate diagnostic possibilities early in the encounter guide the interview and examination to "test" each possibility.
Biomedical Scientist	Only biomedical diagnostic possibilities considered.

and benefits of available treatments. In this type of relationship, the physician shares decision making as equally as possible with a patient with the full understanding that it is the patient who must live with the consequences. The patient acknowledges this responsibility and works with the physician as he or she shares the uncertainty inherent in medicine by frankly discussing with the patient what could be wrong, diagnostic and therapeutic possibilities, and potential risks and benefits of these options. With the sharing of knowledge and responsibility between the partners, decisions are reached mutually and then implemented by those with the technical expertise required.

In between these two extremes is the guidance-cooperation model in which the patient is expected to follow the physician's advice but may assert some level of independent decision making. The physician provides information, but feels that the patient is not entirely capable of autonomous adult decision making and acceptance of consequences. In this relationship there is a dynamic tension between the physician's desire to do what is in the best interest of the patient and the patient's need for independent decision making.

Individual doctor-patient relationship models do not remain static over time but move among the three different types, depending upon the clinical problem, the stage of the relationship over time, and the clinical setting. The usefulness of classifying the doctor-patient relationship in this way and reflecting upon it during an encounter is that models can be switched as needed to accomplish the mutual goals of the doctor-patient encounter.

It also is useful to identify what decision policies, rules, or protocols were operating in the clinical encounter. Each physician develops policies regarding the diagnostic process and therapeutic management. Some of these policies may be related to the goals of diagnosis and therapy. For example, some physicians feel that they must rule out all organic problems before considering a psychosocial diagnosis; some feel they should maximally evaluate problems with diagnostic tests regardless of the cost; some focus diagnostic evaluation on treatable or serious conditions, with more unusual or less severe conditions receiving less priority; and so forth. With regard to management, physicians will develop policies for therapeutic goals, for example, "tight" versus "loose" diabetic control, aggressiveness regarding life-sustaining interventions, emphasis on curative versus preventive care, and so forth.

In addition to these goal-related policies, clinicians may adopt protocol-related policies developed by others, such as diagnostic protocols or algorithms that branch depending upon various test results. They may also adopt therapeutic protocols with standard duration and sequencing of interventions and standard evalua-

tion procedures to monitor the effectiveness of therapy and to detect side effects or complications. In the treatment of hypertension, for example, step therapy and sequential monotherapy are examples of two alternative treatment protocols for this condition. Finally, physicians have developed formal decision rules for determining obstetrical risk scores or diagnosing particular conditions (for example, Jones criteria for diagnosis of rheumatic fever). Sophisticated mathematical decision rules for diagnosing coronary ischemia or deciding whether or not to perform lymph node biopsy are also readily available (Pozen et al., Slap et al.). These rules, however, contain a number of hidden assumptions, which may negate their applicability in certain situations.

By reflecting on the clinical encounter, the physician can determine whether any "standard operating procedures" were followed, whether the policies and protocols were appropriate in the particular clinical situation, and whether the procedures and rules may need to be revised in the light of new research and experience. A key learning task throughout the physician's career is to determine what "standard operating procedures" experts are recommending and how these recommendations are being revised on a continual basis. By reviewing the clinical encounter in these terms, one can determine whether an individual's practice of medicine is state-of-the-art or behind the times.

Finally, once this reflective self-assessment is completed, the physician must declare his or her intention for behavioral change. Consciously making a statement about intentions, whether general or specific, increases the likelihood that the physician will actually change his or her mode of interactions with patients.

SUMMARY: THE AMBULATORY ENCOUNTER CHECKLIST

These five tasks—constructing a problem list, assessing the patient's expectations, developing a therapeutic relationship, negotiating a management plan, and learning from the encounter—and their component parts, constitute a checklist to guide young clinicians through encounters (Table 18–1). As noted at the beginning, this list does not constitute everything that must be accomplished in a competent manner during an ambulatory clinical encounter, but does describe the key decisions and thought processes that must occur for optimal encounters. The clinical illustrations in this text are intended to provide further guidance in future patient encounters. Only with further experience will medical students learn how to incorporate these steps with more ease.

REFERENCES

Elstein AS, Shulman LC, Sprafka SA (Eds.): Medical Problem-Solving: An Analysis of Clinical Reasoning. Cambridge, Harvard University Press, 1978.

Griner PF, Panzer RJ, Greenland P. Clinical Diagnosis and the Laboratory—Logical Strategies for Common Medical Problems. Chicago, Year Book Medical Publishers, 1986.

Holmes TH, Rahe RH. The Social Readjustments Rating Scale. J Psychosom Res 1967; 11:213–218.

Kahneman D, Slovic P, Tversky A (Eds.): Judgment Under Uncertainty. Heuristics and Biases. New York, Cambridge University Press, 1982.

Kleinman A. Patients and Healers in the Context of Culture. Berkeley, University of California Press, 1980, p. 106.

Like R, Steiner RP. Medical anthropology and the family physician. Fam Med 1986; 18:87–92.

Like R, Zyzanski S. Patient requests in family practice: A focal point for clinical negotiations. Fam Prac 1986; 3:216–227.

Llewellyn-Thomas H, Sutherland HJ, Tibshirani R, Ciampi A, Till JE, Boyd NF. The measurement of patients' values in medicine. Med Decis Making 1982; 2:449–462.

Pozen MW, D'Agostino RB, Selker HP, Sykowski PA, Hood WB, Jr. A predictive instrument to improve coronary care unit admission practices in acute ischemic heart disease: A prospective multicenter clinical trial. N Engl J Med 1984; 310:1273–1278.

Rakel RE (Ed.): Textbook of Family Practice. 4th ed. Philadelphia, W.B. Saunders, 1990.

Rosenblatt RA, Chetkin OC, et al. The structure and content of family practice: Current status and future trends. J Fam Pract 1982; 15:681–722.

Sackett DC, Haynes RB, Tugwell P. Clinical Epidemiology—A Basic Science for Clinical Medicine. Boston, Little, Brown, 1985.

Schmidt HG, Norman GR, Boshuizen HPA. A cognitive perspective on medical expertise: Theory and implications. Acad Med 1990; 65:611–621.

Slap GB, Conner JL, Wigton RS, Schwartz JS. Validation of a model to identify young patients for lymph node biopsy. JAMA 1986; 255:2768–2773.

Stuart MR, Lieberman JA. The Fifteen Minute Hour—Applied Psychotherapy for the Primary Care Physician. New York, Praeger, 1986.

Szasz TS, Hollender MH. A contribution to the philosophy of medicine. The basic models of the doctor-patient relationship. Arch Intern Med 1956; 97:585–592.

Weinstein MC, Fineberg HU, Elstein AS, Frazier HS, Neuhauser D, Neutra RR, McNeil BJ. Clinical Decision Analysis. Philadelphia, W.B. Saunders, 1980.

White RL, Williams F, Greenberg B. Ecology of medical care. N Engl J Med 1961; 265:885.

QUESTIONS

1. Which of the following is true? An "illness script" describes
   a. The symptoms of a malingering patient.
   b. The prototypic clinical features of a disease
   c. The standard protocol to work up a disease.
   d. The manner in which an ill patient acts in front of his physician.

2. Which of the following is found more frequently in ambulatory care visits than on daily hospital rounds?
   a. Physician control of the patient
   b. Rapid access to ancillary services and consults
   c. Undifferentiated problems
   d. Patient readily available for reevaluation.

3. According to White et al., out of the approximately 750 adults of 1000 who get ill or become injured during a given month, a physician will see _____ of them as outpatients, _____ will be admitted to a hospital, and _____ will be admitted to university teaching hospital.
   a. 500, 20, 5
   b. 250, 9, 1
   c. 150, 15, 7
   d. 450, 9, 5

4. Which of the following should be included in a problem list for a patient who is a 45-year-old woman with hypertension and whose father had an MI at age 57?
   a. Hypertension
   b. Health maintenance
   c. Family history of CAD

   d. a and c only
   e. All of the above

5. How many hypotheses should you consider at one time while formulating a differential diagnosis during a patient encounter?
   a. Only one—more than that is too confusing.
   b. Three or four—a nice number that attendings usually ask.
   c. More than five—the more the better.
   d. Being a medical student, you should keep *all* of the possible hypotheses in mind *all* of the time.

6. A pathognomonic cue is one that
   a. Is 100% specific.
   b. Is seen consistently with the condition and helps rule it in.
   c. Indicates the patient definitely has the disease.
   d. All of the above.

7. When a patient has a sign, symptom, or abnormal test consistent with a disease, the positive likelihood ratio is
   a. TPR/TNR
   b. FPR/FNR
   c. TPR/FPR
   d. FPR/TPR

8. When your Native American patient states that her illness is caused by offending the spirits of her forefathers, you have elicited the patient's
   a. Delusional break.
   b. Anger toward Western medicine.

    c. Cultural bias.
    d. Explanatory model.

9. Which of the following is not a type of coping mechanism?
    a. Change the problematic situation
    b. Decrease one's responsibility for the problem by blaming others
    c. Decrease the mental stress related to the problem if it cannot be changed
    d. Change one's attitude about the problem

10. Category rating, time tradeoff, and standard gamble
    a. Should be used every time when discussing treatment options with a patient.
    b. Are unbiased approaches to finding patient's preferences for treatments.
    c. Help provide relative values for patients' preferences.
    d. Can only be used formally to get absolute values for patients' preferences.

11. After being told the evaluation and treatment options for an ulcer, your patient, a 64-year-old male business executive, states, "I'll do whatever you think is best, Doctor." The doctor–patient model this patient best fits is the
    a. Guidance-cooperation.
    b. Mutual-participation.
    c. Active-passive.
    d. Guidance-participation.

12. For a medical student, the most important part of the "doctor–patient" encounter is
    a. To find the cure for the patient.
    b. To establish good rapport.
    c. To rigidly follow a standard operating procedure.
    d. To reflect afterward and learn from the encounter.

Answers appear on page 448.

INTERPRETING LABORATORY TESTS

PAUL M. FISCHER and LOIS A. ADDISON

At one time, there was an expectation that laboratory testing would greatly simplify clinical medicine. The hope was that you could order a large number of tests on patients, even those who were asymptomatic, and find out what diseases they had. This fanciful approach fell into disfavor as we learned more about the limitations of testing. There are only a few tests that are good enough to be used for mass screening. All of the rest require a good clinician to judiciously pick the right test for the right patient at the right time, and then to interpret the test result in light of all of the information known about that patient. Laboratory tests do not make clinician's lives simpler. They do, however, have the potential to make clinical care better.

One widely acclaimed model for diagnostic test use is referred to as "decision analysis." This is a method of mathematically analyzing the probabilities that are involved in clinical decisions. It is based on a test's sensitivity, specificity, and predictive value. It is our experience that such an extremely formal approach to testing is not possible in the real world. There is too much ambiguity in most clinical data for physicians to practice in a purely "rational" manner. Much of medicine is intuitive.

In this chapter, we first review some of the limitations inherent in a decision analysis approach to testing. This is followed by short sections on 26 tests. We have tried to choose common tests and to base the descriptions on strategies that clinicians might actually use in clinical situations. It is our hope that students will use these short sections to better understand the laboratory test results that they obtain on their patients.

LIMITATIONS OF DECISION ANALYSIS

The Problem of a "Gold Standard"

The starting point in decision analysis is the identification of a test's sensitivity and specificity. Sensitivity is defined as the percentage of individuals with the disease who have a positive test. Specificity is defined as the percentage of people without the disease who have a negative test. Both concepts depend on a reference or "gold standard" method to identify whether a person is diseased. The problem is that most gold standards are imperfect. If a gold standard misclassifies individuals, then the sensitivity and specificity of a second comparison test will be artificially altered.

This issue has been discussed for tests of ischemic heart disease (Boyko et al.). Coronary angiography has been used as the gold standard for this illness. Several studies have now shown that this test frequently misclassifies both the presence and the absence of significant coronary artery stenosis.

The inadequacy of a gold standard is a problem for such common diseases as group A streptococcal pharyngitis and urinary tract infections. Rapid tests which detect group A streptococcal cell wall antigens are now widely available. Many microbiologists complain that these tests are relatively insensitive because they have a 10% false negative rate compared to cultures. This means that 10% of patients with a negative antigen test have a positive throat culture. However, the culture colony count in these "false negative" cases is usually low. Is the patient infected or just a noninfected strep carrier?

As another example, consider the diagnosis of urinary tract infections. Until recently, it was not uncommon to tell a woman with urinary frequency, urgency, and dysuria that she was "not infected" because her urine culture grew only 50,000 colonies. This was based on time-honored diagnostic level of 100,000 colonies/ml of urine as a cutoff for "significant bacteriuria." This diagnostic level failed to consider the patient's symptoms, how long the urine had incubated in the bladder, or the specimen's specific gravity. More recent studies have indicated that a colony count as low as 100 may indicate infection in a female patient with dysuria. It is impossible to identify a single level of bacteriuria as a gold standard for diagnosing urinary tract infections.

Clinicians must be cautious in interpreting the published performance characteristics of any test. Sensitivity and specificity are not the accurate and precise calculations that we have often supposed them to be. Unfortunately, there is no precise way to adjust for the errors of an imperfect gold standard. Clinicians must rely on common sense.

Spectrum of Disease

The traditional decision analysis model assumes that you either have a disease or you do not. This simplistic ideal is complicated by the "spectrum" of disease (Ransohoff and Feinstein). Any illness is characterized by variation in chronicity and severity. Test results may vary accordingly. The usual pattern is that a test is more likely to be positive when the disease is of a longer duration or greater severity. Many of the sensitivities/specificities reported in the literature are high because of the tendency of researchers to ignore this issue of spectrum of disease.

An example is the literature on carcinoembryonic antigen (CEA) testing for colon cancer. Early studies indicated a 90% sensitivity and 90% specificity for this test. In these early studies the patients usually had extensive disease. Later studies with more representative samples of colon cancer patients (i.e., some with localized disease) showed that the test was sensitive only in patients with extensive cancer.

A test's specificity can be inaccurate because of the character of the nondiseased patients studied. The nondiseased individuals in the early studies on CEA and colon cancer were healthy and asymptomatic. Later studies used individuals with nonmalignant colon diseases or with cancers other than those of the colon. This is the patient population for whom the test would most likely be ordered. In these later studies, the specificity of the CEA test was greatly reduced.

The Problem of Prevalence

Another concept in the decision analysis mathematical equation is that of disease prevalence. This is the number of individuals with a disease in a population at a given time. Unfortunately there are almost no prevalence figures that can be easily "plugged into" a decision analysis formula for actual clinical situations. In real-world situations, the best prevalence information is usually an estimate of "common," "uncommon," or "rare."

What about the prevalence figures that appear in the literature? Of the two typical kinds, the first is derived from case series that are seen in referral centers. What percentage of patients in an endocrinology clinic with the chief complaint of fatigue have hypothyroidism? This prevalence figure would be irrelevant to the primary care clinician seeing patients with fatigue.

The second common type of prevalence is taken from population studies. In this type of research, a sample of individuals in a geographic area is tested (e.g., What is the prevalence of brain cancer in the United States?). This figure will tell you about the general population,

but not necessarily about the patients who come to your office with a specific complaint (e.g., What is the prevalence of brain cancer in individuals who present with headache and have a normal neurologic examination?).

Prevalence may vary from one practice site to another and from month to month (e.g., the difference in prevalence of HIV disease in San Francisco and Omaha, the prevalence of influenza in February compared with July).

Therapeutic Goals

It is often assumed that knowing the positive predictive value of a test is the most important factor in appropriate test ordering. However, even when this is known, there can be great debate about how to use the test. This phenomenon has been described for the tests used to diagnose group A streptococcal pharyngitis (DeNeef). DeNeef looked at 21 different strategies for treating adults with pharyngitis. These included the use of empiric antibiotics, culturing, or using a rapid test. In the end, it was not so much the characteristics of the tests that determined "appropriate" test ordering, but rather the physician's treatment goals. These could be to minimize total cost, minimize adverse outcomes, or minimize both adverse outcomes and unnecessary antibiotics. Two physicians may agree on how good a test is and then come to opposite decisions about when to order it.

Clinicians and Testing

If sensitivity, specificity, prevalence, and predictive value are not practically useful, then how do clinicians interpret tests? It is our observation that they usually ask two questions:

1. Is the test normal or abnormal?
2. If abnormal, is it a little abnormal or very abnormal?

The degree to which the test result is abnormal has often been overlooked in discussions about test interpretation (Statland). It is, however, what clinicians have intuitively used for a long time in deciding whether they should act on a test result. A serum calcium of 10.5 mg/dl, although outside the usual reference range, will often not catch a clinician's attention. A level of 13 mg/dl, on the other hand is impossible to ignore.

Despite the increasing interest in establishing rules for "appropriate" test ordering, the best that can be said is that there are a few instances when a test is clearly appropriate, a few when a test is clearly inappropriate, and many other instances that are open to debate. Clinicians live in a sea of uncertainty.

Tests

Each of the following sections includes background information about a test, the most common causes of an "abnormal" value, and some of the common pitfalls in the test's interpretation.

A table of "normal" values is included. We use the word "normal" rather than "reference range," since it is the term clinicians use. "Reference range" is a statistical concept used by laboratories. "Normal" is a clinical concept used by physicians ("Mr. Jones, your cholesterol is normal"). When appropriate, differences are indicated between the normal values for adults and children, males and females.

Values are given in both conventional (listed first) and System International (SI) units. Conversion factors from conventional to SI units are also given.

We have tried to identify the important diagnoses to consider when interpreting an abnormally high or low test value. When interpretation is aided by the degree of abnormality, we have listed the useful diagnostic ranges. These should be viewed as guides and not fixed rules.

We have also indicated actions (e.g., patient history, physical examination findings, or further laboratory testing) that should be considered in helping to interpret an abnormal test. These are ranked in order to indicate a common-sense plan for further evaluation.

Serum Albumin

Albumin is produced by the liver and released into the plasma, where it accounts for 90% of the intravascular oncotic pressure. The body's production of albumin is reduced with advanced age, poor nutrition, or hepatic disease. Only small amounts are normally lost through the urine or the gastrointestinal mucosa. Hypoalbuminemia develops when there is a reduction in synthesis or increased albumin loss. This is often associated with edema.

Serum albumin is not a useful test for general screening of healthy individuals. When such routine testing is done, most of the abnormal results are mildly elevated or decreased. These represent the extremes of the normal distribution of values and can usually be ignored. The test is extremely useful in evaluating patients with edema, liver disease, or suspected malnutrition.

An elevated albumin is of no clinical significance. It is most commonly seen in the face of dehydration (Table 19–1).

Serum Alkaline Phosphatase

Alkaline phosphatase (ALP) is a family of enzymes found in nearly all body tissues but which have no known function. In normal adults about one-half of the measured serum ALP is produced by the liver and one-half by bone. Children and adolescents have serum ALP levels two to four times that of a normal adult. This is due to rapid bone growth. Pregnant women in the third trimester also have elevated ALP, due to placental production. This increased level returns to normal by 1 month postpartum.

Liver diseases are usually divided into those which are primarily hepatic and those which are cholestatic. Elevation in aminotransferase is the usual marker for direct hepatocyte insult. ALP, on the other hand, is the usual marker for a cholestatic illness. This includes any pro-

TABLE 19–1. NORMAL VALUES FOR ALBUMIN

Diagnostic Units: gm/dl (gm/liter). SI conversion factor = 10
Normal 4.0–6.0 gm/dl (40–60 gm/liter)

Decreased	Diagnoses to Consider	Actions to Consider
<4.0 (40)	Decreased synthesis 　Liver insufficiency 　Malnutrition 　Malignancy Increased loss 　Nephrotic 　　syndrome 　Extensive burns 　Protein-losing 　　enteropathy Pregnancy Inflammatory illness	1. Dietary history 2. Urinalysis 3. 24-hour urine 　　protein 4. Bilirubin 5. Creatinine 6. Hemoglobin

Values in parentheses are SI units.
Source: Rakel RE. Textbook of Family Practice. 4th ed. Philadelphia, W.B. Saunders, 1990, with permission.

cess that causes an obstruction in the bile ducts (e.g., stone, cancer, pancreatitis, primary biliary cirrhosis). In these illnesses, the ALP and conjugated bilirubin levels are moderately to greatly elevated, while the aminotransferase levels are normal or only mildly elevated. In illnesses that are directly hepatotoxic (e.g., viral hepatitis), the aminotransferase and conjugated bilirubin are greatly elevated, while the ALP may be normal or only mildly elevated. Alcohol ingestion is often cited as a cause for elevated ALP; this is rarely the case, unless there is advanced cirrhosis or severe alcoholic hepatitis.

ALP levels are also elevated in disorders associated with osteoblastic activity (i.e., new bone formation). Paget's disease of bone is the prototypical illness. Ninety percent of these patients have an elevated ALP even though most are asymptomatic. Osteoporosis and fractures do not commonly lead to elevated ALP levels.

A gamma glutamyltransferase test (GGT) is useful in differentiating between biliary and bony sources of an elevated ALP. GGT is usually elevated when the ALP is derived from the liver.

ALP is not a useful screening test in asymptomatic individuals. Values less than the normal range are of no clinical significance.

Since more than 200 different medications can cause an elevated ALP, a good first step in anyone with an unexplained ALP elevation is a thorough medication review (Table 19–2).

Aminotransferases

Aminotransferases (or transaminases) are enzymes primarily located within hepatocytes. Alanine aminotransferase (ALAT) used to be referred to as serum glutamic phosphoracetic transaminase (SGPT). Aspartate aminotransferase (ASAT) used to be referred to as serum glutamic oxaloacetic transferase (SGOT). Increased levels of both enzymes are due to liver injury and the subsequent leaking of the enzymes from the

TABLE 19–2. NORMAL VALUES FOR ALKALINE PHOSPHATASE

Diagnostic Units: Units/liter
Normal Adults: 30–120
 Children: 50–400
 Pregnant women: 30–200

Increased	Diagnoses to Consider	Actions to Consider
120–200	Nonfasting patient specimen Drug effect	1. Repeat test with patient fasting 2. Review patient medications

>200	Increased from bone:
	 Paget's disease
	 Osteomalacia
	 Bony metastasis
	 Hyperparathyroidism
	Increased from liver:
	 Bile duct stone
	 Biliary cancer
	 Pancreatic cancer
	 Pancreatitis
	 Liver infiltration
	  (sarcoid)
	 Primary biliary
	  cirrhosis
	 Viral hepatitis
	 Severe cirrhosis
	Other causes:
	 Drug effect
	 Heart failure
	 Hyperthyroidism
	 Lymphoma
	 Leukemia
		1. Review patient medications
		2. Serum bilirubin, GGT, and aminotransferases
		3. RUQ abdominal ultrasound
		4. Pelvis or femur x-rays
		5. Serum calcium
		6. Bone scan

Source: Rakel RE. Textbook of Family Practice. 4th ed. Philadelphia, W.B. Saunders, 1990, with permission.

TABLE 19–3. NORMAL VALUES FOR AMINOTRANSFERASES

Diagnostic Units: Units/liter
Normal 0–35

Increased	Diagnoses to Consider	Actions to Consider
35–400	Both ALAT and ASAT elevated: Infectious hepatitis Toxic hepatitis Alcoholic hepatitis Shock liver Biliary obstruction Only ASAT elevated: Myocardial infarction Hemolysis (in vivo) Pulmonary infarction Muscular dystrophy	1. Review patient medication 2. Review foreign travel, needle sticks, chemical exposures, and transfusion history 3. Alcohol history 4. Serum bilirubin, alkaline phosphatase 5. Test for viral hepatitis 6. Peripheral smear for hemolysis
>400	Both ALAT and ASAT elevated: Infectious hepatitis Toxic hepatitis Shock liver	

Source: Rakel RE. Textbook of Family Practice. 4th ed. Philadelphia, W.B. Saunders, 1990, with permission.

serum amylase is from the pancreas while two-thirds comes from salivary glands. Most pancreatic amylase goes directly into the gut. A small fraction is then absorbed into the circulation.

There are few diseases that are diagnosed with as much certainty, based on a single test, as is pancreatitis from the finding of an elevated amylase. With very few exceptions, an elevated amylase indicates pancreatitis and a normal amylase rules out this diagnosis (Table 19–4). It is important to remember that the degree of amylase elevation does not always correlate with the sever-

cells. In general, the level of the aminotransferases reflects the severity of the hepatic damage. Elevations often occur prior to an increase in bilirubin in hepatic disease (Table 19–3).

ALAT is fairly specific for liver injury. In contrast, ASAT is also increased in cardiac and skeletal muscle diseases. This fact is clinically useful, since if both enzymes are elevated, a hepatic source is very likely. In most illnesses the ALAT value is greater than the ASAT. The only common exception to this rule is in alcoholic hepatitis, in which the ASAT is higher.

ALAT and ASAT testing are not useful in screening healthy individuals. They are, however, extremely useful in diagnosing and monitoring all forms of liver disease and are used as screening tests in patients on medications that can produce liver injury (e.g., INH).

ALAT and ASAT values below the normal limit are infrequently seen and are of little clinical significance. The exceptions to this rule are in advanced cirrhosis and fulminant hepatitis. In these cases a normal or low level may indicate that the disease is so advanced that few hepatocytes remain.

Serum Amylase

Amylase is produced by the pancreas, salivary glands, and some tumors (lung). About one-third of normal

TABLE 19–4. NORMAL VALUES FOR AMYLASE

Diagnostic Units: Somogyi units/dl (Units/liter)
Normal 50–150 (0–130)

Increased	Diagnoses to Consider	Actions to Consider
>150 (130)	Pancreatitis: Alcoholic Gallstone Trauma Hyperlipidemia Infectious Drug-induced Familial ERCP Perforating ulcer Mesenteric infarction Salivary gland disease Chronic renal failure Amylase-secreting cancer	1. Alcohol history 2. Abdominal examination 3. Complete drug history 4. RUQ ultrasound 5. Urinary amylase 6. Amylase/creatinine clearance 7. Lipase or amylase isoenzyme

Values in parentheses are SI units.
Source: Rakel RE. Textbook of Family Practice. 4th ed. Philadelphia, W.B. Saunders, 1990, with permission.

ity of the pancreatic injury. This is particularly true in chronic pancreatitis in which serum levels may be normal despite ongoing pancreatic injury. In such cases, a urinary amylase or an amylase to creatinine clearance ratio may be helpful.

In addition to pancreatitis, patients with abdominal pain and an elevated amylase should be evaluated for a perforated peptic ulcer or mesenteric infarction.

The amylase in the circulation is excreted primarily by the kidneys. Modest elevations in the serum amylase can therefore be seen in patients with chronic renal failure. In unexplained hyperamylasemia, serum lipase may be a helpful test, since lipase is produced by the pancreas, but not by salivary glands. Low serum amylase levels are rarely of clinical significance.

Bilirubin (Total)

Bilirubin is formed from the heme ring as senescent red blood cells are degraded. It is transported in blood attached to albumin and then delivered to the liver, where it is conjugated and excreted in the bile. The common causes for hyperbilirubinemia are increased red cell destruction, liver diseases, and biliary tract obstruction.

Laboratories measure total bilirubin and conjugated (i.e., direct) bilirubin (Table 19–5). The unconjugated (i.e., indirect) fraction is then obtained by subtraction. In normal serum, less than 15% of the total bilirubin is conjugated. The various causes for hyperbilirubinemia have traditionally been divided into those associated with elevations of conjugated or unconjugated bilirubin. However, many diseases are associated with elevations of both.

In hepatic diseases, the bilirubin level is usually proportional to the level of hepatocyte injury. Jaundice is detectable only when the total bilirubin exceeds 3.0 mg/dl. Low serum bilirubin levels are of no clinical significance.

Blood Urea Nitrogen (BUN)

BUN is commonly used to measure renal function. However, the serum creatinine is a much more reliable indicator of the glomerular filtration rate (GFR). This is because BUN is affected by the nitrogen load, water intake, and urine flow. If you want to know about the kidney, order a creatinine.

An elevated BUN is seen with renal insufficiency, but it is not a specific indicator of renal function. It is more useful to calculate the BUN to creatinine ratio (Table 19–6). This ratio can serve as a useful indicator of whether the BUN elevation is due to a high nitrogen load, low urine flow, or high water intake.

The normal BUN is 8 to 26 mg/dl (2.9–9.3 mmol/liter). The SI conversion factor is 0.357.

Serum Calcium

Calcium is essential for maintenance of the skeleton and for normal neuromuscular function. The usual

TABLE 19–5. NORMAL VALUES FOR BILIRUBIN

Diagnostic Units: mg/dl (μ mol/liter). SI conversion factor = 17.1
Normal 0.1–1.0 (2–17)

Increased in Newborns	Diagnoses to Consider	Actions to Consider
1.0–10 (17–171)	Direct < 15% of total: Physiologic Breast feeding ABO incompatibility Rh incompatibility Hemorrhage Maternal diabetes Direct > 15% of total: Sepsis TORCH infections Hepatitis Biliary atresia	1. Mother and infant blood type 2. Direct Coombs' tests 3. Hct
10–20 (171–342)	Kernicterus possible	1. Phototherapy or exchange transfusion (base decision on days of age, weight, maturity)

Increased in Adults	Diagnoses to Consider	Actions to Consider
> 1.0 (17)	Hepatic insufficiency Biliary obstruction Hemolysis Postoperative complications	1. Alcohol history 2. Complete drug history 3. Travel, dietary, and needle stick history 4. Peripheral blood smear 5. Conjugated bilirubin, AST, ALP 6. Reticulocyte count 7. Viral hepatitis tests 8. Direct Coombs' tests 9. RUQ ultrasound

Values in parentheses are SI units.
Source: Rakel RE. Textbook of Family Practice. 4th ed. Philadelphia, W.B. Saunders, 1990, with permission.

serum calcium test measures total calcium (Table 19–7). About half of the total calcium is bound to albumin. The rest is present in serum in the ionized form. The measurement of ionized calcium can be separately ordered.

The serum calcium level is under the complex control of the parathyroid hormone (PTH) and calcitonin. These and other hormones control the rate at which calcium is absorbed from the gastrointestinal tract, excreted in the urine, and gained or lost to bone.

The most common "abnormality" is a low total calcium in a patient with low serum albumin. This is primarily a serum albumin disorder and not a calcium problem, since the ionized calcium remains unchanged. It is possible to mathematically correct the calcium value when the albumin is decreased (1 gm/dl reduction in albumin leads to 1 mg/dl reduction in calcium).

Hypercalcemia is associated with fatigue, depression,

TABLE 19-6. NORMAL VALUES FOR BLOOD UREA NITROGEN/CREATININE RATIO

Normal 10:1 (BUN to Cr)

Increased Ratio	Diagnoses to Consider	Actions to Consider
>10	High nitrogen load: GI bleeding High-protein diet High catabolism (burns) Low urine flow: Dehydration Congestive heart failure Urinary tract obstruction	1. Examine for hydration status 2. Examine for CHF 3. Dietary history 4. Drug history (steroids) 5. Stool occult blood

Decreased Ratio	Diagnoses to Consider	Actions to Consider
<10	High urine flow: Water intoxication SIADH Low-protein diet Protein malnutrition Liver insufficiency	1. Check serum and urine osmolality 2. Check serum sodium 3. Dietary history 4. Bilirubin

Source: Rakel RE. Textbook of Family Practice. 4th ed. Philadelphia, W.B. Saunders, 1990, with permission.

constipation, polydipsia, ulcers, and hypertension. The most common cause of hypercalcemia in outpatients is hyperparathyroidism. Many of these patients are asymptomatic. Malignancies are the most common cause for hypercalcemia in the inpatient setting. The most common cancers producing hypercalcemia are lung, breast, and kidney.

Hypocalcemia produces symptoms that result from neuromuscular excitability. These include carpal pedal spasm, seizures, tetany, stiffness, fatigue, memory loss, and confusion.

There is debate about whether serum calcium is an appropriate screening test for asymptomatic individuals. It is frequently included in screening panels. The rationale for this usage has been that hyperparathyroidism is frequently asymptomatic. This argument has recently come into question because of the uncertainty whether asymptomatic hyperparathyroidism requires any specific therapy.

Chloride

Chloride is the major extracellular anion in the body, yet it is a relatively uninteresting analyte and rarely clinically useful (Table 19–8).

Most dietary chloride is absorbed and the serum level is then controlled by renal excretion of the ion. The primary cause for an abnormal chloride is a response to a shift in serum CO_2 content. The CO_2 level decreases in metabolic acidosis and in the metabolic compensation for a respiratory alkalosis. In these situations, chloride increases in response to the reduction in CO_2 content.

In metabolic alkalosis or the metabolic response to respiratory acidosis, the CO_2 level increases. In these conditions, chloride is reduced to compensate for the increased CO_2.

Chloride can be depleted by either gastrointestinal losses (e.g., vomiting) or renal losses (e.g., salt-losing renal diseases). Such depletion may result in a persistent metabolic alkalosis.

The most frequent use of the chloride test is in calculating the anion gap. This is calculated by subtracting the total measured anions (chloride + bicarbonate) from the total cations (sodium + potassium). The normal range for the anion gap is 16 ± 4 mEq/liter. Increases in the anion gap indicate the presence of unmeasured anions such as ketoacids, lactic acids, and methanol.

Cholesterol

The NIH has established a National Cholesterol Education Program. One goal is to have all adults screened

TABLE 19-7. NORMAL VALUES FOR CALCIUM

Diagnostic Units: mg/dl (mmol/liter). SI conversion factor = 0.2495
Normal 8.8–10.3 (2.20–2.57)

Increased	Diagnoses to Consider	Actions to Consider
10.3–13.0 (2.57–3.24)	Hyperparathyroidism Metastatic cancer Thiazide diuretics Immobilization Vitamin D intoxication Milk-alkali syndrome Multiple myeloma Sarcoidosis Thyrotoxicosis	1. Repeat serum calcium 2. Complete diet and drug history 3. Ionized calcium, albumin, phosphorus, PTH, T_4 4. Chest x-ray 5. Hand x-rays 6. Evaluation for malignancy
>13.0 (3.24)	Hypercalcemic coma	1. Vigorous hydration 2. Furosemide 3. Close monitoring

Decreased	Diagnoses to Consider	Actions to Consider
7.0–8.8 (1.75–2.20)	Hypoalbuminemia Chronic renal failure Hypoparathyroidism (neck surgery) Malnutrition Vitamin D deficiency: Nutritional Anticonvulsants Malabsorption Liver disease Hypomagnesemia Pancreatitis	1. Serum albumin 2. Complete drug history 3. Alcohol history 4. Serum creatinine, phosphate, magnesium, PTH
<7.0 (1.75)	Hypocalcemic seizures Hypocalcemic arrhythmias	1. IV calcium gluconate 2. Serum ionized calcium 3. Serum magnesium

Values in parentheses are SI units.
Source: Rakel RE. Textbook of Family Practice. 4th ed. Philadelphia, W.B. Saunders, 1990, with permission.

TABLE 19–8.   NORMAL VALUES FOR CHLORIDE

Diagnostic Units: mEq/liter (mmol/liter). SI conversion factor = 1
Normal 95–105 (95–105)

Increased	Diagnoses to Consider	Actions to Consider
>105	Metabolic acidosis: 　Loss of bicarbonate 　Production of 　　metabolic acids Respiratory alkalosis with 　metabolic 　compensation Dehydration Head injury Primary aldosteronism	1. HCO_3, Na, K, 　pH, BUN, Cl 2. Calculate anion 　gap

Decreased	Diagnoses to Consider	Actions to Consider
<95	Metabolic alkalosis: 　Hydrogen ion loss 　　(vomiting) 　HCO_3 retention Respiratory acidosis with 　metabolic 　compensation Salt-losing renal disease Thiazide diuretics Addison's disease	1. Urinalysis 2. HCO_3, Na, K, 　pH, BUN, Cl

Values in parentheses are SI units.
Source: Rakel RE. Textbook of Family Practice. 4th ed. Philadelphia, W.B. Saunders, 1990, with permission.

TABLE 19–9.   NORMAL VALUES FOR CHOLESTEROL

Diagnostic Units: mg/dl (mmol/liter). SI conversion factor = 0.02586
Normal <200 (5.2)

Increased	Diagnoses to Consider	Actions to Consider
200–239 (5.2–6.2)	Borderline risk for CHD: 　Familial 　　hypercholesterolemia 　High cholesterol diet 　Biliary obstruction 　Nephrotic syndrome 　Hypothyroidism	1. Repeat cholesterol 　test 2. Evaluate for CAD 　risks 　a. Male sex 　b. Smoking 　c. Family history of 　　CHD 　d. Hypertension 　e. Diabetes mellitus 　f. Severe obesity 　g. History of 　　vascular disease 　h. HDL less than 　　35 mg/dl 3. If patient has known 　CAD or 2 or more 　risk factors, order 　lipoprotein analysis
≥240 (≥ 6.2)	High risk for CHD: 　As above	1. Repeat cholesterol 2. Fasting lipoprotein 　analysis 3. Classify based on 　LDL 　a. <130 = 　　desirable 　b. 130–159 = 　　borderline risk 　c. ≥160 = high 　　risk

Decreased	Diagnoses to Consider	Actions to Consider
<140 (< 3.6)	Low risk for CHD: 　Hyperthyroidism 　Hepatic insufficiency	1. Dietary history 2. Bilirubin 3. T_4, T_3U

Values in parentheses are SI units.
Source: Rakel RE. Textbook of Family Practice. 4th ed. Philadelphia, W.B. Saunders, 1990, with permission.

for hypercholesterolemia. While there is considerable debate about which cholesterol levels require treatment and the optimal approach to treatment, most people now agree that the screening of adults is probably indicated (Table 19–9). Epidemiologic studies have shown that a 1% decrease in total cholesterol is associated with a 2% decrease in coronary heart disease (CHD) risk.

There can be considerable variation in repeated cholesterol levels for the same patient. This is due to test accuracy errors ($\pm 3\%$), test imprecision ($\pm 3\%$), and day-to-day patient variation ($\pm 7\%$). Cholesterol has also been shown to have a seasonal variation. Limited studies have shown that total cholesterol does not appear to be affected by patient fasting. Fasting is, however, essential in measuring triglycerides and the cholesterol lipoprotein fractions.

Cholesterol measurements should be used to diagnose hypercholesterolemia much as blood pressure readings are used to diagnose hypertension. Several readings over a period of time are required before a diagnosis can be made.

If the total cholesterol indicates that the patient is at risk for hypercholesterolemia, the NIH recommends that a fasting lipoprotein analysis be done (total cholesterol, HDL cholesterol, and triglycerides). LDL cholesterol can then be calculated by the formula:

$$\text{LDL cholesterol} = \text{Total cholesterol} - \text{HDL cholesterol} - \frac{\text{triglycerides}}{5}$$

If the LDL cholesterol is between 130 and 160 mg/dl, the patient is considered at a borderline high risk for CHD. If the LDL is greater than 160 mg/dl, the patient is considered at high risk for CHD. LDL values less than 130 mg/dl are desirable.

The NIH recommends that the decision to treat should be based on a patient's risk factors for CHD and the LDL value. Total cholesterol measurements should be used only for case finding and to follow the response to therapy.

CO_2 Content

The CO_2 content of blood is made up of bicarbonate, carbonic acid, and dissolved CO_2. Ninety-five percent of the total CO_2 content is bicarbonate (HCO_3). Bicarbonate is the second most important anion in serum and is

TABLE 19–10. NORMAL VALUES FOR CO_2

Diagnostic Units: mEq/liter (mmol/liter). SI conversion factor = 1
Normal 22–28 (22–28)

Decreased	Diagnoses to Consider	Actions to Consider
<22	Metabolic acidosis:	1. Full drug history
	Bicarbonate loss:	2. Serum electrolytes
	Diarrhea	3. Blood gas
	Renal tubular acidosis	4. Calculate anion
	Primary	gap
	hyperparathyroidism	
	Failure to reabsorb	
	bicarbonate:	
	Triamterene,	
	spironolactone	
	Renal tubular acidosis	
	Production of metabolic	
	acids:	
	Renal failure	
	Diabetic ketoacidosis	
	Lactic acidosis	
	Methanol	
	Ethylene glycol	
	Salicylates	
	Alcoholic ketoacidosis	
	Respiratory alkalosis with	
	compensation:	
	Anxiety	
	Sepsis	
	Salicylates	
	CNS injury	

Increased	Diagnoses to Consider	Actions to Consider
>28	Metabolic alkalosis:	1. Serum electrolytes
	Volume contraction	2. Blood gas
	NG suction	3. Urine electrolytes
	Vomiting	
	Potassium depletion	
	Furosemide	
	Cushing's syndrome	
	Chronic respiratory acidosis	
	with compensation	

Values in parentheses are SI units.
Source: Rakel RE. Textbook of Family Practice. 4th ed. Philadelphia, W.B. Saunders, 1990, with permission.

the most available base to buffer a metabolic acid load. This role in the acid–base balance is its principal clinical function (Table 19–10).

The two physiologic mechanisms for the control of CO_2 content are the respiration of CO_2 gas and renal reabsorption of filtered bicarbonate. Bicarbonate can also be lost pathologically through the gastrointestinal tract.

The most common CO_2 content abnormality is a decreased level due to metabolic acidosis. In this setting it is useful to calculate the anion gap. This value may provide a clue to the cause of the acidosis.

A metabolic alkalosis may be set off by the loss of hydrogen ions (e.g., nasogastric suction). The maintenance of a metabolic alkalosis requires that there be a greater than normal reabsorption of bicarbonate by the kidneys. In patients with an elevated CO_2 content, look for diseases that affect bicarbonate handling by the renal tubules.

Creatinine

Creatinine is released from skeletal muscle and is excreted unchanged in the urine. There are few factors other than renal function which affect its serum level. It is the best of the common tests for monitoring renal insufficiency. A rise in creatinine indicates a falling glomerular filtration rate.

However, a serum creatinine is a relatively insensitive marker of renal disease. A 50% reduction in renal function from normal leads to an increase in creatinine of only 1 to 2.0 mg/dl (Table 19–11). Considerable renal damage may therefore occur before it becomes apparent by a rising creatinine.

A second difficulty with interpreting serum creatinine is that it is slow in reacting to sudden changes in renal failure. In sudden and severe renal failure (e.g., acute tubular necrosis following shock), the creatinine will rise only 1 mg/dl/day. This is despite a creatinine clearance of zero!

A patient's creatinine clearance can be estimated from the following formula:

CR clearance = [(140 − age) (weight in kg)]/(72 × CR in mg/dl)

As a rough guideline, a creatinine of 2 mg/dl is equivalent to a creatinine clearance of 50 ml/min; a creatinine of 4 mg/dl is equal to a clearance of 20 ml/min; and a creatinine of 6 mg/dl is equivalent to a clearance of 10 ml/min.

TABLE 19–11. NORMAL VALUES FOR CREATININE

Diagnostic Units: mg/dl (μmol/liter), SI conversion factor = 88.4
Normal 0.6–1.2 (50–110)

Increased	Diagnoses to Consider	Actions to Consider
1.2–1.6 (110–141)	Mild renal impairment Muscle injury	1. Repeat test 2. Urinalysis 3. Creatinine clearance
>1.6 (141)	Prerenal failure:	1. Urinalysis
	Dehydration	2. Creatinine clearance
	Blood loss	3. Bladder catheterization
	Heart failure	4. Renal imaging
	Liver failure	
	Intrinsic renal failure:	
	Diabetes mellitus	
	Hypertension	
	SLE	
	Nephrotoxins	
	Glomerulonephritis	
	Acute tubular necrosis	
	Postrenal failure:	
	Urethral obstruction	
	Upper tract obstruction	
>6.0 (530)	Severe renal failure	1. HCO_3 (metabolic acidosis) 2. Serum potassium (hyperkalemia)

Values in parentheses are SI units.
Source: Rakel RE. Textbook of Family Practice. 4th ed. Philadelpia, W.B. Saunders, 1990, with permission.

Serum creatinine is a useful screening test in patients at risk for renal injury (e.g., those with hypertension or diabetes). Because of the low prevalence of chronic renal failure in the general population and the low sensitivity of the test, it is NOT a useful test in asymptomatic patients without significant risk factors. A low serum creatinine has no clinical significance.

Digoxin

Various forms of digitalis have been used to treat heart failure for more than 200 years. Digoxin is the drug form most commonly prescribed today. In addition to treating heart failure, it is frequently used to block the A-V node in atrial tachyarrhythmias. Digoxin has a very narrow therapeutic window. Levels below 0.5 ng/ml are generally not therapeutic; levels over 2.2 ng/ml are often associated with toxicity. The ability to properly use digoxin has been enhanced by the availability of therapeutic drug monitoring (Table 19–12).

When used in tablet form, 60% to 80% of digoxin is absorbed. Gelatin capsules (Lanoxicaps) are associated with a 90% to 100% absorption. The peak effect for the drug ranges from 2 to 6 hours after oral administration. It is, therefore, impossible to accurately interpret a digoxin level drawn within 6 hours of an oral dose. During this time, the levels will be high and do not reliably correlate with the steady-state level.

Digoxin is primarily metabolized by the kidney. The half-life of the drug in patients with normal renal function is 1½ days. This increases to 4 or 5 days in anuric patients. The drug's very long half-life means that a steady-state level is not reached until 1 week following a change in dosage of the oral preparation.

Digitalis toxicity is associated with nausea, vomiting, fatigue, confusion, blurred vision, and cardiac disturbances (ventricular ectopy, A-V block, paroxysmal atrial tachycardia, atrial fibrillation, and ventricular fibrillation). The incidence of digoxin toxicity increases with increasing serum levels. Toxicity is found at lower digoxin levels in patients with hypokalemia, alkalosis, hypercalcemia, or hypomagnesemia.

The most common mistake in using serum digoxin levels is "treating the level" instead of the patient. One-third of patients with digoxin toxicity have levels that are within the normal therapeutic range. Levels greater than the normal upper therapeutic limit may be required in some clinical situations (e.g., to slow the ventricular rate in atrial fibrillation). A wide range of medications interact with digoxin. Some are indicated in Table 19–12.

Erythrocyte Sedimentation Rate (ESR) (Westergren Method)

Anticoagulated whole blood is made up of blood cells suspended in plasma. When the blood is allowed to stand for a period of time, the cells settle out. The rate of settling is affected by both red blood cell factors (i.e., shape, size, hematocrit) and plasma factors (fibrinogen and globulins). The ESR is a measure of the rate of blood cell settling (Table 19–13).

The ESR is a nonspecific test used to diagnose and follow the clinical course of a wide variety of diseases which are characterized by tissue inflammation, infection, or malignancy.

The Westergren or Modified Westergren is the preferred test methodology. Most of the relevant research on this test has used one of these two methods.

The most common cause of an elevated ESR is anemia. A hematocrit or hemoglobin should be done on patients with elevated ESRs. It is impossible to accurately correct the ESR value for the degree of anemia.

Any abnormality in RBC shape or size can result in a reduced ESR. Peripheral smears should be done on all patients to check that the RBC morphology is normal.

The ESR is not a useful screening test in asymptomatic patients. It is of limited usefulness in evaluating patients with vague complaints (e.g., fatigue, abdominal pain). It is extremely useful in evaluating patients with suspected temporal arteritis or polymyalgia rheumatica. It is also useful in following the clinical course of patients who have other connective tissue disorders (e.g., rheumatoid arthritis). The ESR will start to decrease within days of the initiation of steroid therapy. Treatment with nonsteroidal anti-inflammatory drugs does not normalize the ESR.

Glucose

Interpreting glucose values can be extremely difficult. The usual reasons for ordering the test are to diagnose

TABLE 19–12. NORMAL VALUES FOR DIGOXIN

Diagnostic Units: ng/ml (nmol/liter). SI conversion factor = 1.281
Therapeutic 0.5–2.2 (0.6–2.8)

Decreased	Diagnoses to Consider	Actions to Consider

<0.5 (0.6)	Inadequate dose
	Noncompliance
	Poor GI absorption
	Absorption interference:
	  Kaolin-pectin
	  Antacids
	  Cholestyramine
		1. Review medication compliance
		2. Review other medications
		3. Increase digoxin dose

Increased	**Diagnoses to Consider**	**Actions to Consider**

2.2–3.0 (2.8–3.8)	Excessive digoxin dose
	Decreased creatinine clearance
	Level taken prior to 6 hours after a dose
	Drug interaction:
	  Quinidine
	  Verapamil
	  Antibiotics
	  Nifedipine
	  Amiodarone
		1. Evaluate for toxicity
		2. Serum K, Ca, Mg, HCO_3
		3. Review medication dosing
		4. Serum Cr or BUN
		5. Review other medications

>3.0 (3.8)	Toxicity very likely	1. Stop digoxin 2. ECG monitoring 3. Correct electrolyte abnormalities

Values in parentheses are SI units.
Source: Rakel RE. Textbook of Family Practice. 4th ed. Philadelpia, W.B. Saunders, 1990, with permission.

TABLE 19–13. NORMAL VALUES FOR THE WESTERGREN ERYTHROCYTE SEDIMENTATION RATE

Diagnostic Units: (mm/hour)

Normal		Male	Female
	Children	0–10	0–10
	<50 years old	0–15	0–20
	50 to 65 years old	0–20	0–30
	>65 years old	0–38	0–53

Increased	Diagnoses to Consider	Actions to Consider
> 100	Temporal arthritis Polymyalgia rheumatica Multiple myeloma Lymphoma/leukemia Metastatic cancer Sepsis Ulcerative colitis Biliary cirrhosis	1. Serum protein electrophoresis 2. CBC
40–100	Anemia Rheumatoid arthritis Malignancy Viral hepatitis Tuberculosis Ectopic prenancy Myocardial infarction Rheumatic fever Hyperthyroidism Hypothyroidism Normal pregnancy Oral contraceptives Macrocytosis	1. Evaluate Hb/Hct and RBC morphology 2. Repeat ESR 3. Evaluate thyroid function

Decreased	Diagnoses to Consider	Actions to Consider
	Polycythemia Congestive heart failure Hemoglobinopathy Spherocytosis RBC abnormalities	1. Evaluate Hb/Hct and RBC morphology 2. Ignore isolated low values in asymptomatic patients

Source: Rakel RE. Textbook of Family Practice. 4th ed. Philadelphia, W.B. Saunders, 1990, with permission.

diabetes, follow the course of diabetic treatment, or diagnose hypoglycemia (Table 19–14).

The American Diabetes Association has defined seven different disorders of glucose metabolism [Physician's Guide to Non-Insulin Dependent (Type II) Diabetes: Diagnosis and Treatment, 1988]:

1. Type I diabetes mellitus. These patients require insulin to prevent ketoacidosis.

2. Type II diabetes mellitus. These patients are usually obese adults and can be treated with diet or oral hypoglycemic agents.

3. Impaired glucose tolerance. These patients have higher than normal glucose values but less than required to be diagnostic for diabetes.

4. Gestational diabetes mellitus. This is hyperglycemia only during pregnancy.

5. Previous abnormality of glucose tolerance. This includes patients who have had diabetes under stress, when obese or pregnant, but who now have normal glucose tolerance.

6. Potential abnormality of glucose tolerance. This includes patients with close relatives who are diabetic.

7. Other types of diabetes mellitus. This includes patients whose diabetes is caused by conditions such as pancreatic disease, Cushing's syndrome, acromegaly, thyrotoxicosis, or drugs (steroids, estrogen, or thiazide diuretics).

Two common reasons for an abnormally elevated glucose value are drawing specimens soon after a patient has eaten and drawing the blood specimen from a vein above an IV infusion.

There are two types of hypoglycemia. One is postprandial or "reactive" hypoglycemia. It is most commonly seen in patients with a history of gastric surgery who have very rapid stomach emptying times. Their symptoms (e.g., sweating, weakness, anxiety, irritability) occur several hours after eating.

The other type, fasting hypoglycemia, is seen primarily in diabetics and alcoholics. The symptoms (e.g., mental confusion, bizarre behavior, seizures) are more gradual in onset and occur after a long period of fasting.

Other disorders associated with hypoglycemia are insulinoma, adrenal insufficiency, hypopituitarism, and drug-induced hypoglycemia (insulin, sulfonylureas, and salicylates).

It is essential to remember that not all glucose specimens are the same. A random glucose taken 2 hours after lunch should not be interpreted the same as a fasting sample. In addition, there are differences between whole blood, serum, and plasma values. Venous plasma and serum glucose values are 15% higher than venous whole blood values. Capillary whole blood values are 10% higher than VENOUS whole blood. Venous plasma and serum values are 5% to 7% higher than those found in capillary whole blood. (The values given in Table 19–14 are for venous plasma and serum. The values for other types of specimens should be adjusted accordingly.)

Table 19–14 differentiates screening tests from diagnostic tests. The usual screening test is a fasting glucose. The results of this test may indicate that the patient is normal, may suggest that a diagnostic test (i.e., glucose tolerance test) be done, or may be diagnostic of diabetes. Note that there are different screening and diagnostic tests for gestational diabetes (i.e., the O'Sullivan test).

Glycosylated Hemoglobin

The glycosylation of hemoglobin occurs continuously during a red blood cell's life and is directly related to the average glucose concentration. Measurement of glycosylated hemoglobin has become a useful clinical test to assess the "average" glucose control in diabetic patients during the previous 1 to 3 months (Table 19–15). Increased percentages of glycosylated hemoglobin reflect increased hyperglycemia [Physicians' Guide to Non-Insulin dependent (Type II) Diabetes: Diagnosis and Treatment, 1988].

TABLE 19–14. NORMAL VALUES FOR VENOUS GLUCOSE

Diagnostic Units: mg/dl (mmol/liter). SI conversion factor = 0.05551

SCREENING TEST: FASTING GLUCOSE

	Normal	*Requires GTT*	*Diagnostic of Diabetes*
Adult	< 115 (6.38)	115–140 (6.38–7.77)	> 140 (7.7) (two tests)
Child	< 130 (7.22)	130–140 (7.22–7.77)	> 140 (7.77) (two tests)

CONFIRMATORY TESTS: GLUCOSE TOLERANCE TESTS

Adult: 75 gram oral glucose dose

	Normal	*Impaired Glucose Tolerance*	*Diabetes*
Fasting	< 115 (6.38)	< 140 (7.77), and	< 140 (7.77), and
30 minutes	< 200 (11.1)		
60 minutes	< 200 (11.1)	1 of 3 > 200 (11.1), and	1 of 3 > 200 (11.1), and
90 minutes	< 200 (11.1)		
120 minutes	< 140 (7.77)	140–200 (7.77–11.1)	> 200 (11.1)

Child: 1.75 grams glucose per kilogram body weight up to 75 grams

	Normal	*Impaired Glucose Tolerance*	*Diabetes*
Fasting	< 130 (7.22)	< 140 (7.77)	> 140 (7.77), and
30 minutes	< 200 (11.1)	< 200 (11.1)	
60 minutes	< 200 (11.1)	< 200 (11.1)	1 of 3 > 200 (11.1), and
90 minutes	< 200 (11.1)	< 200 (11.1)	
120 minutes	< 140 (7.77)	140–200 (7.77–11.1)	> 200 (11.1)

PREGNANCY
   Screening: O'Sullivan screen
        50 grams glucose (patient can be nonfasting)
        "Positive" if ≥ 140 (7.77) at 1 hour

   Confirmation: O'Sullivan 3 hour GTT
     100 grams oral glucose in a fasting patient
     The patient is positive for gestational diabetes if two or more of the   values are:
        Fasting: ≥ 105 (5.79)
        1 hour: ≥ 190 (10.55)
        2 hour: ≥ 165 (9.16)
        3 hour: ≥ 145 (8.05)

HYPOGLYCEMIA
  Males: < 55 (3.05) at the same time as patient has symptoms
  Females: < 40 (2.22) at the same time as patient has symptoms

Values in parentheses are SI units.
Source: Rakel RE. Textbook of Family Practice. 4th ed. Philadelphia, W.B. Saunders, 1990, with permission.

TABLE 19–15. NORMAL VALUES FOR GLYCOSYLATED HEMOGLOBIN

Diagnostic Units: percentage of total hemoglobin
Normal 5–7% (varies by laboratory)

Increased	*Diagnoses to Consider*	*Actions to Consider*
< 9%	Good diabetic control (most glucoses < 200 mg/dl)	1. No change in therapy
9–14%	Average diabetic control (most glucoses < 300 mg/dl)	1. Consider home glucose monitoring
> 14%	Poor diabetic control (i.e., persistent hyperglycemia)	1. Evaluate for causes of poor diabetic control

Source: Rakel RE. Textbook of Family Practice. 4th ed. Philadelpia, W.B. Saunders, 1990, with permission.

Hyperglycemia is associated with the glycosylation of other body proteins, and this glycosylation may be the basis for the angiopathic and neuropathic changes seen in diabetes. Some clinicians, therefore, use the glycosylation hemoglobin test as an assessment of a patient's risk for diabetic complications.

The glycosylation hemoglobin value does not change with rapid hour-to-hour or day-to-day variations in serum glucose. It is therefore not appropriate to use this test in making decisions about insulin dosage in either acutely ill hospitalized patients or ambulatory diabetics on insulin. Home glucose monitoring is a better source of data for these decisions.

There is great variation between laboratories on both the "normal" range of values as well as the degree of elevation associated with various levels of hyperglycemia. It is therefore important to know the characteristics of your specific laboratory's test.

TABLE 19–16. NORMAL VALUES FOR HEMOGLOBIN

Diagnostic Units: Hemoglobin: gm/dl (gm/liter). SI conversion factor = 10.0

			Hemoglobin
Normal	Males	Birth	18.5–21.5 (185–215)
		1 month	15.5–18.5 (155–185)
		3 months	13.5–16.5 (135–165)
		6 months	13.0–16.0 (130–160)
		9 months	12.0–14.0 (120–140)
		1 year	10.0–14.0 (100–140)
		2 years	10.5–14.2 (105–142)
		4 years	11.2–14.3 (112–143)
		8 years	12.0–14.8 (120–148)
		14 years	12.5–15.0 (125–150)
		Adult	13.9–16.3 (139–163)
	Females	Birth	18.0–21.0 (180–210)
		1 month	15.8–18.9 (158–189)
		3 months	13.3–16.4 (133–164)
		6 months	12.8–14.8 (128–148)
		9 months	11.7–13.9 (117–139)
		1 year	10.0–14.0 (100–140)
		2 years	10.5–14.2 (105–142)
		4 years	11.3–14.2 (113–142)
		8 years	11.5–14.5 (115–145)
		14 years	11.6–14.8 (116–148)
		Adult	12.0–15.0 (120–150)

Increased	*Diagnoses to Consider*	*Actions to Consider*

Hb > 16.5 (165)	Dehydration
	Diuretic use
	Polycythemia vera
	Secondary polycythemia:
	  High altitude
	  Pulmonarydisease
	  Cardiac disease
	  Renal tumor
		1. Smoking history
		2. Check volume status
		3. Splenomegaly
		4. Urinalysis
		5. CBC
		6. Platelet count
		7. Alkaline phosphatase

Hb > 22 (220)	Severe polycythemia	1. Consider phlebotomy

Decreased	*Diagnoses to Consider*	*Actions to Consider*
Hb < 11 (110)	Blood loss Decreased blood cell survival Decrased marrow production RBC sequestration (spleen)	1. History of chronic disease 2. Menstrual history 3. Stool for occult blood 4. Splenomegaly 5. RBC indices 6. Reticulocyte count 7. Trial on iron therapy 8. Iron, TIBC, ferritin 9. Folate, B_{12}
Hb < 8 (80)	Severe anemia	1. Consider transfusion

Values in parentheses are SI units.
Source: Rakel RE. Textbook of Family Practice. 4th ed. Philadelphia, W.B. Saunders, 1990, with permission.

The test may be falsely elevated in patients with uremia, alcoholism, or aspirin use. It may be falsely lowered in anemia, hemoglobinopathies, and pregnancy.

Hemoglobin and Hematocrit

These two tests are often used interchangeably in clinical practice to measure the oxygen-carrying capacity of a volume of blood. It is important to remember that they are NOT measures of either total blood volume or red cell mass. Table 19–16 gives the range of values for hemoglobin. The equivalent hematocrit percentage can be obtained by multiplying the gm/dl value by 3 or the gm/liter value by 0.3.

Most automated hematology instruments measure the hemoglobin and calculate the hematocrit from the RBC count and the mean corpuscular volume (MCV). The hematocrit can be measured by centrifuging a microcapillary tube filled with whole blood. The "spun" hematocrit is defined as the percent volume of RBCs after maximal packing has occurred.

These two tests provide comparable information except in patients with abnormally shaped RBCs (e.g., sick-led cells). In such patients, the "spun" hematocrit is ar-tificially high because the RBCs trap plasma as they are packed. A hemoglobin is the test of choice for these pa-tients.

There is little evidence that the general population benefits from routine hemoglobin or hematocrit screen-ing. Screening may, however, be indicated in groups at high risk for anemia, such as infants, pregnant or men-struating females, and the institutionalized elderly. It is also customary to screen patients undergoing a proce-dure that could be associated with blood loss as well as all hospitalized patients on admission.

The most common abnormal finding is a mild, unsus-pected anemia. The patient is usually asymptomatic. The importance of the finding is not based on the need to treat the anemia but rather the need to discover the anemia's cause. The cause is frequently a clinically im-portant diagnosis (e.g., poor nutrition, menorrhagia, pernicious anemia, colon cancer).

In addition to screening, a hemoglobin or hematocrit is an essential test when an anemia is suspected, when there is abnormal bleeding, or when polycythemia is part of the differential diagnosis.

The most common error in interpreting a hemoglo-bin or hematocrit value is to rely on it as an indicator of acute blood loss. These tests are not good measures of total blood volume! Twelve to 24 hours are required after acute blood loss before fluid equilibration has fi-nalized. It is only then that the hemoglobin or hemato-crit can be used to indicate the extent of blood loss.

Mean Corpuscular Volume (MCV)

The MCV is the most important of the red blood cell indices. Its primary use is to differentiate anemias into macrocytic, normocytic, or microcytic (Table 19–17).

Reticulocytes and other very young RBCs are round macrocytes. A rapid marrow release of RBCs will there-fore produce an increased MCV. This should not be confused with other causes of macrocytosis.

It is important to remember that the MCV is an av-erage size of all RBC populations. Mixed populations of macrocytic and microcytic cells may produce a normo-cytic MCV. This is seen in the early treatment of iron de-ficiency anemia (i.e., macrocytic reticulocytes plus mi-crocytic cells) as well as in alcoholic patients who are both folate and iron deficient. It is useful to examine a peripheral blood smear for RBC morphology in an ane-mic patient.

Platelet Count

The normal adult platelet count ranges from 140 to 400×10^9 per liter. Counts below 140×10^9 per liter indicate thrombocytopenia. Counts greater than 400×10^9 per liter indicate thrombocytosis (Table 19–18).

Because most automated blood cell counters rou-tinely count platelets along with the other cells, platelet counts are reported on most specimens sent for a CBC. Thus, the most common platelet count abnormality is a

TABLE 19–17. NORMAL VALUES FOR MEAN CORPUSCULAR VOLUME

Diagnostic Units: cubic microns (fL). SI conversion factor = 1
Normal 76–100

Increased	Diagnoses to Consider	Actions to Consider
100–120	Reticulocytosis Folate deficiency B_{12} deficiency Hypothyroidism Response to chemotherapy	1. Reticulocyte count 2. Serum B_{12} 3. Serum or RBC folate 4. T_4
> 120	Folate deficiency B_{12} deficiency	1. Serum B_{12} 2. Serum or RBC folate

Decreased	Diagnoses to Consider	Actions to Consider
70–76	Iron deficiency Thalassemia Anemia of chronic disease Hereditary sideroblastic anemia Lead poisoning RBC fragmentation (burns)	1. Reticulocyte count 2. Peripheral smear 3. Serum iron, TIBC, or ferritin 4. Hb electrophoresis
< 70	Severe iron deficiency Thalassemia	1. Reticulocyte count 2. Peripheral smear 3. Serum iron, TIBC, or ferritin 4. Hb electrophoresis

Source: Rakel RE. Textbook of Family Practice. 4th ed. Philadelphia, W.B. Saunders, 1990, with permission.

small increase or decrease from normal in an otherwise asymptomatic individual. There is usually no benefit from further evaluation (including repeating the test) of these cases.

The platelet count is useful as a screening test in pa-tients undergoing a major surgical procedure and in the evaluation of patients with abnormal bleeding, bruising, purpura, petechiae, or splenomegaly. It is of little use in testing asymptomatic outpatients, or in admission test-ing for nonsurgical hospitalized patients.

Thrombocytopenia can be caused by a reduction in the marrow's production of platelets (from marrow sup-pression or infiltration), increased platelet destruction, or sequestration of platelets in the spleen. A platelet count is a very useful indicator of marrow sensitivity to cytotoxic medications in the treatment of cancer.

It should be remembered that platelets may be ade-quate in number but defective in function. Medications are the most common cause of abnormal platelet func-tion (e.g., aspirin, other nonsteroidal anti-inflammatory drugs, alcohol, and penicillins).

Potassium

Potassium is the major cation in the intracellular fluid. Ninety-eight percent of the total body potassium is contained within the cells. The kidneys are responsible for regulating the level of extracellular potassium. Hy-

TABLE 19–18. NORMAL VALUES FOR PLATELET COUNT

Diagnostic Units: platelets $\times 10^9$/liter
First week of life: 84–478
After first week of life: 140–400

Decreased	Diagnoses to Consider	Actions to Consider
100–400	Response to viral illness Response to bacterial illness	1. Repeat test
50–100 (may have bleeding with major surgery)	Thrombocytopenia purpura Post transfusion Spleen sequestration Marrow infiltration (i.e., leukemia) Response to cytotoxic drugs	1. History of all medications 2. Alcohol history 3. Examine for splenomegaly 4. CBC 5. Trial off all medications 6. Bone marrow biopsy
20–50 (may have bleeding with minor procedure)	Thrombocytopenia Marrow infiltration DIC	1. Platelet transfusion for any procedure
< 20 (may have spontaneous GI or CNS hemorrhage)	Severe thrombocytopenia	1. Platelet transfusion to prevent spontaneous bleeding
Increased	**Diagnoses to Consider**	**Actions to Consider**
400–600	Splenectomy Infection Blood loss Inflammatory bowel disease Collagen vascular disease	1. Repeat test
600–1000	Malignancy Polycythemia vera	1. Evaluate for malignancy
> 1000 (may have spontaneous thrombosis and bleeding)	Severe thrombocytosis	1. Administer antiplatelet drugs

Source: Rakel RE. Textbook of Family Practice. 4th ed. Philadelphia, W.B. Saunders, 1990, with permission.

pokalemia and hyperkalemia are primarily due to renal disorders or to abnormalities in the intake of potassium.

It is not useful to test healthy outpatients for this electrolyte. However, the test is very useful for patients with renal disease, those on diuretics, and those who complain of weakness (Table 19–19). It is customary to obtain a serum potassium on all acutely ill hospitalized patients. Potassium disorders are common in hospitalized patients because of the frequent use of IVs and nasogastric suction.

The most commonly seen potassium disorder is a mild hypokalemia in patients on a thiazide or loop diuretic. These patients are often asymptomatic and may not require treatment. Mild hypokalemia can be associated with vague complaints such as weakness, muscle cramps, or paresthesias. More severe hypokalemia may cause arrhythmias, paralytic ileus, or paralysis. All hypokalemic patients on digoxin require treatment because of the increased risk for digoxin toxicity with even mild hypokalemia.

The most common reason for hyperkalemia is hemolysis of red cells during blood collection or processing. In some cases, these specimens have red serum. If in doubt, retest the patient prior to initiating a long workup for hyperkalemia.

Hyperkalemia is associated with patient complaints of weakness or paralysis. Severe hyperkalemia (greater than 8) is associated with bradycardia, hypotension, ventricular fibrillation, and cardiac arrest.

When there is suspicion of laboratory error, a quick and useful maneuver is to do an electrocardiogram (ECG). Clinically significant hyperkalemia or hypokalemia is usually associated with the ECG findings cited in Table 19–19.

Protein

The "total" serum protein measured by the laboratory includes albumin plus the various globulins (Table 19–20). Fibrinogen, another blood protein, is not measured since it is depleted when serum clots.

Decreased levels of total protein are seen in a wide variety of illnesses. In most cases, these diseases are better followed by serum albumin tests, since it is the albumin fraction which is usually reduced. A reduction in albumin is also a better guide to edematous states, since it is responsible for 90% of the oncotic pressure.

Increased levels of protein are occasionally seen and usually lead to an evaluation for multiple myeloma. However, myeloma can be associated with increased, normal, or decreased total protein levels.

When there is a question about the interpretation of

TABLE 19–19. NORMAL VALUES FOR POTASSIUM

Diagnostic Units: mEq/liter (mmol/liter). SI conversion factor = 1
Normal 3.5–5.0 (3.5–5.0)

Increased	Diagnoses to Consider	Actions to Consider

5.0–7.5	Hemolyzed specimen
	Drugs:
	  Potassium-sparing diuretics
	  NSAID
	  ACE inhibitors
	  Potassium
	    supplementation
	Decreased renal excretion:
	  Acute renal failure
	  Chronic renal failure
	  Addison's disease
	Acidosis
	Tissue destruction
		1. Repeat K on new
		   specimen
		2. Drug and diet history
		3. Check ECG for
		   peaked T
		4. Creatinine
		5. Serum electrolytes
		6. Urine electrolytes

> 7.5	Hyperkalemic arrhythmias
	Hyperkalemic paralysis
		1. ECG for peaked T,
		   wide QRS, absent P
		2. Calcium gluconate
		3. Glucose/insulin
		   infusion
		4. Bicarbonate
		5. Ion exchange resins

Decreased	Diagnoses to Consider	Actions to Consider

3.5–2.5	Renal loss:
	  Thiazide or loop diuretics
	  Renal tubular acidosis
	  Hyperaldosteronism
	Gastrointestinal loss:
	  Vomiting
	  Diarrhea
	Inadequate dietary potassium
	Inadequate IV potassium
	Insulin therapy
	Metabolic alkalosis
		1. Drug and diet history
		2. Serum electrolytes
		3. Urine electrolytes
		4. ECG for ST sagging,
		   T depression, and U
		   waves
		5. Monitor for digoxin
		   toxicity
		6. Administer oral
		   potassium

< 2.5	Hypokalemic arrhythmias	1. Monitor closely for
		   arrhythmias and
		   paralysis
		2. Administer IV and
		   oral potassium

Values in parentheses are SI units.
Source: Rakel RE. Textbook of Family Practice. 4th ed. Philadelphia, W.B. Saunders, 1990, with permission.

any abnormal total protein, it is useful to obtain a protein electrophoresis. This test separates albumin from the various globulins. The electrophoretic pattern may be diagnostically helpful. Immunologic typing should be done for any electrophoretic "spike" to further test for multiple myeloma.

Prothrombin

The prothrombin time (PT) is the only coagulation test commonly used in the outpatient setting (Table 19–21). PT is the time required to initiate clotting when tissue thromboplastin is mixed with blood. It measures the extrinsic clotting system (i.e., Factor VII) as well those factors common to both intrinsic and extrinsic system (i.e., Factor X, Factor V, prothrombin, and fibrinogen) (Hirsh and Levine).

A PT is not a useful screening test for asymptomatic patients, even those undergoing a surgical procedure. It is most commonly used in monitoring the anticoagulation effects of warfarin (Coumadin). It is also a useful test in evaluating patients with abnormal bleeding. It is important to note that the PT is normal in patients with classic hemophilia (i.e., Factor VIII deficiency) and those with von Willebrand's disease.

There has been much confusion about PT testing. A broad range of values have been called "normal" by different laboratories. There has also been disagreement about appropriate therapeutic PT levels in patients on warfarin. Many of these problems are due to the fact that the test procedure relies on thromboplastin reagents which vary considerably in their clotting activity. The reagents used today are less active than those used in the early studies on therapeutic anticoagulation. This has led some clinicians to over-anticoagulate their patients.

Table 19–21 gives values for these different PT reporting systems. PT results may be reported in seconds, as a ratio compared with normal controls, or as an International Normalized Ratio (INR). The INR is standardized to the World Health Organization's reference thromboplastin. It is essential to know which of these reporting systems is being used to assure adequate anticoagulation without risking unnecessary bleeding.

Sodium

Sodium is the major cation in extracellular fluid. To interpret this test properly it is necessary to think about it not as a measure of total body sodium, but rather as a measure of both the total body water and the effective

TABLE 19–20. NORMAL VALUES FOR PROTEIN

Diagnostic Units: gm/dl (gm/liter). SI conversion factor = 10.0
Normal 6–8 (60–80)

Decreased	Diagnoses to Consider	Actions to Consider

< 6 (60)	Decreased synthesis:
	  Liver insufficiency
	  Malnutrition
	  Malignancy
	Increased loss:
	  Nephrotic syndrome
	  Extensive burns
	  Protein-losing
	   enteropathy
	Inflammatory illness
	Myeloma
	Overhydration
		1. Dietary history
		2. Urinalysis
		3. 24-hour urine
		   protein
		4. Bilirubin
		5. Creatinine
		6. Protein
		   electrophoresis

Increased	Diagnoses to Consider	Actions to Consider
> 8 (80)	Dehydration Multiple myeloma Sarcoidosis Monoclonal gammopathy Chronic inflammation	1. Creatinine, BUN 2. Protein electrophoresis 3. Chest x-ray

Values in parentheses are SI units.
Source: Rakel RE. Textbook of Family Practice. 4th ed. Philadelphia, W.B. Saunders Company, 1990, with permission.

TABLE 19–21. THERAPEUTIC VALUES FOR PROTHROMBIN TIME

Normal	Seconds	Patient/Control Ratio (Rabbit Brain Thromboplastin)	INR*
	11–13	0.9–1.1	0.8–1.3

Increased Due to Disease	Diagnoses to Consider	Actions to Consider
>12 seconds	Liver disease Malabsorption DIC Warfarin therapy Factor II, V, VII, X deficiency Vitamin K deficiency	1. Liver enzymes, bilirubin 2. PTT 3. Clotting factor assays 4. Serum carotene 5. 72-hour stool fat 6. Administer vitamin K

Optimal Anticoagulation Therapy	Seconds	Patient/Control Ratio (Rabbit Brain Thromboplastin)	INR*
Treatment of deep vein thrombosis	15–18.5	1.3–1.6	2.0–3.0
Treatment of pulmonary embolism	15–18.5	1.3–1.6	2.0–3.0
Prevention of embolism in atrial fibrillation or tissue heart valves	15–18.5	1.3–1.6	2.0–3.0
Prevention of embolism in patients with prosthetic heart valves	18.5–21	1.6–1.8	3.0–4.5
Prevention of embolism in patients with recurrent emboli	18.5–21	1.6–1.8	3.0–4.5

*INR: International Normalization Ratio.
Source: Rakel RE. Textbook of Family Practice. 4th ed. Philadelphia, W.B. Saunders, 1990, with permission.

circulatory volume (Table 19–22). In normal situations the serum osmolality is used by the body to adjust the serum sodium. When osmolality increases, thirst increases, more water is taken in, and the antidiuretic hormone (ADH) is secreted, so that less free water is lost by the kidneys. When osmolality decreases, thirst is turned off and ADH secretion is suppressed. In situations where the effective circulatory volume is reduced (e.g., heart failure), the body may sacrifice a normal osmolality in an effort to maintain the circulatory volume. In this case, sodium falls as free water is retained.

A serum sodium cannot be properly interpreted without a physical examination of the patient's volume status. In hypovolemic states there will be an orthostatic blood pressure drop, decreased skin turgor, dry mucous membranes, and weight loss. Hypovolemia can be associated with a normal, increased, or decreased serum sodium. To a large extent, the sodium value in the face of dehydration depends on a patient's access to free water. Hypovolemia leads to thirst. If this results in drinking low-sodium fluids, hyponatremia follows.

Heart failure, cirrhosis, and nephrotic syndrome are frequent causes of hypervolemia (e.g., edematous states). In each case, the total body water is increased but the effective circulating volume is decreased. Therefore, ADH is stimulated and free water is retained. This leads to hyponatremia.

Pseudohyponatremia is seen with hyperglycemia, severe hyperlipidemia, or hyperproteinemia. In these conditions, the presence of other solutes in the serum results in an artificially low serum sodium value when measured by flame photometry.

Serum sodium is not a useful test in the routine screening of healthy individuals. It is very useful in patients with heart failure, liver disease, chronic renal failure, and other edematous states. All acutely ill hospitalized patients should be tested, since serum sodium is often altered by IV therapy or nasogastric suction. Patients on lithium therapy should be tested because this drug can lead to nephrogenic diabetes insipidus.

Theophylline

Therapeutic drug level monitoring is extremely important when using medications that have serious toxic effects and that display wide variations in absorption or metabolism. Theophylline is such a drug, so its measurement has become a common practice (Table 19–23).

The bioavailability of theophylline is the fraction of drug absorbed. Following absorption, the blood level reaches a peak, which is the highest drug concentration. For currently available theophylline preparations, the dose-to-peak time varies from 2 to 12 hours. Theophylline is then metabolized by the liver and excreted by the kidneys. The time required to decrease the drug's blood concentration by 50% is referred to as its half-life. Theophylline's half-life is 8 to 9 hours and does not vary with the preparation type. After four to five consecutive doses have been taken, the drug reaches a steady state level. A drug level drawn just before the next dose is the

TABLE 19–22. NORMAL VALUES FOR SODIUM

Diagnostic Units: mEq/liter (mmol/liter). SI conversion factor = 1
Normal: 135–147 (135–147)

Increased	Diagnoses to Consider	Actions to Consider

> 147	Fluid loss in excess of salt:
	  Sweating
	  Diarrhea
	  Diabetes mellitus (osmotic diuresis)
	  Diabetes insipidus
	  Hyperaldosteronism
	Reduced fluid intake:
	  Altered mental status (unable to drink)
	  Vomiting
	Excessive salt intake:
	  Infant formula
	  Hypertonic NG feeding
	  Salt poisoning
		1. Clinical assessment of fluid status
		2. Serum electrolytes
		3. Serum BUN/creatinine
		4. Serum glucose
		5. Urine specific gravity
		6. Give PO fluids

> 160	CNS symptoms if an acute change	1. Slow hydration with isotonic saline (reduce serum sodium no faster than 10 mEq/liter each day)

Decreased	Diagnoses to Consider	Actions to Consider

< 135	Excess water:
	  Psychogenic polydipsia
	  Excessive IV hydration
	Decreased effective circulatory volume:
	  Diuretic therapy
	  Congestive heart failure
	  Cirrhosis
	  Nephrotic syndrome
	  Dehydration with free water access
	Inability to excrete water:
	  Renal failure (Cr Cl < 15)
	  SIADH
	Sodium depletion:
	  Gastrointestinal loss
	  Excessive sweating
	  Adrenal insufficiency
	Pseudohyponatremia
		1. Clinical assessment of fluid status
		2. Urine/serum osmolality
		3. Urine protein
		4. BUN, creatinine
		5. Urine specific gravity
		6. Serum albumin
		7. Serum electrolyte
		8. Water restriction

< 120	CNS symptoms are likely due to brain swelling	1. Administer hypertonic saline (3%) until sodium is 125 mEq/liter.

Values in parentheses are SI units.
Source: Rakel RE. Textbook of Family Practice. 4th ed. Philadelphia, W.B. Saunders, 1990, with permission.

lowest steady-state level and is referred to as a "trough" level.

Theophylline levels are affected by a variety of factors, including the type of drug preparation, frequency of dosing, and the patient's size and age. The body's metabolism of theophylline can be decreased by liver disease, pulmonary disease, heart failure, and the concomitant use of erythromycin or cimetidine. Smoking, on the other hand, increases theophylline metabolism.

There is debate about whether a peak or trough level is better in managing a patient on theophylline. The answer depends on what information is needed. In general, the peak level is used to assess toxicity, while the trough is a useful measure of dosing adequacy.

High theophylline levels are associated with nausea, vomiting, diarrhea, headache, insomnia, agitation, tachycardia, seizures, tremor, and fever. The occurrence of toxic side effects tends to be very individual. Some patients will have seizures, tachyarrhythmias, or circulatory collapse at a theophylline level of 50. Others remain asymptomatic at this level.

It is essential that a complete dosing history be taken whenever a theophylline level is drawn. It is impossible to interpret a value without knowing which preparation is being taken, if the patient has been compliant, and the timing of the last dose.

Thyroxin (T_4)

Thyroxin is the principal hormone secreted by the thyroid gland. It is almost completely bound to proteins in the circulation. Most of the binding is to thyroxin-binding globulin (TBG), but a small amount is also bound to albumin. The active form of the hormone is free thyroxin (i.e., not bound to protein). The body uses thyroxin to regulate tissue metabolism.

The most common screening thyroid test is a serum thyroxin. Unfortunately, this test measures *total* thy-

TABLE 19–23. VALUES FOR THEOPHYLLINE

Diagnostic Units: μg/ml (μmol/liter). SI conversion factor = 5.55
Therapeutic: 10–20 (56–111)

Decreased	Diagnoses to Consider	Actions to Consider

< 10 (56)	Noncompliance
	Inadequate dosage
	Change in drug
	  metabolism
	Trough level
	Use of short half-
	  life theophylline
		1. Review drug compliance
		2. Check time of last dose
		3. Is patient a new smoker?
		4. Is drug being absorbed?
		5. Increase dose or frequency
		  by 100% if level is < 5
		  by 50% if level is 5–8
		  by 20% if level is 8–10

Increased	Diagnoses to Consider	Actions to Consider

20–35
(111–
194)
	Excessive dose
	Excessive dosing
	  frequency
	Erythromycin alters
	  drug metabolism
	Cimetidine alters
	  drug metabolism
	Liver disease
	Heart failure
		1. Complete drug history
		2. Examine for side effects
		3. Decrease dose

> 35
(194)
	Dosing error
	Intentional
	  overdose
		1. Examine for side effects
		2. Hospitalize to monitor
		3. Administer activated
		  charcoal

> 50	Seizures or
	  arrhythmias very
	  likely	

Values in parentheses are SI units.
Source: Rakel RE. Textbook of Family Practice. 4th ed. Philadelphia, W.B. Saunders, 1990, with permission.

TABLE 19–24. NORMAL VALUES FOR THYROXIN

Diagnostic Units: μg/dl (nmol/liter). SI conversion factor = 13.0
Normal: 5.5–12.5 (72–163)

Increased	Diagnoses to Consider	Actions to Consider

> 12.5 (163)	Hyperthyroidism
	Elevated TBG:
	  Birth control pills
	  Pregnancy
	  Estrogens
	Liver disease
	Drugs:
	  Propranolol
	  Amphetamines
	  Contrast media
	  Amiodarone
	  Heparin
		1. Complete drug
		  history
		2. T$_4$ index
		3. Sensitive TSH
		4. Free T$_3$
		5. Thyroid uptake scan

Decreased	Diagnoses to Consider	Actions to Consider

< 5.5 (72)	Hypothyroidism
	Decreased TBG:
	  Malnutrition
	  Liver diseases
	  Nephrotic syndrome
	  Androgens
	  Glucocorticoids
	Sick thyroid syndrome
		1. T$_4$ index
		2. TSH
		3. Albumin
		4. Urinary protein

Values in parentheses are SI units.
Source: Rakel RE. Textbook of Family Practice. 4th ed. Philadelphia, W.B. Saunders, 1990, with permission.

roxin and not just the active free T$_4$. Many of the test abnormalities that are seen are due to abnormal levels of thyroid-binding globulin, not that of active T$_4$.

The free T$_4$ level can be approximated by ordering a T$_3$ uptake test and calculating the free T$_4$ index (Table 19–24). This index approximates the free T$_4$. If it is increased, it suggests hyperthyroidism. If it is decreased, it suggests hypothyroidism.

When using the T$_4$ or the T$_4$ index as screening tests, there frequently remain cases in which the diagnosis is uncertain. If hypothyroidism is the concern, a thyroid-stimulating hormone (TSH) test is usually helpful. If hyperthyroidism is the concern, the free T$_3$ on a sensitive TSH test can be helpful.

Thyroxin-binding globulin and free T$_4$ levels are available, but are rarely used diagnostically. In difficult cases, the response to thyrotropin-releasing hormone (TRH) can be studied to sort out both hyperthyroid and hypothyroid diagnoses.

Uric Acid

The serum level of uric acid is based on the balance between the rate at which purines are absorbed or produced by the body and their rate of metabolism and excretion (Table 19–25). Increased levels can be due to increased purine absorption (e.g., high-protein diet), increased production (e.g., leukemia), or reduced excretion (e.g., chronic renal failure).

There is no evidence that uric acid in solution causes any disease. All the diseases associated with hyperuricemia are due to the deposition of uric acid crystals. These illnesses include acute gouty arthritis, gouty tophi, gouty nephropathy, and urolithiasis. Low uric acid levels are occasionally seen in patients with renal tubular defects and are otherwise of no clinical significance.

The most common test abnormality is mild hyperuricemia in asymptomatic patients. The frequency of this

TABLE 19–25. NORMAL VALUES FOR URIC ACID

Diagnostic Units: mg/dl (μmol/liter). SI conversion factor = 60
Normal: 2.5–7.0 (150–420)

Increased	Diagnoses to Consider	Actions to Consider

> 7.0
(420)
	Gout
	Diuretics
	Chronic renal failure
	High protein diet
	Leukemia,
	  lymphoma
		1. Tap inflamed joint
		2. Complete dietary history
		3. Complete drug history
		4. Serum creatinine
		5. 24-hour urinary uric
		  acid
		6. Colchicine trial
		7. CBC

Values in parentheses are SI units.
Source: Rakel RE. Textbook of Family Practice. 4th ed. Philadelphia, W.B. Saunders, 1990, with permission.

finding is due to the presence of uric acid on screening panels. There is wide agreement that in the absence of acute gouty arthritis, tophi, renal disease or renal stones, these patients require no treatment. Most patients with renal failure will have hyperuricemia due to the kidney's reduced ability to excrete uric acid. Such patients' levels are usually less than 10 and do not require treatment if asymptomatic.

A uric acid less than 7 is sometimes seen in patients with acute gout. This is believed due to a urate diuresis that occurs in response to joint inflammation. The diagnosis of acute gouty arthritis must be based on the microscopic identification of urate crystals in synovial fluid. Many patients have been misdiagnosed as having gout when they had another form of arthritis (e.g., os-

teoarthritis) but also had incidental, asymptomatic hyperuricemia.

White Blood Cell Count (WBC Count)

Changes in the WBC count are seen in many infectious, hematologic, inflammatory, and neoplastic diseases. This variety of diseases makes the WBC count a nonspecific test. However, the WBC can be a sensitive indicator of disease in some clinical situations. Its degree of increase or decrease often correlates with the severity of the disease process. Following changes in the WBC count over time can provide useful information about the course of an illness (Table 19–26).

Leukopenia usually indicates neutropenia. This is de-

TABLE 19–26. NORMAL RANGES FOR WHITE BLOOD CELL COUNT

Diagnostic Units: cells/mm^3 (cells $\times$ 10^9/liter.) SI conversion factor = 0.001

Age	Average	95% Range
Birth	18,100	9,000–30,000
12 hours	22,800	13,000–38,000
24 hours	18,900	9,400–34,000
1 week	12,200	5,000–21,000
2 months	11,000	5,500–18,000
1 year	11,400	6,000–17,500
2 years	10,600	6,000–17,000
6 years	8,500	5,000–14,500
10 years	8,100	4,500–13,500
20 years	7,500	4,500–11,500
Adult	6,500	3,200–9,800

Decreased	Diagnoses to Consider	Actions to Consider
500–3200 (0.5–32) in adults	Infections: 　Severe bacterial infection 　Influenza 　Infectious mononucleosis 　Typhoid fever Drugs: 　Cytotoxic 　Idiosyncratic Congestive splenomegaly Felty's syndrome SLE Megaloblastic anemia Aplastic anemia Congenital neutropenia	1. Complete drug history 2. Peripheral smear 3. Platelet count 4. CBC 5. Mono test 6. ANA 7. Folate, B$_{12}$ levels 8. Bone marrow biopsy
< 500 (0.5)	At risk for severe bacterial infections	1. Frequent examinations 2. Antibiotics for fever

Increased	Diagnoses to Consider	Actions to Consider
9800–30,000 (9.8–30) in adults	Physiologic reaction to stress Infection Tissue destruction Leukemia Cancer Hemorrhage Splenectomy	1. Symptom-directed physical examination 2. Peripheral smear
> 30,000 (30)	Leukemia Leukemoid reaction	1. Peripheral smear 2. Examine for hepatomegaly and splenomegaly

Values in parentheses are SI units.
Source: Rakel RE. Textbook of Family Practice. 4th ed. Philadelphia, W.B. Saunders, 1990, with permission.

TABLE 19–27. NORMAL VALUES FOR WHITE BLOOD CELL DIFFERENTIAL COUNT BY AGE

Age	Segmented Neutrophils %	Band Neutrophils %	Eosinophils %	Basophils %	Lymphocytes %	Monocytes %
Birth	47	14	2.2	0.6	31	5.8
1 week	34	11.8	4.1	0.4	41	9.1
1 year	23	8.1	2.6	0.4	61	4.8
4 years	34	8.0	2.8	0.6	50	5.0
12 years	47	8.0	2.5	0.5	38	4.4
20 years	51	8.0	2.7	0.5	33	5.0

Source: Rakel RE. Textbook of Family Practice. 4th ed. Philadelphia, W.B. Saunders, 1990, with permission.

fined as fewer than 2×10^9 neutrophils per liter in white patients or 1.5×10^9 per liter in blacks. In patients receiving chemotherapy, neutropenia of fewer than 0.5×10^9 per liter is often associated with severe infection.

Lymphopenia is defined as fewer than 1.5×10^9 lymphocytes per liter. It is seen in association with a wide variety of physiologic stresses and is of no clinical significance. Reductions in monocytes, eosinophils, and ba-

sophils are occasionally seen and are not clinically useful.

An increased WBC count can be seen in many diseases. The average WBC count tends to be higher in children than adults (see Table 19–26). Most elevated outpatient WBC counts are below 30×10^9 per liter. Counts greater than 30×10^9 are usually due to leukemia or a leukemoid reaction. It is obviously crucial to differentiate between these two diagnoses.

REFERENCES

Boyko EJ, Alderman BW, Barron, AE. Reference test errors bias the evaluation of diagnostic tests for ischemic heart disease. J Gen Intern Med 1988; 3:476–481.

DeNeef P. Selective testing for streptococcal pharyngitis in adults. J Fam Pract 1987; 25:347–351.

Hirsh J, Levine MN. The optimal intensity of oral anticoagulant therapy. JAMA 1987; 258:2723–2726.

National Institutes of Health. Lowering blood cholesterol to prevent heart disease, consensus conference. JAMA 1985; 253:2080–2086.

Physician's Guide to Non-Insulin Dependent (Type II) Diabetes: Diagnosis and Treatment. American Diabetes Association, Alexandria, Virginia, 1988.

Ransohoff DF, Feinstein AR. Problems of spectrum and bias in evaluating the efficacy of diagnostic tests. N Engl J Med 1978; 299:926–929.

Statland BE. Clinical Decision Levels for Lab Tests. Oradell, N.J., Medical Economics Books, 1987.

QUESTIONS

1. For which of the following clinical problems is a serum albumin an important test to order?
   a. Obesity
   b. Edema
   c. Hypothyroidism
   d. Constipation
   e. Diabetes mellitus

2. A 70-year-old asymptomatic white male is found to have an elevated alkaline phosphatase (320 units per liter). The best test to determine from where the alkaline phosphatase originated is a(n)
   a. Ionized calcium.
   b. Hand x-ray.
   c. GGT.
   d. ALAT.
   e. ASAT.

3. Clinicians most commonly use which of the following in their test interpretation?
   a. Sensitivity
   b. Decision analysis
   c. Decision levels
   d. Prevalence
   e. Predictive value

4. In a patient with an elevated ASAT, but a normal ALAT, it is important to consider each of the following EXCEPT
   a. Myocardial infarction.
   b. Bowel infarction.
   c. Skeletal muscle injury.
   d. Hemolysis.
   e. Pulmonary infarction.

5. A 40-year-old male with known alcoholism presents to the emergency room with nausea, vomiting, and abdominal pain. The serum amylase is 730. In addition to alcoholic pancreatitis, it is important to consider

a. Pneumonia.
b. Hepatitis.
c. Esophageal varices.
d. Perforating ulcer.
e. Myocardial infarction.

6. A patient has a BUN of 45 and a creatinine of 1.3. (BUN to creatinine ratio = 34). This is least consistent with
a. Drug-induced acute tubular necrosis.
b. Dehydration.
c. Congestive heart failure.
d. GI bleeding in a burn patient.
e. Urine obstruction from prostate hypertrophy.

7. A patient with nephrotic syndrome is found to have a serum total calcium of 6.3. His ionized calcium
a. Is probably abnormally low.
b. Is probably abnormally high.
c. Is probably normal.
d. May be low, high, or normal.

8. Which of the following is NOT considered a risk for coronary artery disease by the National Cholesterol Education Program?
a. HDL cholesterol less than 35 mg/dl
b. Male sex
c. Obesity
d. Smoking
e. An LDL cholesterol less than 130 mg/dl

9. A patient with Type I diabetes mellitus is brought to the emergency room because of confusion and agitation. The serum bicarbonate is 12 mEq/liter. The most likely explanation is
a. Metabolic acidosis.
b. Metabolic alkalosis.
c. Respiratory acidosis.
d. Respiratory alkalosis.

10. Diabetic patients are known to be at risk for renal damage from IVP dye. The most useful test to follow in such a patient who receives this dye would be
a. Creatinine.
b. BUN.
c. Urine electrolytes.
d. Urinalysis.
e. Serum sodium.

11. A 67-year-old asymptomatic female is found to have an erythrocyte sedimentation rate (Westergren) of 50 mm/hr. The most likely diagnosis in this patient is
a. Cancer.
b. Temporal arteritis.
c. Multiple myeloma.
d. Polymyalgia rheumatica.
e. Normal.

12. Which of the following patients can be diagnosed as having diabetes?
a. An adult with two fasting venous glucose values of 135 and 145 mg/dl
b. A child with two fasting venous glucose values of 135 and 145 mg/dl
c. A pregnant patient with an O'Sullivan screening value of 145 mg/dl
d. An adult whose glucose tolerance test results in a fasting venous glucose of 135, a 1 hour of 220, and a 2 hour of 160 mg/dl

13. A glycosylated hemoglobin is most useful for
a. Deciding when to change a patient from oral hypoglycemic therapy to insulin.
b. Diagnosing diabetes.
c. Adjusting insulin dosing.
d. Predicting diabetic retinopathy.
e. Evaluating month-to-month diabetic control.

14. The most useful test to evaluate the volume of blood loss in a patient with an acute gastrointestinal bleed is
a. Supine and standing blood pressure.
b. Hemoglobin.
c. Hematocrit.
d. Tagged red blood cell volume.
e. Reticulocyte count.

15. In a patient with a hemoglobin of 10 gm/dl and an MCV of 90, the next best test to evaluate the anemia is
a. Serum ferritin.
b. Vitamin B_{12}.
c. Folate.
d. Hemoglobin electrophoresis.
e. Peripheral blood smear.

16. The optimal prothrombin time in seconds in a patient with a prosthetic heart valve is
a. 14.
b. 16.
c. 18.
d. 20.
e. 22.

17. The most common reason for an ambulatory patient to have a serum potassium of 3.0 mEq/liter is
a. Inadequate dietary potassium.
b. Hypertensive therapy.
c. Renal tubular acidosis.
d. Hyperaldosteronism.
e. Specimen hemolysis.

18. In a patient with asthma on a long-acting theophylline preparation (200 mg b.i.d.), the serum theophylline is found to be 6 micrograms/mL. The theophylline dosage is increased to 300 mg b.i.d. The most appropriate next theophylline level to obtain would be

a. A trough level in one day.
b. A peak level in one day.
c. A trough level in three days.
d. A peak level in three days.

19. The single most useful test in evaluating a patient suspected of having hypothyroidism is
a. TSH.
b. Free T_3.
c. Total T_4.

d. T_3 uptake.
e. T_4 index.

20. The most likely explanation for a newborn to have a WBC cell count of 25,000 cells/mm^3 is
a. Sepsis.
b. ABO incompatibility.
c. Pneumonia.
d. Birth asphyxia.
e. Normal.

Answers appear on page 448.

CLINICAL CASE STUDIES

Weight Loss and Diarrhea

SUSAN M. MILLER

INITIAL VISIT

SUBJECTIVE

Patient Identification. Robert is a 37-year-old divorced Caucasian attorney who has come to the office for a new patient visit because of a change in his group insurance policy.

Presenting Problem. Robert had been in good health until 3 months ago, when he noticed unintentional weight loss, persistent diarrhea, and fatigue.

Present Illness. After a camping trip to Colorado Springs, Robert experienced crampy, watery diarrhea four to five times a day. His diarrhea was not melanotic, and it was not exacerbated by eating. He has not experienced incontinence, nausea, vomiting, or abdominal pain. The stool is semisolid to watery, malodorous, and not relieved with Pepto-Bismol or over-the-counter Imodium A-D. He complains of a dry mouth, halitosis, and soreness of the tongue when he drinks orange juice. He estimates that he has lost 15 pounds in the last 6 weeks, although his appetite is ravenous. He notes early satiety.

For the last month he has had to take a nap when he arrives home from work. Instead of sleeping 6 hours per night, he now needs 8 to 10 hours to feel rested the next morning.

Past Medical History. Robert had an appendectomy at age 11. At age 24 he was in a motor vehicle accident and underwent a splenectomy. He also sustained multiple rib fractures without pneumothorax. He received 4 units of blood. He does not remember his last tetanus immunization, nor does he remember a pneumococcal vaccination after his splenectomy. He is allergic to sulfa drugs (rash). He takes multiple vitamins and denies using laxatives or cathartics routinely. He received treatment for syphilis and gonorrhea 10 years ago. He may have had a herpes infection of the penis. He has been treated for hemorrhoids. He denies hepatitis. He

drinks two six-packs of beer per week. He has never used intravenous drugs, but he does smoke marijuana occasionally. He has borrowed sleeping pills and Xanax from friends when he feels "stressed out." He tried "crack" once but felt his heart race and did not enjoy it. Upon further questioning, he admits to the use of "poppers."

Family History. His father, a retired attorney, is in good health and is on no medications at age 77. His mother, age 67, works for an insurance company and is in good health. She had a hysterectomy 20 years ago for bleeding. His paternal grandfather died in World War I, and his paternal grandmother died in 1938 of tuberculosis. His material grandparents both died in their eighties from natural causes. Robert is an only child.

Social History. Robert divorced his wife 7 years ago after being married less than 1 year. They had met while he was in law school. She lives in another state, and they had no children. He is currently involved in a monogamous relationship of 6 months' duration. He has had over 20 sexual partners, and he has performed both receptive and insertive anal intercourse. Although he and his current partner are practicing safe sex, neither is aware of their HIV antibody status.

His last heterosexual contact was with his wife 7 years ago. She was his only female sexual partner.

He just made partner in his law firm and earns in excess of $500,000 per year. His area of expertise is discrimination.

Review of Systems. Robert notes that two to three nights per week he has to change his bedding because of night sweats. In the afternoon he frequently has a low-grade fever. He denies headache, scotomata, cough, shortness of breath, dyspnea on exertion, nausea, vomiting, abdominal pain, dysuria, or paresthesias. He notes that his skin is drier and that he has had a scaling rash on his forehead, scalp, and chest for the last 9 months. He has two pet cats in good health. He travels overseas one to two times yearly. His most recent trip was to Thailand. He notes increasing insomnia, even though he is sleeping more hours per night. He has been having nightmares about death, and his friends have been teasing him about his memory lapses. He runs three to four times per week and lifts weights at the gym 2 to 3 days per week. He enjoys swimming, racquetball, and tennis. Last year he ran a half-marathon.

OBJECTIVE

Physical Examination. Robert is a muscular 195-lb man. His blood pressure is 105/60, pulse 58, respiratory rate 12, temperature 99.5°F. *HEENT:* PERRL, EOMI, cotton wool spot O.S., and oral candidiasis. *Lymphadenopathy:* He has anterior and posterior chain cervical adenopathy. *Thyroid:* Normal. *Lungs:* Clear to auscultation. *CV:* Sinus bradycardia without a murmur. *Abdomen:* Well-healed midline and McBurney incisions without hepatomegaly. Bowel sounds are present and normoactive. No guarding or rebound. No CVAT. *Rectal:* Decreased rectal tone with hemorrhoids. Guaiac negative. *GU:* Circumcised male with condyloma on the glans. *Skin:* Xerosis and seborrheic dermatitis of the face and scalp. Tinea cruris and pedis are present. Onychomycosis of the left hallux. *Neuro:* Normal. No cognitive deficit noted on screening exam.

ASSESSMENT

Differential Diagnoses

1. *Hyperthyroidism* is unlikely given the presence of bradycardia and a normal thyroid gland.

2. *Lipid storage disease* as an etiology of his lymphadenopathy, such as Gaucher's or Niemann-Pick disease, is unlikely secondary to the acute onset of symptomatology and age of presentation.

3. *Diabetes mellitus* could be considered. Robert's complaints of weight loss, voracious appetite, and dry mouth are consistent with hyperglycemia. His halitosis may represent ketosis. In fact, the diarrhea may have precipitated the clinical onset of diabetes mellitus. A serum glucose determination would be helpful.

4. An essential aspect of this patient's evaluation was obtaining the sexual history. This information has provided clues to various high-risk sexual and social behaviors. His clinical examination provides findings suggestive of *immunosuppression*, such as oral candidiasis, seborrheic dermatitis, and atypical lymphadenopathy. An infectious etiology of his diarrhea and weight loss should be considered.

5. *Lymphoma* also must be considered and is consistent with weight loss, fatigue, night sweats, fever, and atypical lymphadenopathy. Lymphoma of the gastrointestinal tract also may cause protracted diarrhea. The types of lymphoma may include Hodgkin's lymphoma and T- or B-cell lymphoma. The location of his lymphadenopathy provides an important clue to the differential diagnosis. In cases of lymphadenopathy, it is important to assess the node location, patient's age, associated clinical symptoms, and physical characteristics of the lymph node (asymmetry, size, tenderness, texture, mobility). Under normal conditions in an adult patient, the inguinal nodes can range in size from 0.5 to 2.0 cm. Particular attention must be paid to anterior cervical, posterior cervical, occipital, axillary, and supraclavicular adenopathy.

In addition to a malignant etiology of his lymphadenopathy, infectious causes also must be considered. These can include (a) viral (HBV, HIV, CMV, EBV), (b) bacterial (*Salmonella*, cat-scratch disease), (c) fungal (histoplasmosis, coccidiodomycosis), (d) mycobacterial (MTB, MAC), and (e) parasitic (toxoplasmosis) infections.

Not all lymph node enlargement is associated with local inflammation. However, Robert's clinical findings are not consistent with immunologic diseases such as rheumatoid arthritis, serum sickness, drug reactions, or systemic lupus erythematosus (although he does have a facial rash).

6. Based on his sexual and clinical history, *HIV infection* must be considered. All his clinical and physical findings are consistent with HIV infection. In addition, he could have lymphoma in the presence of HIV infection, more specifically B- and T-cell lymphomas (versus Hodgkin's lymphoma). Furthermore, although he does not have suggestive cutaneous or mucocutaneous findings, Kaposi's sarcoma also may present as lymphadenopathy. In HIV infection, it is the presence of extra-inguinal adenopathy that is considered clinically significant.

PLAN

Laboratory and Special Tests

1. During the initial patient visit, it is reasonable to obtain stool studies for ova and parasites, stool guaiac, and culture and sensitivities to look for a treatable cause of his diarrhea.

2. A complete blood count, chemistry profile, and urinalysis would be helpful. Anemia may be present secondary to malabsorption, hemolysis, lymphoma, or HIV infection. In patients with advanced HIV infection or lymphoma, an absolute lymphocytopenia can be present. Eosinophila can occur in parasitic infections or malignancies. The chemistry profile might reveal hyperglycemia, azotemia, hypokalemia, hypo- or hypernatremia, hyperuricemia, hypergammaglobulinemia, or liver enzyme elevation.

3. HIV antibody testing should be obtained in a confidential manner (Table 20–1). Before a serologic sample is drawn, Robert must be informed about the consequences of serologic testing and be assured of confidentiality. Pretest counseling includes a review of his risk behaviors, virus transmission, the incubation and latency period(s) of HIV infection, what positive and negative tests mean, reasons for false-positive and false-negative test results (Table 20–2), and how to reduce high-risk behaviors. At some testing sites, an informed consent and demographic form are completed. Finally, a follow-up appointment is made for release of the test results.

TABLE 20–1. ADULT HIV SEROLOGIC TESTING: UNITED STATES RECOMMENDATIONS

Pretest and Posttest Counseling

Pretest and posttest counseling must address the following issues: determination of individual potential risk status (past, current, future); implications of positive, negative, and indeterminate test results; pregnancy and contraception issues; behavior modification to reduce risk; low-risk sexual activities; and referral to appropriate agencies for follow-up.

Note: Pretest and posttest counseling provides an opportunity to tailor risk-reduction education. Health care providers may wish to consider the use of an informed consent form. Finally, a sample that is repetitively positive needs to be confirmed by an independent antibody assay.

Anonymous or Confidential Testing

A system must be implemented that has the ability to protect the anonymity and confidentiality of test specimens and results. Preferably, results of testing are given in a face-to-face encounter.

Note: If testing is performed in a private office, the physician may wish to use numerically coded samples. If this is not feasible, use of alternative testing sites may be advisable.

Voluntary versus Mandatory Testing

Although voluntary testing is preferable, in certain situations, mandatory testing is performed.

Mandatory testing: Testing of blood, plasma, sperm, and organ donation. Mandatory testing also occurs within the military and in specific legal interactions.

Voluntary testing: Previous or current high-risk behavior, prior blood transfusion, occupational exposure, new-onset tuberculosis, syphilis, and public health surveillance. Voluntary testing is also used to confirm a clinical diagnosis.

Interpretation of Results

A negative enzyme-linked immunosorbent assay screen and absence of antibody bands on the Western immunoblot test at 3, 6, 9, and 12 months provide evidence that no immune response to HIV has occurred. Indeterminate test results need to be followed closely. Polymerase chain reaction testing may have a role in confirmation.

Source: From Rakel RE. Textbook of Family Practice. Philadelphia, W.B. Saunders, 1990, with permission.

TABLE 20–2. POTENTIAL SOURCES OF FALSE-POSITIVE OR FALSE-NEGATIVE ANTIBODY TESTS

FALSE POSITIVE	FALSE NEGATIVE
Populations with low seroprevalence	Prior to host antibody response (i.e., "window period")
Passive transfer of antibody in immunoglobulin preparations	Late infection, resulting from deterioration of host antibody response
Cross reactive antibodies secondary to multiple blood transfusions, serum proteins (cryoglobulins, rheumatoid factor), other retroviruses, or human leukocyte antigens	Laboratory error
Transplacental transfer of maternal antibody	
Laboratory error	

Source: From Rakel RE. Textbook of Family Practice. Philadelphia, W.B. Saunders, 1990, with permission.

If referral is needed for community services, this information can then be provided. At this time the patient may experience significant anxiety and a sense of fatality. Support services are essential. Risk assessment for potential suicide may be warranted.

Disposition. Stool studies, a complete blood count, a chemistry profile, and HIV antibody testing (ELISA and Western blot) were obtained. The patient was scheduled for a follow-up visit within the week.

FIRST FOLLOW-UP VISIT

SUBJECTIVE

Robert's diarrhea persisted. He was extremely anxious to know the test results and had brought his significant other to the clinic to hear the findings.

OBJECTIVE

Robert has lost an additional 2 lb. His stool studies revealed the presence of *Giardia lamblia*. His WBC was 8200; Hg/Hct were 11.7/34.1; his platelet count was 94,000. His serum glucose was 104; potassium, 3.4; total protein, 9.1; and cholesterol, 108. Both the ELISA and Western blot tests were positive.

ASSESSMENT

1. *Giardia lamblia* infection
2. Mild hypokalemia secondary to diarrhea
3. Decreased serum cholesterol
4. HIV infection with probable decreased CD4 lymphocyte counts
5. Elevated total protein probably secondary to B-cell activation as a result of HIV infection.

PLAN

1. Metronidazole 500 mg PO t.i.d. for 7 to 10 days.
2. A chest radiograph to rule out occult tuberculosis and to serve as a baseline should future pulmonary symptoms develop.
3. Placement of a purified protein derivative (ppd) skin test and candida control.
4. Assessment of his immunologic status. This can be achieved by obtaining CD4 lymphocyte subsets. A p24 antigen, β_2 microglobulin, and CMV/EBV serology are not necessary at this time.
5. Updating his immunization status. Tetanus toxoid, pneumovax, and annual influenza vaccines are considered standard. Hepatitis B vaccine may be considered if continued high-risk behavior is anticipated or if the patient is a health care worker. The HIB vaccine also should be administered. Live vaccines are generally avoided.
6. Toxoplasmosis IGG antibody. An HIV-infected person who is IGG seropositive has a 20% to 33% chance of disease reactivation. Robert is at risk for exposure secondary to his travel and pet history.
7. A patient with positive serology for syphilis requires aggressive follow-up. Syphilis may be a cofactor for disease progression in HIV infection. In addition, syphilis is difficult to treat in the presence of immunosuppression and may more rapidly progress to the tertiary stage.
8. Female patients may require a pregnancy test

TABLE 20–3. SUGGESTED PROTOCOL FOR AMBULATORY MANAGEMENT OF HIV INFECTION

Establish an index of suspicion.

Evaluate past and current transmission risk.

Accurate assessment of HIV serology (e.g., sequential ELISA and Western blot testing).

Determine stage of infection.

Document baseline physical examination.

Record HIV-directed review of systems.

Update immunization status (dT, pneumovax, annual influenza vaccine; consider HBV and HIB vaccines) *Note:* Prior BCG vaccination is *not* a contraindication to placement of a ppd. *Review childhood infections and immunizations.*

Laboratory evaluation:

  Baseline: Complete blood count, chemistry profile, chest radiograph, ppd with control, toxoplasmosis IgG antibody, RPR, absolute T4 lymphocyte count and percent

  Other (based on clinical presentation): Hepatitis serology, cryptococcal antigen, p24 antigen, stool for O & P or cultures, sputum for AFB, Pap smear, pregnancy tests, STD tests, drug screening, biopsy

Document drug allergies.

Consider zidovudine and PCP prophylaxis therapy.

Safe-sex counseling.

Consider research protocols.

Document unconventional therapies.

Document living will and power of attorney status.

Obtain illicit drug history.

Refer to community resources.

Aggressive workup of symptoms.

and Pap smear. HIV infection is often overlooked in female patients and should be considered part of a differential diagnosis for sexually transmitted diseases (STDs), atypical Pap smears, unresolving gynecologic infections, pregnancy, atypical dermatologic problems, multiple sexual partners, history of blood transfusions (or spouse with a blood transfusion), rape, or substance abuse.

9. Safe-sex guidelines must be reviewed. Contact tracing of known sexual partners (including his former wife) should be initiated.

10. Robert may need re-referral to community support groups. He also may wish to consider updating his will and power of attorney and obtaining a living will.

Disposition. The preceding were obtained (see Table 20–3). A follow-up visit was scheduled for 1 week. Metronidazole and Mycelex troches were prescribed. Alcohol was prohibited. Reassurance and support were provided.

SECOND FOLLOW-UP VISIT

SUBJECTIVE

Robert's diarrhea had resolved, although the metronidazole imparted a metallic taste to his food. His anxiety was diminished, but he still had not told his ex-wife about his serologic status.

His thrush was better. He noted mild fatigue, myalgias, and fever after receiving his vaccinations.

OBJECTIVE

Chest x-ray, RPR, toxo titer, and hepatitis B surface antigen/antibody were all negative. His total WBC was 8300, with a differential of 45% polymorphonuclear lymphocytes (PMNs), 40% lymphocytes, 0% atypical lymphocytes, 3% monocytes, 1% eosinophils, and 1% basophils. His Hg/Hct were 11.4/34.6. His platelet count was 94,000. His percentage CD4 lymphocyte count was 14% and percentage CD8 lymphocyte count was 37%. His ppd skin test was measured at 6-mm induration.

ASSESSMENT

1. The anemia and thrombocytopenia are probably related to his HIV infection. The thrombocytopenia likely has an autoimmune etiology and is occurring in the presence of an asplenic patient. His WBC of 8300/mm^3 does not reflect acute infection, since his differential is normal and the count is relatively elevated for a patient with HIV infection. This "spuriously high" WBC is most likely secondary to asplenia. Therefore, his CD4 lymphocyte count of 465 is relatively high for the number of clinical symptoms he is having; hence his CD4 percentage is a better surrogate marker for the degree of immunosuppression present.

2. Robert is a candidate for zidovudine therapy (Table 20–4). His CD4 lymphocyte count is between 200 and 500, and he is symptomatic for immunosuppression. His thrombocytopenia might improve with zidovudine.

3. In addition, Robert is also a candidate for PCP prophylaxis (Table 20–5), since his CD4 percentage is less than 20%. Since he is allergic to sulfa (e.g., Bactrim/Septra), Robert should receive aerosolized pentamidine (300 mg every month). He should tolerate this fairly well, although his tobacco and marijuana use need to be curtailed, since these increase his risk of bronchospasm. Aerosolized pentamidine is associated with the following side effects (Table 20–6). An alternative therapy might be dapsone (50 mg/day), although Robert may be cross-allergic to dapsone if he is allergic to trimethoprim-sulfamethoxazole.

Disposition. Zidovudine therapy was initiated at 500 mg per day. Robert was educated about potential side effects of the medications and what clinical symptoms warranted a return visit to the clinic. He also was educated about local research study sites and potential medications. Alternative treatment regimens were dis-

TABLE 20–4. INDICATIONS FOR ZIDOVUDINE (RETROVIR, AZT) THERAPY

Prior opportunistic infection or AIDS-defining illness

An absolute CD4 lymphocyte count less than 200 cells/mm^3

An absolute CD4 lymphocyte count between 200 and 500 cells/mm^3

TABLE 20–5. INDICATIONS FOR *PNEUMOCYSTIS CARINII* PNEUMONIA PROPHYLAXIS

An absolute CD4 lymphocyte count less than 200 cells/mm^3 (or CD4 percentage less than 20%)

Prior *Pneumocystis carinii* pneumonia

TABLE 20–6. ADVERSE EFFECTS OF AEROSOLIZED PENTAMIDINE THERAPY

Cough
Bronchospasm
Elevated triglycerides
Metallic taste
Extrapulmonic pneumocystosis
Dissemination of *Mycobacterium* tuberculosis
Pneumothorax
Rarely: dermatitis, conjunctivitis, renal insufficiency, pancreatitis

cussed. He was asked to keep a question diary of things he heard or read so that they could be discussed during his clinic visits. Arrangements were made for his ex-wife to receive serologic testing.

DISCUSSION

HIV infection is a chronic viral infection. The average length of time from infection to the onset of an AIDS-defining illness is approximately 10 years. Frequently, patients feel that HIV infection implies that they have AIDS and that death is imminent. This fear of death supersedes the concept of HIV being a chronic disease and contributes to a state of acute, severe anxiety. An individual's coping mechanisms may be strained at the time of (1) HIV diagnosis, (2) initiation of zidovudine therapy, (3) AIDS diagnosis, or (4) in the terminal stages of infection. Physician sensitivity to these crisis events can help smooth the transition and facilitate individual coping skills. A relatively unique aspect of HIV infection is that the physician may treat both partners or family members in the relationship. This is further complicated by who survives whom and for how long. If one member of the couple is a hemophiliac, for example, guilt over the perceived role of transmission must be addressed.

Zidovudine (Retrovir) is a thymidine analogue that inhibits HIV replication at the level of the reverse transcriptase enzyme. For zidovudine to be active, it undergoes phosphorylation by the host's cellular enzymes into a 5'-triphosphate form. The rate of this phosphorylation will vary between T-lymphocytes and monocyte/macrophage cells. The intracellular triphosphate form of zidovudine is active against HIV, not the extracellular analogue.

Studies by Fischl et al. and Volberding et al. suggest that zidovudine therapy should be initiated when the CD4 lymphocyte count is below 500 cells/mm³. Initiating therapy earlier in disease appears to delay the progression to AIDS. Additional studies by Fischl et al. show that a reduced dose of zidovudine is at least as effective as the previous standard dose, with a significant reduction in toxicity. In the short term, anemia and neutropenia are still seen, but at a much reduced frequency. Nausea, anorexia, myalgias, and headache also may occur during the first few weeks of therapy. Only rarely are patients allergic to zidovudine. Furthermore, a recent study by Collier et al. suggests that 300 mg per day of zidovudine showed similar effects to higher daily doses. The long-term efficacy and potential appearance of HIV resistance still need to be determined.

The long-term toxicities and antepartum effects of zidovudine are still being studied. A recent observation includes the appearance of a myopathy after being on zidovudine for more than six months. Patients typically complain of fatigue, proximal muscle wasting, difficulty climbing or descending stairs, and pain with palpation. The creatinine phosphokinase level may be extremely elevated. At this point it is prudent to discontinue zidovudine therapy and initiate a trial of nonsteroidal anti-inflammatory agents. If zidovudine is reintroduced, a lower dose is suggested (300 mg/day). This toxicity appears to be due to a direct mitochondrial toxicity by zidovudine. Furthermore, the clinician may consider switching to another reverse transcriptase analogue, such as dideoxyinosine (didanosine, Videx), or dideoxycytidine (HIVID).

Macrocytosis secondary to zidovudine administration does not require a cessation of therapy. The clinician should look for concomitant B_{12} or folate deficiency and correct it if it is present. If the patient is receiving a sulfa compound for PCP prophylaxis, leucovorin may be considered.

The lack of curative therapy is frequently discussed in the examination room. It may be helpful to compare the chronicity of HIV infection with hypertension or diabetes mellitus. In neither illness does curative therapy exist, but effective therapy does exist that prolongs the life of these individuals. A strong emphasis on patient education, patient autonomy, and patient responsibility regarding health is important. A medical treatment program may be divided into three components: (1) HIV infection, (2) opportunistic infections and malignancies, and (3) immune reconstitution. Categories 1 and 2 have had the most clinical success to date. Category 1 includes such medications as zidovudine, dideoxyinosine, and dideoxycytidine. Category 2 includes such medications as ganciclovir, foscarnet, fluconazole, alpha-interferon, combination therapy for mycobacterial infections, aggressive management of herpes and syphilis infections, discernment and description of types of infections and malignancies seen in HIV infection, PCP prophylaxis, and preventive immunizations. Category 3 includes such therapy as alpha-interferon, GM-CSF, EPO, and HIV vaccinations (before and after exposure). Passive immunotherapy is being studied.

Finally, management of substance abuse is essential. This includes not only the use of street drugs, but also the overprescribing of benzodiazepenes and painkillers. These medications may cloud an individual's ability to think. Judicious use of antidepressants should be considered. Referral to Alcoholics Anonymous or drug-treatment programs must be considered. It is extremely difficult to treat HIV infection in a person actively abusing drugs.

SUGGESTED READING

Collier AC, Bozzette S, Coombs RW, et al. A pilot study of low-dose zidovudine in human immunodeficiency virus infection. N Engl J Med 1990; 323:1015–1021.

Fischl MA, Parker CB, Pettinelli C, et al. A randomized controlled trial of a reduced daily dose of zidovudine in patients with the acquired immunodeficiency syndrome. N Engl J Med 1990; 323:1009–1014.

Fischl MA, Richman DD, Hansen N, et al. The safety and efficacy of zidovudine (AZT) in the treatment of subjects with mildly symptomatic human immunodeficiency virus type 1 (HIV) infection. Ann Intern Med 1990; 112:727–737.

Miller SM. Infectious disease: Ambulatory management of AIDS. In Rakel RE (ed.): Textbook of Family Practice, 4th ed. Philadelphia, W.B. Saunders, 1990, pp. 487–495.

Miller SM. Treatment of opportunistic infections associated with acquired immune deficiency syndrome (AIDS). In Carter B (ed.), Primary Care: Pharmacotherapy. Philadelphia, W.B. Saunders, 1990, pp. 543–564.

Volberding PA, Lagakos SW, Koch MA, et al. Zidovudine in asymptomatic human immunodeficiency virus infection: A controlled trial in persons with fewer than 500 CD4-positive cells per cubic millimeter. N Engl J Med 1990; 322:941–949.

QUESTIONS

1. What is this patient's absolute CD4 lymphocyte count?

   a. 1162
   b. 592
   c. 464
   d. 3320

2. Would this patient be a candidate for zidovudine therapy?

   a. No, he does not have a diagnosis of AIDS.
   b. Yes, because his T4 count is between 200 and 500 cells/mm³.
   c. No, his T4 count is not less than 200 cells/mm³.
   d. Yes, because his percent T4 is less than his percent T8.

3. Is this patient a candidate for PCP prophylaxis?

   a. Yes, because of the presence of oral candidiasis.
   b. No, because he has not had PCP.
   c. Yes, because his percent CD4 lymphocyte is less than 20%.
   d. No, because his CD4 lymphocyte count is not less than 200 cells/mm³.

4. What would be an indication for isoniazid prophylaxis?

   a. Induration greater than 15 mm
   b. Induration greater than 10 mm
   c. Induration greater than 5 mm
   d. Induration greater than 1 mm

Answers appear on page 448.

Cough

JOHN G. PRICHARD

INITIAL VISIT

SUBJECTIVE

Patient Identification. Devin H. is a 28-year-old Irish woman who is an equine broker and who was seen for a complaint of persistent cough.

Present Illness. She was in excellent health until 10 weeks ago. During the month of January, she developed a febrile illness characterized by a cough that was only minimally productive, upper anterior chest pain, and mild to moderate dyspnea, for which she received treatment by another physician who prescribed erythromycin. Other symptoms noted at that time included a frontal headache, a right earache, myalgia, and anorexia. Despite the occurrence of gastric discomfort with erythromycin, Devin completed 2 weeks of therapy. After 2 weeks, she was able to return to work, but since that time she has had a persistent cough that is much worse in the early evening to late night hours. Presently, her cough is nonproductive, and all other symptoms noted during the acute illness have resolved.

Past Medical History. At age 4, while living in Ireland, Devin was hospitalized for pneumonia. She had been treated for asthma with several hospitalizations, but this largely remitted by age 13. A breast biopsy on the right side was done for a solitary lesion at age 21. It was found to be a benign cyst. Otherwise, Devin has had no other surgery, takes no medications, and has no allergies or drug sensitivities.

Family History. Devin has two older siblings, a mother, and a father, all of whom are in perfectly good health. There is no family history of respiratory disease.

Health Habits. Devin smoked cigarettes, one package per day, from age 15 through 20, but not since. She drinks two glasses of wine per week. She has not been concerned about diet, and she has never been overweight. She drives extensively and always uses seat belts.

Social History. Devin was raised in Ireland until age 12, at which time her family immigrated to Barbados, where the family was involved in ranching. Subsequently, Devin completed college and received an MBA at a small southern university. Since then, she has been self-employed and successful as an independent broker. She considers herself to be well adjusted, and she has had no significant complaints about her health. She considers herself to have an active social life and is involved romantically with two men.

Review of Systems. During her acute illness several weeks ago, Devin lost 5 lb in weight, but since then, it has been regained. She is otherwise well and has no complaints on review of systems.

OBJECTIVE

Physical Examination. Vital signs were found as follows: Devin is 68 in tall, 118 lb. Blood pressure is 100/60, and heart rate is 55. She appeared clinically well, and the only abnormalities noted on physical examination were end-expiratory wheezing with forced expirations. Specifically, there were no abnormalities of the skin, and no nasal polyps were found.

Laboratory Tests. An x-ray report that the patient provided was compared with an x-ray taken today. The previous report showed bilateral, predominantly lower lobe alveolar infiltrates that were homogeneous in density. The current x-ray showed complete clearing of all previously described abnormalities.

ASSESSMENT

This young woman presents with an isolated complaint of persistent cough. This follows on an acute lower respiratory tract infection, documented by infiltrates on x-ray that are now resolved. The only other abnormality noted at the present time is the presence of wheezing.

Cough is an extremely common problem. As with most common complaints, the causes are of a benign nature in the vast majority. In most instances, a cough will have an immediately apparent cause, such as that associated with viral respiratory tract infections. A more challenging difficulty is the patient whose cough has proved persistent following a definable inciting event or, less commonly, where the etiology is simply not apparent.

Cough may be elicited by stimulating receptors at such sites as the sinuses, nose, ears, larynx, trachea, and large airways. A large number of conditions may affect any of these sites and produce cough. The pleura and peripheral lung parenchyma do not contain cough receptors. This accounts for the absence of cough with isolated pleural effusions or even pneumonia involving the periphery of the lung. In cases of persistent cough, the review of systems and physical examination should focus on dysfunction or abnormalities of these cough receptor–bearing areas. Furthermore, inquiries should be made regarding possible precipitants of cough not obvious to the patient, such as environmental factors (e.g., use of a new hairspray, working in a new environment) or use of a new medication such as beta-blockers or an angiotensin-converting enzyme (ACE) inhibitor. Coughs that are psychogenic in origin may be precipitated by a variety of stresses and may seem to occur de novo or follow a respiratory illness of which cough was a part. In most instances, the very nature of the cough suggests its origin, in addition to such factors as absence during sleep.

In this patient, there are two immediately apparent factors that may explain the persistent cough: a recent episode of pneumonia and a history of asthma. In studies that have examined the cause of persistent cough, asthma, allergies producing postnasal discharge, and recent respiratory infections have been found to be the most common causes of persistent cough. The lower respiratory tract infection Devin experienced was likely due to *Mycoplasma*. A viral infection such as influenza or an infection due to *Chlamydia* is less likely. The features of her illness did not suggest typical bacterial pneumonia. In this case, the chest x-ray was helpful in two respects: First, the abnormalities noted in the previous x-ray had cleared, confirming that one was dealing with pneumonia rather than a noninfectious cause of pulmonary disease. Second, the x-ray gave some reassurance that a new process was not producing the present symptoms. Examples of the latter would include neoplasms, adenopathy, or cardiac disease.

The patient's history of asthma is important from two points of view; postinfectious cough appears to be more common and prolonged in patients with a history of reactive airways. Many are more susceptible to environmental factors that may produce clinical bronchospasm, such as chemical pollutants or changes in environmental temperatures or humidity. Additionally, the present illness may, in fact, represent a recurrence of asthma. Asthma is the most common chronic illness of childhood. Both its prevalence and severity tend to decrease with age. It sometimes occurs, however, that an apparent remission in preadolescence or about the time of puberty may be temporary, with symptoms returning in young adulthood or indeed even late in life.

It has been found in several studies that patients with postinfectious cough can be demonstrated to have hyperreactive airways. The supposition then would be that this patient's history of asthma predisposed her to the development of persistent postinfectious cough.

PLAN

Diagnostic. With regard to the present illness, further tests are not necessary.

Therapeutic. Reassurance is of therapeutic benefit in this instance. The present thinking about the nature of the persistent cough should be explained. Because the symptoms are felt to be sufficiently disruptive, both a bronchodilator (beta-2-agonist) and a cough suppressant should be prescribed. The recommended cough suppressant can be an over-the-counter preparation with dextromethorphan, a drug somewhat less effective than codeine but with fewer side effects.

Patient Education. Since the patient voiced concerns about recurrence of asthma, reassurance, to the extent possible, should be given. The use of the metered-dose inhaler should be demonstrated, and a plan should be jointly developed for future evaluation if the symptoms do not remit promptly. A need for developing a source of ongoing care that would provide continuity should be emphasized.

Disposition. All the preceeding was done. The patient was asked to call at the end of 10 days to report on symptoms.

FOLLOW-UP

The patient did call the office and reported that after 48 hours of use of both the inhaled bronchodilator and the dextromethorphan, her symptoms largely remitted. After 1 week she discontinued use of the metered-dose inhaler and found that the cough could be managed by using the dextromethorphan in the late afternoon and evening. She also made arrangements at a later date for health maintenance, which would include Pap smear, breast examination, and blood pressure determination.

DISCUSSION

A postinfectious cough may persist for as long as 10 weeks following the initial respiratory tract infection. In many instances, multiple factors may conspire to irritate cough receptors. Attempting to define these factors and eliminate them becomes part of the treatment if empiric therapy fails. The best approach is then to go back over the history and exclude the numerous potential inciting factors at the various sites of cough receptors and focus the physical examination on these areas. Spirometric studies eventually may have disclosed that this young woman did indeed have reactive airways disease and was experiencing a relatively mild recurrence of asthma. It would not be an unusual scenario that the recurrence of asthma in adulthood is heralded by persistent chest symptoms following a lower respiratory tract infection.

SUGGESTED READING

Rakel RE. Textbook of Family Practice, 4th ed. Philadelphia, W.B. Saunders, 1990, pp. 496–530.
Rodnick JE, Gude JK, Diagnosis and antibiotic treatment of community-acquired pneumonia. West J Med 1991; 154:405–409.
Stulbarg M. Evaluation and treating intractable cough. West J Med 1985; 143:223–228.

QUESTIONS

1. What are the x-ray signs most strongly suggestive of typical bacterial pneumonia as opposed to atypical pneumonia?
2. List features that suggest that a persistent cough is habitual or of psychogenic origin?
3. What are the four most common causes of persistent cough?

Answers appear on page 448.

Fever and Chest Pain

JOHN G. PRICHARD

INITIAL VISIT

SUBJECTIVE

Patient Identification. This is a 42-year-old self-employed dentist who is a single father of two children ages 8 and 11.

Present Illness. The patient was in excellent health until 4 days ago when he noted the abrupt onset of myalgias, low-grade fever, sore throat, and substernal chest pain. On the second day of his illness, he was unable to work, but he remained ambulatory. At the end of the third day of his illness, he began to feel improved, but during the early morning hours on the fourth day, he awoke with a sudden chill and development of a rather marked right anterior pleuritic chest pain. His cough worsened but remained nonproductive. He recorded his temperature at 102.5°F. Tylenol improved the anterior chest pain, but it remained of moderate severity. Although he was not dyspneic at rest, ambulating occasioned deeper respirations with more severe chest pain. He had not had severe respiratory illnesses in the past, he did not smoke, and he had not recently traveled away from his home in southern California.

Past Medical History. An appendectomy had been performed at age 19. The patient took no medications, and no other serious illnesses have occurred.

Family History. The patient has no siblings. His father died during a motor vehicle accident 10 years ago. His mother is alive and well, living in another state.

Health Habits. The patient drinks 4 to 6 oz of alcohol per week, has never been overweight, and engages in vigorous tennis three to four times weekly.

Social History. The patient separated from his wife 5 years ago when she became habituated to cocaine. There has been no further contact with his wife since their separation, and the patient is presently not involved in a significant relationship. He has been able to adjust his office practice so that he can care for his two young sons during their school year.

Review of Systems. Apart from the immediate illness, the review of systems was noncontributory. In his practice of dentistry, the patient uses standard barrier methods, including gloves and masks, and he has done so for the last 4½ years.

OBJECTIVE

Physical Examination. The patient appeared moderately ill and uncomfortable from his anterior chest pain. The pain was clearly pleuritic in nature, aggravated by lying supine and improved by leaning forward with his upper body leaning to the right. His temperature was 101.2°F, pulse was 90 and regular, respirations were guarded and shallow at 20, and blood pressure was 110/65. The pharynx was mildly injected; other mucous membranes and conjunctiva were normal. His neck was supple, and there was no adenopathy. The lungs were clear to percussion, but faint rales were heard over the low anterior chest without a friction rub. He coughed only intermittently during the examination. Cardiac examination gave normal findings, and the abdominal examination was unrevealing. The extremities were normal in all respects. On neurologic examination, he was alert and awake and could communicate clearly. There were no focal findings, and the remainder of the physical examination was normal.

Laboratory Tests. The patient was referred to a nearby emergency room, and the following tests were performed. The chest x-ray showed that there were air bronchograms and an obscured right heart border. The WBC showed a total count of 15,000, with 70% segmented forms, 7 bands, and 23 lymphocytes. Oxygen saturation was 96%. An induced sputum yielded scant material, and a Gram's stain showed lancet-shaped diplococci. Two blood cultures were obtained.

ASSESSMENT

Since this episode occurred during the winter months, it seemed likely that the initial illness was a relatively mild case of influenza. As the patient was beginning to improve, the clincial course changed, with the development of pleuritic chest pains, increasing fever, and findings of rales, pulmonary infiltrates, and leukocytosis. The most likely diagnosis is that of acute bacterial pneumonia complicating a resolving lower respiratory tract viral infection. Although nonbacterial pneumonia or pulmonary embolus are considerations, they are not issues to be entertained seriously because the clinical syndrome is not compatible.

Non-hospital-acquired pneumonia occurs in 3 million Americans yearly. About 500,000 persons are admitted to hospital with this diagnosis each year. In most instances, the cause of community-acquired pneumonia is not etiologically diagnosed with certainty. Even among hospitalized patients, studies have shown that despite aggressive and thorough investigation of each case of pneumonia, an unequivocable etiologic diagnosis can only be achieved in 60% of cases. In ambulatory practice, there are numerous constraints on achieving etiologic diagnoses, including the need for invasive studies, the lack of long-term follow-up for serologic testing, and the unreasonable costs attendant to achieving a specific diagnosis when empiric therapy is often satisfactory. The principal causes, apart from viruses, of community-acquired pneumonia include the following organisms, roughly, by their frequency: *Streptococcus pneumoniae, Mycoplasma pneumoniae, Haemophilus influenzae, Chlamydia pneumoniae,* and *Branhamella catarrhalis. Staphylococcus aureus* causes a very small proportion of cases but is more frequent following influenza outbreaks. Pneumonia due to mouth anaerobes is a common cause of pneumonia in the elderly, particularly those who are not edentulous and have difficulty managing secretions either because of previous strokes or altered levels of consciousness.

The clinical features of this patient's illness strongly suggest a bacterial etiology (typical pneumonia) as opposed to pneumonia caused by *Chlamydia* or *Mycoplasma* (atypical pneumonia). The differential features of both types are listed in Table 20–7. In this patient's case, there was a short prodromal illness, probably influenza, with sudden worsening. The chest pain was pleuritic in origin, the WBC was elevated, and there was a lobar dis-

TABLE 20–7. FEATURES DIFFERENTIATING TYPICAL AND ATYPICAL PNEUMONIA

FEATURE	TYPICAL	ATYPICAL
Prodromal illness	+ +	+ + +
Sudden onset (or sudden worsening of prodrome)	+ + +	+
Rigors	+ + + +	+ to + +
Chest pain	+ + + +	+ to + +
Fever (>102°F)	+ + + +	+ +
Purulent sputum	+ + + +	+ +
White cell count with left shift	+ + + +	+ +
Dyspnea	+ + +	+ to + +
Degree of illness	+ + +	+ to + +
X-ray worse than anticipated	+ to + +	+ + + to + + + +
Lobar distribution of infiltrate	+ + + +	+
Pleural effusion	+ + + +	+

tribution of the pulmonary infiltrates. Although purulent sputum was not produced spontaneously, as is often the case in the early course of bacterial pneumonia, purulent sputum could be induced and demonstrated a predominant organism consistent with S. pneumoniae.

Most patients with community-acquired bacterial pneumonia are managed satisactorily as outpatients. The decision to admit a patient to hospital is not based solely on the severity of the illness at the time of presentation, but also on the patient's ability to care for himself or herself, his or her insight into the nature of the illness, and the likelihood that it might become further complicated. Both the predisposition to and the ability to resolve acute bacterial pneumonia depend in part on having intact mucociliary transport. The latter may be impaired by the use of alcohol and/or cigarettes, old age, and severe ongoing viral respiratory tract infection. Patients with chronic bronchitis or chronic bronchiectasis may have impaired clearing of secretions. Those with chronic lung disease (emphysema, chronic bronchitis, or asthma) not only develop pneumonia more commonly but resolve their disease more slowly as well. Functional respiratory reserve is impaired, increasing the likelihood that hospitalization with supplemental oxygen may be required. Certain underlying conditions may not only increase the rate with which pneumonia occurs but also limit its resolution: diabetes mellitus, hypospleenism (prior splenectomy, lymphoma, sickle-cell disease), alterations of cell-mediated immunity (corticosteroid therapy, underlying lymphoma, or infection with HIV), and finally, defects of humoral immunity (such as those seen with multiple myeloma, chronic lymphocytic leukemia, or congenital hypogammaglobulinemia).

This patient had no history of any of these illnesses, nor was support for their presence found either on physical examination or in laboratory testing.

PLAN

Diagnostic. A sputum culture should be obtained on the induced sample. Blood cultures should be drawn because in the cases of S. pneumoniae, bacteremia may occur in as many as 25% of cases.

Therapeutic. Hospitalization should be recommended. Since the patient had not been exposed to beta-lactam antibiotics within the last 3 months, nor was he an inpatient during that period of time, and he presented with only single-lobe disease, the likelihood of penicillin-resistant S. pneumoniae is small.

Disposition. The patient, however, declined admission because he had a large deductible on his health insurance. He felt that he could manage himself at home, and he had no one at present who could supervise his children. A long-acting cephalosporin was given by intramuscular injection along with a nonnarcotic analgesic for relief of his chest pain. With respect to the immediate illness, the patient was counseled to call at the end of the day, and the physician would call his home

and check on him that evening. He was to be seen the next day in the office for repeat injection of the long-acting antibiotic.

FOLLOW-UP

Eight hours after being seen in the office, the patient began to produce purulent sputum, some of which was rust colored. Upon telephone consultation, he was found to be alert and did not sound to be more than moderately uncomfortable. The following morning, the patient was seen in the office. His physical examination showed increasing rales over the middle interior chest, although his clinical appearance was one of improvement. He was afebrile. Blood cultures were negative at 24 hours. A repeat dose of the cephalosporin was given, and the patient returned home. At 48 hours, the patient was again seen in the office complaining of fatigue, but overall, he felt considerably improved. Rales persisted over the right middle lung field, and no clinical signs of pleural effusion could be elicited. The chest pain had lessened. Parenteral antibiotics were continued for 4 days, at which time oral penicillin was substituted. At the end of a 10-day period, the patient was clinically well.

DISCUSSION

For a variety of social and (increasingly) economic reasons, hospitalization is simply not possible even though the physician may consider it in the patient's best interest. The availability of outpatient infusion of antibiotics and the ability to follow the patient in the home, office, or emergency room will allow satisfactory treatment of many patients on an ambulatory basis. In this instance, the patient was highly reliable, and outpatient therapy proved satisfactory, although doubtlessly anxiety provoking for the clinician.

In most instances, the initial therapy for community-acquired pneumonia is based on the known frequency with which various pathogens occur and the likelihood that one is dealing with a bacterial, mycoplasmic, or chlamydial infection.

In this instance, the sputum Gram's stain and, subsequently, the sputum culture proved that pneumonia was due to S. pneumoniae. The parenteral second-generation cephalosporin proved to be satisfactory therapy. It was recommended to the patient that he receive annual immunization with influenza vaccine insofar as his profession brought him into close contact with patients throughout the year.

SUGGESTED READING

Douglas RG. Prophylaxis and treatment of influenza. N Engl J Med 1990; 322:443–450.

Rakel RE. Textbook of Family Practice, 4th ed. Philadelphia, W.B. Saunders, 1990, pp. 496–530.

Rodnick JE, Gude JK. Diagnosis and antibiotic treatment of community-acquired pneumonia. West J Med 1991; 154:405–409.

QUESTIONS

1. What are the clinical signs that most strongly suggest the presence of a bacterial pneumonia as opposed to an atypical pneumonia?
2. What are the principal causes of atypical pneumonia?
3. Which underlying diseases increase the likelihood that a pneumonia will be complicated by a prolonged course or increase the likelihood of respiratory insufficiency?

Answers appear on page 448.

Fever and Runny Nose

RICHARD D. CLOVER and STEPHEN J. SPANN

INITIAL VISIT

SUBJECTIVE

Patient Identification and Presenting Problem. Kristin C. is a 15-month-old girl who presents for fever and pulling at her ears. Her mother, Mrs. C., states that Kristin was in her usual good health until approximately 3 days ago, when she developed a running nose and a low-grade fever. Yesterday, Kristin became less playful and slightly irritable. Her appetite also has been decreased. Mrs. C. denies Kristin has had a cough, difficulty breathing, vomiting, or diarrhea.

Past Medical History. Kristin was a product of a term gestation to a 27-year-old white female, P11001. Pregnancy and delivery were uneventful. Kristin has been treated successfully twice previously for otitis media with amoxicillin. Growth and development have been normal. Her immunization record is as follows: DTP and OPV at 7 weeks of age; DTP and OPV at 4 months of age; and DTP at 6 months of age.

Family History. Kristin's father, a physician, is in good health at age 28. Her mother, a teacher, is in good health. Her maternal grandmother died at age 32 from lymphoma. Her other grandparents are in their fifties with no major medical problems.

OBJECTIVE

Physical Examination. Kristin's vital signs are temperature of 39°C, respirations 20, heart rate 100, and weight 25 lb. Generally, Kristin was alert and active, although slightly irritable. Her tympanic membranes were red, dull, and bulging bilaterally. Her nose had purulent rhinorrhea, and her throat was mildly injected but without exudate. Her neck was supple with small anterior cervical lymphadenopathy. Lung, heart, and abdominal examinations were within normal limits. Her neurologic examination was appropriate for age. Her skin was without rashes.

ASSESSMENT

Working Diagnosis

1. Upper respiratory infection, probably viral in origin.
2. Bilateral otitis media. A frequent complication of viral upper respiratory infections, it is impossible to distinguish on physical examination a viral versus bacterial etiology for the otitis.
3. Immunization deficient. Kristin is up-to-date on DTP and OPV but deficient on measles, mumps, rubella and *Haemophilus influenzae* vaccinations.

Differential Diagnosis

1. Acute sinusitis—a difficult diagnosis in young children, since the maxillary and frontal sinuses are not fully developed at this age. Ethmoid sinusitis can occur at this age and is associated with orbital cellulitis. Children with sinusitis usually present with purulent rhinorrhea, cough, and halitosis.
2. Allergic rhinitis—usually associated with clear rhinorrhea, a more chronic history, and without fever.
3. Pneumonia—should be in the differential diagnosis of a febrile child with respiratory symptoms. The usual signs of consolidation are frequently not present in infants and young children. With an obvious source for the fever in this child and without tachypnea (the most sensitive sign for pneumonia), pneumonia is unlikely in Kristin.
4. Bacteremia—may be present in 3% to 5% of highly febrile children with otitis media, with the most frequent organism isolated being *Streptococcus pneumoniae*. The majority of children with otitis media and bacteremia respond well to oral antibiotics and outpatient management.

PLAN

Diagnostic. No diagnostic tests are appropriate at this time. A WBC is of little to no predictive value in the clinical situation described. A tympanogram would simply be confirmatory and not of any value for changing the management. Sinus x-rays may be beneficial in confirming or excluding acute sinusitis; however, the management would be the same as that of otitis media. More invasive tests, including blood culture or tympanocentesis, are not indicated in this clinical situation.

Therapeutic

1. Amoxicillin 50 mg/kg/day divided in three doses daily for 10 days.
2. Decongestants have not been found beneficial in helping otitis media.
3. Antihistamines should be avoided because of possible thickening of secretions and the delay of resolution of symptoms.
4. Tylenol at dosages of 10 mg/kg of body weight every 4 to 6 hours as needed for discomfort.

Patient Education

1. Mrs. C. will be advised that the child's symptoms should improve remarkably within the next 48 hours. If the child's temperature persists, or if the child's clinical appearance worsens, she is to return to the clinic. Otherwise, she is to return to the clinic for follow-up of the otitis in approximately 2 to 3 weeks.
2. The mother will be advised that fever is an individual's normal defense mechanism in fighting infections. A temperature of less than 40°C in a child is not harmful to the child; however, for the child's comfort, Tylenol may be given as described above.

Disposition. Mrs. C. was asked to return in 2 to 3 weeks for follow-up or sooner if the child's condition does not improve or deteriorates.

FOLLOW-UP VISIT

SUBJECTIVE

Mrs. C. brings Kristin back in and states that the child became afebrile after the first day on antibiotics. The child's appetite and activity have returned to normal. The mother reports no new complaints.

OBJECTIVE

Generally, Kristin is alert, active, and playful and in no acute distress. Examination of the ears reveals the right tympanic membrane to be normal; however the left tympanic membrane is dull and has decreased mobility. The remainder of the physical examination is within normal limits.

ASSESSMENT

1. Resolving left middle ear effusion
2. Immunization deficiency

PLAN

Diagnostic. No tests are necessary at this time.

Therapeutic

1. Observation. The persistence of fluid in the middle ear is common at a 2- to 3-week follow-up visit. There is great debate in the literature about the best therapy for resolving effusions. Generally, greater than 90% of ear effusions will resolve by 6 weeks without any further intervention. For those children who do develop recurrent symptoms, investigators have found that the effusion is usually due to a different organism than the one that caused the initial infection. Decongestants have no role in the management of persistent ear effusions.
2. Immunization deficiency. The child will be given her MMR and HBOC vaccines today.

Patient Education

1. The mother is advised that the fluid in Kristin's left middle ear should continue to resolve. However, if Kristin develops any of the signs that she initially presented with, the mother is to call the clinic for evaluation.
2. The mother is advised of the potential development of fever and soreness at the spot of injection of the vaccines and of the potential for the child to develop a low-grade fever and a rash in about 2 to 3 weeks following vaccination.

Disposition. The patient is to return to clinic in 4 weeks for follow-up of the middle ear effusion.

DISCUSSION

Acute otitis media is second only to viral upper respiratory tract infections in prevalence during childhood. At least two-thirds of all children will have at least one episode of otitis media. The etiologic agents for acute otitis media are indicated in Table 20–8. It is important to note that although *Haemophilus influenzae* is a frequent cause of otitis media, it is usually an untypable *Haemophilus influenzae* organism, in contrast to the *Haemophilus influenzae* type B that produces such invasive diseases as pneumonia, epiglottitis, and meningitis. Therapy should be directed toward the most common

TABLE 20–8. BACTERIAL PATHOGENS ISOLATED FROM MIDDLE EAR FLUID IN 4675 CHILDREN WITH ACUTE OTITIS MEDIA*

MICROORGANISM	MEAN PERCENTAGE OF CHILDREN WITH PATHOGEN
Streptococcus pneumoniae	33
Haemophilus influenzae	21
Streptococcus, group A	8
Staphylococcus aureus	2
Branhamella catarrhalis	3
Gram-negative enteric bacilli	1
Miscellaneous bacteria	1
None or nonpathogens	31

*Twelve reports from centers in the United States, Finland, and Sweden, 1952–1981 (Blueston and Klein).

organisms. The drug of choice for the initial treatment of acute otitis media is amoxicillin at 50 mg/kg of body weight per day divided into three equal doses. For persistence of infection or relapse, there are multiple antibiotics from which to choose and none has demonstrated a clear superiority over the others. These antibiotics include erythromycin combined with sulfamethoxazole, trimethoprim and sulfisoxazole, cefaclor, cefuroxime, amoxicillin with clavulinic acid, and cefixime. The most serious complication of or coexisting disease with acute otitis media is meningitis. Although children presenting with meningitis frequently have otitis, the vast majority of children presenting with acute otitis media do not have meningitis. Meningitis should be considered when the child is lethargic, inconsolable, or appears toxic. Meningitis should be expected when children present with fever, stiff neck, and/or acute neurologic deficit.

There have been numerous changes in the recommendations for immunizations during infancy and childhood. The reader is referred to publications from the ACIP, the American Academy of Pediatrics, and the American Academy of Family Physicians for the exact guidelines. However, this case does illustrate a common misconception in the administration of immunizations. A mild upper respiratory infection without fever is not a contraindication to the administration of immunizations. Immunizations were withheld from this child during the first visit because of the presence of the fever. However, on the subsequent examination, the child had recovered from this infection and immunizations were indicated.

SUGGESTED READING

Blueston CD, Klein JO (eds.). Otits Media in Infants and Children. Philadelphia, W.B. Saunders, 1987.
Hess GH (ed.). Immunization Guidelines. St. Louis, Mo., American Academy of Family Physicians, 1988.
Peter G (ed.). Report of the Committee on Infectious Diseases, 21st ed. Chicago, American Academy of Pediatrics, 1988.
Rakel RE. Textbook of Family Practice, 4th ed. Philadelphia, W.B. Saunders, 1990.
Schutzman SA, Petrycki S, Fleisher GR. Bacteremia with otitis media. Pediatrics 1991; 87:48–53.

QUESTIONS

1. The most common bacterial etiology for acute otitis media in children is
   a. *Mycoplasma pneumoniae.*
   b. *Haemophilis influenzae* type b.
   c. *Haemophilis influenzae* untypable.
   d. *Streptococcus pneumoniae.*
   e. *Branhamella catarrhalis.*

2. Bullous myringitis has been associated with which of the following organisms?
   a. *Mycoplasma pneumoniae*
   b. *Haemophilus influenzae*
   c. *Streptococcus pneumoniae*
   d. Respiratory viruses.
   e. All the above.

3. The most frequent cause of bacteremia in children with acute otitis media and high fever is
   a. *Haemophilus influenzae* type b.
   b. *Nisseria* meningitis.
   c. *Branhamella catarrhalis.*
   d. *Streptococcus pneumoniae.*

4. In a child who presents with a mild upper respiratory infection without fever and is behind on his or her immunizations, the physician should
   a. Administer the appropriate immunizations.
   b. Wait at least 2 weeks until the respiratory infection is resolved.
   c. Wait at least 6 weeks until the body has made the appropriate immune response to the initial respiratory infection.
   d. Administer the killed vaccines but not the live attenuated vaccines.

Answers appear on page 448.

Sinus Congestion

STEPHEN J. SPANN and RICHARD D. CLOVER

INITIAL VISIT

SUBJECTIVE

Patient Identification. Mary B. is a 30-year-old, married, Caucasian secretary, mother of two, who is being seen for the first time for facial pain, sinus congestion, and dental pain.

Present Illness. Mary has been experiencing pain in the right side of her face and right upper teeth for 48 hours. She has been suffering from "nasal and sinus" congestion for about 2 weeks, as she does every spring. She has noticed a greenish coloration to her nasal discharge over the last 2 days. She has felt mildly ill over the past 48 hours and has felt feverish, although she has not taken her temperature. She has had no chills or sweats. The pain in her face is on the right side over the cheekbone, and it is made worse by bending over. She also has noticed pain in the upper teeth on the right side of her mouth. She denies earache or sore throat. She has had a slight cough but has not been coughing up any phlegm. She has had no pain in her chest. She denies any neurologic symptoms.

Past Medical History. Mary has been generally healthy all her life. She has had no surgery, serious illnesses, or serious injuries. Her only hospitalizations have been for the birth of her two children, now ages 3 and 5, who were delivered vaginally. She has no known medication allergies. She takes no medications regularly, other than terfenadine (Seldane), which she takes occasionally as needed for "sinus problems," with good relief of her symptoms.

Family History. Both of Mary's parents are in their late fifties and healthy. One younger sister is healthy. Both her father and sister also have "sinus problems." Mary's husband is healthy, and the children are basically healthy—both have had recurrent problems with otitis media, however.

Health Habits. Mary has smoked a pack of cigarettes daily for 10 years. She denies alcohol consumption or use of illicit drugs. She wears seat belts when she drives or rides in a car. She participates in "jazzercise" at a local health club for 30 minutes three times a week. She tries to eat "healthy."

Social History. Mary has been married for 8 years and states that she has a happy, stable, monogamous sexual relationship with her husband. They use barrier contraception. Her husband is a certified public accountant, and she works as a secretary for a local oil and gas firm. She identifies no unusual stressors in her life and notes that she and her husband are involved in a local church and have a number of close friends.

Review of Systems. Mary denies ear problems, recurring sore throats, or history of asthma or bronchitis.

OBJECTIVE

Physical Examination. Blood pressure is 120/80, normal heart rate of 80, respiration 16, temperature 98.6°F. *Head:* Right maxillary sinus is tender to palpation and percussion. *Ears:* Tympanic membranes are clear and mobile bilaterally. *Nose:* The nasal mucosa is somewhat inflamed and edematous. Speculum examination shows a purulent discharge exuding from the middle meatus on the right. *Mouth and throat:* Teeth are in good repair, and there is no periodontal disease. The throat is not inflamed. There is some cobblestoning of the posterior oropharynx. *Neck:* Without adenopathy. *Lungs:* Resonant to percussion, clear to auscultation. Transillumination of the sinuses is performed and reveals opacification of the right maxillary sinus.

Laboratory Tests. No laboratory tests were performed.

ASSESSMENT

Working Diagnoses. Two likely diagnoses best explain Mary's symptoms and findings:

1. *Seasonal allergic rhinitis* would explain the recurring symptoms of nasal congestion, responsive to antihistamines, occurring each spring and the cobblestoned appearance of the posterior oropharynx.
2. *Acute right maxillary sinusitis* is suggested by the constellation of the patient's symptoms and physical findings. Acute sinusitis is a common complication of allergic rhinitis.

Differential Diagnoses. Mary's symptoms and findings suggest a few other possibilities, which include

1. *Allergic rhinitis/sinusitis.* The presence of facial and dental pain, purulent nasal discharge, and sinus tenderness and the decreased transillumination suggest that this is more than allergic rhinitis/sinusitis and that there is a complicating bacterial sinusitis.
2. *Viral upper respiratory infection.* While a viral upper respiratory infection can cause nasal and sinus congestion and, occasionally, purulent rhinorrhea, the presence of the facial and dental pain, the tender right maxillary sinus, and the decreased transillumination suggest a bacterial sinus infection.

PLAN

Diagnostic Laboratory and Special Tests. The symptoms and physical findings are highly suggestive of a diagnosis of acute right maxillary sinusitis. The physician does not need additional diagnostic confirmation before instituting treatment for this problem.

Treatment

1. Amoxicillin 500 mg every 8 hours for 14 days was prescribed.
2. The patient was advised to use oxymetazoline 0.05% (Afrin), an over-the-counter nasal spray, in the following manner: Spray each side of the nose twice, 5 minutes apart, every 6 hours for 3 days. If, at the end of this time, nasal and sinus congestion is still a problem, begin taking pseudoephedrine (Sudafed), 60 mg orally every 6 hours, until symptoms of congestion have subsided.
3. The patient was advised that she might want to perform steam inhalations two or three times daily to help liquefy the nasal secretions.
4. The patient was advised to take acetominophen by mouth as needed for pain relief.

Patient Education

1. The patient was educated about the pathophysiology of acute sinusitis and the importance of taking all the antibiotics as prescribed. She also was educated about the importance of decongestants and the impor-

tance of not using topical decongestant nasal spray for more than 3 days at one time. She was told that her seasonal allergic rhinitis may have precipitated the acute sinusitis and that a treatment plan for this more chronic problem would be discussed at the next visit.

2. The patient was advised that smoking was not only dangerous to her general health but also might be a contributing factor to the cause of her sinus infections. She was encouraged to stop smoking and told that whenever she desired to do so, she could be counseled on effective smoking cessation methods.

Disposition. The patient was asked to return for follow-up in 3 weeks' time.

FIRST FOLLOW-UP VISIT

Mary returned 3 weeks after her initial visit as scheduled. She had completed her course of antibiotics as prescribed. Her facial and dental pain and purulent nasal discharge had resolved after 5 days of prescribed therapy. She was now feeling well, although she was still having some intermittent nasal stuffiness and clear nasal discharge, along with intermittent sneezing, as was usual for this time of the year. She was still smoking and expressed no desire to quit.

OBJECTIVE

Vital signs were normal. *Nose:* Nasal mucosa somewhat violaceous and boggy. Clear rhinorrhea. *Throat:* Cobblestoning of the posterior oropharynx.

ASSESSMENT

1. Persistent seasonal allergic rhinitis.
2. Acute maxillary sinusitis resolved.

PLAN

Diagnostic. A nasal smear was submitted for Wright's stain and showed multiple eosinophils per microscopic high-power field.

Therapeutic. Mary was started on topical nasal beclomethzone spray, one puff in each nostril three times daily, to be used during the months of the year when she usually had allergic rhinitis symptoms.

Patient Education. Mary was advised that it would take 2 to 3 weeks before she noted an improvement in her allergic rhinitis symptoms from the topical beclomethzone spray. She was advised that she should use this three times daily everyday during the months of the year when she was prone to allergic rhinitis symptoms. She was again reminded of the adverse effects of smoking on her health.

Disposition. Mary was asked to return in 6 weeks for follow-up of her allergic rhinitis symptoms.

DISCUSSION

Seasonal allergic rhinitis is a common affliction, caused by respiratory allergens, that is manifest by nasal congestion, sneezing, and clear rhinorrhea, which occur on a seasonal basis. Common physical findings include nasal mucosa that is edematous and violaceous in appearance and a cobblestoned appearance to the posterior oropharynx. Nasal smears usually show many eosinophils. Symptomatic treatment includes antihistamines. Prophylactic treatment can include topical nasal steroids or topical nasal cromolyn sodium (Nasalcrom). Patients who do not respond to these therapies are candidates for allergic desensitization therapy.

Acute sinusitis is a common problem in primary medical practice. Acute sinusitis is usually preceded by a viral upper respiratory infection or an exacerbation of allergic rhinitis. The pathophysiology of acute sinusitis involves obstruction of the osteomeatal complex. The most common infecting organisms include *Streptococcus pneumoniae, Haemophilus influenzae,* and *Moraxella catarrhalis.* There is not one single symptom or sign that is pathognomonic for acute sinusitis. Common findings include a history of sinus pain, purulent nasal discharge, and generalized malaise in the presence of preceding acute upper respiratory infection or allergic rhinitis symptoms. Tenderness over the frontal and/or maxillary sinuses and decreased transillumination of the involved sinuses may be present. While plain x-ray films of the sinuses may be helpful as diagnostic aids in equivocal situations, these are neither very sensitive nor very specific tests. While computed tomography (CT) and nuclear magnetic resonance (NMR) imaging studies are more sensitive tests, these probably have no place in the primary-care management of the patient with sinusitis. Therapy is aimed at treating the bacterial infection with appropriate antibiotics, relieving obstruction through the use of topical and systemic decongestants, and providing adjunctive symptomatic measures of relief.

Suboptimal management of acute sinusitis can lead to the development of chronic sinusitis. Patients who either have suffered more than three bouts of acute sinusitis in a year or have developed chronic sinusitis should be referred to an otorhinolaryngologist for further evaluation and treatment.

The most likely explanation for the failure of the current therapeutic regimen would be infection with a beta-lactamase–producing organism such as *H. influenzae* or *M. catarrhalis.* This would be an indication for broadening the spectrum of antibiotic coverage by using something like amoxicillin with clavulinic acid (Augmentin) or cefuroxime axetil (Cefitin). Changing the antibiotic to Augmentin (amoxicillin with clavulinic acid) would achieve this goal.

Acute sinusitis frequently involves more than one sinus. However, the classic symptoms may be helpful in localizing the involved sinus. Ethmoid and sphenoid sinusitis are more difficult to diagnose clinically than maxillary and frontal sinusitis. Plain x-ray films or even CT images may be necessary to confirm these diagnoses.

SUGGESTED READING

Rakel RE. Textbook of Family Practice, 4th ed. Philadelphia, W.B. Saunders, 1990, pp. 552–554.

Winther B, Gwaltney JM. Therapeutic approach to sinusitis: Antiinfectious therapy as the baseline of management. Otolaryngol Head Neck Surg 1990; 103:876.

QUESTIONS

1. Mary returns after 5 days of therapy and is no better. Your next step would be
   a. To change the antibiotic from amoxicillin to amoxicillin and clavulinic acid (Augmentin).
   b. To change the antibiotic from amoxicillin to doxycycline.
   c. To change the antibiotic from amoxicillin to erythromycin.
   d. To refer Mary to an otorhinolaryngologist for antralpuncture to obtain material for culture and precise identification of the organism.

2. Match each of the following types of sinusitis with the typical clinical presentation.
   a. Frontal sinusitis
   b. Maxillary sinusitis
   c. Ethmoid sinusitis
   d. Sphenoid sinusitis
      (1) Retro-orbital pain, occipital headache
      (2) Pain over the bridge of the nose and behind the eye
      (3) Pain radiating to the teeth
      (4) Causes generalized headache, may progress rapidly.

Answers appear on page 448.

Recurrent Ear Infections

GREG L. LEDGERWOOD

INITIAL VISIT

SUBJECTIVE

Patient Identification. William is a 7-year-old Caucasian boy currently in the second grade.

Presenting Problems. William presents with his mother with a history of recurrent nasal stuffiness and frequent ear infections.

Present Illness. William began experiencing ear infections at age 6 months. According to his mother, he has had "continuous" ear infections, clearing with antibiotic therapy. As soon as antibiotics are completed, his ear infections return. Currently, his general care has been delivered by a family practitioner, and he has not yet been seen by an ear, nose, and throat specialist. His mother states that during the past school year he has missed 3 weeks of school because of these infections.

William is the product of a gravida II, para II, born without complications at 40 weeks of gestation. His mother's prenatal history is noncontributory to this current problem. With his last ear infection, William also developed a cough, and when he was seen by his family physician, he was noted to have some wheezing.

On further questioning, it is discovered that most of the infections have occurred during the winter months, but he has always had a stuffy nose. During the months of May and June and again in August and September he seems to have had a great deal of nasal stuffiness with periods of sneezing, sometimes sneezing 7 to 10 times in a row. His mother relates that during these times, his eyes seem red, and he is constantly rubbing his nose. The home is heated by an electric central heating system using forced air. The home was insulated using fiberglass insulation. During the winter months, the family also has used a wood stove. The carpets in the home are made of synthetic material, and the mother states that the previous owners did have animals, specifically a cat and dog. Both frequented the house. William's bedroom is of conventional design. He sleeps in a single bed with standard mattress and box springs and uses synthetic bedding and a synthetic pillow. A cat does live with the family, and his mother states that it is William's pet and frequently sleeps on his bed. There is one member of the family, William's father, who smokes and does so inside the house. William's mother relates that she has carefully watched certain foods. At one time, early in his life, she felt that milk created a problem for William. He has been on multiple medications, primarily antibiotics and over-the-counter antihistamines/decongestants. The latter seemed to cause a fair amount of sedation and frequently did not relieve his symptoms. The mother states that other than his ear and nose problems, William's health has been good. To her knowledge, he has never had any significant problems with his skin, except a rash in the diaper area developing after one particular lengthy course of antibiotic therapy.

Past Medical History. William is the product of a gravida II, para II. His birth and development have been normal. His immunizations were delayed primarily due to recurrent infections. He has had no previous surgery. He is not allergic to any medications. He has been using an antihistamine–decongestant combination purchased over the counter on an intermittent basis.

Family History. William's father is a dairy farmer. Both the mother and the father had recurrent ear disease as infants; however, they seemed to "grow" out of it. The father has had problems with nasal stuffiness, particularly when working with his cattle. A maternal grandfather had asthma as an adult, but the rest of the family history is negative for chronic respiratory illnesses, including cystic fibrosis.

Health Habits. William has missed a great deal of school because of respiratory illness. He seems to be fatigued a great deal of the time, even though his mother feels that he gets plenty of sleep. He has not had any hospitalizations for these illnesses.

Social History. William is enrolled in the second grade. When feeling well, he participates in all school activities. Last year he was involved in a school soccer league until coughing after exercise prohibited his activity.

Review of Systems. As stated, other than his chronic respiratory illnesses, William has been in good health. He has not had any other significant problems.

OBJECTIVE

Physical Examination. General: Appearance is of a well-nourished male child. *HEENT:* There is a "bluish" discoloration below both eyes, with a pleat present below the lower lids. Likewise, a nasal pleat is present. William appears to be a mouth breather. His ears appear normal externally. His ear canals are slightly erythematous. The tympanic membranes show scarring. There is some erythema running along the short process of the malleus bilaterally. The light reflex is dull bilaterally. The nasal membranes show a pale, bluish discoloration. The middle and inferior turbinates are markedly swollen and obstruct the nasal passages approximately 90% on each side. Purulent material is present in each naris. The oropharynx is moist. The posterior pharynx shows lymphoid hyperplasia along the pharyngeal gutters bilaterally. Mucopurulent material is present. *Neck:* Normal. *Respiratory:* Chest is symmetrical and clear to percussion and auscultation. *Cardiovascular:* Normal sinus rhythm without murmur, rub, or gallop. *Abdomen:* Normal. There is no palpable organomegaly, mass, or tenderness. Bowel tones are normal. *Skin:* There are several areas of dry, scaly maculae, somewhat hypopigmented, located on both upper extremities and on the face. *Extremities:* Normal. *Neurologic:* Normal.

Laboratory Tests. A nasal smear for eosinophils, using Hansel stain, is positive, showing 4+ eosinophils present. CBC shows a hematocrit of 41%, a hemoglobin level of 14.6, WBC count is 6700, with 12% eosinophils. Spirometry examination is done and is normal for age. Total serum IgE is 200 (normal 1–120 IU/ml). Sinus x-rays show an air–fluid level in the left maxillary sinus.

ASSESSMENT

Working Diagnosis

1. *Allergic rhinitis with nasal obstruction.* A seasonal history or an association with an inhaled allergen is helpful. It is often difficult to associate specific allergens with perennial rhinitis. Occasionally, a change in environment, such as a vacation, may point to the existence of environmental allergens. In perennial allergic rhinitis, nasal congestion, itching, obstruction, and the need to constantly "sniff" may be associated with a loss of sense of taste or smell and a feeling of being "stuffed up" with decreased hearing and a popping sensation in the ears.

2. *Chronic, recurrent otitis media.* Although patients with chronic otitis media and serous otitis are not all allergic, children who present with this condition have a higher evidence of inhaled and, rarely, ingested IgE-mediated disease.

3. *Reactive airway disease, exertionally induced.* Asthma following exercise is common in atopic children and young adults. It is usually brief and indistinguishable from asthma due to other causes.

4. *Sinusitis, occult.* Over the past several years, it has been shown that the atopic child/adult with recurrent upper respiratory infections usually has radiologic evidence of sinusitis. The child with recurrent otitis media and an "atopic" history frequently will have radiographic evidence that either one or both maxillary or ethmoid sinuses are involved. Sinusitis alone does not imply allergy.

5. *Mild atopic dermatitis.* The clinical features vary with age. In infants, the lesions often appear on the face first and may extend to the scalp, trunk, and extensor aspects of the extremities. Vesiculation, oozing, and crusting are prominent, and secondary infection is common. In older children, the lesions tend to localize in flexural sites. Vesiculation is less prominent; the lesions are maculopapular and with time become lichenified. Generalized dryness of the skin is a common problem.

Differential Diagnosis. William's problems suggest several other possibilities, including

1. *Subclass IgG deficiency.* Recent evidence has suggested that subclass IgG (particularly IgG_2 and IgG_4) deficiency predisposes children to increased problems with recurrent bacterial otitis media and sinusitis.

2. *Nasal polyposis.* Nasal polyps often develop in the absence of or coincidentally with allergy. They arise from infected sinus areas and can be seen in the nasal

cavity. They can cause obstruction and aggravate the preexisting sinus disease.

3. *Cystic fibrosis.* Any child with recurrent upper chronic respiratory disease should have this disease excluded. This is highly unlikely in this patient because of the presenting history and physical findings.

PLAN

Laboratory Tests

1. Nasal smear for eosinophils. Although a positive smear done with Hansel staining showing eosinophils is not diagnostic for allergic disease, it is supportive. A smear showing polyps has been associated with infection, either bacterial or viral.

2. Sinus x-rays. The diagnosis of sinusitis can be confirmed objectively.

3. CBC. Eosinophil counts greater than 10% are supportive of, but not diagnostic of, allergic rhinitis.

4. Subclass IgG levels. Not always indicated, but in a child with recurrent upper respiratory infections (URIs), this should be considered.

5. Peak flow rates. Will help document exertional induced asthma.

6. Total serum IgE levels may or may not be helpful. Normal levels of serum IgE can be seen in patients with allergic rhinitis, depending on the season of year and the degree of "allergic" exposure.

Treatment

1. Start antibiotics for infectious component. Amoxicillin (125–250 mg q8h) is still considered the drug of choice. Sulfamethoxazole–trimethoprim and cefaclor are alternatives.

2. Consider intranasal steroids. Topical steroids such as beclomethasone, in an aqueous base, are effective in reducing turbinate size and improving aeration of paranasal sinuses. Steroids also are effective in reducing the inflammatory response mediated by allergic reactions.

3. Antihistamine and/or antihistamine/decongestants. For years these have been the foundation of therapy for allergic rhinitis. Unfortunately, almost all except terfenadine and astemizole have side effects that may preclude their use in school-age children, and they have limited value in an allergic child with an infectious problem. The newer, nonsedating antihistamines are not cleared for use in children under age 10.

Patient Education

1. Dust and dander control. Environmental control is the foundation of treatment in allergic disease. House dust mites are the chief allergen found in houses, particularly where humidity levels are high. Animal dander, likewise, adds to the "antigenic load."

2. Tobacco smoke exposure. Allergic and nonallergic children with chronic URIs are definitely made more symptomatic in homes where one or both parents smoke.

3. Symptom diary. Keeping a diary of the patient's symptoms in response to exposures to food groups and activities may substantiate the role of a particular "allergen."

FIRST FOLLOW-UP VISIT

SUBJECTIVE

William returns having completed a 2-week course of antibiotics and presents with his mother. There has been a marked improvement in his nocturnal coughing and his sleeping pattern.

OBJECTIVE

The facial features still show mild discoloration below both eyes. Ear examination shows the ear canals to be normal. There is still scarring bilaterally on the tympanic membranes, but the eardrums no longer appear retracted and tympanograms show normal curves. The erythema along the long process of the malleus is no longer present. Nasal examination shows the turbinates to be reduced in size (approximately 50%) with only a mild amount of clear discharge present. The posterior pharynx is normal. The chest is clear to percussion and auscultation, and the rest of the examination is unchanged. Repeat sinus series, specifically the Water's view, shows absence of air–fluid levels in the maxillary antrums with only minimal membranous thickening present.

ASSESSMENT

1. Occult sinusitis resolved.
2. Allergic rhinitis improved.

PLAN

Patient education is reviewed. Dietary diary will be continued. Dust control in the home will continue.

Future Considerations

1. Standard allergy testing to scratch and prick will be considered if rebound allergic problems persist.

2. Continued use of antihistamines and/or decongestants on an as-needed basis.

3. Use of an inhaled β_2-agonist (Albuterol) if exertional asthma prohibits the patient's participation in school and/or recreational activities.

4. Use of intranasal steroids.
5. Use of intranasal cromolyn sodium.

DISCUSSION

The primary care physician is in a unique position to help diagnose and manage the allergic child. Many of the problems that the allergic patient experiences can be handled appropriately by the primary care physician, and only at such a time when conservative management fails should referral to an allergist be considered. The history is usually the most important component in the evaluation of a patient suspected of having an allergic problem. In interviewing a new patient, the physician takes care to identify any previous allergy problems in the patient and also the presence of allergy in close family members. This is particularly helpful in providing support for the diagnosis of atopic disease. Environmental factors and variations in symptoms with seasons and with changes in locations should be recorded carefully.

Most allergic problems involve the skin or respiratory tract, and these should receive the most attention on physical examination. The nose is often overlooked or given only a cursory examination. The color and degree of swelling of its mucus membranes, the amount and consistency of secretions, and the presence or absence of polyps should be noted. The lungs, if free of rales, should be examined during forced expiration, which may bring out asthmatic wheezing.

The atopic child may have dark circles under the eyes ("allergic shiners") and a transverse crease above the tip of the nose from frequent nasal rubbing. Of particular importance in children is observation of the tympanic membrane and its mobility using a tympanometer, a pneumatic otoscope, or both.

A few general laboratory procedures may be helpful, such as a nasal or sputum smear, looking for eosinophils. Blood eosinophilia is helpful, if present, but its absence does not exclude allergic disease. The measurement of total serum IgE is of limited value and frequently is not worth its expense.

For further evaluation of obstructive airway disease, several recording spirometers are simple, durable, and accurate. They can be used for the purpose of confirming or ruling out airway disease, establishing the degree of response to an inhaled bronchodilator, and monitoring the progress of the patient. Several inexpensive peak flowmeters are also available for monitoring the patient's progress.

Provocation testing involves the measurement of ventilatory function before and after some inhaled stimulant. It can be used by most physicians as an aid in diagnosing exercise bronchospasm.

Skin testing should be selective and based on clues provided by the history, whenever possible. In adults, testing is limited to pollens, house dust, feathers, animal danders, and mold spores. If a history is suggestive, skin tests to some foods also may be done. Food testing is more useful in young children.

Specific IgE antibodies to a variety of antigens can be measured using the radioallergosorbent (RAST) test, but this test is expensive and provides no more information than skin testing.

Some other procedures purported to identify allergy, particularly food allergies, have received considerable attention in recent years in the lay press. These are cytotoxic testing, subcutaneous or sublingual provocative testing, and neutralization testing. None of these has been established as reliable in properly controlled trials.

The primary care physician is diluged with new information about diagnosis and treatment of allergic disease on a daily basis. With new information, the primary care physician's role in diagnosing and treating allergic conditions has expanded greatly. Reference laboratories have provided "kits" for allergy testing and "inhouse evaluation studies" utilizing RAST methods. It becomes important for the primary care physician to understand the limitations of these testing techniques when applied to the allergic patient. Even in qualified hands, these tests alone are not diagnostic, since they are subject to interpretation by the person performing the test and can lead most well-meaning physicians astray.

Infectious disease in the allergic or atopic child is most commonplace. The child presenting with recurrent upper respiratory tract infections without an obvious cause should be evaluated for the possibility of allergic disease. Recurrent otitis media, with or without a secretory component, and particularly recurrent purulent rhinitis, is often a characteristic of the atopic child. Transillumination and percussion of the sinuses often are subjective to the examiner's experience, and without radiographs, one cannot ascertain objectively whether or not sinusitis is present. Baseline sinus films not only are extremely helpful in determining the extent of sinus disease in the atopic child but also help, in an objective fashion, the treating physician to make appropriate therapeutic decisions regarding length of therapy and/or referral to appropriate specialists. Use of long-term antibiotics, particularly drugs such as sulfisoxazole, using even a "prophylactic" dose at bedtime for 30 to 60 days, often is extremely helpful in preventing a recurrence of infection in the atopic child.

A number of studies have supported the fact that antihistamine–decongestant combinations are marginally effective in treating the infectious problems seen in the atopic child, particularly those with chronic secretory otitis. More recently, the use of intranasal steroids, particularly flunisolide and beclomethasone, has added another treatment regimen. Most of the antihistamine–decongestant combinations that are available and approved for use in children, unfortunately, have side effects that preclude their use on a regular daily basis. The newer, nonsedating antihistamines, in particular terfenadine and astemizole, have not been cleared by the FDA for use in children under age 10. These drugs, when used on a regular basis, not only have few side effects but also seem particularly effective in the management of patients with both seasonal and perennial allergic rhinitis. Cromolyn sodium has received new attention, and it has been found to be effective when used on a regular basis both intranasally and intraocularly in controlling symptoms related to those organ systems. Unfortunately, its maximum effect is achieved only if it used on a three to four times a day basis. Patient compliance often comes into play in this situation. Children with exercise-induced asthma respond very nicely with use of the newer β_2-agonists such as metaproterenol and albuterol. The delivery of these drugs through a metered-dose inhaler often requires a great deal of hand–eye coordination. This can be eliminated with use of "spacing" devices. Using the medication 15 to 20 minutes prior to a planned exercise often blocks completely any exercise-induced response.

The treatment of "house dust" allergy is primarily based on avoidance of allergens. Providing the proper amount of humidity in a home, avoiding animals in the home, and avoiding tobacco smoke will greatly enhance a positive response.

If food allergies are suspected, a very carefully kept diary often will pinpoint a specific food group. Food allergies, once thought to be quite common, have been shown to be, in fact, rare, and often an intolerance is mistakenly referred to as an allergy. If a specific food group is suspected of causing or reproducing allergic symptoms, then withdrawing this food group for a period of time, up to 10 days, and rechallenging should reproduce the symptoms. Immunotherapy has been shown to be quite effective, particularly for control of pollen symptoms, in 80% of the patients and in up to 60% patients who show, on skin testing, a sensitivity to molds or house dust. It is therefore more effective in seasonal allergic rhinitis than in perennial allergic rhinitis. When considering the use of immunotherapy, the ease of control using other methods should be weighed with respect to the frequency and severity of problems.

SUGGESTED READING

Eisenberg MS, Copass MK (eds.). Emergency Medical Therapy, 3d ed. Philadelphia, W.B. Saunders, 1988, p. 454.

Rakel RE. Textbook of Family Practice, 4th ed. Philadelphia, W.B. Saunders, 1990, chap. 34.

VanArsdale PP Jr, Larson EB. Diagnostic tests for patients with suspected allergic disease: Utility and limitations. Ann Intern Med 1989; 110:304.

QUESTIONS

1. In evaluating the allergic patient, the history is the most important component. All the following are considered important *except*
   a. Family history of allergic disease.
   b. Seasonal variation.
   c. Recurrent upper respiratory infections.
   d. Normal serum total IgE levels.
   e. Episodic sneezing.

2. In seasonal allergic rhinitis, exposure is followed by all the following *except*
   a. Paroxysmal sneezing.
   b. Watery nasal discharge.
   c. Nasal itching.
   d. Conjunctival irritation.
   e. Purulent nasal discharge.

Answer true (T) or false (F) to each of the following options.

3. In seasonal allergic rhinitis,
   a. Antihistamines are the foundation of therapy.
   b. Skin testing (prick) should be performed as a "first line" diagnostic procedure.
   c. Environmental control of dust and dander is important only after "allergy shots" have been started.

4. Complications of allergic disease might include
   a. Recurrent otitis media.
   b. Exercise-induced bronchospasm.
   c. Occult sinusitis.
   d. Postoccipital headaches.

Answers appear on page 448.

Multiple Allergies

GREG L. LEDGERWOOD

INITIAL VISIT

SUBJECTIVE

Patient Identification. Sharon L. is a 29-year-old white woman who presents with problems of allergic nasal disease, atopic dermatitis, and asthma.

Presenting Problems. Sharon has had problems with "allergies" since childhood. They have been manifested by atopic dermatitis and asthma, and prior to her presentation, Sharon had been seen by an allergist. Positive skin tests to pollen and dust resulted in immunotherapy for an extended period of time. Sharon stated that she is not sure that her "allergic condition" is any better and has some questions about continuing immunotherapy. She states that she has had allergic rhinitis for most of her life. Previously, she had a diagnosis of a nasal septal deviation, and subsequently, she underwent nasal surgery with some significant improvement with regard to her nasal obstruction. She did not feel, however, that this resulted in any benefit with regard to her asthma. Her course has been complicated by recurrent otitis media as well. Since the surgery, she feels that there has been an improvement as far as the number of infections she has experienced. She states that since her senior year in high school she has had more difficulty with the asthma. She feels that perhaps it is worse in the fall, but her asthma symptoms are present throughout the year. Over the past month or so, Sharon has, in general, been awakening once a night with difficulty breathing. She has been using a metered-dose inhaler more frequently, about one canister every 2 weeks. Her other medications include a slow-release theophylline preparation, 300 mg twice a day. She notices that her asthma is exacerbated by emotional upset, such as crying or laughing. She has cold-induced and exertional wheezing. Her husband is a smoker, but he smokes outside the house. In childhood, her father also was a smoker. Sharon does not smoke. She works in a day-care center now and is exposed to frequent upper respiratory infections and feels that she has had a cold ever since fall began. She lives in a mobile home that was built in the 1970s. Urea formaldehyde may have been used in the wall construction, but Sharon is unaware of any odors in her home at this time. Sharon has no pets, and she and her husband have lived in this current home for 2 years. The previous owners had pets, including dogs that were kept indoors. The carpeting is intermediate nap with foam backing. Sharon is planning to replace the carpet soon. Electric forced-air heat is used with a wall unit air conditioner. There is no humidification. Sharon denies any hospitalizations for her asthma. She states that she is able to use aspirin-containing products without any exacerbation of her symptoms.

Past Medical History. Other than the chronic respiratory problems she relates, Sharon has otherwise been in good health and is on birth control pills in addition to the medications already mentioned. She denies any medicine allergies.

Family History. Sharon has two children, ages 4 and 8, who are alive and well without chronic respiratory disease. One sibling, age 27, had "mild asthma." Both parents are in their fifties with no medical problems. Sharon has a maternal grandmother with adult-onset diabetes.

Health Habits. Sharon works in a day-care center 5 days a week and on weekends enjoys outdoor activities, including gardening and, during the winter months, skiing. She states that her outdoor activities have been limited recently because of increased wheezing and shortness of breath any time the wind blows or she overexerts herself. She does not smoke and does not use perfumes or hairsprays, stating that they often "choke her up."

Social History. Sharon has been happily married for 10 years, and of those 10 years, 8 have been spent working outside the home. She describes her marital life as excellent, and at this time she denies any current stressful situations other than those related to her illness. She admits that she has frequently been discouraged about her health. She does not feel better and often cannot participate with her family in some of their outdoor activities.

Review of Systems. Sharon has noticed no change in appetite or weight, but she does note that her energy level seems to have dropped off over the past several years and relates this to her respiratory problems. She denies any headaches or change in vision. She states that she has frequently experienced "rawness" in her throat on awakening in the morning. She has significant dyspnea on exertion with any vigorous activity, including swimming and bicycling. She denies any cardiac problems. *Gastrointestinal:* She denies any problems. *Musculoskeletal:* Noncontributory. *Neurologic:* Noncontributory. *Endocrinologic:* Noncontributory.

OBJECTIVE

Physical Examination. Sharon is a pleasant, well-appearing white woman who is alert and cooperative and gives a good medical history. Her blood pressure is 112/70 in the left arm, sitting. She weighs 146 lb; her pulse is 78 and regular; and respirations are 15 and labored. She does describe frequently during the history and physical the frustration of having to use the inhaler and not wanting to "live like this." Her physical examination is significant for the following. *Skin:* She has dry, lichenified areas on the flexor surfaces of her forearms with an erythematous base. *Neck:* There is no cervical or supraclavicular adenopathy and no thyroid enlargement. *ENT:* Examination is unremarkable, with the exception of clear rhinorrhea with good nasal patency. *Chest:* Symmetrical, expanding symmetrically with respiration. There is a certain coarseness to the breath sounds, but no rales, rhonchi, or rubs. Wheezing and a prolonged expiratory phase at rest are present in both lung fields bilaterally. *Cardiac:* Rhythm is regular, and there are no murmurs, rubs, or gallops. The rest of her examination is normal.

Laboratory Tests. A CBC shows 8200 white blood cells, with a differential showing 13% eosinophils; otherwise, it is normal. Nasal cytology is absent for eosinophils, but a sputum cytology shows 2+ eosinophils. Spirometry is significant, showing a decrease in FEV-1 and an FEF 25/75 (10% below normal). These both return to near-normal levels after a bronchodilator is used. Chest x-ray is interpreted as normal.

ASSESSMENT

Working Diagnoses

1. *Reactive airway disease.* This is demonstrated by the abnormal pulmonary function tests returning to "normal" after bronchodilation therapy and a normal chest x-ray.
2. *Allergic nasal disease.* Previous "allergy tests" showed positive reactions to pollen and "dust."
3. *History of nasal obstruction* secondary to nasal septal deviation.

Differential Diagnosis

1. *Hyperventilation syndrome.* This is generally associated with anxiety and nonpulmonary symptoms, and

its relief through relaxation with reassurance often differentiates it from "asthma."

2. *Pulmonary emboli.* In older patients this can be differentiated by a history of predisposing factors (thrombophlebitis, cardiac failure, oral contraceptive use, prolonged bed rest, or malignancy).

3. *"Cardiac" asthma.* History of cardiac disease, moist rales in the chest, and a third heart sound distinguish it from extrinsic asthma. Cardiac asthma is usually exhibited as such in a patient with underlying obstructive lung disease who develops heart failure.

4. *Chronic bronchitis.* Although patients with this condition do have wheezing and coughing as part of their symptoms, purulent sputum production, particularly in the morning, is the hallmark of this disease.

5. *Allergic bronchopulmonary aspergillosis.* See Discussion.

PLAN

Therapeutic

1. Discussion of etiology and expectations of her disease.

2. Demonstrate to patient the proper use of a metered-dose inhaler with a "spacer" device. Many patients are given metered-dose inhalers without proper instruction and frequently are not getting the prescribed dose. Using a "spacer" eliminates the problems of "timing with breathing" associated with metered-dose inhalers.

3. Add cromolyn sodium metered-dose inhaler. Used after a β_2-agonist, this gives additional stability to reactive airways disease.

4. Continue use of long-acting theophylline. Continuing this with a β_2-agonist and cromolyn sodium frequently will prevent the nocturnal asthma flares.

5. Consider CT scan of sinuses. Standard radiographs of the sinus cavities are of limited value after nasal surgery because of secondary scarring often associated with the procedure. Untreated sinusitis, often severe, is a frequent, often-missed problem in the adult asthmatic. A naturally mediated reflex can occur when infection of the sinus is present, resulting in bronchospasm. The mechanisms of this reflex are unknown. If this problem is not addressed, control of "asthma" symptoms is much more difficult.

Patient Education

1. Instruct the patient to recognize secondary respiratory infections and get prompt treatment. Some "steroid-dependent" asthmatics should have antibiotics available at home (i.e., tetracycline, amoxicillin) and use them at the earliest sign of infection.

2. Counsel the patient on the need for yearly influenza vaccine and a one-time pneumococcal vaccine.

3. Instruct the patient on the avoidance of areas high in pollution, such as smoke-filled rooms, and so on.

4. Encourage the patient to become an "active" participant in treating her disease.

Disposition. The patient was instructed to begin the new medications and return for follow-up in 2 weeks.

FIRST FOLLOW-UP VISIT

SUBJECTIVE

Sharon returns after 2 weeks for a visit, noticing not only an improvement in her resting respiratory state, but also a decrease in the amount of nocturnal shortness of breath. She states that she finds it difficult using the medications on as regular a basis as prescribed and admits to having missed some of the doses during the day. She does relate, however, that she seems to be able to do more without developing shortness of breath and that she is pleased with what has happened so far.

OBJECTIVE

Physical Examination. This date reveals a normal examination. Repeat spirometry without bronchodilator therapy shows an improvement in her FEV-1 and FEF 25/75 compared with her first visit. CT scan of the sinuses shows no evidence of active sinus disease. Mild thickening of the membranes lining the maxillary cavities is seen bilaterally.

ASSESSMENT

The patient has appeared to stabilize.

PLAN

1. Continued patient education about the importance of regular use of metered-dose inhalers.

2. Early intervention with antibiotics when infection arises.

3. Consider other medications if treatment failure occurs, including inhaled steroids (beclomethasone), inhaled atropine-like medications (i.e., ipratropium, Atrovent), and a short burst of systemic steroids (i.e., prednisone).

4. Reassess the efficacy of immunotherapy.

DISCUSSION

Asthma is a reversible obstructive disorder of the tracheobronchial tree characterized by paroxysmal episodes of respiratory distress often interspersed with periods of apparent well-being. Asthma can begin at any age, but it most often appears in childhood, commonly with a familial predisposition. When the onset is early, prognosis is excellent, and most patients improve at puberty. Until puberty, asthma is twice as common among males as among females. This distribution reverses between puberty and early adulthood so that, among adults with asthma, females are affected more frequently than males. Asthma can be conveniently divided by etiologic factors into two main groups, as seen in Table 20–9.

In "intrinsic" asthma, most commonly seen in adults, symptoms are provoked and worsened by infection, exertion, emotion, and nonspecific environmental factors and are not related to allergen exposure. The majority of "extrinsic" asthma patients are atopic with symptoms related to environmental allergens.

TABLE 20–9. CLINICAL FEATURES OF EXTRINSIC AND INTRINSIC ASTHMA

	EXTRINSIC ASTHMA		INTRINSIC ASTHMA (IDIOPATHIC)
	Atopic	*Nonatopic*	
Age of onset	Usually childhood	Adult	Usually after age 25
Symptoms	Variable with environment and season	Usually occupation related	Unpredictable fluctuations, often chronic
Associated conditions	Allergic rhinitis, atopic dermatitis	None	Bronchitis, sinusitis, nasal polyps
Family history of atopic disease	Strong	Minor	Asthma only (?)
Skin tests (wheal-erythema)	Several positive, related to history	Negative, or one reaction only	Usually negative
Total IgE	High	Usually normal	Normal
Eosinophilia	High during allergen exposure	Sometimes high during allergen exposure	High
Prognosis	Good, especially with allergen avoidance	Good, especially with allergen avoidance	Fair, remissions uncommon

The characteristic physiologic change in asthma is airway obstruction due to bronchial smooth-muscle spasm, mucous plugging, edema, and inflammation of the bronchial wall. As a result of such airway narrowing, inspiration and expiration are impeded. Obstruction of airflow results in air trapping and hyperinflation of the lungs. Smooth-muscle spasm can occur in large, medium, or small airways. When large airways are involved, wheezing predominates. When small airways are involved, the predominant symptoms are dyspnea and cough rather than wheeze.

It is becoming increasingly clear that asthma has both immediate (bronchospastic) and late (inflammatory) phases in response to inhaled allergens and certain other provoking agents. The occurrence of this dual asthmatic response has important therapeutic implications.

The history often provides a diagnosis. Asthma should be suspected in any person with unexplained episodes of dyspnea, cough, repeated chest colds, or bronchitis, particularly in children. Even cough by itself may be a symptom of asthma. In evaluation of the acute attack, severity is related to frequency, duration, intensity, and response to previous medications with side effects, as well as symptom-free intervals. When symptoms are chronic or continuous, the condition may be confused with irreversible chronic obstructive pulmonary disease (COPD). A family history may be positive for asthma or atopy, and a search for provocative environmental factors, including occupational exposures, smoking, stress, infection, exercise, and medication (aspirin, propranolol), may yield important information.

In assessing the patient physically, recording blood pressure is important, since steroids, adrenergic agents, and theophylline may elevate blood pressure. During an asthmatic episode, the patient presents with difficulty in respiration with an increased respiratory rate using accessory muscles and suprasternal retraction, pursed-lip expiration, and flaring of the nostrils. Expiration is prolonged, with intercostal retraction. Cardiac dullness may be present, and the liver edge may be palpable owing to a lower diaphragm from pulmonary hyperexpansion.

To supplement the history and physical examination, the response to a bronchodilator may be used to establish the presence of reversible obstructive lung disease. Measurements of FEV-1 and FEF 25/75 often are extremely helpful before and after bronchodilation. Sputum analysis likewise is helpful in assessing in general terms potential etiology. Care should be taken to note the type of cells, either lymphocytic, neutrophilic, or eosinophilic. Worsening of asthma symptoms is usually accompanied by an increase in the total-blood eosinophil and sputum eosinophil counts. Both are decreased when glucocorticoid therapy is instituted.

A chest x-ray is often not helpful in evaluation of the noncomplicated asthmatic patient, since it is usually normal. However, it does provide a baseline for future comparisons. A majority of asthmatics will show hyperinflation with increased bronchial markings and flattening of the diaphragm during an acute episode.

The total serum IgE level is not particularly useful information for the management of asthma. It is normal in intrinsic asthma but not always elevated in extrinsic asthma. Its main significance is as an aid in diagnosing bronchopulmonary aspergillosis, which commonly has markedly elevated serum IgE levels and is a treatable cause of "asthma." Baseline pulmonary function studies are extremely helpful not only in defining the type of lung disease that is present but also in serving as a reference source for future episodes and as a way of measuring medication efficacy. In patients who do not have abnormal pulmonary function studies when examined but complain of symptoms occurring at other times that suggest asthma, a bronchochallenge with histamine or metacholine may be useful. These procedures, however, should be done by properly trained personnel because they can be potentially dangerous.

The aim of management is to keep the patient as symptom-free as possible with minimal medication. It is essential that the patient understand the disease and its precipitating and aggravating factors and recognize its early manifestations so that an acute episode can be treated early in order to prevent hospitalization. Recognition of the impact of emotional factors on asthma from a personal, family, and work standpoint can facilitate an acceptance of the limitations of the disease without overreaction and frustration. Patients can be taught

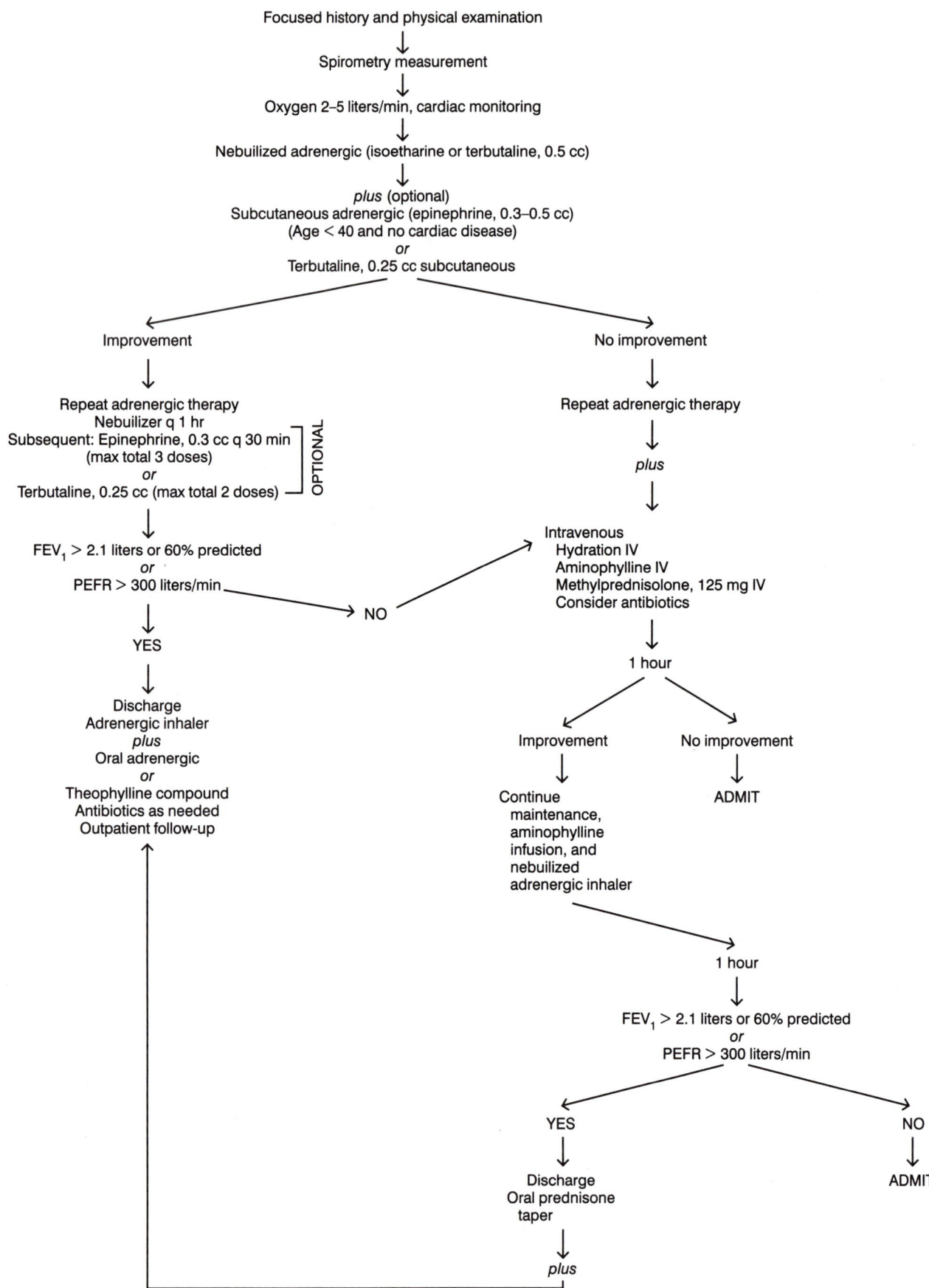

Figure 20–1. Algorithm for management of status asthmaticus.

to practice relaxed breathing to help prevent the panic that is often associated with the onset of acute symptoms.

For a patient with mild paroxysmal asthma, a β_2-adrenergic bronchodilator such as metaproterenol or albuterol, administered by a metered-dose inhaler, one to three inhalations spaced 5 minutes apart, usually provides relief for at least 6 hours. More sustained relief, especially at night, can be provided with long-acting (8–12 h) theophylline preparations given around the clock. An oral β_2-adrenergic drug may provide some additional benefit but usually has no advantage over, and more side effects than, the same drug given by inhalation.

Status asthmaticus must be treated aggressively in order to promote rapid reversibility. Oxygen, nebulized β-adrenergic agents, and the use of subcutaneous epinephrine, if needed, often result in the rapid reversal of status asthmaticus. Please refer to the flowsheet in Figure 20–1.

The management of chronic asthma presents a different challenge, again with the goal being to maintain the patient as symptom-free as possible around the clock. It is generally agreed that β_2-adrenergic agents delivered through a metered-dose inhaler with a spacer are the first line of therapy. In addition, cromolyn sodium used with a β_2-adrenergic medication has been shown to be effective in ongoing therapy. Cromolyn sodium, however, should be discontinued if an acute attack occurs because it is irritating and not effective in acute asthma. In the patient who is resistant to bronchodilator therapy and threatened with steroid dependence, a trial of inhaled steroids can be effective if they are given when ventilatory function is still fairly good. Rinsing of the mouth and gargling with water after inhalation of steroids can decrease the risk of oropharyngeal candidiasis. If continuous oral glucocorticoid therapy is necessary, giving the drug on alternate days will minimize the side effects. Unfortunately, most patients who require steroid therapy often find that they have a flare of bronchospasm during their "off" day. Ipratropium bromide, an anticholinergic bronchodilator, has been shown to be effective in bronchospasm associated with chronic bronchitis and emphysema. Its effectiveness in asthmatic patients is variable; generally, it is less effective than a β-adrenergic agent, and it has no effect on the late-phase asthmatic reaction. Cromolyn sodium and inhaled glucocorticoids, however, appear to be very effective in the late-phase reaction.

Several other medications are under investigation for the treatment of patients who have severe, chronic, steroid-dependent asthma. These include troleandomycin, methotrexate and gold salts. Their use is beyond the scope of this discussion.

Few patients present with the primary problem of asthma only, and one needs to consider the possibility of extenuating processes, such as infection and occupational irritants, when evaluating patients with this disease process.

SUGGESTED READING

Eisenberg MS, Copass MK (eds.). Emergency Medical Therapy, 3d ed. Philadelphia, W.B. Saunders, 1988, p. 454.

Rakel, RE. Textbook of Family Practice, 4th ed. Philadelphia, W.B. Saunders, 1990, chap. 34.

VanArsdale PP Jr, Larson EB. Diagnostic tests for patients with suspected allergic disease: Utility and limitations. Ann Intern Med 1989; 110:304.

QUESTIONS

1. Asthma has which of the following characteristics?
    a. Characterized as a restrictive lung disease
    b. Is irreversible
    c. Often interspersed with periods of apparent well-being
    d. Generally only occurs after puberty

2. Physiologic changes in asthma include all the following *except*
    a. Bronchial smooth-muscle spasm.
    b. Mucous plugging.
    c. Edema.
    d. Hemoptysis.
    e. Inflammation of the bronchial wall.

Answer true (T) or false (F) to each of the following options.

3. The differential diagnoses of respiratory distress in children include
    a. Bronchiolitis.
    b. Croup.
    c. Epiglottitis.
    d. Aspiration.

4. Therapeutic modalities used in the treatment of an acute asthma attack include
    a. β_2-agonists via nebulizer.
    b. Subcutaneous epinephrine.
    c. Oxygen.
    d. Cromolyn sodium.
    e. Beclomethasone via metered-dose inhaler.

Answers appear on page 449.

Diarrhea

JERRY E. JONES

INITIAL VISIT

SUBJECTIVE

Patient Identification. Melva H. is a 32-year-old Caucasian woman, mother of two active boys, who presents complaining of watery stools for the last 3 days.

Present Illness. Melva states that she was in her usual state of good health prior to 3 days ago. The onset of diarrhea was sudden and was associated with slight abdominal cramping, some nausea, but no vomiting. Melva has felt generalized malaise, but she denies fever, chills, or night sweats. She denies seeing blood or mucus in her stools. She states that the number of stools has been as high as six to eight per 24-hour period, with the last stool being a few hours before her office visit. She has been able to tolerate her usual diet but has not felt hungry.

Past Medical History. Melva has had no surgeries, accidents, or serious injuries. She was hospitalized once 6 years ago for a renal stone but has had no further difficulty. She has no known medication allergies.

Family History. Both of Melva's parents are living and in good health. There is a history of diabetes mellitus in a grandmother and a history of hypertension in both grandfathers. Melva's only sister is alive and well. No one else in the family has been ill.

Health Habits. Melva does not smoke cigarettes or drink alcohol. She does not actively exercise, but she states that keeping up with two small children keeps her active.

Social History. Melva is married to a third-year dental student. They have two children, ages 2 and 5 years. Melva works part time outside the home as a visiting nurse. She has not traveled recently and has no known exposure to hepatitis. She lives in a community of 2500 and is on city water.

Review of Systems. Melva's appetite has decreased the last several days. She has had an occasional headache and has noted some increase in "gas." She has had difficulty sleeping because of the diarrhea. She has no skin rash.

OBJECTIVE

Physical Examination. Melva appears comfortable, with a blood pressure of 118/72, a heart rate of 88, and a temperature of 99°F. Her weight is 142 lb, and her height 68 in. Her mucous membranes appear moist. On physical examination, bowel sounds are active, and there is slight upper abdominal and left lower quadrant tenderness. She is somewhat flushed. Her rectal vault was empty.

Laboratory Tests. The fecal occult blood test was negative. Microscopic examination of the stool showed no red blood cells and only a few white cells. The urinalysis was negative for ketones. WBC count and liver enzyme studies were normal. No parasitic ova or cysts were identified in the digital rectal examination.

ASSESSMENT

Working Diagnosis. A diagnosis of *viral gastroenteritis* is most likely in this patient (rotavirus or Norwalk agent). Additional considerations could be early viral hepatitis, which may present with diarrhea before the onset of liver involvement and infection with *Giardia lamblia*.

Differential Diagnoses. With the stool negative for red and white cells, a *bacterial cause* is unlikely. There are multiple bacterial causes of acute diarrhea, including *Campylobacter jejuni*, enteroinvasive *Escherichia coli*, *Salmonella spp.*, *Shigella spp.*, and *Yersinia enterocolitica*. With the negative exposure history, diarrhea due to *drugs* or *toxins* is unlikely. Since no one else in the immediate family is ill, *food poisoning* is also unlikely. Food poisoning associated with staphylococci or mushrooms produces vomiting as well. *Protozoan infections* with *Entamoeba histolytica* and *Balantidium coli* present with blood and mucus in the stools.

PLAN

Diagnostic. Since this patient is a health care worker, she is at high risk for hepatitis exposure. With two small children at home, this possibility needs to be evaluated.

Therapeutic. The patient has continued to tolerate her usual diet. A discussion of replacing fluids orally will be helpful, along with symptomatic treatment of the diarrhea. Effective replacement solutions include carbonated beverages and the commercially available drink Gatorade. Therapeutic use of bismuth subsalicylate (Pepto-Bismol) in volunteers with gastroenteritis caused by Norwalk virus has produced some reduction in abdominal cramps without affecting the rate of virus excretion.

Patient Education. A review of the most likely causes will be helpful in educating the patient regarding "viral gastroenteritis." It will be important to discuss the fact that antibiotics are not indicated in a viral illness. Careful handwashing is indicated.

Disposition. The patient was told to return for re-evaluation if the number and frequency of stools did not improve. Otherwise, the natural course of the illness would be that of gradual improvement and return of normal function.

FIRST FOLLOW-UP VISIT

SUBJECTIVE

The patient returned in 2 weeks, stating that the initial bout of diarrhea seemed to clear. However, 2 days ago there was a second bout of foul-smelling diarrhea associated with epigastric discomfort and increasing gas. The patient noted increasing nausea without vomiting and experienced a 10-lb weight loss over the past 2 weeks, accompanied by generalized fatigue. Her oldest son has also started having loose stools.

OBJECTIVE

The patient appears fatigued. Blood pressure was 110/68, pulse 90, respirations 20, and temperature 98.8°F. Her weight is 136 lb. Her abdominal examination has changed little. There is slight epigastric tenderness and diffuse active bowel sounds. A digital rectal examination reveals soft stool in the ampula and is again negative for occult blood. A microscopic examination of the stool reveals cysts of *Giardia lamblia.*

ASSESSMENT

Giardiasis.

PLAN

1. The patient is started on metronidazole, 250 mg PO three times a day for 5 days.
2. Stool examinations are obtained on the remaining family members, and both children are found to have cysts of *Giardia.*
3. Upon further investigation, the patient's community water supply had recently experienced problems, with a breakdown in water treatment. The community at large had experienced bouts of diarrhea, and local health officials were notified of the clustering of these cases. The patient was instructed to use bottled water for drinking and cooking until the community water supply problem could be corrected.
4. The children are not involved in day care and are treated with furazolidone suspension, 5 mg/kg in four equally divided doses during a 24-hour period for 7 days.
5. Repeat stool examinations are requested for all family members in 4 weeks.

DISCUSSION

Giardiasis is the human infection caused by the flagellated protozoan *Giardia lamblia.* It occurs in all age groups and can present to the physician with a range of symptoms. In the acute phase, it will present with diarrhea, abdominal pain, bloating, and flatulence. As in this patient, it may present initially as the "garden variety" gastroenteritis. Cyst passage is variable and can be overlooked easily in the stools. Even without treatment, the natural course of giardiasis is to spontaneously improve. Following the initial bout, the host may then recover without further problems or become a chronic carrier with intermittent episodes of recurrent diarrhea.

The "chronic" phase of giardiasis may be prolonged and last several years after the first contact with this organism. The chronic phase presents with flatulence, upper abdominal pain, epigastric gnawing, nervousness, and weight loss. Diagnosis is at times difficult. The cyst passage is variable, with high numbers being passed initially during the "acute" phase. Stool examinations for ova and parasites are helpful but frequently are not obtained during the acute episode. Digital rectal examination is one way to obtain samples for microscopic examination in the office setting. This also will provide a method for examining for red and white cells in the stool.

It will be helpful to catagorize the presenting signs and symptoms into an "acute" episode or a "chronic" episode. If it appears that the symptoms represent a chronic infection (duration of recurrent symptoms greater than 3 months), it may be necessary to use the "string test" to obtain duodenal samples for diagnosis. In this case, the "trophozoite" phase is identified. This procedure can be used in the office setting and is a fairly simple method for upper intestinal sampling. Figure 20–2 outlines a diagnostic approach to giardiasis.

Since any intestinal protozoan infection indicates that the patient has experienced fecal contamination, it is important to explore the possible sources of this contamination. This patient has several possible sources, including her young children (giardiasis is a major cause of day-care epidemics), her part-time job (working as a home health care nurse places her in situations of chronic care), and the breakdown of her community water supply. In this situation, the local health department identified solutions that were helpful in correcting the community outbreak.

The collection of fecal specimens is often embarrassing and frequently difficult to accomplish in the office setting. Stool collection kits are available and helpful in improving compliance. It is important to check other family members for possible infections, since many infections may be asymptomatic and provide a source for reinfection. Careful instructions on how to collect a stool sample at home will be necessary. The use of plastic kitchen wrap under the toilet seat is a helpful way to instruct individuals in the collection of a specimen. By placing this wrap beneath the toilet seat, one can obtain a sample of stool without having to dip into the toilet bowl or try to pass stool into a container. The sample is place into a prepared kit containing two vials, one with polyvinyl alcohol (PVA) and the other with buffered Formalin. These kits are available commercially (Meridian Diagnostics, Inc., Cincinnati, Ohio).

Morphologic characteristics that distinguish the cyst

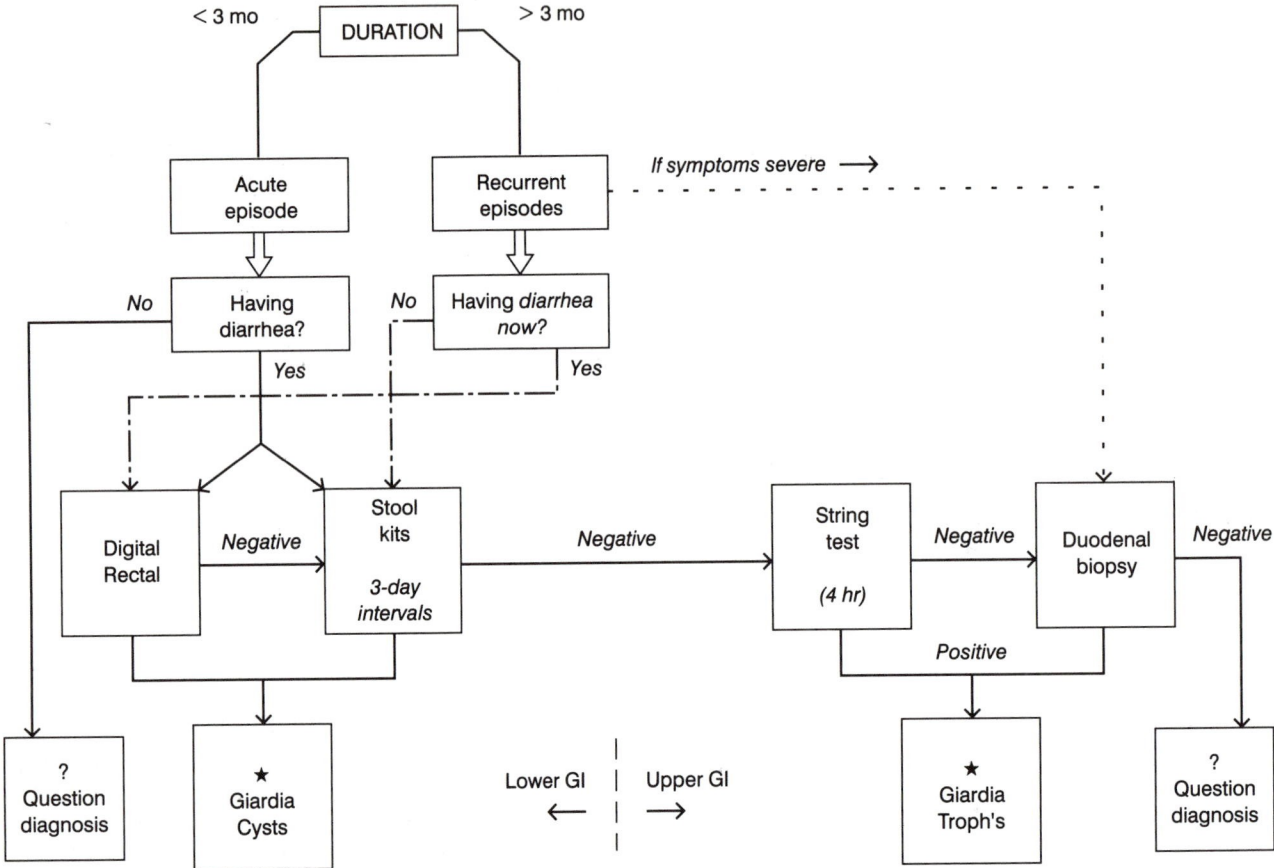

Figure 20–2. A flowchart for the diagnosis of *Giardia lamblia* infection. (From Jones JE. Giardiasis. In Balows A, Hausler WJ, Lennette EH (eds.): Laboratory Diagnosis of Infectious Diseases: Principles and Practice, vol. 1. New York, Springer-Verlag, 1988, pp. 872–882, with permission.)

are its shape, size, and intracytoplasmic structures. The cyst has a distinctive oval shape and is approximately the size of a white blood cell. On wet preparation, a refractile body called the "axoneme" will be seen obliquely within the cytoplasm. One to two of the four nuclei are usually seen in any one field of focus. A drop of dilute iodine placed on the edge of the cover slip will help outline the nuclear characteristics of the cysts.

TABLE 20–10. DRUG TREATMENT OF GIARDIASIS

ADULTS

Quinacrine HCl, 100 mg t.i.d. for 5 days
Metronidazole, 250 mg t.i.d. for 5 days
Furazolidone, 100 mg q.i.d. for 7–10 days
Paromomycin,* 25–30 mg/kg in three divided doses over 7–10 days

CHILDREN

Quinacrine HCl, 2 mg/kg t.i.d. for 5 days (max. 300 mg/day)
Metronidazole, 5 mg/kg t.i.d. for 5 days
Furazolidone, 1.25 mg/kg q.i.d. for 7 days

*For first trimester of pregnancy if treatment is deemed necessary.
Source: Modified from Jones JE. Parasitology. In Rakel RE (ed.): Textbook of Family Practice, 4th ed. Philadelphia, W.B. Saunders, 1990, pp. 591–601.

Trophozoites are easily recognized on wet preparations by their irregular motion and activity. The trophozoite is pear-shaped, and on special stains the two large nuclei give it its characteristic "monkey face" appearance.

Treatment with metronidazole is generally effective, although some treatment failures have been reported. Quinacrine is equally effective. Table 20–10 outlines the drugs available for the treatment of giardiasis. Special consideration is needed for the pregnant patient because metronidazole is contraindicated during the first trimester.

SUGGESTED READING

Jones JE. String test for diagnosing giardiasis. Am Fam Physician 1986; 34:123–126.
Jones JE. Giardiasis. In Balows A, Hausler WJ, Lennette EH (eds.): Laboratory Diagnosis of Infectious Disease: Principles and Practice, vol. 1. New York, Springer-Verlag, 1988, pp. 872–882.
Jones JE. Parasitology. In Rakel RE (ed.): Textbook of Family Practice, 4th ed. Philadelphia, W.B. Saunders, 1990, pp. 591–601.
Jones JE. Giardiasis. Primary Care 1991; 18(1):43–52.
Tietze PE, Jones JE. Parasites during pregnancy. Primary Care 1991; 18(1):75–100.

QUESTIONS

1. The acute phase of giardiasis is characterized by
   a. Constipation.
   b. Fever.
   c. Vomiting.
   d. Diarrhea.
   e. Blood in stools.

2. The chronic phase of giardiasis is characterized by
   a. Vomiting.
   b. Flatulence.
   c. Blood in stools.
   d. Mucus in stools.
   e. Fever.

3. A simple office procedure for obtaining trophozoites in suspected cases of chronic giardiasis is
   a. Digital rectal examination.
   b. Iodine stain.
   c. String test.
   d. Sputum examination.
   e. Fecal Gram stain.

4. The drug of choice for treating giardiasis during the first trimester of pregnancy is
   a. Quinacrine.
   b. Metronidazole.
   c. Furazolidone.
   d. Paromomycin.
   e. Iodoquinol.

Answers appear on page 449.

Normal Pregnancy

MARSHA C. HOLLEMAN

INITIAL VISIT

SUBJECTIVE

Patient Identification and Presenting Problems. Charlotte, a 27-year-old woman, presents with a 2-week history of fatigue, nausea, and breast tenderness. She requires up to 10 hours of sleep per night and even naps during the day to combat her ever-present fatigue. She feels nauseated almost every afternoon but has not vomited. Her last menstrual period was June 11 (today is July 28), but her menstrual cycles are often long and irregular, particularly in the summer. She has had no pelvic pain or vaginal spotting. For contraception she uses a diaphragm with contraceptive cream, except for an occasional lapse. She and her husband, married for 1 year, had planned to delay conception for several years because of career demands, but she is concerned that she might be pregnant. She has not seen a doctor in over a year and asks for a full physical examination to evaluate her fatigue.

Past Medical History. Charlotte had an appendectomy at age 14. She has no drug allergies. She occasionally takes aspirin for tension headaches.

Family History. Charlotte's mother, age 57, has hypertension. Her father, age 58, has a history of peptic ulcer disease. Cancer is prominent in the family: lung cancer (paternal uncle), endometrial cancer (paternal grandmother), and prostatic cancer (maternal grandfather).

Health Habits. Charlotte has one or two glasses of wine a week. She does not smoke or use illicit drugs. She runs 3 miles five times a week.

Social History. Charlotte has been an attorney for 1 year in a large law firm where long hours and weekend work are expected. Her husband travels frequently on business trips. Both extended families live nearby.

Review of Systems. Charlotte is myopic and wears soft contact lenses, which occasionally irritate her eyes. During college, she weighed 30 lb more than her current weight; she works hard at diet and exercise to keep her weight down.

OBJECTIVE

Physical Examination. On examination, Charlotte is a quiet, tense woman. Blood pressure is 100/68; pulse rate is 60; and temperature is 97.8°F. Pertinent to her examination is a normal thyroid, heart with regular rate and rhythm without murmurs, breasts without mass or discharge, and abdomen with well-healed right lower quadrant scar, without mass or tenderness. On pelvic examination, the vulva and vagina are normal with a white mucous discharge. The cervix is slightly blue-tinged and is closed, long and posterior. The uterus is anteverted and slightly enlarged to an approximate 6-week gestational size. The examination of the adnexae reveals bilateral ovaries of approximately 3 × 3 cm size without other masses.

Laboratory Tests. The urine pregnancy test is positive.

ASSESSMENT

The diagnosis is *intrauterine pregnancy* at 6¾ weeks' gestation. The patient's typical symptoms of fatigue and breast tenderness, along with the presence of Chadwick's sign (blue-tinged cervix) and an enlarged uterus, point clearly to the diagnosis. Although ectopic pregnancy is remotely possible, the lack of pelvic pain, vaginal spotting, and adnexal masses make it very unlikely, and no further testing need be done to ensure that the pregnancy is intrauterine.

At this point, the patient and her husband, unless they opt for abortion, are embarking on the long, life-changing, sometimes wonderful, sometimes difficult course of pregnancy, childbirth, and parenting. As long as the pregnancy remains normal, the physician's role is to watch carefully for developing problems and to prepare the patient and her husband for what lies ahead. Certain specific prenatal care tasks for the physician include the following:

1. *Establish the diagnosis and estimated due date.* A urine pregnancy test, based on the binding of human chorionic gonadotrophin (hCG) by an antibody–enzyme complex, may be positive at hCG levels as low as 25 mIU/ml. This correlates to a pregnancy of approximately 10 days' duration or less. Since menses usually occurs approximately 14 days after ovulation, the urine pregnancy test can diagnose a pregnancy prior to the missed menses.

The "estimated due date" (EDD) or "estimated date of confinement" (EDC) is, by Knaegele's rule, the date of the first day of the last menstrual period (LMP) plus 1 year and 7 days minus 3 months. For example, in Charlotte's case, her LMP is 6/11/91, so her EDD is 3/18/92. The length of human gestation is 280 days, or 40 weeks, as counted from the first day of the LMP to the EDD. A "term pregnancy" may extend from 37 to 42 weeks' gestation.

The best, most accurate way to date a pregnancy is by an accurate date of LMP. If the patient is unsure of her LMP, an ultrasound examination can date the pregnancy with a first-trimester accuracy of plus or minus 4 days. Pregnancy milestones, such as hearing fetal heart tones with the Doppler by 12 weeks' gestation or measuring the fundus (top of the uterus) at the umbilicus at 20 weeks' gestation, can either confirm an accurate pregnancy date or indicate an inaccurate date, thereby necessitating an ultrasound examination to discover the correct EDC.

Establishing an accurate EDC is critically important for correlating the growth of the fetus during the pregnancy and for determining when a patient in labor is preterm (before 37 weeks' gestation), term, or postdates (after 42 weeks' gestation).

2. *Diagnose and treat prenatal disease.* The physician thoroughly questions the patient regarding her past obstetrical experiences, past medical illnesses, surgical procedures, exposures to infection, and risk of genetic diseases. Specifically, the physician asks about previous pregnancies, including the type of delivery (vaginal, whether or not forceps or vacuum was needed, cesarean section), the baby's weight, and—of utmost importance—whether or not the patient had preterm labor. (A history of preterm labor is the most important risk factor for its development in subsequent pregnancies.)

Some of the most important medical illnesses that cause problems in pregnancy include heart disease, since some heart conditions, particularly valvular diseases, worsen with the stress of pregnancy; and diabetes mellitus, since altered glucose levels may result in congenital malformations or in a difficult birth because of a large baby. Troublesome habits during pregnancy are use of cigarettes, which results in an increased incidence of intrauterine growth retardation, preterm labor, and abruptio placentae; ethanol use, which may result in the fetal alcohol syndrome, especially among daily drinkers; and illicit drug use, with its potential for numerous congenital defects and HIV infection.

Sexually transmitted and other infectious diseases that put the fetus at risk for infection are herpes simplex type II, syphilis, gonorrhea, *Chlamydia,* HIV, hepatitis B, and tuberculosis. A history of any genetic disease among the patient, the father, or both extended families should be sought, particularly of the diseases that are diagnosable during pregnancy, such as sickle-cell disease or Tay-Sachs disease. The risk of Down syndrome increases with maternal age, and patients of "advanced maternal age" (35 years or greater) are advised of serum and amniotic fluid tests available for its prenatal diagnosis.

The physician performs a complete physical examination early in the pregnancy, paying special attention to the thyroid, in which abnormalities can create fetal hyperthyroidism or hypothyroidism resulting in decreased intellectual function; the breasts, in which abnormal masses may grow quickly under the influence of gestational hormones; and the heart, in which abnormal sounds may indicate a heart disease that causes difficulty during pregnancy (e.g., Marfan's syndrome or mitral stenosis). The pelvic examination is performed carefully, with special attention to cervical dilation and effacement (size of its opening and length), uterine size, and adnexal masses. The size of the uterus during early pregnancy correlates well with the gestational age of the pregnancy and is invaluable for estimating, corroborating, or contradicting the pregnancy dates.

Laboratory data obtained routinely during pregnancy include (1) a complete blood count (CBC), to determine the presence of anemia and to obtain a baseline platelet count; (2) blood type and Rh, to identify Rh-negative patients; (3) an indirect Coombs' test (or unexpected antibody), to identify antibodies that might harm the fetus, especially anti-Rh, anti-Kell, anti-Duffy; (4) urine culture, to identify patients with asymptomatic bacteriuria, with its attendant risks of pyelonephritis and preterm labor; (5) rubella screen, to determine the patient's rubella status (if no antibody is present, the patient is advised to avoid sick children during the pregnancy and to obtain the rubella immunization during the postpartum period); (6) Papanicolaou smear, to identify patients with dysplasia, who need treatment during pregnancy; and (7) RPR, gonorrhea cervical culture, and hepatitis B surface antigen, to identify patients whose infants are at risk for prenatal or perinatal transmission. Other laboratory examinations should be added as indicated, such as sickle-cell screen, HIV antibody, or *Chlamydia* culture. Some physicians routinely perform these last two tests.

3. *Promote a healthy pregnancy.* The physician emphasizes to the patient her responsibilities in providing as healthy an environment for the fetus as possible and often asks the patient to read further on the subject, such as *What to Expect When You're Expecting,* by Arlene Eisenberg et al., or *The Well-Pregnancy Book,* by Michael Samuels and Nancy Samuels. Specific health-promotion topics to be reviewed with each patient include stopping cigarette smoking and illicit drug use by means of such steps as setting a stop date and scheduling frequent follow-up visits, avoiding moderate to heavy ethanol intake (some groups such as the FDA advise no ethanol intake at all during pregnancy), and avoiding medications not prescribed by the physician. In Charlotte's case, the physician would probably recommend acetaminophen rather than aspirin for pain because of aspirin's role in decreased coagulation and in fetal ductus arteriosus closure.

Good nutrition during pregnancy includes gaining at least 20 lb, increasing the protein intake (75–100 gm/day), and taking in adequate calcium (1200 mg/day), iron (30–60 mg/day), and folic acid (200–400 μg/day). This translates into a diet of four servings each of protein, dairy, and grain foods, two vitamin C fruit or vegetable servings, two other fruit or vegetable servings, and at least one leafy green vegetable. The physician encourages aerobic, low-impact exercise during pregnancy, advising that peak-level exercising last 15 minutes or less, that the heart rate not exceed 140 beats/minute to avoid placental shunting, that lying supine be avoided after the 4th month of gestation, and that the patient remain well-hydrated.

The patient should realize that pregnancy brings an increased sleep requirement and that she should sleep and rest enough to avoid fatigue. Research does not substantiate the fear that women in demanding, time-consuming jobs have worse pregnancy outcomes; however, reducing work demands in order to incorporate healthy sleep, nutritional, and exercise habits can only benefit the pregnancy.

Encouraging breast-feeding begins early in pregnancy so that the physician may identify patients who do not plan to breast-feed. When the physician understands the patient's reluctance to breast-feed, he or she may be able to address the patient's concerns, perhaps via having the patient consult with the La Leche League or by discussing the advantages of breast-feeding with family members who discourage it.

4. *Examine personal and family issues surrounding the pregnancy.* Personal issues may include whether the pregnancy is by choice or not, what anxiety the mother has regarding whether the baby will be normal, and what changes are and will be occurring in the relationship with her spouse. Family issues to discuss include the father's involvement in pregnancy and child-care responsibilities, the couple's reason for having a child, what work interruptions will occur as a result of the pregnancy, the inevitable lifestyle changes after the birth (no more sleep!), and how relationships with the extended family may change after the infant's arrival.

PLAN

Charlotte is stunned by the news of her pregnancy, mostly because she is surprised, but also because she is uncertain about how she will accommodate the demands of both her job and the pregnancy. She is sure, however, that she will not get an abortion, and she asks the physician to proceed with the prenatal evaluation.

Diagnostic. The physician orders the routine prenatal laboratory examinations described above.

Therapeutic. The physician prescribes daily prenatal vitamins.

Patient Education. The physician explains what Charlotte can do to promote a healthy pregnancy.

Disposition. Charlotte will return in 4 weeks for evaluation of uterine growth and fetal heart tones (FHTs). If at that point FHTs are not heard by Doppler (10 weeks' gestation), Charlotte will return weekly through 12 weeks' gestation until the physician hears them in order to confirm the pregnancy's dates and continued viability. She is to call if she develops lower abdominal pain or vaginal spotting, which might indicate a spontaneous abortion or ectopic pregnancy.

FIRST FOLLOW-UP VISIT

SUBJECTIVE

Charlotte returns 4 weeks later at 10⅝ weeks' gestation. She continues to have nausea and fatigue. She has had no pelvic pain or vaginal spotting. She has been trying to change her diet but finds it difficult to get four dairy servings a day. Since she does not like milk, she has found some low-fat yogurts and cottage cheese that she likes. She has quit running because she feels as if she has a "rock shaking around" in her pelvis when she runs, but she has found an exercise videotape for pregnant women that she enjoys.

She and her husband have adjusted to the idea of the pregnancy, and he is with her today in the office. He wants to come to the office visits as much as his business travel allows. They both realize that their knowledge is minimal regarding how the demand of a pregnancy and a child will change their relationship, their leisure time, and their ability to work hard at their jobs, but they want to learn as much as they can in order to be prepared. They are beginning to be excited about the prospect of a baby in their family.

OBJECTIVE

Charlotte is a talkative, smiling woman in no acute distress. Her blood pressure is 105/72; her temperature is 98°F; her pulse rate is 64; and her respiratory rate is 18. Her weight has increased by 1 lb. The abdominal examination reveals no masses, and the fetal heart tones are present by Doppler, which both she and her husband hear.

Laboratory results are normal. She is not anemic, has blood type A+, is rubella immune, and has a negative indirect Coombs' test, urine culture, RPR, gonorrhea culture, hepatitis B surface antigen, and Papanicolaou smear.

ASSESSMENT

The presence of FHTs further confirms a viable pregnancy. As much as 50% of pregnancies spontaneously abort, most often due to genetic abnormalities. Once FHTs are heard, the possibility of a spontaneous abortion becomes less than 5% to 10%.

The presence of FHTs also confirms Charlotte's dates of 11 weeks' gestation. Documenting FHTs at 10 to 12 weeks' gestation, along with other pregnancy milestones, such as the measure of the uterine height in centimeters equaling the gestational age in weeks between 20 and 32 weeks' gestation, helps to confirm the patient's menstrual dates and to avoid the need for ultrasound to establish dates.

Charlotte has no developing medical problems. She has done well in her efforts to be healthy for her pregnancy. She and her husband are adjusting admirably well, with amazingly good insight into the further adjustments ahead of them. Some signs that the family will do well include the husband's high level of interest and their flexible approach to what lies ahead.

PLAN

Diagnostic. No tests are needed at this time.

Therapeutic. Charlotte is to continue with her current strategies.

Patient Education. Charlotte and her husband plan to read a book about pregnancy.

Disposition. Charlotte is to return monthly. Should she develop lower abdominal pain, vaginal spotting, or any unusual symptoms, she is to call.

SUGGESTED READING

Creasy RK, Resnik R (eds.). Maternal–Fetal Medicine: Principles and Practice. Philadelphia, W.B. Saunders: 1989.
Rakel RE (ed.). Textbook of Family Practice, 4th ed. Philadelphia, W.B. Saunders, 1990, chap. 36, pp. 602–635.

QUESTIONS

1. When are fetal heart tones first established by Doppler?
   a. 8 to 10 weeks' gestation
   b. 10 to 12 weeks' gestation
   c. 12 to 14 weeks' gestation
   d. 14 to 16 weeks' gestation

2. When does the measurement of the uterine height from the symphysis pubis to the fundus in centimeters equal the gestational age in weeks?
   a. 28 to 40 weeks
   b. 20 to 32 weeks
   c. 16 to 28 weeks
   d. 12 to 24 weeks

3. The optimal weight gain during pregnancy is at least how many pounds?
   a. 15
   b. 20
   c. 25
   d. 30

4. True or false: Knaegele's rule states that the estimated due date is established by adding 1 year and 7 days to and subtracting 3 months from the first day of the last menstrual period.

Answers appear on page 449.

Newborn Care

ROBERT H. SPRINKLE

INITIAL VISIT

SUBJECTIVE

Patient Identification and Presenting Problems. Baby Z. is a 2134-gm boy, a product of a 36-week (by dates) pregnancy in a now $16\frac{11}{12}$-year-old $G_1P_1Ab_0$ unmarried Caucasian female whose pregnancy was unplanned but, by her own report, uncomplicated. The last normal menstrual period date was well remembered. Prenatal care had been sought at a "women's clinic" about 3 months after recognition of amenorrhea, but prepayment requirements had precluded professional evaluation; thereafter, public hospital presentation was anticipated "just as soon as the baby dropped." About 2 hours prior to delivery, the mother experienced rapidly worsening abdominal pain and cramping. Her former employer brought her to the hospital's emergency room door. The woman was assumed by ER staff to be in active labor. She also was found to be without private insurance. While being readied for taxicab transfer to the county hospital, her blood pressure was recorded as 88/46 mmHg and her pulse was 124 beats/minute; fetoscopy was not performed. The hospital administrator on call was contacted at home; he encouraged rapid disposition but suggested that plans be revised to provide an IV saline infusion and a licensed practical nurse to accompany the patient, and he reminded the staff to notify the county hospital ER clerk of the intention to transfer.

The charge nurse, however, grew increasingly concerned. Noticing the presence of a member of the obstetrics and gynecology staff, she asked privately for a nonadministrative opinion. This opinion having been rendered, the patient was phlebotomized immediately for routine preoperative and obstetrical studies plus a coagulation profile; volume repletion orders were accepted verbally; and the operative delivery room was staffed. The patient was wheeled through the radiology suite, where a placental abruption was quickly demonstrated ultrasonographically. In due course, the patient's baby was delivered by cesarean section. A large, concealed retroplacental hemorrhage was evacuated. Amniotic fluid was clear. Apgar scores were 5 at 1 minute, 7 at 5 minutes, and 8 at 10 minutes (-1 for color and -1 for reflex stimulation). The mother responded well to crystalloid, colloid, and 3 units of packed red blood cells.

The baby was taken to the intermediate-care nursery, where pulse oximetry in room air showed oxygen saturation levels in the 88% to 89% range. The baby was placed in 30% oxygen under a radiant warmer; within 5 minutes, SaO_2 by oximetry had risen to the 91% to 92% range. (At all times, oximeter heart rate measurement correlated closely with heart rate as monitored electrocardiographically by chest-wall impedance leads.) Blood glucose level by chemical-strip analysis was well above 40 mg/dl. Initial spun hematocrit was 51%. CBC with differential WBC count was within normal limits. First urination and passage of a small meconium stool were noted.

Mild expiratory grunting was noted at 1 hour, at which time the baby's respiratory rate had increased to 64 breaths/minute and his SaO_2 had fallen to the 89% to 90% range. Inspired oxygen fraction was increased to 40%. A chest radiogram showed mild haziness, some central perihilar streaking, and a generous cardiac shadow. Treatment with artificial surfactant was discussed, as was the prospect of mechanical ventilation, but neither was thought warranted. By 6 hours of age, hematocrit had fallen to 43%; by 12 hours, to 41%. By 18 hours of age, hematocrit had stabilized, and the baby was breathing room air comfortably, with pulse oximetry consistently showing SaO_2 levels in the 93% to 94% range. Hematocrit and blood glucose surveillance orders and feed-as-tolerated orders were written by nursery staff.

OBJECTIVE

Baby Z. is examined at 20 hours of age and found to be stable and remarkable only for signs of mild prematurity and relatively (though not "diagnostically") small size, his weight, length, and head circumference all being about the 15th percentile for estimated gestational age (EGA).

ASSESSMENT

The problem list is as follows:

1. Prematurity (estimated gestational age 36 weeks)
2. Perinatal stress
   a. Placental abruption with maternal hypotension
   b. Emergent delivery by cesarean section
3. Perinatal distress and depression, mild (Apgars 5, 7, 8)
4. Transient tachypnea of the newborn, resolved
5. Maternal adolescence

Each of these problems is common individually, and their pathophysiologic interdependence is well described, if not at every level well understood. *Transient tachypnea of the newborn* (TTN), a syndrome lasting, by convention, no more than 24 hours, must be distinguished expeditiously from more dangerous illnesses that also cause respiratory distress, such as *hyaline membrane disease* (presenting as the "respiratory distress syndrome"), *bacterial pneumonia* (e.g., group B beta-hemolytic streptococcal pneumonia), *spontaneous pneumothorax* or *pneumomediastinum, aspiration pneumonitis, congenital anomalies affecting cardiopulmonary function* (e.g., cardiovascular malformations, pulmonary malformations, diaphragmatic herniation), *serious disorders of transition* (e.g., persistent pulmonary hypertension of the newborn), and *central neurologic insult*. TTN is thought to be caused by slow resorption of fetal lung fluid, and it is somewhat more common following cesarean than vaginal deliveries, presumably because cesarean delivery bypasses the physiologic "vaginal squeeze." However, Baby Z. was delivered through cesarean section because of maternal hypovolemic shock; therefore, he was at higher than usual risk for various other pathophysiologies affecting respiratory function, especially ischemic damage to surfactant-producing cells lining the alveoli.

Particularly intriguing—though not particularly unusual—in Baby Z's history is the coincidence of placental abruption and maternal adolescence.

PLAN

Diagnostic. The following supplemental studies are obtained:

1. Urine for drug screen (newborn)
2. Urine for drug screen (mother)
3. Meconium for drug screen

Therapeutic. The nursery staff is asked to observe Baby Z. especially for signs of drug withdrawal (e.g., jitteriness, seizures), intracranial hemorrhage (e.g., apnea), cardiovascular instability (e.g., cyanosis), or gut ischemia (e.g., vomiting, increasing abdominal girth, failure to defecate, blood in feces). The maternal and family histories are reviewed, as are the antecedents of the mother's placental abruption.

FIRST REEVALUATION

SUBJECTIVE

Baby Z's mother has had no contact with her parents in over a year. She left her hometown and came to the city with her 19-year-old boyfriend, with whom she is no longer associated. She was befriended and later "employed" by a man for whom she has occasionally performed sexual favors and at whose request and direction she has also functioned from time to time as a prostitute. Most recent intercourse was 3 days ago. She never used condoms until her pregnancy began "showing," after which time she became concerned that intercourse "without protection" might harm her baby. On the night of her presentation, a "customer" had suggested precoital smoking of "crack" cocaine, some minutes after which she began complaining first of abdominal pain and then of cramping. Since she thought she had begun laboring, she asked her "employer" to take her to a hospital. She denies alcohol, tobacco, and intravenous drug use but does admit to frequent marijuana and much less frequent "crack" smoking. She has, to her knowledge, never had a sexually transmitted disease. The maternal family history is medically noncontributory. The identity of Baby Z's father is indeterminate; personal and family histories of candidate fathers are unknown.

She asks about her baby's condition, asks to see her baby as soon as possible, and asks whether he should "drink" homogenized or low-fat milk. Her day sheet records the initiation of bromocriptine mesylate 2.5 mg with meals twice daily to be continued for 14 days.

OBJECTIVE

Late on day-of-life 2, the following laboratory values are reported:

1. Urine screen for (or for metabolites of) amphetamines, barbiturates, benzodiazepines, and opioids (mother): negative
2. Urine screen for cocaine and cannabinoid metabolites (mother): positive
3. Urine screen for (or for metabolites of) amphetamines, barbiturates, benzodiazepines, cocaine, and opioids (newborn): negative
4. Urine screen for cannabinoid metabolites (newborn): positive
5. Meconium screen for (or for metabolites of) amphetamines, barbiturates, benzodiazepines, and opioids: negative
6. Meconium screen for cocaine and cannabinoid metabolites: positive
7. RPR, serum (mother): positive

ASSESSMENT

Maternal cocaine self-intoxication is now common in pregnancy and has in several series been recognized as an immediate antecedent of placental abruption and premature labor. In an age group and in social circumstances favoring cocaine use, gestational cocaine exposure should be suspected. Although it ordinarily raises systemic blood pressure, cocaine intoxication has presented in this case as hypovolemic shock, presumably through the mechanism of placental abruption.

Cocaine is rapidly metabolized, usually disappearing from blood and urine within 12 hours, but its inactive metabolites, benzoylecgonine and ecgonine methyl ester, may persist in urine for up to 6 days. Therefore, despite the delay in evaluation and the urinary dilution enforced on this mother by vigorous volume repletion, a positive maternal urine screen for cocaine metabolites should be expected.

Cocaine reduces placental perfusion in a dose-dependent manner; therefore, the fetus is to some extent "protected" from immediate drug exposure, especially in the occasional patient in whom cocaine-induced placental vasoconstriction has actually caused the ripping away of some part of the placenta from the uterine wall. Although a first-voided newborn urine might contain cocaine even under these circumstances, Baby Z. voided many hours before his urine was sampled.

That said, the mother has admitted smoking "crack" previously during her pregnancy. This "older" cocaine would have been metabolized by fetal serum and hepatic cholinesterases, and its metabolites would have been excreted in the fetal bile and, accordingly, stored in meconium, a substance that may persist in newborn feces for days and which is more suited to screening for certain drugs of interest than is urine. Baby Z's positive meconium cocaine screen, then, confirms the mother's history of cocaine use earlier in pregnancy but does not speak to events immediately preceding ER presentation. Gestational cocaine exposure has been linked to decreased newborn weight, length, and head circumference.

Cannabinoid detection in both maternal and newborn urine and in meconium is likely with a history of frequent marijuana use. In regular (perhaps weekly or biweekly) marijuana users who are pregnant, fetal exposure to cannabinoids released from fatty stores may be constant. Gestational marijuana exposure has been linked to decreased newborn weight and length.

Syphilis is increasingly common in promiscuous heterosexual populations, and a "crack"-to-prostitution-to-syphilis sequence has been described. In the absence of a history of adequate parenteral penicillin treatment (*not* spectinomycin treatment) at least 30 days prior to delivery, a positive maternal nontreponemal screening test, such as the venereal disease research laboratory (VDRL) test or the rapid plasma reagin (RPR) test, implies, but does not prove, both maternal and congenital syphilis.

PLAN

Congenital infection precautions are instituted, and then Baby Z. is examined with particular attention to skin, mucosal surfaces (especially the nasal mucosa), lymph nodes, eyes, liver, spleen, and neurologic findings (including those elicited by transillumination). A lumbar puncture is performed, plus the following studies:

1. Cerebrospinal fluid (CSF) for routine CSF studies (cell count, glucose, protein, Gram's stain, and culture), VDRL, and IgM antibodies (if available on CSF)
2. RPR (with titer) on newborn serum
3. FTA-ABS (fluorescent treponemal antibody test absorbed with nonpallidum treponemes) on maternal serum
4. FTA-ABS on newborn serum (*Note:* FTA-ABS performed on the 19S IgM fraction of newborn serum is preferable but is not widely available.)
5. Dark-field microscopic examination or direct fluorescent antibody staining of the placenta and umbilical cord for *Treponema pallidum*
6. Long-bone radiograms
7. Human immunodeficiency virus (HIV) antibody test on saved cord blood (*Note:* This last study is requested only after obtaining maternal approval in a manner consistent with the state's relevant statutes and only after confirming that the hospital is staffed with well-prepared professional counselors.)
8. Head ultrasound (*Note:* This study is ordered because of cocaine exposure, not as part of a congenital syphilis workup.)

SECOND REEVALUATION

SUBJECTIVE

Inapplicable.

OBJECTIVE

1. Cerebrospinal fluid examination results:
   a. Cells 64/mm^3, 7 polymorphonuclear and 57 mononuclear
   b. Glucose 53 mg/dl
   c. Protein 81 mg/dl
   d. Gram's stain: negative; culture pending
   e. VDRL: negative
   f. IgM antibodies: canceled (sample discarded inadvertently)
2. RPR, serum (newborn): positive, but at a titer less than that found in maternal serum
3. FTA-ABS, serum (maternal): positive
4. FTA-ABS, serum (newborn): negative
5. Dark-field examination of the placenta and umbilical cord for spirochetes: positive
6. Long-bone radiograms show metaphyseal dystrophy (osteochondritis) and diaphyseal periostitis
7. HIV antibody test, cord blood: positive
8. Head ultrasonography shows a small right lateral intraventricular hemorrhage and abnormal echodensities in the left basal ganglion, the frontal lobe, and the posterior fossa.

ASSESSMENT

Baby Z's problem list is expanded and now is as follows:

1. Prematurity (estimated gestational age 36 weeks)
2. Perinatal stress:
   a. Placental abruption with maternal hypotension
   b. Emergent delivery by cesarean section
3. Perinatal distress and depression, mild (Apgars 5, 7, 8)
4. Transient tachypnea of the newborn, resolved
5. Maternal adolescence
6. Maternal social problems, severe
7. Gestational substance exposure problems:
   a. Gestational cocaine exposure
   b. Gestational marijuana exposure
8. Neurologic problems:
   a. Right lateral intraventricular hemorrhage, small
   b. Abnormal echodensities:
      (1) Left basal ganglion
      (2) Frontal lobe
      (3) Posterior fossa
   c. CSF mononuclear pleocytosis

9. Congenital syphilis, untreated

10. Anti-HIV IgG, cord blood

Interpretation of CSF findings early in the newborn period can be difficult. Normal ranges for cell count (0–20 or 25 cells/mm^3) and protein level (as high as 150–170 mg/dl) are wider and their medians higher than in babies just several weeks older, and in CSF differential cell counts, polymorphonuclear forms may even outnumber mononuclear forms. Baby Z's CSF cell count, though, is distinctly elevated, showing a mononuclear pleocytosis (a finding whose differential explanation is *not* limited to neurosyphilis). CSF glucose level is normal, even as it would be in neurosyphilis. While it is highly specific for neurosyphilis, a CSF VDRL test is not highly sensitive (22% to 69% positive in patients known by other criteria to have neurosyphilis); a negative result is not informative.

Long-bone radiograms are helpful only if distinctly abnormal (which, supposedly, they should be in 80% to 90% of infants with syphilis). Side-by-side comparison with known-normal films is important, especially for nonsenior radiologic consultants inexperienced with congenital syphilis. Baby Z's films, as read, are highly suggestive of congenital syphilis.

Promiscuity, prostitution, and, classically for heterosexuals, ulcerative genital lesions (such as syphilitic chancres, noticed or unnoticed) are risk factors for HIV acquisition. Assuming true test positivity, the presence of HIV antibody in cord blood indicates maternal HIV infection. It does not, however, indicate congenital HIV infection; anti-HIV IgG crosses the placenta and persists for months. Reported HIV vertical transmission rates range widely—from less than 20% to more than 50%. Unless and until a subsequent study or the onset of an AIDS-defining illness demonstrates that the HIV has already been acquired, Baby Z should not be breastfed by his mother.

Congenitally syphilitic babies co-infected with HIV may be at increased risk for antitreponemal treatment failure; higher doses and longer treatment schedules are prudent choices.

Ultrasonographic examination of Baby Z's head demonstrates findings typical of—though not specific for—perinatal cocaine encephalopathy, a disease frequently (or even usually) asymptomatic in the newborn period but sometimes behaviorally provocative and intellectually limiting in later childhood.

PLAN

1. Full and confidential disclosure of the findings and their implications to Baby Z's mother and to her attending physicians

2. Bottle feeding only

3. Antitreponemal penicillin treatment:

   a. Crystalline penicillin G 100,000 to 150,000 units/kg/day IV divided q8–12h for 10 to 14 days, *or*

   b. Procaine penicillin G 50,000 units/kg/day IM qd for 10 to 14 days

4. Notification (and, where appropriate, involvement) of the following:

   a. Health Department (syphilis and HIV infection are reportable diagnoses)

   b. Adult AIDS clinic in this or another hospital

   c. Pediatric AIDS clinic in this or another hospital

   d. Social Services

   e. Child Protective Services or its equivalent

   f. An "early infant stimulation program," if available

   g. Baby Z's maternal grandparents if contact is authorized by Baby Z's mother

SUGGESTED READING

Baucher H, Zuckerman B. Cocaine, sudden infant death syndrome, and home monitoring. J Pediatr 1990; 117(6):904–906.

Dixon SD, Bejar R. Echoencephalographic findings in neonates associated with maternal cocaine and methamphetamine use: Incidence and clinical correlates. J Pediatr 1989; 115(5):770–778.

Durand DJ, Espinoza AM, Nickerson BG. Association between prenatal cocaine exposure and sudden infant death syndrome. J Pediatr 1990; 117(6):909–911.

Hicks DA, Anas NG. Oxygen saturation monitoring. In Levin DL, Morriss FC (eds.): Essentials of Pediatric Intensive Care. St. Louis: Quality Medical Publishing, 1990, pp. 864–868.

Ikeda MK, Jenson HB. Evaluation and treatment of congenital syphilis. J Pediatr 1990; 117(6):843–852.

Noller KL, Avant RF. Obstetrics. In Rakel R (ed.): Textbook of Family Practice, 4th ed. Philadelphia, W.B. Saunders, 1990, pp. 602–635.

Ostrea EM, Brady MJ, Parks PM, et al. Drug screening in infants of drug-dependent mothers: An alternative to urine testing. J Pediatr 1989; 115(3):474–477.

Parks WP, Scott GB. Pediatric AIDS. In Oski F, DeAngelis CD, Feigin RD, Warshaw JB (eds.): Principles and Practice of Pediatrics. Philadelphia, Lippincott, 1990, pp. 192–195.

Rolfs RT, Goldberg M, Sharrar RG. Risk factors for syphilis: Cocaine use and prostitution. Am J Public Health 1990; 80(7):853–857.

Sprinkle R. Care of the newborn. In Rakel R (ed.): Textbook of Family Practice, 4th ed. Philadelphia, W.B. Saunders, 1990, pp. 636–673.

Tramont EC. Syphilis in the AIDS era. N Engl J Med 1987; 316(25):1600–1601.

Ward SLD, Bautista D, Chan L, et al. Sudden infant death syndrome in infants of substance-abusing mothers. J Pediatr 1990; 117(6):876–881.

Zuckerman B, Frank DA, Hingson R, et al. Effects of maternal marijuana and cocaine use on fetal growth. N Engl J Med 1989; 320(12):762–768.

QUESTIONS

1. Its inherent limitations acknowledged, continuous pulse oximetry is a significant technical advance, and despite its inability to report pH, PaO_2, $PaCO_2$, and base excess and its unreliability when SaO_2 falls below 50%, continuous pulse oximetry has in large part supplanted direct arterial blood gas tension measurement in newborns. However, even in motionless babies being monitored with well-calibrated equipment away from sources of "light contamination," SaO_2 pulse oximetry readouts can be misleading in settings of hypotension, hypothermia, and peripheral vasoconstriction. What is the mechanism of mismeasurement common to these three settings?

a. Insufficient time spent "arterializing" blood flow peripherally
b. Significant reduction in vascular pulsation peripherally
c. Exaggerated left shift of the oxygen–fetal hemoglobin dissociation curve in peripheral tissues.
d. Right shift of the oxygen–fetal hemoglobin dissociation curve in peripheral tissues.

2. When neurosyphilis is suspected, CSF is submitted for a VDRL, even though it is a relatively insensitive test in this application. Why not use the RPR or FTA-ABS instead or in addition?
a. When used for CSF evaluation, the RPR and FTA-ABS are even less sensitive than the VDRL.
b. When used for CSF evaluation, the RPR and FTA-ABS are too sensitive, yielding many false-positive results.
c. When used for CSF evaluation, the RPR and FTA-ABS are too sensitive, yielding many false-positive results, and false-positive results are particularly troublesome in this setting, since treatment and follow-up for syphilis are much more expensive and extensive with central nervous system involvement than without it.
d. When used for CSF evaluation, the RPR and FTA-ABS are too sensitive, yielding many

false-positive results, and false-positive results are particularly troublesome in this setting, since treatment and follow-up for syphilis are much more expensive and extensive with central nervous system involvement than without it, and since neurosyphilis can be diagnosed on the basis of other criteria even if the CSF VDRL is falsely negative.

3. Perinatal cocaine encephalopathy is thought by some, but not by others, to be a risk factor for the sudden infant death syndrome (SIDS). Should Baby Z. be sent home—or sent somewhere—with an apnea monitor?
a. Yes; the link to SIDS is clear.
b. No; the link to SIDS is not well supported.
c. Maybe, depending on the mother's physician-guided analysis of risks, costs, and benefits as inferred from data published in peer-reviewed journals.
d. Maybe, depending first on Baby Z's observed course during in-hospital antitreponemal therapy, depending second on a review of best-available published data and analysis, depending third on the feasibility of accurate monitoring and effective response in the best-available discharge setting, and depending fourth on the mother's (or the guardian's) physician-assisted assessment of Baby Z's best interest.

Answers appear on page 449.

Short Child

SANFORD R. KIMMEL

INITIAL VISIT

SUBJECTIVE

Patient Identification. Johnny J. is a 5-year-old Caucasian boy seen for a prekindergarten "well-child" physical examination.

Presenting Problem. Johnny's mother notes that he is smaller than other boys his age. His 3-year-old sister is almost as tall.

Present Illness. Johnny's only recent illness has been a cold, which was treated with an over-the-counter antihistamine–decongestant medicine. His appetite and physical activity are normal. Although a picky eater, he generally eats foods from the four basic food groups. He plays and keeps up with other boys his age.

Past Medical History. Johnny was the product of a full-term, uncomplicated pregnancy. His birth weight was 7 lb 8 oz (3.4 kg), and his length was 20 in (51 cm). A chart of his growth is presented in Figure 20–3.

His developmental milestones include the following: He smiled at 2 months, sat without support at 6 months, said "dada" specifically at 11 months, walked alone at 13 months, and now dresses himself without supervision.

Immunizations include diphtheria, pertussis, and tetanus (DPT) at 2, 4, 6, and 18 months of age; oral polio vaccine (OPV) at 2, 4, 18 months of age; a measles, mumps, rubella vaccine (MMR) at 15 months; and a conjugate *Haemophilus influenzae* B vaccine (HbCV) at 18 months of age.

Johnny has had four to five upper respiratory infections per year and three lifetime episodes of otitis media. He has not been hospitalized nor required major surgery.

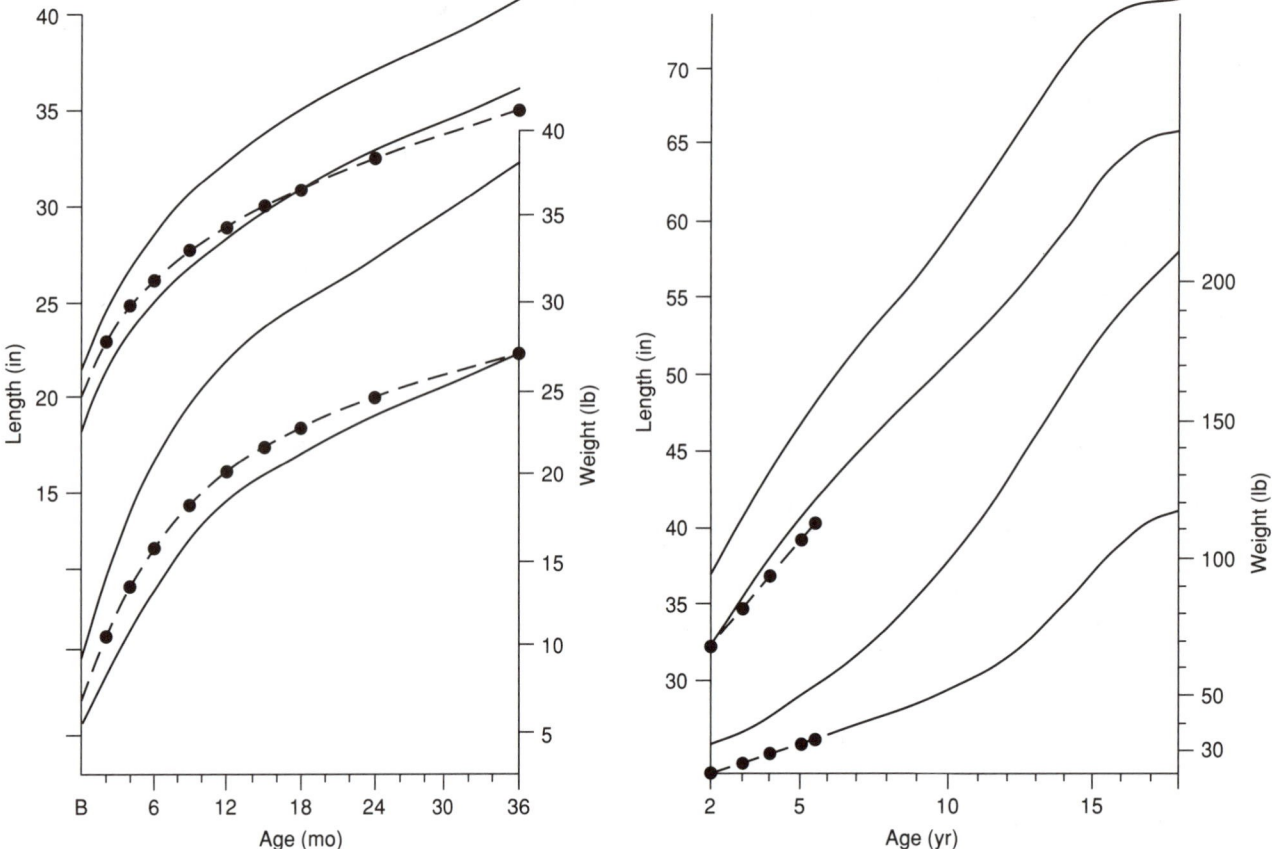

Figure 20–3. Growth curves for Johnny J. for length/height (top curve) and weight (lower curve). The 95th and 5th percentiles for each parameter are also outlined.

Family History. Johnny's mother is 26 years old and in good health. She is 5 ft 4 in tall and weighs 132 lb. His 30-year-old father is 5 ft 8 in tall and weighs 150 lb. Johnny's father recalls being smaller than his peers as a child and being a "late bloomer." Johnny's 57-year-old paternal grandfather had a heart attack 2 years ago. His other grandparents are also in their fifties and in good health. Johnny's 3-year-old sister is 37 in tall and weighs 33 lb.

Health Habits. Johnny wears his seat belt when traveling in the car. His parents limit television viewing to 2 hours per day.

Social History. Johnny is currently in nursery school but will be starting kindergarten next year. His mother, who is a teacher, reports that he interacts well with other children his age. However, she and her physician husband are concerned that his small size may place him at a disadvantage in school.

Review of Systems. Other than slight rhinorrhea and occasional nonproductive cough, the review of systems is unremarkable.

OBJECTIVE

Physical Examination. Johnny's height is 38½ in; weight is 33 lb; blood pressure is 94/58; and pulse is 76

and regular. He appears normally proportioned and has no detectable deformities. Examination of the head, neck, eyes, ears, nose, and throat is normal. The cardiorespiratory and abdominal examinations are also normal. His genitalia are prepubertal (Tanner state I). He can balance on one foot for 10 seconds, catch a bounced ball, and draw a man with a head, eyes, mouth, body, arms, and legs.

Laboratory Tests. An office hemoglobin determination for this visit was 12.5 gm/dl. A urinalysis demonstrates a specific gravity of 1.020, pH 6.0, with negative dipstick and microscopic examination.

ASSESSMENT

Working Diagnosis. The most likely diagnosis is *constitutional growth delay* in an otherwise well child. Although Johnny's height is below the 5th percentile and his weight is at the 5th percentile, his rate of growth parallels the growth curve. His deceleration in growth occurred prior to age 2 with crossing of percentile lines. Since age 2 his linear growth has averaged 4 to 5 cm per year. This condition is more common in boys who enter puberty and develop later than their peers. Their bone age is correspondingly delayed and approximately equal to their height age. Johnny's family history of delayed physical development also suggests this diagnosis.

Differential Diagnoses

1. *Familial short stature* seems less likely because Johnny was of normal size at birth. His parents also are of average height, and their calculated midparental height is within the normal range. If Johnny has familial short stature, bone-age films of the hands and wrists should approximate his chronologic age.

2. *Environmental conditions* such as adverse nutritional or socioeconomic factors always should be considered in the evaluation of a child's growth. Johnny's background does not suggest emotional or sociocultural deprivation.

3. *Chronic systemic illness* is not suggested by Johnny's history or physical examination. Failure to grow is sometimes the only manifestation of inflammatory bowel disease or renal disease. The normal urinalysis rules out diabetes insipidus or diabetes mellitus. There is no history of loose or foul-smelling stools to suggest malabsorption syndrome.

4. *Endocrinologic causes* of short stature are relatively uncommon but treatable diseases that must be considered. Despite prenatal screening, *hypothyroidism* may present later in childhood, either as an acquired condition or because it was missed in earlier testing. Constipation, slow pulse, dry scaly skin, sluggishness, and developmental delay are signs and symptoms that are not present in Johnny's situation. The excessive production of adrenal androgens in *congenital adrenal hyperplasia* leads to initial rapid growth and even virilizing features. However, the resulting premature closure of the epiphyses produces short stature as an adult. Johnny does not have the truncal obesity, "moon" facies, violet striae, hypertension, or cataracts seen in *Cushing's syndrome.* *Congenital* or *acquired growth-hormone deficiency* causes severe retardation of skeletal and overall growth that may be accompanied by central adiposity and immature facies. A history of neonatal hypoglycemia may accompany the poor growth that is usually apparent by 6 to 12 months of age in the congenital form of this disorder.

PLAN

Diagnostic

1. Proper evaluation of the growth curve is the most important consideration. A normal rate of growth excludes most organic causes of short stature.

2. A bone-age film differentiates familial short stature from constitutional growth delay and various endocrinologic disorders (Table 20–11).

3. The "upper segment–lower segment ratio" for age is determined by measuring the distance from the top of the symphysis pubis to the floor for the lower segment. The distance subtracted from the total height then equals the upper segment. This ratio decreases from 1.7 at birth to approximately 1.1 at age 6. Osteochondrodystrophies cause a higher than expected ratio, whereas failure of the epiphyses to close in hypogonadism produces longer extremities and a lower than normal ratio.

4. In the underweight child, a CBC with differential

TABLE 20–11. CONDITIONS AFFECTING BONE AGE

Some causes of retarded bone age:
1. Hypopituitarism
2. Hypothyroidism
3. Malnutrition
4. Constitutional dwarfism
5. Chronic disease
6. Severe illness
7. Male hypogonadism
8. Delayed adolescence

Some causes of accelerated bone age:
1. Sexual precocity
2. Obesity

Source: From Kimmel SR, Fay L. Growth and development. In Rakel RE (ed.): Textbook of Family Practice, 4th ed. Philadelphia, W.B. Saunders, 1990, p. 681, with permission.

may reveal anemia or malignancy, whereas an erythrocyte sedimentation rate (ESR) may detect nonspecific inflammatory disorders such as inflammatory bowel disease or collagen–vascular disease.

5. Serum thyroxine (T_4) and thyroid-stimulating hormone (TSH) determinations should be considered, since hypothyroidism is easily detected and treated. The T_4 is often included in a chemistry profile. A low or borderline T_4 and an elevated TSH indicate primary hypothyroidism. Similar T_4 values and a low TSH suggest pituitary or hypothalamic defects.

6. Renal and liver function tests and calcium, phosphorus, and electrolyte determinations are also available in the chemistry panel. Since a panel typically costs less than individual tests, it is useful in ruling out renal disease, hyponatremia, or rickets.

7. A serum cholesterol determination is useful because the family history is suspicious for early cardiac disease.

Therapeutic

1. The parents' concerns were acknowledged. Johnny's satisfactory rate of growth despite his small absolute size was then demonstrated on the growth curve. The parents were told that although some children were going to constitute the lower percentiles of the normal population, the family history suggested that Johnny might be a "late bloomer" like his father. A follow-up visit in 6 months to monitor his growth was recommended.

2. The appropriate preschool immunizations should be given, including a booster DPT, OPV, and MMR.

Patient (Parent) Education

1. Most children with constitutional growth delay will reach their predicted midparental height. Some may remain several inches below their target height. Children with familial short stature will grow up to be short adults, a fact that some families may not accept. Although the administration of human growth hormone (hGH) may initially accelerate linear growth in these

children, it remains to be seen whether this will produce a greater adult height.

2. Anticipatory guidance should include the following: Injury prevention, such as locking up poisons, medicines, dangerous tools, or firearms; teaching children to follow the proper rules of the road when bicycling, wearing a helmet, and modeling this behavior; constantly watching children in or near the water and teaching them to swim; the child should know his or her name, address, and telephone number and to say "no" to strangers. Encourage age-appropriate chores at home as well as quality family time; appropriate and consistent limit setting should balance the child's need for autonomy; and playing well with other children, taking turns, following simple directions, and dressing self may indicate skills appropriate for school entry.

Disposition. Johnny is scheduled to return in 6 months for a follow-up of his growth parameters. Laboratory results and any subsequent necessary action will be communicated by telephone.

FIRST FOLLOW-UP VISIT

SUBJECTIVE

Johnny returned 6 months later accompanied by his mother. He has been in kindergarten several months and is adjusting well.

OBJECTIVE

Johnny's height is now 39¾ in, and his weight is 35 lb. His bone-age film of the wrists done shortly after his first visit approximated 3 years and 6 months. His chemistry panel demonstrated normal electrolytes, calcium, phosphorus, total protein, and albumin. His creatinine was normal at 0.6 mg/dl (53 μmol/liter), as was his BUN at 7 mg/dl (2.50 mmol/liter). His alkaline phosphatase was elevated above the normal adult value at 172 U/liter. Other liver enzymes were normal. Serum T_4 was normal at 8.2 μg/dl (105 nmol/liter), and the TSH was 3.5 μU/liter. The ESR was normal at 4 mm/h. Serum cholesterol is 156 mg/dl (4.04 mmol/liter).

ASSESSMENT

1. The diagnosis of constitutional growth delay is supported by the delayed bone age consistent with height age and a normal growth velocity.

2. An alkaline phosphatase elevated two to three times the adult normal is appropriate for a child with active skeletal growth.

PLAN

Diagnostic

1. Continued monitoring of Johnny's growth at yearly intervals is essential.

2. No further diagnostic testing is necessary at this time. The serum cholesterol determination may be repeated in 5 years.

Therapeutic

1. At this time, Johnny does not seem to be suffering any adverse psychologic effects such as poor self-image or social isolation. Continued reassurance is sufficient.

2. Although human growth hormone has been given to short children who were not growth hormone deficient, the risks and benefits of such therapy are not fully known. If the child is sustaining deleterious psychologic effects, then referral to a pediatric endocrinologist to consider a trial of human growth hormone therapy is in order.

Patient Education. Johnny's mother is reassured that his delayed bone age indicates he has additional time to "catch up" in growth. His family can expect that he will enter puberty later and be a "late bloomer" like his father.

DISCUSSION

Parents are interested in their child's growth. They are often concerned if he or she is smaller than his or her peers. A careful history should include prenatal factors such as nutrition, smoking, and drug use; problems in the perinatal period; and the child's subsequent growth and development. A family history of short stature, delayed maturation, genetic abnormalities, and chronic diseases is also necessary. Accurate measurements of the child's recumbent length should be made prior to age 3 and of shoeless standing height thereafter. The child should be wearing minimal clothing when his or her weight is taken at each visit, preferably on the same scale. After age 2, normal children grow linearly at a rate of 5 cm or more per year and gain approximately 5 lb per year until the adolescent growth spurt (Table 20–12).

If the child's growth rate is normal, then observation is usually all that is required. If the child's growth rate is declining, then further investigation is warranted. If bone age is delayed, then endocrinologic evaluation

TABLE 20–12.   RULES OF THUMB: GROWTH GUIDELINES FOR CHILDREN

AGE	LENGTH OR HEIGHT	WEIGHT
Newborn	50 cm (20 in) average	3.4 kg (7½ lbs) average
NB–3 months		1 kg/month (½–1 oz/day)
4–5 months		Doubles birth weight
6 months		0.5 kg/month
12 months	Increases by 50%	Triples birth weight
12–24 months		0.25 kg/month
>2 years	>5 cm (2 in) per year until adolescent growth spurt	2.3 kg (5 lb) per year until adolescent growth spurt
4 years	Doubles (40 in approximately)	40 lb approximately

Source: Adapted from Keefer CH. Normal growth and development: An overview. In Dershewitz RA (ed.): Ambulatory Pediatric Care. Philadelphia, Lippincott, 1988, p. 24, with permission.

should be carried out. Emotional deprivation can produce functional hypopituitarism with inadequate response of growth hormone to provocative stimuli. Hypothyroidism also must be corrected prior to growth hormone testing or the response to stimuli may be blunted. Children with growth hormone neurosecretory dysfunction may exhibit a normal growth hormone response to the usual provocative tests but demonstrate a marked deficiency of pulsatile secretion of growth hormone over a 24-hour period. Therefore, referral to a pediatric endocrinologist is in order when growth hormone deficiency is suspected.

Turner's syndrome should always be considered in short girls, especially if there is no family history of short stature. Characteristic features such as low birth weight, webbing of the neck, low posterior hairline, broad chest with widely spaced nipples (shieldlike chest), and cubitus valgus indicate the need for chromosomal analysis. However, short stature may be the only manifestation if mosaicism is present.

SUGGESTED READING

Cara JF, Johanson AJ. Growth hormone for short stature not due to classic growth hormone deficiency. Pediatr Clin North Am 1990; 37:1229–1254.

Kimmel SR, Fay L. Growth and development. In Rakel RE (ed.): Textbook of Family Practice, 4th ed. Philadelphia, W.B. Saunders, 1990, pp. 674–696.

LaFranchi S, Hanna CE, Mandel SH. Constitutional delay of growth: Expected versus final adult height. Pediatrics 1991; 87:82–87.

Lipsky MS, Horner JM. The child with short stature. Am Fam Physician 1988; 37:230–241.

Silverstein JH, Rosenbloom AL. Evaluating growth failure: Diagnostic tools. Fam Pract Recertification J 1988; 10:43–69.

QUESTIONS

1. The calculated midparental height for Johnny's parents is
   a. 6 ft.
   b. 5 ft 9 in.
   c. 5 ft 6 in.
   d. 5 ft 3 in.

2. "Height age" is defined as the age when
   a. Maximum height velocity is reached.
   b. Bone age equals chronologic age.
   c. Height plots on the 50th percentile.
   d. Weight and height curves cross.

3. Match the expected bone age with each cause of short stature in items (1) to (4). Each answer may be used once, more than once, or not at all.
   a. Bone age less than chronologic age
   b. Bone age equal to chronologic age
   c. Bone age greater than chronologic age
      (1) Constitutional growth delay
      (2) Familial short stature
      (3) Growth hormone deficiency
      (4) Hypothyroidism

Answers appear on page 449.

Abdominal Pain

MARSHA C. HOLLEMAN

INITIAL VISIT

SUBJECTIVE

Patient Identification and Present Illness. Maria L. is a 12-year-old Hispanic girl with abdominal pain and diarrhea. For the past 3 days she had not felt as well as usual, with decreased energy and mild abdominal discomfort after eating. Today she awoke at 4:00 a.m. with moderately severe, generalized abdominal pain of a dull aching character associated with several watery bowel movements and nausea. When she vomited at 6:00 a.m., she awoke her mother, who brought her to the clinic at 8:00 a.m. She is not hungry. She has not traveled out of the country in the last 5 years. She has had no fever, cough, or dysuria. She has not had similar episodes in the past. No one at home is ill.

Past Medical History. Maria has had no major medical illnesses or surgery. She has no medical allergies. She does not take any medications.

Family History. Maria's maternal grandmother, who lives in El Salvador, has type II diabetes mellitus. Because her parents are separated, Maria is unaware of any illness on the paternal side of the family.

Health Habits. Maria does not smoke, drink alcohol, or use illicit drugs. She enjoys her exercise class at school. Her mother believes her diet is well-balanced.

Social History. Maria lives with her mother, 15-year-old brother, and 10-year-old sister in an apartment. Her parents separated 4 years ago. Her 17-year-old brother lives with her father. She enjoys school and makes A's, B's, and C's. Her favorite activity is reading.

Review of Systems. Maria had a 4-day episode of rhinorrhea 1 week ago. Menarche was at age 11, with menses every 3 to 6 weeks without dysmenorrhea. The last menstrual period was 2 weeks ago.

OBJECTIVE

Physical Examination. Maria is an alert girl who lies quietly on the examining table on her left side with hips flexed. Her blood pressure is 100/75; her temperature is 99°F orally; her respiratory rate is 16; and her pulse is 74 and regular. The physical examination is normal, except for the abdominal examination. Bowel sounds are positive and slightly increased throughout the abdomen. The abdomen is soft, with mild tenderness to palpation, especially in the epigastrium, and without rebound tenderness. There is no mass or hepatosplenomegaly. Rectal examination is not done.

ASSESSMENT

Working Diagnosis. The most likely diagnosis is *gastroenteritis* with abdominal pain, vomiting, and diarrhea. This may be due to the Norwalk agent (a calcivirus) or rotavirus. Bacterial possibilities include early *Salmonella*, *Shigella*, *Campylobacter* or *Yersinia* infections.

Differential Diagnoses. Other possibilities include the following:

1. *Early appendicitis.* In the first few hours of the attack, appendicitis may mimic gastroenteritis. The initial pain due to appendicitis may be generalized and, especially in children, may be accompanied by diarrhea. The onset of pain often awakens the patient with appendicitis in the middle of the night. After the onset of pain, a patient with appendicitis usually experiences nausea, sometimes accompanied by vomiting and anorexia. Then the pain localizes to the right lower quadrant, with maximal point tenderness immediately inferior to the middle of a line from the umbilicus to the anterosuperior iliac spine. Less consistently tender is McBurney's point, located 1.5 to 2 in from the anterosuperior iliac spine directly on the line connecting the anterosuperior iliac spine and the umbilicus. Rebound tenderness or tenderness to percussion may next develop if the overlying peritoneum becomes inflamed. Other signs, which may or may not be present, include hyperesthesia (increased sensitivity to touch or pin prick) in the right lower quadrant or right upper quadrant depending on the location of the appendix, abdominal wall rigidity (especially in the case of peritonitis due to local inflammation or a perforated appendix), and right lower quadrant distension. Fever to 100 or 101°F usually develops next, followed by a leukocytosis, which indicates local peritonitis. To review, the course of events in appendicitis is often predictable: (1) generalized or epigastric abdominal pain, (2) nausea, and possibly anorexia or vomiting, (3) localized abdominal pain, usually to the right lower quadrant, (4) fever, and (5) leukocytosis.

The abdominal pain of appendicitis may occasionally occur differently than described above. If the inflamed appendix is located retrocecally (posterior to the cecum), it may produce minimal abdominal-wall tenderness but major pain on rectal examination. The "iliopsoas test" may be positive in this setting: With the patient lying on the side opposite his or her pain, the examiner extends the leg on the painful side. If the movement causes increased pain, the test is positive, indicating that inflamed tissue is contacting the iliopsoas muscle.

Another test, the "obdurator" or "thigh rotation test," is most often positive in the presence of a perforated appendix or local abscess. With the patient supine and leg flexed, the examiner rotates the hip. If hypogastric pain occurs, especially on internal rotation, the test is positive, indicating inflammation over the obdurator internis fascia.

2. *Influenza.* Often influenza presents with myalgia, fever, and headache, but it may start with gastrointestinal symptoms. Usually, however, the vomiting precedes the abdominal pain rather than vice versa.

3. *Early pneumonia.* Children especially may present with abdominal pain when they have a lower lobe pneumonia. Usually, though, the child has not had vomiting and diarrhea and often will have a temperature of 101°F or above.

Less likely possibilities include the following:

1. *Hepatitis.* Mild abdominal pain, anorexia, and nausea may herald the onset of hepatitis. Diarrhea is usually not present. Eventually, the patient's liver enzymes and bilirubin increase, and the patient becomes jaundiced.

2. *Diabetes mellitus.* A patient may present with abdominal pain as a symptom of ketoacidosis, along with polyuria, polydipsia, and polyphagia. Vomiting may be prominent, but usually there is no diarrhea. The patient will have a markedly elevated glucose level along with other laboratory abnormalities.

3. *Genitourinary disorder.* A spectrum of disorders, including urinary tract infections, pyelonephritis, and nephrolithiasis, may begin as abdominal pain. Dysuria and frequency are generally prominent. With renal abnormalities, the abdominal pain often radiates to the labia or testis. With a urinary tract infection, the abdominal pain is usually suprapubic.

4. *Crohn's disease.* A chronic inflammatory disease of the bowel wall, Crohn's disease presents with recurrent bouts of severe abdominal pain and diarrhea. Although this patient may be having a first bout of Crohn's disease, she should not at this point be subjected to further diagnostic testing, such as a barium enema or intestinal biopsies, unless and until she has had several recurrent bouts of unexplained abdominal pain.

5. *Adenitis.* A nonspecific inflammation of intestinal lymph nodes may cause abdominal pain. The patient usually does not have vomiting or diarrhea. Eventually the pain resolves spontaneously.

6. *Meckel's diverticulum.* A rare occurrence, inflammation of a Meckel's diverticulum may cause ab-

dominal pain, diarrhea, vomiting, and other symptoms similar to appendicitis. Symptoms from Meckel's diverticulum usually occur in the first 2 years of life.

PLAN

Diagnostic. Since the patient most likely has a self-limited illness, no testing is indicated at this point.

Therapeutic. Maria is to go home and rest, drinking small sips of clear liquids every few minutes. If the abdominal pain, diarrhea, and vomiting resolve, she may gradually resume normal activities.

Patient Education. The physician advises that there are many causes for abdominal pain, including some serious ones requiring surgery. The physician asks Maria and her mother to return or call should the abdominal pain change, worsen, or fail to resolve within the next day.

Disposition. No return appointment is scheduled. The patient will call or return if needed.

FIRST FOLLOW-UP VISIT

SUBJECTIVE

Six hours later, Maria returns with worsened symptoms. The pain is more intense and has moved to the right lower quadrant. After several bouts of vomiting and diarrhea, these symptoms have resolved. She is not hungry.

OBJECTIVE

The patient lies immobile on her left side with hips and knees flexed and appears uncomfortable. Blood pressure is 110/75; temperature is 101.2°F orally; respiratory rate is 16; and pulse is 86. The physical examination is normal, except for the abdominal examination. To avoid the abdominal pain produced by lying with legs extended, Maria lies on her back with hips flexed. The abdomen is soft. Bowel sounds are decreased, especially in the right lower quadrant. She has moderately severe tenderness in a small area in the right lower quadrant below the line between the anterosuperior iliac spine and the umbilicus. The rest of the abdomen is nontender. She has rebound tenderness in the right lower quadrant as elicited by percussion. There is a patch of hyperesthesia in the right lower quadrant. The obdurator and iliopsoas tests are negative. There is no inguinal, femoral, or umbilical hernia. Rectal examination shows normal rectal tone without mass, with tenderness of the right rectal wall.

ASSESSMENT

Right lower quadrant abdominal pain. Most patients with severe abdominal pain for 6 hours or more have a condition requiring surgery. The most likely diagnosis is *acute appendicitis,* with the patient developing over a few hours the classical symptoms: generalized or epigastric pain, followed by nausea or anorexia, pain localized to the right lower quadrant, and low-grade fever. Hyperesthesia, especially in the right lower quadrant, is another clue supporting this diagnosis. Perforation seems unlikely because there is not a higher fever or a rigid abdominal wall.

At this stage of the symptoms, important entities to differentiate from appendicitis include some of those discussed above with the initial visit, especially urinary tract problems such as pyelonephritis or nephrolithiasis or an incarcerated hernia. Maria has no evidence of a hernia on physical examination. The symptoms are not typical for a urinary tract problem, but a urinalysis always should be obtained in this setting. Even in the absence of urinary tract disease, the urinalysis in appendicitis may be abnormal, with a few white blood cells or red blood cells.

Disorders of the female genital tract may mimic appendicitis, necessitating consideration of a pelvic examination, including both speculum and bimanual examinations, for each female patient. An ectopic pregnancy in the right fallopian tube produces right lower quadrant pain. Amenorrhea, irregular vaginal bleeding, a right adnexal mass, and a positive pregnancy test may be present. A patient with an ovarian cyst may have a history of cysts, a right adnexal mass, and a negative pregnancy test. Acute salpingitis usually presents with bilateral lower abdominal pain, but on occasion, there is more pain on one side. Implantation and bleeding of endometrial tissue on the ovary may produce severe abdominal pain. Often these patients have a history of endometriosis with severe dysmenorrhea.

PLAN

Diagnostic

1. Complete blood count, especially evaluating for leukocytosis
2. Urinalysis
3. Electrolytes may be obtained, to evaluate for changes due to vomiting or for the unlikely possibility of diabetes mellitus.
4. An ultrasound to measure the appendix is deferred, since the symptoms fit the diagnosis well.

Therapeutic. A general surgeon is consulted, who agrees that acute appendicitis is the most likely diagnosis. Surgery is planned pending results of the laboratory tests.

Patient Education. The family physician and surgeon discuss with Maria and her mother the diagnosis and need for surgery. They discuss the unlikely possibility of perforation of the appendix with abscess, necessitating leaving the wound open and allowing it to heal by secondary intention. Risks of the surgery include infection; bleeding; damage to the intestines, ureter, bladder, or genital tract; and the development of postoperative intestinal obstruction due to adhesions.

Disposition. The WBC count is 13.9×10^3 cells/ mm^3. The urinalysis is normal, with a rare WBC seen per high-power field. Electrolytes are normal.

The patient undergoes an appendectomy without complication. The surgeon finds an inflamed appendix without perforation. The patient recovers smoothly from the surgery.

SUGGESTED READING

Rakel RE. Textbook of Family Practice, 4th ed. Philadelphia, W.B. Saunders, 1990, pp. 754–755, 1251–1253.
Schwartz SI, Shires GT, Spencer FC, et al. Principles of Surgery, 5th ed. New York, McGraw-Hill, 1989, p. 1317.
Silen, W. Cope's Early Diagnosis of the Acute Abdomen, 16th ed. New York, Oxford University Press, 1983.

QUESTIONS

1. The order of development of symptoms and signs in acute appendicitis is
   a. Epigastric or generalized abdominal pain; nausea, vomiting, or diarrhea; right lower quadrant abdominal pain; leukocytosis; and fever.
   b. Nausea, vomiting, or diarrhea; epigastric or generalized abdominal pain; fever; right lower quadrant abdominal pain; and leukocytosis.
   c. Epigastric or generalized abdominal pain; nausea, vomiting, or diarrhea; right lower quadrant abdominal pain; fever; and leukocytosis.
   d. Nausea, vomiting, or diarrhea; epigastric or generalized abdominal pain; right lower quadrant abdominal pain; fever; and leukocytosis.

2. "The general rule can be laid down that the majority of severe abdominal pains which ensue in patients who have been previously well, and which last as long as _____ hours are caused by conditions of surgical import" (Sir Zachary Cope).
   a. 24
   b. 18
   c. 12
   d. 6

3. Early in the course of acute appendicitis, the condition may mimic
   a. Diabetic ketoacidosis.
   b. Gastroenteritis.
   c. Pyelonephritis.
   d. Adenitis.
   e. All the above.

4. In a menstruating female, possible causes for severe abdominal pain in the right lower quadrant (due to disorders in the genital tract) include
   a. Ectopic pregnancy.
   b. Right ovarian cyst.
   c. Acute salpingitis.
   d. Ovarian endometrioma.
   e. All the above.

Answers appear on page 449.

Breast Discomfort

CHRISTINE C. MATSON

INITIAL VISIT

SUBJECTIVE

Patient Identification. Mrs. Smith is a 56-year-old married Caucasian homemaker, mother of two adult children, who presents for her annual physical examination.

Presenting Problem. Because of a recent family illness and resulting stress for her, Mrs. Smith has become more concerned for her own health and wants to have her annual cancer screening tests performed. She also has noted a small thickening in the right breast that she feels is firmer than surrounding tissue.

Present Illness. Mrs. Smith's story begins with a description of her role in caring for her elderly parents, both of whom have been diagnosed with colon cancer in the last 2 years. Her mother, to whom she had been close, died 1 year ago after an 8-month illness, and her father, whose cancer was diagnosed shortly after his wife's death, now seems to be in the terminal stage of his illness. As her parents' only child, Mrs. Smith has assumed the role of primary caretaker for her father, who lives with her and her husband, is confined to bed, and requires assistance in all activities of daily living. Although assisted by her husband and a visiting nurse, Mrs. Smith finds her father's care to be both physically and emotionally exhausting. Nevertheless, she describes no recent physical symptoms other than fatigue. She relates the fatigue to frequent interruption of her sleep because of the need to administer her father's pain medications and reposition him during the night, as well as decreased opportunities for relaxation and enjoyment outside the home. She continues to experience sadness because of her mother's death and the anticipated loss of her father, and she often worries about her own cancer risk.

Mrs. Smith also notes that since she has begun examining her breasts more closely in the last 3 or 4 months, she has noted a small area in the upper outer quadrant of her right breast that seems more firm than the surrounding area, not movable, and not painful. She noted it because of a vague discomfort that drew her attention to the area. She remembers no trauma or inflammation in the region.

Past Medical History. Mrs. Smith had a breast biopsy at age 40, with a final diagnosis of fibrocystic changes. Her weight has been approximately 20% over ideal for about 10 years. She had a transabdominal hysterectomy at age 45 for fibroids; until that time she had regular menstrual periods after a menarche at age 11. She has no known allergies to medications. She has taken conjugated estrogens 0.625 mg each day 3 out of every 4 weeks since menopause at age 48 and occasionally uses a mild laxative for constipation. She has never used oral contraceptive pills and has no known exposure to ionizing radiation other than her previous mammograms.

Family History. Parents both had colon cancer (see Present Illness); one paternal great aunt had breast cancer at age 70. Paternal grandparents died of unknown causes after age 70; maternal grandmother died of a stroke at age 75; and maternal grandfather died at age 40 in an accident. Spouse is hypertensive but otherwise well, and two sons, ages 36 and 33, are healthy.

Health Habits. Mrs. Smith has a 25 pack-year smoking history, and her husband also smokes. She and her spouse have one or two alcoholic drinks each evening and a maximum of three on rare occasions. Her diet has included several servings of dairy products each day and three to four servings of red meat each week and has excluded foods prepared with added fat. Until about 2 years ago she did not restrict fat in her diet. Her exercise other than household and garden tasks is limited. She performs self-breast examination every 2 to 3 months, monitoring areas thought to be fibrocystic, and she has had a normal mammogram every 2 to 3 years since age 45, the last one 2 years ago. Flexible sigmoidoscopy performed 2 years previously was negative, as were annual fecal occult blood examinations since age 50.

Social History. Mrs. Smith has been married for 38 years, rearing two children with her husband, in a mutually satisfactory marriage. She attended 2 years of college and worked outside the home for 10 years in her thirties and forties as a secretary. Her husband is a lawyer. She enjoys gardening and volunteering for charitable agencies.

Physical Examination. Mrs. Smith is mildly overweight and moderately anxious in appearance. Her blood pressure is 130/80; her pulse rate is 84 and regular; her respirations are 16/minute; and her temperature is 98.8°F. Her weight 165 lb, and her height is 66 in. Skin examination showed scattered freckling in sun-exposed areas but no darkly pigmented or scaly lesions. Head, ears, eyes, nose, throat, neck, chest, back, and heart examinations were within normal limits. Breast examination showed normal symmetry, no skin abnormalities, no lymphadenopathy, and no nipple discharge. The breasts were mostly soft in texture, except for increased irregular densities suggesting fibroglandular tissue in the upper outer quadrants of both breasts, essentially symmetrical. The area noted by the patient was a 1 $\times$ 1 cm thickening at eleven o'clock in the right breast, approximately 2 cm from the areola; it was nontender, not movable, and minimally discrete from surrounding fibroglandular tissue. The abdominal and genitourinary examinations were unremarkable, except for a surgically absent uterus. Rectal examination was unremarkable, with negative fecal occult blood examination. No abnormality in the examination of the extremities and neurologic or hematopoietic systems were noted.

ASSESSMENT

1. Mrs. Smith is experiencing normal anxiety about her cancer risk in light of her parents' illnesses. This anxiety is functional in that it motivated the current visit and led her to perform self-breast examinations.

2. Fatigue is a problem, which could be attributed in part to frequent disturbance of sleep, increased responsibilities, less relaxation, and the effect of increased worry about her father and her own health.

3. Fibrocystic changes exist in both breasts, documented by physical examination, mammography, and previous biopsy. A new 1-cm area of thickening recently was detected by the patient.

4. The visit is primarily for health maintenance, so all age-appropriate screens are indicated.

PLAN

Diagnostic

1. Age-appropriate cancer screening recommendations, including reinforcing and demonstrating the technique of self-examination, mammography, fecal occult blood testing, and sigmoidoscopy. Smoking as a risk factor for multiple health problems including cancer was discussed, and a recommendation was made to stop smoking.

2. Cholesterol screen (not previously documented), CBC, and urinalysis.

3. Follow-up visit scheduled to discuss results, to further address stress caused by father's illness, and to offer emotional support.

FIRST FOLLOW-UP VISIT

SUBJECTIVE

Mrs. Smith returned 2 weeks after the initial visit and was initially tearful. She stated that her father had been admitted to the hospital and was expected to die any day. She said she was "not taking it well," following as it did so closely after her mother's terminal illness. She described decreased appetite, tearfulness, and sadness alternating with anxiety. She requested something to help her with sleep, saying that she was unable to get the rest she needs at night because she was upset by concern about her father.

After an extended conversation exploring the areas of greatest difficulty that her situation poses for her, as well as available resources and possible sources of support, Mrs. Smith was a little more comfortable and had made a plan for getting through the next few days. However, as her physician began to discuss her laboratory results, she mentioned that she had noted some intermittent, mild, sharp pain in the upper outer aspect of her right breast for about a week. She had stopped all intake of coffee, tea, and cola drinks when the pain started because she had heard caffeine might make benign breast disease worse, but the pain had not improved. She remembered no trauma to the breast, had worn no new brassiere, and had increased neither her dietary xanthine nor her estrogen intake prior to onset of the pain.

OBJECTIVE

The patient wept intermittently during the visit and appeared anxious. Vital signs were within normal limits. Examination of her breasts showed no change from the previous visit, except mild tenderness noted in the area of the 1-cm mass.

The film-screen mammograms performed since the first visit showed moderate fibrocystic changes in the upper outer quadrants of both breast, with more density on the right than on the left. Benign-appearing secretory calcifications were noted in both breasts, unchanged from previous mammograms 2 and 3 years previously. The radiologist's impression was that the breasts were stable radiographically; specifically no radiographic signs were present that were suggestive of breast cancer, such as grouped calcifications, vascular distortion, stellate density, or skin thickening.

Laboratory values, including cholesterol, CBC, and urinalysis, were normal, including a total cholesterol value of 190 mg/dl. Three fecal occult blood determinations were negative. Flexible sigmoidoscopy performed to 60 cm showed no abnormality.

ASSESSMENT

1. The patient's anxiety about risk of cancer was greatly increased by the new symptom of pain in her breast. In addition, she has developed somatic symptoms apparently in response to the stress of her father's imminent death, consistent with the diagnosis of an adjustment disorder. Fatigue continues to be part of her symptom constellation.

2. Well-documented fibrocystic breast changes, with a new symptom of pain in the right breast, but no new findings except tenderness on physical examination. The mammograms showed increased density on the right compared with the left in areas suggestive of fibrocystic changes, but no internal change.

Differential Diagnosis. Fibrocystic changes in the breast are very common, occurring clinically in more than 50% of women. Distinguishing these changes from *neoplastic disease* is often a challenging problem. While fibrocystic disease is not in itself a risk factor for breast cancer, its presence may obscure the emergence of a tumor. Furthermore, the difficulty in examining fibrocystic breasts may discourage women from performing self-breast examination. Cyclical changes in the breasts, especially premenstrual tenderness, and decrease in lumpiness when dietary xanthines (coffee, tea, colas) are withdrawn may help to differentiate fibrocystic changes from malignant disease.

The findings on physical examination of a dominant mass, especially with a hard or gritty texture; fixation to the skin or chest wall; overlying skin changes, including edema or inflammation; or the presence of palpable lymph nodes all suggest the possibility of malignant disease and mandate evaluation of the mass. Sometimes a mass, especially a rapidly emerging one, may suggest a *fluid-filled cyst.* In such a case, if fluid can be aspirated from the cyst, with resolution of the mass, malignancy is very unlikely. Table 20–13 lists the most common types of malignant tumors of the breast and their relative frequency.

Fibroadenomas are smooth, rubbery, well-defined masses in the breast that usually present in the 2nd or 3rd decade of life. While benign, these tumors should be excised for histologic evaluation. *Cystosarcoma phyllodes* is a rapidly growing tumor that may rarely arise from a fibroadenoma, making up 1% of breast tumors. *Inflammatory masses* or *abscesses* are not uncommon in the breast and must be distinguished from *inflammatory carcinoma,* or *Paget's disease,* which can be rapidly progressive. *Fat necrosis,* which usually presents as a tender, ill-defined breast mass, sometimes with overlying bruising or skin retraction, also can be confused with carcinoma. A history of trauma to the breast can be helpful in making this diagnosis but is not reported by the majority of women.

Pain in the breast (*mastalgia*) is most frequently associated with a benign, especially hormonal, cause. Discomfort is associated with malignant breast disorders in only 20% of patients. In a postmenopausal woman on a

TABLE 20–13. CLASSIFICATION OF MOST COMMON TYPES OF BREAST CARCINOMATA

TYPE	PERCENTAGE OF ALL CASES
Noninvasive*	
Comedocarcinoma	1
Ductal papillary (in situ)	5
Lobular (in situ)	3
Invasive	
Infiltrating ductal carcinoma	70–80
Medullary	5–7
Lobular	5–10
Paget's, inflammatory, infiltrating papillary, tubular, mucinous	<5

Source: From Matson CC, et al. General surgery. In Rakel (ed.): Textbook of Family Medicine, 4th ed. Philadelphia, W.B. Saunders, 1990, p. 748, with permission.

steady dose of estrogen replacement, hormonal variation should not be responsible for this symptom.

Pain in the breast may be due to *glandular hypertrophy* (exogenous estrogens, including oral contraceptives or postmenopausal estrogen replacement; endogenous fluctuations, including the menstrual cycle or pregnancy; or stimulation of the adenyl cyclase system by dietary or pharmacologic xanthines) or trauma. More rarely, unrelated causes such as *costochondritis* in a rib underlying the breast, radiation of pain from *ischemic heart disease,* or an incipient outbreak of *herpes zoster* may produce pain in the breast. A decrease in pain threshold because of increased emotional arousal also should be considered.

Many younger women have radiographically dense breasts, as do some older women with fibrocystic changes of the breasts. In these situations, the mammographic sensitivity for neoplasms is decreased. In general, approximately 5% to 10% of cancers in the breast are not identified by x-ray. In this case, the documentation of no radiographic change for nearly 3 years and the lack of suspicious signs would not have been completely reassuring in view of the finding of a new, even though not highly suspicious breast mass in a 56-year-old woman.

The finding of a dominant or suspicious mass on physical examination should always mandate surgical evaluation of the lesion. For this particular patient, her strong family history of cancer, her anxiety about her own risk, and new onset of pain in her breast without other explanation are reasons for further investigation in addition to the development of pain associated with a mass. In addition, her risk factors for breast cancer include her age, early menarche, a history of high-fat diet, regular alcohol use, and obesity more than 30% of ideal body weight. Although she has been on estrogen replacement, its cyclic use should not increase her risk. Pregnancy before the age of 25 is considered to be a protective factor (this patient had two), as is regular vigorous physical activity (not applicable here). Some evidence exists that prolonged stress may decrease levels of immune surveillance, resulting in increased likelihood of emergence of a deregulated clone of neoplastic cells.

PLAN

Diagnostic

1. The alternatives of needle versus excisional biopsy in a one- or two-step procedure were discussed with Mrs. Smith. She elected to have an excisional biopsy first and then to discuss her options after the pathology report was available so that she would have as much information as possible to plan her course. She was referred to a general surgeon with special interest in breast disease for the biopsy.

2. Initial preoperative laboratory tests were ordered, including a CBC, chemistry panel, urinalysis, chest roentgenogram, and ECG.

Patient Education. Mrs. Smith's concern about her cancer risk was addressed, although no categorical reassurance could be offered at this point. Her personal and social resources were explored, and plans were made for contacting friends and family to help her through this difficult time of her father's illness and concern about her own health. An offer was made to meet together with Mr. Smith if that would be helpful.

SECOND FOLLOW-UP VISIT

An excisional biopsy was performed, and the results as reported by telephone to the physician were the findings of both a microinvasive intraductal carcinoma and a lobular carcinoma in situ. Hormone receptor results were still pending. In the meantime, Mrs. Smith's father had died of his cancer. Mrs. Smith reports that her family has rallied around her and is giving her excellent support and that her husband, as her main source of emotional support, has been "like a rock." Despite her stressful events, Mrs. Smith has been successful in stopping smoking. She discussed her treatment options with the surgeon, who recommended a simple mastectomy with axillary dissection of lymph nodes and consideration of a contralateral mastectomy, either at this time or later, in view of the presence of lobular carcinoma.

PLAN

Diagnostic. Preoperative laboratory results revealed no abnormality, including a normal alkaline phosphatase level. Accordingly, no further metastatic evaluation was performed. The palpable tumor size less than 2 cm, absence of palpable nodes, and absence of documented metastases place this patient in stage I for staging purposes, the best prognostic category.

Patient Education. The patient's questions regarding treatment options were discussed, including the indications for simple mastectomy rather than a more conservative approach. The option of contralateral mastectomy because of the tumor type was discussed, and the patient elected to request this procedure simultaneously with initial surgical therapy because of her marked level of anxiety concerning recurrence. A consultation also was arranged with a plastic surgeon to discuss early breast reconstruction, with the plan that tissue expanders could be inserted at the time of surgery, with later insertion of breast implants. Mrs. Smith and her husband also were referred to a family therapist for short-term counseling to assist them with the adjustment required to her father's death and impending loss of her breasts. The support groups available through the American Cancer Society at the local hospital also were offered.

DISCUSSION

Needle biopsy of a suspicious breast mass often can be helpful in planning therapy. Because of the high specificity of a positive needle biopsy, the physician can inform the patient with confidence that cancer is present, and therapeutic options can be discussed. Because the false-negative rate for needle biopsies is 3% to 5%, depending on the experience of the operator and the pathologist, a suspicious mass must still be excised even if the needle biopsy is negative for cancer.

Approximately 40% of women have mixed tumor types when breast cancer is diagnosed, and prognosis tends to be associated with the most aggressive cell type. This patient has the most common type of carcinoma affecting the breast, infiltrating ductal or intraductal (see Table 20–13), which unfortunately has the tendency to metastasize early. The second type, lobular carcinoma, occurs in 5% to 10% of patients and is characterized by a tendency to be multicentric and bilateral.

Subtotal mastectomy (lumpectomy, segmentectomy), when combined with local radiation therapy, produces similar results to more extensive procedures in terms of the patient being disease-free at 5 years postoperatively. Certain conditions, however, contraindicate conservative surgery, including lobular carcinoma (because of its tendency to be multicentric), location of tumor in the midbreast, large tumor size in relation to breast size, and the presence of grave signs (skin involvement such as dimpling, erythema, or lymphatic infiltration or fixation of tumor to skin or chest wall). The success of conservative breast surgery is consistent with the concept that breast cancer is a systemic disease, that is, that prognosis is associated with the likelihood that blood-borne metastasis has already occurred at the time of detection, and not with spread by local extension. The recommendation for conservative therapy combined with local radiation therapy and, in some cases, prophylactic chemotherapy supports the overall goals of breast cancer treatment: to control local disease, treat distant metastases, and achieve maximal quality of life for the patient.

In terms of psychologic adjustment, Mrs. Smith's course is complicated by the stress of her father's death from cancer at the same time that she is dealing with the issues associated with a personal diagnosis of cancer. Because Mrs. Smith's psychologic adjustment prior to these stresses was very good and her marital relationship is stable and supportive, her long-term psychologic adjustment will probably be good with appropriate support from family, friends, and the medical team.

SUGGESTED READING

Beute BJ, Kalisher L, Hutter RVP. Lobular carcinoma in situ of the breast: Clinical, pathologic, and mammographic features. AJR 1991; 157:257–265.
Droegenmueller W. Breast diseases. In Herbst AL, Mishell DR Jr., Stenchever MA, Droegenmueller W, (eds.): Comprehensive Gynecology. St. Louis, Mosby, 1987, pp. 334–357.
Fisher B. Biological prespective of breast cancer: Contributions of the National Surgical Adjunct Breast and Bowel Project clinical trial. CA 1991; 41:97–111.
Fisher B, Redmond C, Fisher ER, et al. Ten-year results of a randomized clinical trial comparing radical mastectomy and total mastectomy with or without radiation. N Engl J Med 1985; 312:674–681.
Kinne DW. The surgical a mangement of primary breast cancer. CA 1991; 41:71–84.
Matson CC, Burch JM, Feliciano DV. General surgery. In Rakel RE (ed.): Textbook of Family Practice, 4th ed. Philadelphia, W.B. Saunders, 1990, p. 748.
Schover LR. The impact of breast cancer on sexuality, body image and intimate relationships. CA 1991; 41:112–120.

QUESTIONS

1. Which of the following are risk factors for breast cancer?
   a. Early menarche
   b. Early menopause
   c. High xanthine diet (e.g., caffeine)
   d. High-fat diet
   e. Obesity (>30% ideal body weight)

2. The presence of carcinoma in a suspicious breast mass can be ruled out by
   a. Physical examination by a skilled, experienced physician.
   b. Film-screen mammography.
   c. Needle biopsy.
   d. None of the above.

3. Match the following.
   a. Tendency to be multicentric 4
   b. Most common breast cancer 3
   c. May be misdiagnosed as eczema 2
   d. Approximately 40% of breast tumors 5
      (1) Cystosarcoma phallodes
      (2) Inflammatory carcinoma
      (3) Infiltrating ductal
      (4) Lobular carcinoma
      (5) Mixed tumor types

4. Reasons to avoid conservative (lumpectomy, quadrantectomy) breast surgery for carcinoma include
   a. Diagnosis of medullary carcinoma.
   b. Fixation of tumor to skin.
   c. Retroareolar position of tumor.
   d. Location of tumor in medial aspect of breast.
   e. Patient's fear of recurrence of tumor in the breast.

Answers appear on page 449.

LOUIS A. KAZAL, Jr.

INITIAL VISIT

SUBJECTIVE

Patient Identification and Presenting Problem. Gus is a 32-year-old white male rancher who drove himself to the emergency room for evaluation of a 4-hour-old lacerated arm injured while he was hunting.

History of Present Illness. Gus had "dressed out" a five-point bull elk, and as he hoisted one of the hindquarters onto the bed of his truck, the broken end of the elk's femur lacerated the inside of his left arm. He applied pressure over the wound with a clean folded bandana, which stopped the bleeding. On arriving home 3 hours later, Gus was not going to seek medical attention, but his wife insisted that he see their family physician.

In the emergency room, his only concern was to make sure that stitches would not be necessary. There was no associated numbness or weakness.

Past Medical History. Gus has no history of a bleeding disorder or other medical illness. He has been immunized against tetanus; his last tetanus booster was 12 years ago. There were no known allergies to or current use of any medications.

Family History. Gus's father died of a myocardial infarction at age 48, as did his paternal grandfather at age 55. Gus's mother and two sisters are in good health.

Health Habits. Gus does not use a seat belt when driving. He has smoked two packs of cigarettes per day for 15 years. He rarely drinks alcohol.

Social History. Gus is a high school graduate who is currently a successful rancher in western Wyoming. He and his wife of 8 years have two healthy children.

Review of Systems. Gus last saw a physician 12 years ago after stepping on a nail. His cholesterol level has never been checked. He coughs up yellowish phlegm every morning. There is no history of hemoptysis.

OBJECTIVE

Physical Examination. Gus was alert, cooperative, and in no apparent distress. Alcohol was not detected on his breath. His vital signs were blood pressure 140/92, pulse 80, respirations 20, and temperature 98.6°F. He weighed 189 lb and was 5 ft 10 in tall. A pack of cigarettes was noticed in his shirt pocket.

Examination of his left arm revealed a jagged 2.5-cm laceration of the midforearm on the flexor surface. There was some dried blood over wound. There was no weakness with resistance to flexion of the left hand at the wrist or to the pronation of the forearm. His biceps and brachioradialis reflexes were normal. The distal sensation and circulation in that extremity were intact.

Laboratory. No tests were ordered.

ASSESSMENT

1. Gus was diagnosed with what appeared to be an uncomplicated 2.5-cm laceration of the left forearm. (The full extent of the injury cannot be determined until it is explored.)

2. Gus does not use a seat belt, which places him at increased risk for traumatic injury or death if he is involved in a motor vehicle accident. (Injuries are the number one cause of death under age 45, and nearly half are related to motor vehicle accidents. It is estimated that crash mortality can be reduced 40% to 50% with the use of lap and shoulder belts.)

3. Gus has a 30 pack-year history of smoking cigarettes (15 years $\times$ 2 packs per day). (Cigarettes are the leading preventable cause of death in the United States.)

4. Gus has an elevated blood pressure reading. (He is not "labeled" as hypertensive because this diagnosis typically requires a confirming elevated blood pressure recorded at a separate time. Repeat blood pressure measurements as an outpatient over a few weeks are helpful and can be averaged, resulting in a more accurate diagnosis.)

5. Gus is obese. (His ideal weight, given his height and medium frame, would be approximately 155 pounds. His 189 pounds is greater than 120% of his ideal weight, and thus he is obese.)

PLAN

1. These findings were reviewed with Gus, and he gave verbal permission to assess and repair his injury. (Lacerations of the body and extremity should not be closed if older than 6 hours because they are prone to infection. An exception is sometimes made for those of the head and neck, which have excellent blood supply and may be repaired up to 12 hours after injury.)

2. Tetanus toxoid was given in his nondominant arm. (Tetanus prophylaxis is a priority in laceration care. If the patient has not been immunized against tetanus, 0.5 ml toxoid is given, repeated in 6 weeks, and again in 6 to 12 months. If the wound is tetanus-prone, 250 units of human tetanus antitoxin also is given at the initial visit. If the patient has been immunized and the wound is tetanus-prone, a booster is recommended when more than 5 years have passed since the last dose. For the immunized patient with a clean wound, a tetanus booster is not necessary unless it has been more than 10 years since the last dose.)

3. Gus's poor health maintenance record will be addressed during the laceration repair.

PROCEDURE

1. Two milliliters of 1% Xylocaine without epinephrine was injected with a sterile 1.5-in 27-gauge needle through the open wound, infiltrating the surrounding tissue in a fanlike fashion.

   a. 1% lidocaine HCl (Xylocaine) is the drug of choice as a local anesthetic in laceration repair. Approximately 1 ml is required for each 2 cm of wound. The maximum adult dose with epinephrine is 7 mg/kg, and without epinephrine it is 4.5 mg/kg. *Note:* Each milliliter of 1% Xylocaine contains 10 mg lidocaine HCl.

   b. Aqueous epinephrine combined with lidocaine is useful in closing lacerations of the scalp and other vascular areas. In tissues with less blood supply, routine use of lidocaine with epinephrine is discouraged because it decreases blood supply, leading to delayed healing and possible infection. Its use is contraindicated in the fingers, toes, penis, and earlobes.

   c. Anesthetic solutions should not be injected into rigid fascial compartments (tamponades neurovascular bundles). Regional blocks are preferred in these circumstances after evaluation of sensation and function.

   d. Important cosmetic landmarks should be marked before injecting, and the least amount of local anesthetic should be used so as not to cause distortion and malalignment of the wound edges.

   e. Pain can be minimized by injecting (1) slowly to avoid rapid distension of the tissue (using a 27-gauge needle assists in this goal), (2) through the opening of the wound in a fanlike fashion rather than repeatedly through the skin, and (3) with a longer needle (1.5 in), minimizing the number of "sticks."

   f. Local anesthetic should be infiltrated 1 cm into the wound margins. (Subcutaneous fat does not need to be anesthetized.)

   g. Small (1–2 cm) superficial lacerations requiring only a couple of sutures may be closed without an anesthetic. Another option is the use of TAC (tetracaine, adrenaline, and cocaine), which is a topical anesthetic that is especially useful in children with minor lacerations.

2. The skin surrounding the wound was scrubbed with Hibiclens antiseptic. The wound was irrigated with sterile saline, after which the field was draped in a sterile fashion and illuminated.

   a. Commonly used surgical preps are chlorhexidine gluconate (Hibiclens), povidone-iodine (Betadine), and hydrogen peroxide. Debate exists about which is the best solution because each has cytotoxic properties that interfere with wound healing and local immune response. Regardless, antiseptics should be kept from entering open wounds.

   b. Irrigation is best accomplished using a large syringe (10–50 ml) with an 18-gauge needle providing jet-stream turbulence.

   c. Avoid shaving any hair about the wound because this increases the rate of infection.

3. There was some oozing of blood easily controlled with sterile 4 × 4's and pressure.

4. The wound edges were ragged and ecchymotic in some areas. The laceration extended through the subcutaneous tissue and fascia without injury to the underlying musculature. No debris was seen. Digital examination using a sterile gloved finger revealed no foreign body or disruption of the underlying structures.

5. Ample skin was present to permit debridement of the wound without resulting in excessive tension. An ellipse was made parallel to the lines of tension with a no. 15 blade scalpel to produce symmetrical, freshly "squared off" wound edges with intact blood supply.

   a. Debridement of devitalized tissue is essential whenever possible, except when it would compromise function or result in greater cosmetic deformity than expected if the crushed edges were closed.

   b. Follow the tension lines or wrinkles in the skin when revising a wound in order to minimize the retractive forces on the wound.

   c. Ellipses require a length-to-width ratio of approximately 3:1 in order to avoid an uneven closure.

6. The new wound edges were bluntly undermined with tissue scissors (Fig. 20–4).

   a. Most wounds require some degree of undermining, especially if there has been loss of tissue.

   b. Undermining the edges 4 to 5 mm reduces tension on the laceration by disrupting the elastic fibers that cause inversion of the skin edges.

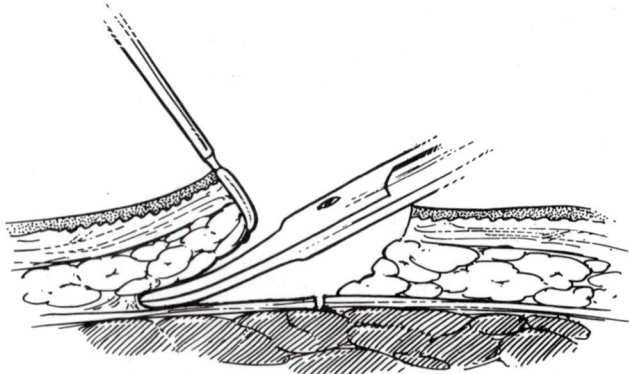

Figure 20–4. Undermining. Preparation of a laceration for repair often requires some undermining of the wound edges. Undermining disrupts elastic fibers that cause inversion of the edges and facilitates placement of deep sutures.

7. The wound was reirrigated copiously with sterile saline.

8. Hemostasis was achieved with steady compression of the wound with a sterile 4 × 4 for 5 minutes. Health maintenance issues were discussed during this time.

   a. Hemostasis usually can be attained in 5 to 10 minutes with compression.

   b. Prevention of hematoma formation is critical for proper wound healing. Hematomas cause wider scars by increasing wound tension and by separating the skin edges. Wound edges also may necrose when capillary ingrowth to the skin is prevented by hematoma formation. Additionally, hematomas promote infection by providing a source of culture medium for bacteria.

9. The revised laceration was closed in layers, the *deep* layer first, with interrupted simple sutures of 4-0 Vicryl with inverted knots (Fig. 20–5).

   a. Closing all ''dead space'' is essential. This reduces tension on the healing skin edges and decreases the chance of hematoma formation.

   b. The size of suture is dependent on the location of the laceration and the degree of tension. The smaller the number, the thicker and stronger is the suture. For the deep layer, a 2-0 or 3-0 absorbable suture is used in the extremities and a 4-0 or 5-0 is used in the face.

   c. Absorbable sutures such as polyglactic acid (Vicryl), polyglycolic acid (Dexon), or chromic catgut swedged on a curved cutting needle are typically used to close the deep and subcutaneous layers.

   d. Knots should be inverted (buried), with the ends of the suture cut closely.

   e. The deeper layers should be approximated so that the skin edges come together evenly and with little tension. These layers include the dermal–fat and fat–fascial junctions, depend-

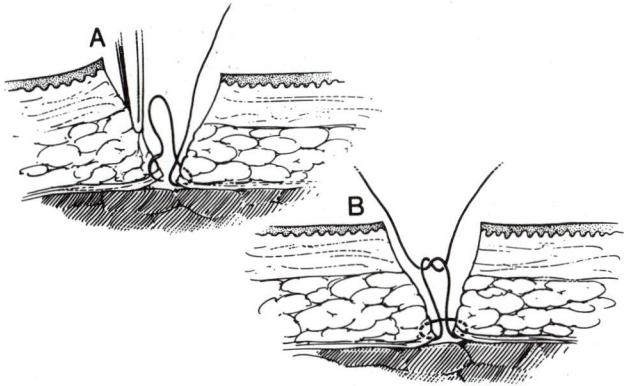

Figure 20–5. The inverted knot. Deep sutures should be tied so that the knots are buried below the layer being closed. This prevents the knots from interfering with the approximation of wound edges and minimizes tissue reaction to suture near the skin's surface. Start from under one edge (*A*) and end underneath on the opposite side (*B*).

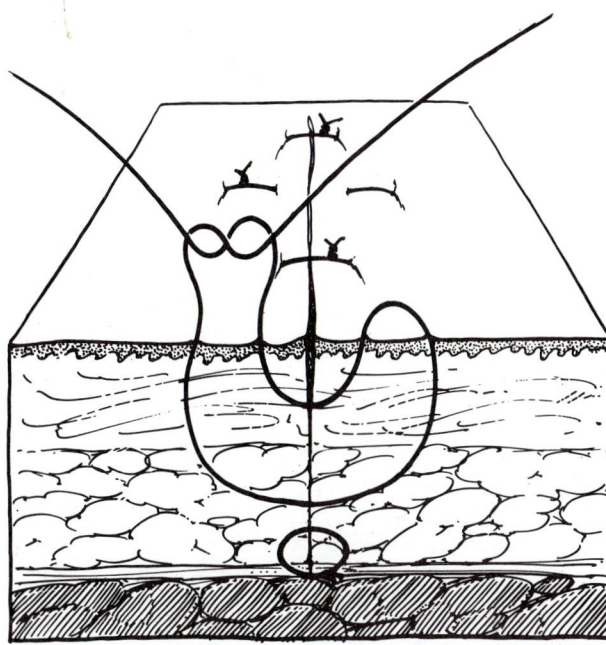

Figure 20–6. Alternating simple and vertical mattress sutures. The vertical mattress suture is an excellent technique to evert wound edges. The increased width of the deep portion of this double-layered suture also provides added wound support.

ing on the depth of the laceration. In this case, the skin on the inside of the forearm was thin, and therefore, the dermal–fat layer was able to be approximated with the skin closure as described below.

10. The skin was closed with a combination of alternating vertical mattress and simple sutures using 4-0 Ethilon (Fig. 20–6).

   a. A major goal in laceration repair is the gentle approximation of everted skin edges, which allows for matching of the regenerating basal layer of skin to produce a thinner scar that heals flatly without a ridge.

   b. Simple sutures will evert the wound edges if (1) the needle enters and exits the skin at identical distances from each edge, (2) they are deeper than they are wide, and (3) the ''base'' of the loop incorporates more tissue than its epidermal counterpart (Fig. 20–7).

   c. In areas of thin skin or increased tension, a vertical mattress suture effectively everts the wound edges. It is stronger than the simple suture and is often used on extremities. Alternating vertical mattress and simple sutures is a common practice. This takes some of the remaining tension off the larger vertical mattress sutures, decreasing stitch scarring.

   d. Use the smallest suture possible: 6-0 on the face, 4-0 or 5-0 on the trunk and extremities, and 4-0 on the back or other thick-skinned areas.

   e. Stitch marks occur when sutures are (1) too heavy a gauge, (2) too long (distance from entrance to exit sites), (3) too tight, (4) left in too

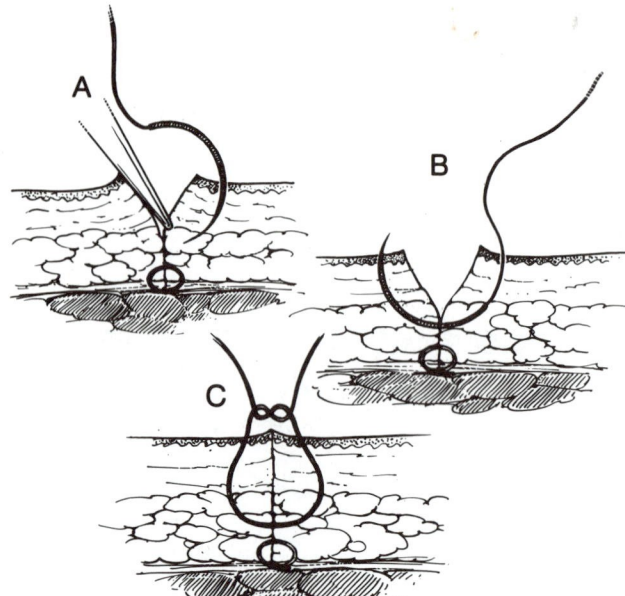

Figure 20–7. The simple suture. This basic suture will evert wound edges when placed correctly. (*A*) Begin by piercing the skin with the needle at a right angle or greater, (*B*) take a bite of subcutaneous tissue that is deeper than it is wide, and (*C*) exit the skin symmetrically on the opposite side of the wound.

long, or (5) when they incorporate too much tissue.

f. The skin layer is usually closed with nonabsorbable monofilament suture, either nylon (Ethilon or Dermalon) or polypropylene (Prolene or Surgilene) on a curved needle.

g. Start the closure at one corner of the wound and work toward the other (unless an anatomic landmark is present, which is then approximated first). The needle should enter and exit the skin at a distance from the edge equal to the skin's thickness, usually about 3 to 4 mm. Sutures should be placed at a distance from each other equal to their length.

h. The skin needs to be handled as atraumatically as possible by using skin hooks or by gently grasping the dermal–fat junction with tissue forceps held parallel to the plane of the skin.

i. The knots are tied with the needle holder by a technique known as the "instrument tie." A surgeon's knot is made, followed by three or four square knots. Remember to approximate, not strangulate, the tissue when tying knots.

11. The repaired laceration was cleansed and dried. Benzoin was applied with a cotton swab to the skin on both sides of the laceration. Steri-Strips were taped across the wound, and the drapes were removed. The repair was covered with Adaptic and a sterile gauze dressing.

  a. Repairs are cleansed with either normal saline or hydrogen peroxide.

  b. Tincture of benzoin is a liquid that makes the skin more adhesive after it dries, which helps the Steri-Strips remain in place longer.

  c. Steri-Strips are sterile microporous tape of various widths that add support to the repair and take some tension off the sutures.

  d. Adaptic is a sterile nonadhering petroleum mesh.

Disposition

1. Gus was asked to keep the wound clean and dry and to rest and elevate his arm over the next 24 hours.

2. Signs of infection (i.e., fever, redness, tenderness, increased local warmth, or purulent discharge) were explained, for which he would need to return earlier than the scheduled follow-up in 2 days.

3. The dressing is to be changed after 24 hours, and any dry blood may be removed from the sutures with hydrogen peroxide.

4. Gus was educated about the need to use a seat belt when driving and advised to stop smoking.

5. Gus's blood pressure will be rechecked at the time of follow-up and again when his sutures are removed. Because of his risk factors for coronary artery disease (cigarette smoking, male sex, positive family history, and obesity), a fasting lipid profile instead of a random screening cholesterol will be ordered.

6. Gus was advised to begin considering a diet and exercise program.

FIRST FOLLOW-UP VISIT

SUBJECTIVE

Gus returned for follow-up and had no concerns about his arm. He was not aware of any fever and had no pain or paresthesias. He was happy to report that he stopped smoking cigarettes and has already started to "watch" what he eats. His wife says he wore his seat belt today.

OBJECTIVE

Gus had no fever, and his blood pressure was 120/80, with a pulse rate of 70. There were no cigarettes in his pocket. The dressing was dry, and no distal edema was noted. His circulation, sensation, and function remained normal. The dressing was removed. The wound was clean and dry without signs of inflammation (i.e., redness, swelling, tenderness, or increased warmth). There was no necrosis of the skin edges or hematoma formation. The wound edges were slightly everted and well approximated.

ASSESSMENT

1. The revised layered repair of Gus's 2.5-cm laceration of the left forearm was healing well without signs of infection.

2. Gus's blood pressure was within normal limits today.

3. Gus has discontinued his cigarette habit.

PLAN

1. Gus will return in 7 days for suture removal.
2. Gus will continue to keep the wound clean and protect it with an adhesive bandage.
3. Gus was congratulated on his cessation of smoking, seat belt use, and attention to diet.
4. Gus's blood pressure will be recorded by a friend (nurse) two times each week for 3 weeks, and he is to return to the office with these readings.
5. Blood for the lipid profile was drawn, and the results will be discussed with him at his next visit. At that time, an appropriate diet and exercise plan will be outlined.

Face 3-5 days
Scalp 5-7
trunk + extremities 7-10
Back hands feet 10-14

DISCUSSION

The schedule for suture removal is approximately 3 to 5 days for the face, 5 to 7 days for the scalp, 7 to 10 days for the trunk and extremities, and 10 to 14 days for the back, hands, and feet. If a patient returns for suture removal and has a slow-healing wound with areas that may separate, partial suture removal should be considered as an option to minimize stitch scarring. Steri-Strips are applied in places where sutures were removed, and the remaining sutures are taken out as soon as possible.

Scars require 2 years to fully mature, during which time they become less erythematous and hypertrophic. Progressive collagen turnover results in retraction and produces a softer scar. Any revision should be delayed until this process of remodeling is complete.

SUGGESTED READING

Baldwin B, Stal S, Matson CC. Plastic and reconstructive surgery. In Rakel RE (ed.). Textbook of Family Practice, 4th ed. Philadelphia, W.B. Saunders, 1990, pp. 782–786.

Breitenbach KL, Bergera JJ. Principles and techniques of primary wound closure. In Snell GF (ed.). Office Surgery. Primary Care Clin Office Pract. Philadelphia, W.B. Saunders, 1986; 13(3):411–431.

Dushoff IM. A stitch in time. Emergency Medicine 1973; 5:21–43.

Leversee JH. Syllabus for Workshop on Office Minor Surgery. Seattle, University of Washington, 1985.

Little DN. Simple and infected lacerations. In Mayhew HE, Rodgers LA (eds.). Basic Procedures in Family Practice. Bethany, Conn., Fleschner Publishing, 1984; pp. 7–12.

Moy RL, Lee A, Zalka A. Commonly used suturing techniques in skin surgery. American Family Physician 1991; 44:1625–1634.

Norton LW. Trauma. In Hill GJ II (ed.). Outpatient Surgery, 2nd ed. Philadelphia, W.B. Saunders, 1980, pp. 112–114.

Report of the U.S. Preventive Services Task Force. Guide to Clinical Preventive Services: An Assessment of the Effectiveness of 169 Interventions. Baltimore, William & Wilkins, 1989.

Smith CW Jr. Surgery. In Driscoll CE, Bope ET, Smith CW Jr, Carter BL. The Family Practice Desk Reference, 2nd ed. St. Louis, Mosby Year Book, 1991, pp. 359–362.

Weatherley-White RCA, Lesavoy MA. The integument. In Hill GJ II (ed.). Outpatient Surgery, 2nd ed. Philadelphia, W.B. Saunders, 1980, pp. 304–308.

Williamson PS. Repair of simple lacerations. In Driscoll CE, Rakel RE (eds.). Patient Care: Procedures for Your Practice. Oradell, N.J., Medical Economics, 1988, pp. 193–198.

QUESTIONS

1. An 18-year-old female whose immunizations are up to date presents to you on Sunday afternoon with a 1-cm laceration of the lower leg caused by a piece of rusted barbed wire. The injury occurred the previous morning. Her last tetanus booster was 2 years ago. Appropriate intervention(s) is/are

   a. Immunoglobulin.
   b. Cleansing of the wound.
   c. Tetanus booster.
   d. Steri-Strip closure of the laceration.
   e. Suture repair of the laceration.

2. A 45-year-old butcher presents to your office immediately after lacerating his left index finger with a clean knife. His tetanus status is current. The wound is located across the radial side of the index finger and is about 1.5 cm in length. The degree of injury is difficult to assess because of bleeding and pain. Pressure on the laceration for a couple of minutes does not successfully stop the bleeding. Proper wound management includes

   a. Injecting the wound with 1% lidocaine with epinephrine to control the bleeding. *NO*
   b. Regional block after sensation distal to the injury is tested.
   c. Continued compression of the wound for 10 minutes to control bleeding. *Yes*
   d. Tetanus booster. *NO*
   e. Removal of the sutures 4 days after the repair. *NO*

3. Scarring from skin sutures is a problem when they remain in place longer than required. Match the ideal time of suture removal with the appropriate wound location.

   a. A 3-cm elliptical excision of a 1-cm melanocytic nevus on the back *3*
   b. A superficial 1.5-cm laceration of the forehead *1*
   c. A 2-cm laceration of the scalp over the external occipital protuberance *2*

      (1) 3 to 5 days
      (2) 7 days
      (3) 10 to 14 days
      (4) 21 days

Answers appear on page 449.

Vaginitis

JOHN E. SUTHERLAND

INITIAL VISIT

SUBJECTIVE

Patient Identification. Sandra J. is a 23-year-old divorced female being seen for an irritating vaginal discharge.

Presenting Problem. Leukorrhea for the past 2 days that has become progressively profuse and odorous.

Presenting Illness. Sandra began noticing a vaginal discharge about 3 to 4 days after her last coitus 2 weeks ago. Initially, it was only mildly irritating, but now it is accompanied by vaginal burning, some terminal dysuria, and a bothersome odor. She has been afraid of dyspareunia, so she has not had coitus again. She has had a mild discharge once before, about 2 years ago, which occurred while she was on antibiotics for bronchitis. It caused some perineal pruritus, but it seemed to clear up on its own about a week after discontinuing the antibiotic.

Sandra is on oral contraception at present and having no problems. She is gravida 2 para 1011 (1 full term pregnancy, 0 premature births, 1 abortion, 1 living child). She had a normal spontaneous vaginal delivery 4 years ago and a spontaneous abortion 2 years ago. She has never had any pelvic pain or infections.

Past Medical History. Sandra had tympanostomy tubes placed at age 4 for chronic serous otitis media. She was hospitalized for childbirth 4 years ago.

Family History. Sandra's father is 48 years old and in good health. Her mother is 45 years old and in good health, but she needed a hysterectomy for "chronic infection" at age 36. Sandra has an older brother and a younger sister, both without medical problems. Her 75-year-old paternal grandmother has diabetes and hypertension. Her 70-year-old maternal grandmother has osteoarthritis. Both her grandfathers died in their mid-seventies of heart attacks. Her son is in good health.

Health Habits. Sandra smoked from the ages of 16 to 18 but stopped with her first pregnancy. She drinks alcohol "moderately" on weekends in a social context. She wears seat belts. Her diet is balanced. She occasionally runs and takes aerobics classes.

Social History. Sandra has been divorced for a year and was separated from her husband for 6 months before that. She has had a few dating relationships these past 18 months, and she just started seeing her most recent boyfriend 1 month ago. Her last relationship terminated about 2 months ago. She works as a computer programmer, and her 4-year-old boy is in day care.

Review of Systems. Except for occasional respiratory infections, this patient has no complaints. She has never had a urinary tract infection.

OBJECTIVE

Physical Examination. Sandra's blood pressure is 110/70; she weighs 125 lb; her height is 65 in; and her temperature is 98.6°F. The examination was limited to the abdomen and pelvis. Her abdomen and costovertebral angles were not tender. No masses were palpable. Her perineum was normal, without inflammation. A vaginal speculum examination revealed a bubbly pool of greenish yellow discharge with a pH of 5.5. The cervix had some petechiae on it, but there was no discharge from the os. A bimanual examination of the pelvis was normal, with no adnexal tenderness.

Laboratory Tests. A normal saline wet smear and potassium hydroxide (KOH) preparation were performed. The KOH prep was negative. The wet mount was positive for motile pear-shaped parasites, but negative for "clue cells." A urinalysis was normal.

ASSESSMENT

Working Diagnosis. Trichomoniasis. Vaginal wet mount revealed classic *Trichomonas vaginalis* organisms.

Differential Diagnoses. Sandra's symptoms and history suggest other causes of leukorrhea also:

1. *Monilial vaginitis* (candidiasis, moniliasis). The history suggests that Sandra might have had this before while on antibiotics, and she currently is on oral contraceptives, which also make her susceptible. However, the KOH vaginal preparation is negative for yeast and mycelia and her vaginal pH is abnormal.

2. *Bacterial vaginosis* (formerly *Gardnerella vaginalis*, *Haemophilus vaginalis*, and nonspecific vaginitis). This is also a common cause of vaginal discharge. However, "clue cells," typical of this disorder, are not seen. The vaginal pH is compatible with this diagnosis, as are the symptoms of vaginal burning.

3. *Cervicitis* from *Chlamydia trachomatis* or *Neisseria gonorrhoeae*. These sexually transmitted diseases can cause leukorrhea, but there is usually a cervical discharge and/or adnexal tenderness present on pelvic examination.

PLAN

Diagnostic. No other tests are necessary at this time.

Therapeutic. Metronidazole (Flagyl), 2 gm in a single oral dose.

Patient Education. Trichomoniasis is explained to the patient as being one of the common vaginal infections that does not spread into the uterus or pelvis. The importance of treating her sexual partner is explained because trichomoniasis is sexually transmitted and can recur with reexposure.

Disposition. This patient was told to return if her symptoms did not clear within a couple of weeks or if they recurred later. Her annual periodic health examination is due in 1 month, and this condition will be reevaluated then.

DISCUSSION

"Vaginitis," defined as any inflammatory process involving the vagina, consists of a common group of unrelated diseases with diverse symptoms and causes. Taking time to make a specific diagnosis will help prevent recurrence. Generally benign and local, its predominant symptoms are leukorrhea, perineal pruritis, and external dysuria. The overwhelmingly most common etiologic agents in descending order of frequency are bacterial vaginosis, moniliasis, and trichomoniasis. Other causes of vaginitis include reactive vaginitis, atrophic vaginitis, herpes simplex virus type 2, and vulvovaginitis associated with upper respiratory tract infections.

It is possible to confuse a normal physiologic discharge with vaginitis. A clear mucoid discharge with some leukocytes and epithelial cells and a pH of less than 5 is normal. Normal bacterial flora include *Streptococous, Staphylococcus, Lactobacillus,* Doderlein's bacillus, diphtheroids, *Klebsiella,* and *Escherichia coli.* It is unusual for a physiologic discharge to be accompanied by discomfort and odor.

The necessary basic diagnostic materials are isotonic saline and 10% potassium hydroxide for wet mounts, a microscope, nitrazene paper for determination of pH level, slides, and a vaginal speculum. Some people also recommend routine use of a Gram-stain preparation.

Characteristics and findings of various organisms that cause vulvovaginitis are displayed in Table 20–14. Sexually transmitted diseases that cause cervicitis that can be confused with simple vulvovaginitis are *Chlamydia trachomatis, Neisseria gonorrhoeae,* and herpes simplex virus type 2.

Sandra's symptoms are compatible with more than one cause. The burning sensation, terminal dysuria, bothersome odor, and elevated vaginal pH make it more likely to be bacterial vaginosis or trichomonal vaginitis than moniliasis. The petechiae present on the cervix, giving it a "strawberry" appearance, also may be present on the vagina and are pathognomonic for trichomoniasis, as is the greenish color of the discharge. Trichomoniasis is not as common as bacterial vaginosis or moniliasis. It is sexually transmitted.

Trichomoniasis symptoms include foul-smelling leukorrhea, often accompanied by a burning sensation, pruritis, and dysuria. Patients may be asymptomatic carriers. The diagnosis is customarily made by observing motile pear-shaped parasites with flagella on the wet smear, a procedure first described in 1836. The pH is 5 to 6.5. Sometimes the diagnosis is made on Papanicolaou (Pap) stained gynecologic smears. Both the vaginal wet mount and Pap smears have shortcomings as diagnostic tools. Direct immunofluorescence with monoclo-

TABLE 20–14. DIFFERENTIAL DIAGNOSIS OF VULVOVAGINITIS

DIAGNOSIS	HISTORY	PHYSICAL FEATURES	LABORATORY FINDINGS AND DIAGNOSTIC METHODS	TREATMENT
Bacterial vaginosis	Mildly odorous discharge	Gray, mucoid, pasty discharge; pH 5 to 6	Saline preparation studded with "clue cells"; culture as needed	Metronidazole, 500 mg b.i.d. for 7 days
Candidiasis	Recurrent pruritic discharge	Creamy, curdly discharge; pH 4 to 5	Potassium hydroxide preparation, mycelia, buds; culture as needed	Terconazole, clotrimazole, miconazole, butoconazole or another antifungal
Trichomonal vaginitis	Odorous leukorrhea; dysuria	Greenish yellow discharge; pH 5 to 6.5; friable hyperemic cervix	Saline preparation, motile flagellate protozoa; culture as needed	Metronidazole, 2 gm in a single dose
Reactive vaginitis	Use of hygienic sprays and douches; odorous discharge	Foreign bodies; erythema	None	Elimination of offensive agent, corticosteroids
Atrophic vaginitis	Dyspareunia; burning	Sticky brown discharge, thin vaginal tissue	None	Topical estrogen
Normal cervical or vaginal discharge vaginitis	Minimal discharge	Clear mucoid discharge, pH 4.5; ectropion	Saline preparation, a few leukocytes and epithelial cells	None or povidone-iodine

nal antibodies and/or culture media are sensitive and specific alternatives that are not currently widely available to clinicians.

Treatment with a single 2-gm dose of metronidazole provides therapy with an acceptable failure rate and good patient compliance. Other metronidazole regimens such as 250 mg t.i.d. for 7 days or 500 mg b.i.d. for 7 days have the advantage of fewer gastrointestinal complaints. The partner must be treated for this sexually transmitted disease. Furazolidine or povidone-iodine may be useful when metronidazole is contraindicated.

Bacteria is the most common cause of vaginitis. It has gone by many different names over the past several years including *Gardnerella* vaginitis, Haemophilus vaginalis vaginitis, *Corynebacterium vaginale* vaginitis, and nonspecific vaginitis. It is a superficial polymicrobial vaginal infection caused by an increase in anaerobic organisms and a concomitant decrease in lactobacilli. *Gardnerella* is one of several endogenous members of the vaginal flora that overgrow in this condition. Symptoms remain unreliable but include a profuse gray homogeneous discharge that may have a "fishy" odor. Patients may be asymptomatic. They sometimes have external dysuria and mild vaginal burning.

The diagnosis of bacterial vaginosis is made by wet preparation of the vaginal secretions with normal saline. One will see bacteria embedded in the epithelial cells, so-called clue cells. One also may perform a "whiff test" by adding a drop of KOH to a slide with the discharge on it. A characteristic fishy odor will be emitted. The pH of the leukorrhea is 5 to 6.

Metronidazole is the treatment of choice, with the most common and standard current regimen being 500 mg twice a day for 7 days, although a single 2-gm dose has been shown to be nearly as effective. Other antibiotics, including ampicillin, cephalosporins, and tetracycline, are also effective. The issue of sexual partner treatment is controversial, although most authorities recommend it.

Monilial vaginitis is the second most common cause of leukorrhea. Yeast is ubiquitous and part of the normal flora of the vagina. Under conditions that may increase the pH of the vagina or disturb its normal flora, yeast will flourish and cause vulvovaginitis. Pregnancy, diabetes mellitus, antibiotics, oral contraceptives, and the premenstrual phase may be at fault. The most common symptoms are intense itching and a white, curdly discharge with a pH of 4 to 5. There may be vaginal and vulvar edema and erythema.

Candida albicans is the most frequent pathogenic strain, but *Candida tropicales* or *Torulopsis glabrata* can be problematic. When tested, discharge material prepared with KOH shows branching mycelia, pseudohyphae, and yeast buds. If necessary, a culture may be done on Nickerson's or Sabaroud's medium.

Treatment consists of topical cream with one of several agents, including terconazole, miconazole, clotrimazole, butoconazole, and genitian violet. Both cream and suppository forms are available, and patients may be treated from 1 to 7 days. This condition is often re-

current and needs retreating. In some patients, a monthly prophylactic dose is necessary.

Patients with persistent and/or recurrent infections can be treated with maintenance prophylactic therapy with oral ketoconazole for 6 to 10 days. Male patients are routinely treated by some, whereas others just treat symptomatic topical lesions of balantitis and inguinal intertrigo.

FIRST FOLLOW-UP VISIT

SUBJECTIVE

Sandra returned 1 month after her initial visit for her periodic health examination. Her symptoms had completely cleared within about 1 week after the dose of metronidazole. Her sexual partner also had been treated. They had resumed sexual activity 2 weeks ago and had no problems. Her review of systems was unremarkable. She stated that she wanted to renew her oral contraceptive prescription. She did not know if she had ever had a cholesterol level drawn.

OBJECTIVE

A physical examination was performed, and no abnormalities were detected. The cholesterol level was determined and found to be 185. The pelvic examination revealed a normal-appearing amount of clear vaginal discharge. A Pap smear was done and later was reported as normal.

ASSESSMENT

1. Normal periodic health examination
2. Resolved trichomoniasis
3. Contraceptive planning

PLAN

Diagnostic. None. It is not necessary to retest the vaginal secretions for evidence of cure.

Therapeutic. The oral contraceptive prescription was renewed.

Patient Education. The physician advised Sandra again that the trichomoniasis was probably cured because treatment efficacy is about 90% and she was free of symptoms. She also was advised that the incidence of moniliasis was higher than normal while on the "pill" and that she should take the precautions of daily bathing and avoidance of tight and synthetic fabric undergarments if any early symptoms of discharge or itching developed.

Disposition. Sandra was advised to return in a year for a periodic health examination or earlier if her vaginitis symptoms recurred.

DISCUSSION

The modern management of vaginitis involves the identification of the causative organism, appropriate specific therapy, and selective treatment of the male sexual partner(s). Specific symptoms are notoriously unreliable in the differential diagnosis of these conditions. The term "nonspecific vaginitis" should rarely, if ever, be used in modern gynecology. When in doubt, cultures can be used to supplement information from wet mounts and KOH preps. With the exception of motile trichomonads in vaginal discharge, no single finding demands treatment.

Trichmonas vaginalis is a sexually transmitted anaerobic parasite that infests the periurethral glands of both men and women. Most men are asymptomatic and more resistant to postexposure infection than are women. It is very important to educate and treat the male partner, even when he is asymptomatic.

Metronidazole is the standard and only effective treatment for trichomoniasis. Treatment of recurrent or persistent trichomoniasis begins with an inquiry about and treatment of sexual partners. Retreatment can be with either the single dose or a week-long regimen of 250 mg t.i.d. In resistent cases, a higher dose may be helpful.

It must be noted that metronidazole is contraindicated in pregnant women in their 1st trimester because the drug crosses the placenta and its safety to the fetus has not been established. Local treatment such as povidone-iodine may alleviate symptoms and also should be tried first in the 2nd and 3rd trimesters. Clotrimazole has antitrichomonal activity and may be used during pregnancy, curing about 50% of infections.

Atrophic vaginitis should be mentioned, although not a consideration in this patient. It is caused by diminished estrogen stimulation that results in dry, shiny vaginal mucosa. The symptoms are dyspareunia and burning. Physical findings include a sticky brown discharge and thin vaginal tissue. Topical estrogen therapy, initially daily and later two to three times a week, is very effective.

Reactive contact vaginitis, which is a consideration in this age group, may be caused by a variety of hygiene sprays, douche powders, and foreign bodies. Removal of the irritating agent or foreign body and topical corticosteroid therapy are usually effective.

SUGGESTED READING

Gobel JD. Recurrent vulvovaginal candidiasis. N Eng J Med 1986; 315:1455–1458.
Krieger JN, Tarn MR, Stevens CE, et al. Diagnosis of trichomoniasis. JAMA 1988; 259:1223–1227.
Rakel RE. Textbook of Family Practice, 4th ed. Philadelphia, W.B. Saunders, 1990, pp. 796–817.
Weaver CH, Mengel MB. Bacterial vaginosis. J Fam Pract 1988; 27(2):207–215.

QUESTIONS

1. The most prominent symptom(s) of trichomonal vaginitis is
   a. Pruritus.
   b. Odorous leukorrhea.
   c. Profuse leukorrhea.
   d. Recurrence.

2. All the following conditions are associated with a vaginal pH of 5 or less *except*
   a. Monilial vaginitis.
   b. Normal physiologic discharge.
   c. Bacterial vaginosis.
   d. Reactive vaginitis.

3. Match each of the following causes of leukorrhea with the clinical manifestations listed.
   a. Bacterial vaginosis
   b. Monilial vaginitis
   c. Trichomonal vaginitis
   d. Cervicitis
   (1) Pruritus, frequent recurrence, creamy discharge
   (2) Odorous, greenish color, vaginal petechiae
   (3) Internal dysuria, mucoid yellow discharge, friable mucosa
   (4) Mild "fishy" odor, profuse discharge, external dysuria

4. Non-sexually-transmitted episodes of vaginitis may be associated with which of the following?
   a. Bacterial vaginosis
   b. Monilial vaginitis
   c. Trichomonial vaginitis
   d. Atrophic vaginitis

Answers appear on page 449.

Amenorrhea

ALAN G. MOORE

INITIAL VISIT

SUBJECTIVE

Patient Identification and Presenting Problem. Beth, a 28-year-old white woman, presents for routine Papanicolaou smear. She has not had a menstrual period for the last 6 months, since stopping her birth control pills.

History of Present Illness. Beth stopped her birth control pills 6 months ago when she and her fiancé broke up after calling off their engagement. She is not currently sexually active.

Past Medical History. Menarche was at age 13. Beth's menstrual cycle is every 28 to 30 days, with 4 days of flow and mild cramps on the first 2 days of her period. Beth became sexually active at age 18 and has had only two sexual partners. *Contraception:* Initially Beth used condoms and foam; then she switched to birth control pills and has taken them off and on for the last 7 years. Beth only takes pills when she is sexually active and took her last birth control pill for 1 year before stopping for the reasons mentioned above. There are no contraindications to birth control pill use. *Papanicolaou smear history:* Beth has had yearly Pap smears since 18 years of age, and all have been within normal limits.

Family History. Both of Beth's parents are alive and well. Beth has one male sibling, 27 years old, alive and well. There is no family history of birth defects or chromosome abnormalities and no history of cancer on either side of the family.

Health Habits. Beth has never used tobacco and abstains from alcohol, except for a rare glass of wine with dinner. Beth has run 2 to 3 miles a day three to five times a week for the past 2 years.

Social History. Beth is single and has never married; she works as a bank teller and likes her work. She broke up with her fiancé 6 months ago, is no longer seeing him, and is still upset about it. She is not currently dating anyone else.

Review of Systems. Beth denies headache, vision changes, loss of smell, skin or hair changes, galactorrhea, pelvic pain, dyspareunia, or dysmenorrhea. Her appetite is normal. She eats three meals a day regularly. She lost approximately 30 lb when she started running with her fiancé 2 years ago, but her weight has been stable over the past 12 months.

OBJECTIVE

Physical Examination. Beth's height is 66 in; her weight is 110 lb. She is a well-developed, well-nourished Caucasian female in no acute distress who appears to be in excellent condition with good muscle tone. She has normal breast development and pubic hair. Her pelvic examination is within normal limits, except for scant cervical mucus and slight atrophy of the rugae of the vagina. The remainder of the physical examination is normal. A Pap smear is performed. A urine beta human chorionic gonadotropin (β-HCG) test done in the office is negative. Serum thyroid-stimulating hormone (TSH), prolactin, follicle-stimulating hormone (FSH), and leutenizing hormone (LH) screens are all drawn and sent to the laboratory along with the Pap smear.

ASSESSMENT

Differential Diagnoses. (1) *Secondary amenorrhea,* most likely hypothalamic amenorrhea secondary to a combination of stress, weight loss, and exercise, (2) *premature ovarian failure,* (3) *pituitary lesion,* (4) *end-organ (uterus) failure.* Hypothalamic amenorrhea, however, is a diagnosis of exclusion, and a full workup to rule out other possibilities in the differential diagnosis of secondary amenorrhea is mandatory.

Amenorrhea can occur at any of the four levels necessary for normal menstrual cycling: (1) hypothalamic, (2) pituitary, (3) ovarian, and (4) end-organ or outflow tract. The first obvious cause of amenorrhea (i.e., pregnancy) has been ruled out with a negative pregnancy test. The diagnosis of "postpill amenorrhea" is an imprecise diagnosis and does not adequately explain the etiology of the patient's amenorrhea or provide a guidance for therapy. The vast majority of patients stopping birth control pills resume normal menses within 3 to 6 months after stopping the birth control pills. Any amenorrhea that persists longer than this demands complete evaluation because of the potential seriousness of the etiologies involved. Since Beth has had normal periods beginning at a normal-age menarche and has had normal periods associated with her birth control pills, it is unlikely that she has congenital anomalies of her uterus such as mullerian agenesis, testicular feminization, and gonadal dysgenesis (Turner's and other syndromes). Therefore, the source of her amenorrhea is most likely either simple anovulation or a failure at the level of the hypothalamus, pituitary, or ovary.

PLAN

Diagnostic. In addition to the blood tests drawn, Beth will be given a progestin challenge test to see if there is enough circulating estrogen to cause a normal withdrawal period. If withdrawal bleeding occurs, this establishes that the hypothalamus, pituitary, and ovary have produced sufficient estrogen to cause withdrawal bleeding but suggests anovulation, since no period has occurred. If the patient experiences normal withdrawal bleeding to this simple test, the diagnosis of anovulation is confirmed and no further workup is necessary. The leading cause of anovulation is polycystic ovarian syndrome, but this patient has none of the classic signs or symptoms of this disorder (such as obesity and hirsutism), so it is unlikely, but not impossible, that she has this disorder.

If no withdrawal occurs to the progestin challenge, Beth will be given an estrogen and a progestin (such as Premarin 2.5 mg PO q.d. for 25 days with Provera 10 mg PO q.d. on days 16 through 25). If withdrawal bleeding occurs with this combination (as it should, since she also withdrew to birth control pills, which is another form of combination of estrogen and progestin), this proves that her uterus and outflow tract are functioning normally and are responsive to exogenous hormone stimulation but that there is failure at some other level of the hypothalamus–pituitary–ovarian axis. Results of the hormone test should give an indication at what level this failure is occurring. If the prolactin is elevated, a CT scan of the sella turcica would be indicated to rule out either a pituitary microadenoma or macroadenoma. Most, but not all, of these patients will have galactorrhea. If the TSH level is elevated, this would be consistent with hypothyroidism as the etiology for the amenorrhea and would respond to simple thyroid replacement therapy. Again, Beth has no signs or symptoms of hypothyroidism, so this diagnosis is also unlikely. Some patients with hypothyroidism are euthyroid chemically only as a result of the markedly elevated TSH, which is stimulating the failing thyroid gland to produce normal circulating levels of thyroid hormone. This clinical situation also can cause amenorrhea. If the LH and FSH levels are elevated, this is consistent with ovarian failure, and at Beth's age, which is distant from the normal menopausal age of 50, a workup for autoimmune disease would be in order to rule out an autoimmune etiology for her premature ovarian failure. A karyotype also would be in order, since she could be a Turner's mosaic. If the LH and FSH levels are normal or low, this implies hypothalamic or pituitary failure as the etiology of her amenorrhea. A CT of the sella turcica will rule out pituitary tumors or the empty sella syndrome (Sheehan's syndrome). If the CT scan is negative, then the diagnosis, by exclusion, is hypothalamic amenorrhea, which is in fact the most common etiology and can only be confidently diagnosed after all other causes have been ruled out. The etiology of this disorder is failure of the regular pulsatile gonadotropin-releasing hormone (GnRH) secretion from the hypothalamus and is usually caused by combinations of anorexia, weight loss, bulimia, stress, or excessive exercise.

Therapeutic. The treatment will depend on which etiology is found for Beth's amenorrhea. If Beth is anovulatory, she will need regular progestin withdrawal to prevent the hyperplasia of the endometrium or even cancer that can occur in the face of chronic unopposed estrogen stimulation. Monthly progestin withdrawal (Provera 10 mg PO q.d. × 10 days each month, for example) is not contraception, however, and if the patient needs contraception, birth control pills are in order to counter the unopposed estrogen and restore her normal periods. If the anovulatory patient wishes to become pregnant, she is a good candidate for induction of ovulation using clomiphene or other agents. If a diagnosis of ovarian failure is made, the patient needs estrogen replacement therapy to prevent osteoporosis and the adverse lipid state associated with hypoestrogenic states. She also should be told that it is unlikely she will be able to get pregnant on her own but may be a candidate for the new assisted reproductive technologies. If an elevated prolactin level is found and the CT of the sella turcica reveals either a microadenoma or a macroadenoma, Beth is a candidate for either surgery or bromocriptine therapy. If an elevated TSH level is found, Beth can simply be treated with thyroid replacement therapy. If Beth is found to be suffering from hypothalamic amenorrhea, her hypoestrogenic state again places her at risk for osteoporosis and she needs estrogen replacement therapy. This can be provided either by an estrogen and progestin regimen similar to that described above or, if the patient is sexually active, she also can be placed on birth control pills. It is not unusual for hypothalamic amenorrhea to resolve spontaneously when some of the underlying etiologies such as weight loss, excessive exercise, stress, anorexia, or bulimia are treated or resolved. Therefore, these patients must be advised that they can in fact get pregnant without warning. If pregnancy is desired, these patients are candidates for ovulation induction as well, but not by clomiphene, which requires an intact and functioning pituitary.

Patient Education. Beth must be informed of the reasons for the evaluation and the differential diagnosis being entertained. She should be told that the likely source at this juncture is hypothalamic amenorrhea, possibly secondary to a combination of the stress of her recent breakup with her fiancé, her weight loss over the past 2 years, and her strenuous exercise. She needs to be told the importance of the workup, since she will need treatment for either anovulation (to prevent endometrial cancer) or hypoestrogenism (to prevent osteoporosis). If in fact the tentative diagnosis of hypothalamic amenorrhea is confirmed, she also can be told that occasionally mild modifications of strenuous exercise and stress-reduction techniques and slight weight gain often can induce a spontaneous return of normal menses.

Disposition. A prescription was given for Provera 10 mg q.d. × 5 days for a progestin challenge test. Beth was instructed to call the office if no bleeding occurred within 7 days, and if so, she will then be instructed to take Premarin 2.5 mg during days 1 to 25 of the next month, with Provera 10 mg on days 16 to 25 of the next month, and to report if no bleeding occurs within 7 days of the last pill of that regimen. A follow-up visit will be set up after completion of these tests.

FIRST FOLLOW-UP VISIT

SUBJECTIVE

Beth called the office to say that she had no withdrawal bleeding after the Provera and therefore took the Premarin and Provera as prescribed. She had a normal period after completion of this regimen. An outpatient CT of the sella turcica was ordered at this point. Beth has started dating again and has met someone in whom she is very interested and feels better about breaking up with her fiancé. She is considering becoming sexually active with her new boyfriend and desires contraception.

OBJECTIVE

The Pap smear report shows a maturation index with a shift to the left consistent with the weak estrogen effect: The TSH level is less than 5; the prolactin level is 5 (within normal limits); the LH level is 5; the FSH level is 5; and CT of the sella turcica is within normal limits.

ASSESSMENT

There is no evidence of hypothyroidism, hyperprolactinemia, or pituitary disorders. Her LH and FSH levels are low normal to low, and therefore, the diagnosis, by exclusion, is hypothalamic amenorrhea, probably secondary to this patient's combination of stress, weight loss, and exercise.

PLAN

Since Beth is at risk for osteoporosis, she needs estrogen replacement therapy. However, she also needs contraception; therefore, birth control pills will provide her both a suitable source of estrogen and contraception. If she ever stops her birth control pills, however, and amenorrhea recurs, she will need to be placed back on either estrogen replacement therapy or birth control pills. If she desires pregnancy in the future and her periods do not return spontaneously after stopping hormone replacement therapy or birth control pills, she will need ovulation induction. She is told to return in 3 months for follow-up.

DISCUSSION

Amenorrhea is a challenging problem occurring in an outpatient family practice setting. It demands a thorough evaluation and therapy in every case, since amenorrhea is either hypoestrogenic, which requires estrogen replacement therapy to prevent osteoporosis, or represents chronic unopposed estrogen stimulation, as in the case of anovulation, which requires progestin

withdrawal to prevent endometrial cancer. Amenorrhea cannot simply be ignored or written off to "postpill amenorrhea." With the simple scheme and tests described here, a complete evaluation and therapy can be performed with a minimum of testing in a very short time.

SUGGESTED READING

Speroff L, Glass RH, Kase NG. Clinical Gynecologic Endocrinology and Infertility, 4th ed. Baltimore, Williams & Wilkins, 1989, chap. 5, pp. 165–212; chap. 6, pp. 213–232.

QUESTIONS

1. In the evaluation of amenorrhea, no withdrawal bleeding to either a progestin challenge or to a combination of estrogen and progestin characterizes failure of which system?
   a. Hypothalamus
   b. Pituitary
   c. Ovary
   d. Uterus/outflow tract
   e. Thyroid

2. In the evaluation of amenorrhea, a normal withdrawal to the initial progestin challenge test is consistent with a diagnosis of
   a. Anovulation.
   b. Pituitary failure.
   c. Hypothalamic amenorrhea.
   d. Outflow tract obstruction.
   e. Turner's syndrome.

3. In the evaluation of amenorrhea, a negative withdrawal to progestin but a positive withdrawal to estrogen and progestin with normal TSH, prolactin, LH, and FSH levels and a normal CT scan of the sella turcica is consistent with a diagnosis of
   a. Anovulation.
   b. Microadenoma of the pituitary.
   c. Hypothalamic amenorrhea.
   d. End-organ failure or outflow tract obstruction.
   e. Ovarian failure.

4. In the same situation as Question 3, if the LH and FSH levels were both greater than 40, this would be consistent with
   a. Anovulation.
   b. Microadenoma of pituitary.
   c. Hypothalamic amenorrhea.
   d. End-organ/outflow tract obstruction.
   e. Ovarian failure.

5. Match the clinical situation with the most appropriate therapy described.
   a. Amenorrhea secondary to anovulation in a 30-year-old patient not currently sexually active
   b. Amenorrhea secondary to premature ovarian failure in a 38-year-old gravida 3, para 3 patient who has had a tubal ligation.

c. Hypothalamic amenorrhea in a 20-year-old cross-country runner who is currently sexually active.

   (1) Oral contraceptive pills

   (2) Estrogen replacement therapy

   (3) Monthly progestin withdrawal

   (4) Ovulation induction

Answers appear on page 449.

Vaginal Bleeding

ALAN G. MOORE

INITIAL VISIT

SUBJECTIVE

Patient Identification and Presenting Problem. Susan is a 22-year-old Caucasian woman who presents because of cramping and vaginal bleeding.

Present Illness. Susan's last menstrual period was 6 weeks ago. She complains of 2 days of vaginal bleeding without passage of tissue and lower abdominal cramping greater on the left than on the right. She denies any lightheadedness, dizziness, shoulder pain, dysuria, or change in bowel habits.

Past Medical History. Susan had asthma until age 12 years and had an appendectomy at 8 years of age. She is otherwise healthy, with no chronic medical problems. Her menarche was at age 13. Her periods are 28 to 40 days in interval, 4 days in length, with cramps for the first 2 days. *Contraception:* Susan has used oral contraceptives since 17 years of age and stopped them to achieve her two pregnancies. Her last use of birth control pills was 2 months ago. There is no history of IUD use. *OB history:* Susan had one normal spontaneous vaginal delivery 2 years ago. Her antepartum, intrapartum, and postpartum course was uncomplicated, except for some spotting in the 1st trimester that resolved. *Gynecologic history:* One episode of pelvic inflammatory disease was treated on an outpatient basis when Susan was 18 years old. *Papanicolaou smears:* Human papillomavirus was identified on her Pap smear at the time of her last pregnancy. Colposcopic examination at that time was within normal limits. Her Pap smear last year showed squamous atypia, and Susan was supposed to return for another colposcopy but has not kept that appointment. There is no history of DES exposure, infertility, or uterine abnormality.

Family History. Susan's parents are alive and well. There are no siblings. There is no family history of birth defects, chromosome disorders, or mental retardation.

Health Habits. Susan has smoked one-half pack of cigarettes per day for the last 5 years and occasionally drinks alcohol socially.

Social History. Susan has been married 3 years and denies any marital problems. Her husband is a construction worker, and she does not work outside the home. The highest level of education Susan achieved was high school.

Review of Systems. Noncontributory.

OBJECTIVE

Physical Examination. Susan's height is 63 inches; her weight is 105 lb; her blood pressure is 110/60 with a pulse rate of 78 lying down and 105/60 with a pulse rate of 85 sitting; and her temperature is 98.9°F. Susan is a well-developed, well-nourished Caucasian female in no acute distress. The physical examination is unremarkable, except for the abdominal examination, which reveals a soft abdomen without masses, some tenderness in both lower quadrants, left greater than the right, without rebound or guarding. *Pelvic examination:* The external genitalia are within normal limits; there is a small amount of blood in the posterior fornix and no bulge in the cul-de-sac. The cervix is closed to ring forceps, with a slight trickle of blood, and parous in appearance. The uterus is 4 to 6 weeks in size and anteverted. The adnexa are slightly tender; the right is $1 \times 2 \times 2$ cm and minimally tender; the left is $2 \times 3 \times 2$ cm and slightly more tender. Rectovaginal examination is confirmatory.

Laboratory Tests: Urine HCG positive, hematocrit 36, hemoglobin 12, WBC count 8.9. Quantitative β-HCG performed stat is 926 mIU. Susan's blood type is O negative. A vaginal probe ultrasound is reported as a probable empty uterus, no identifiable gestational sac or fetal pole, but a decidual reaction is identified with a small amount of blood or fluid in the uterine cavity consistent with early pregnancy or a pseudosac with possible ectopic pregnancy. No adnexal masses are identified, and there is no fluid in the cul-de-sac. There is a 3-cm cyst on the left ovary that probably represents a corpus luteum cyst.

ASSESSMENT

Working Diagnosis. Susan most likely has either a potential miscarriage or an unruptured ectopic pregnancy. While there is a small chance that Susan could have an early normal intrauterine pregnancy with implantation bleeding, the fact that no clear-cut, identifiable gestational sac can be seen on vaginal probe ultrasound makes this diagnosis unlikely. Susan could be undergoing a spontaneous abortion, which would account for her bleeding, cramping, and empty uterus on ultrasound, assuming that she has unknowingly passed some of or all her products of conception. Of course, the most worrisome diagnosis would be an ectopic pregnancy, probably unruptured, since Susan is clinically stable. Susan's history of pelvic inflammatory disease makes the possibility of ectopic pregnancy even more likely, since the frequency is associated with a history of prior tubal damage from pelvic inflammatory disease. Susan's left-sided pain is worrisome as well, but it could be due to the corpus luteum cyst identified on the left by ultrasound.

Differential Diagnoses. (1) *Intrauterine pregnancy*, (2) *spontaneous abortion*, (3) *ectopic pregnancy*.

Bleeding with or without cramping occurs in approximately 30% of all pregnancies. Roughly half of these go into a spontaneous miscarriage, and the other half go on to term pregnancy. However, a clinician must always be on the alert for the 1% to 2% of these patients who bleed and who will turn out to have an ectopic pregnancy. With ultrasound and quantitative β-HCG determination, early diagnosis should be facilitated to rule out an ectopic pregnancy versus a viable intrauterine pregnancy versus a spontaneous abortion. The first step in the evaluation is, of course, to perform an examination. If the patient is hemodynamically unstable or has a surgical abdomen, then, of course, the diagnosis of a ruptured ectopic pregnancy is easy and the patient will be taken directly to the operating room. Susan is clinically stable, however, and further evaluation is in order. If Susan had passed tissue or tissue had been seen in an open cervical os, it could be sent for pathology to identify products of conception, thus confirming intrauterine pregnancy and spontaneous abortion. Material that appears to be tissue occasionally can represent a decidual cast that is passed in the setting of an ectopic pregnancy, however, and this is why all tissue that is passed must undergo pathologic diagnosis to confirm intrauterine products of conception versus the decidual cast of an ectopic pregnancy. If the cervix is closed, the evaluation must proceed further to rule out an ectopic pregnancy or, if an intrauterine pregnancy is found, to determine the viability of the intrauterine pregnancy to rule out spontaneous abortion.

When ruling out an ectopic pregnancy, the goal is to clearly identify an intrauterine pregnancy on the vaginal sonogram, since a simultaneous ectopic pregnancy and intrauterine pregnancy is a rare event, occurring somewhere between 1 in 5000 to 35,000 pregnancies. The vaginal sonogram has made it easier to identify fetal structures at earlier gestations. In a viable pregnancy, a gestational sac should be identified by 4 to 5 weeks of gestation, a yolk sac by 5 to 6 weeks, and a fetal pole with cardiac motion by 6 to 7 weeks. Fortunately, most episodes of bleeding and cramping in either threatened abortion or ectopic pregnancy occur at 6 to 9 weeks, so in the vast majority of cases you should be able to see an intrauterine pregnancy to rule out an ectopic pregnancy. Once intrauterine products of conception are identified, the task then is to determine the viability of the pregnancy by visualizing cardiac motion. Once cardiac motion has been established, the chance of a spontaneous miscarriage occurring is only 3% to 7%, and the patient can be given a great deal of reassurance that the bleeding will stop and a miscarriage will not occur. For a patient to present with bleeding and cramping at 6 to 7 weeks' gestational age, the best prognosis is to see the cervical os closed and to perform vaginal probe ultrasound that shows a clear-cut intrauterine fetal pole with positive cardiac motion. With this simple test the patient can be reassured that she has an intrauterine pregnancy, that an ectopic pregnancy has essentially been ruled out, and that there is a 93% to 97% chance that the bleeding will stop and she will not abort.

The problem arises because in both an ectopic pregnancy and in an abortion in process, often an intrauterine pregnancy or products of conception cannot be visualized. In this setting, a quantitative β-HCG determination often can be of help. Knowing that the β-HCG normally doubles every 48 to 72 hours in a viable pregnancy, studies have been done to determine at what level an intrauterine pregnancy can be identified in virtually 100% of cases. With the older abdominal ultrasound and the older method of preparation for β-HCG determination, this "discriminatory zone," as it has come to be called, originally turned out to be 6000 to 6500 mIU of β-HCG. That is, once the β-HCG was above 6000 to 6500 mIU, one should have been able to see an intrauterine gestational sac on ultrasound and, if not, this implied an ectopic pregnancy. If, on the other hand, the level was less than 6000 to 6500 mIU and the uterus was empty, this was nondiagnostic, and the recommendation was to calculate the number of days it would take for the actual level to climb above this "discriminatory zone" and then repeat the β-HCG determination and the sonogram. The problem with this older "discriminatory zone" was that the levels were so high that the majority of ectopics fell well below the "discriminatory zone," and therefore, the scheme was of little clinical utility. Vaginal sonography and the refined β-HCG technique have allowed us to move the "discriminatory zone" down to 1000 to 1500 mIU. The same principles apply, but now the majority of ectopics will be in this range, and the scheme is very helpful to rule out ectopics earlier in less clinically obvious situations such as Susan represents. If the repeat β-HCG determination is now above the zone and still no intrauterine pregnancy is seen, again, an ectopic pregnancy is suggested. If an intrauterine pregnancy is seen, an ectopic pregnancy is ruled out. If the rise is abnormal or falls, an abnormal pregnancy is diagnosed. If the suspicion is more likely a spontaneous miscarriage, a D&C can be performed, and if products of conception are seen on the pathology report, a spontaneous miscarriage is confirmed. If no products of conception can be identified by D&C, however, the clinician has the choice of performing a laparoscopy to rule out an ectopic pregnancy, or if the patient is completely asymptomatic and it is likely the patient has had a complete spontaneous miscarriage as the reason no products of conception are identified at D&C, then the patient's β-HCG level can simply be followed until it comes down to zero, with laparoscopy reserved for the occasional patient who becomes symptomatic again or in whom the titers do not fall completely to zero.

PLAN

Diagnostic. In Susan there is a questionable intrauterine pregnancy, and the β-HCG on the first level is below the "discriminatory zone." Susan has irregular periods, so she could be as little as 4 to 5 weeks pregnant with physiologic bleeding from implantation, and her pain could be secondary to the left corpus luteum cyst that produced the pregnancy. These findings also could represent a spontaneous miscarriage in progress, with most or all of the tissue having been passed. In this case, the β-HCG level would likely be falling, and the uterus would be almost empty on ultrasound, except for the blood in the cavity, which can create a "pseudosac" effect. Lastly, of course, it could represent an ectopic pregnancy, with this "pseudosac" again being the effect of the β-HCG on the endometrium and the associated bleeding. Since the initial level of β-HCG is 926, however, we will have to wait the 48 to 72 hours for the β-HCG to double over the "discriminatory zone" of 1000 to 1500. If the level rises to the expected range of about 1800 in that time period, we should be able to see a clear-cut intrauterine pregnancy by vaginal sonogram if, in fact, this is an early normal pregnancy. If the level rises but no pregnancy is seen, this will confirm the suspicion of an ectopic pregnancy, and laparoscopy is indicated. If the levels rise abnormally or fall, an abnormal pregnancy is diagnosed, and either a D&C or laparoscopy are performed, depending on the clinical picture at the time.

Therapeutic. Susan is told to rest as her symptoms dictate and to return in 48 hours for a repeat β-HCG determination.

Patient Education. It is extremely important to give Susan ectopic precautions, that is, to call as soon as possible if there is increased bleeding, increased cramping, orthostatic symptoms, or increased pain, since an ectopic pregnancy has not been ruled out. One must emphasize the potentially serious consequences of a rupture of an ectopic pregnancy to reinforce compliance. Susan should be instructed to save any tissue that she passes and should be given a sterile cup in which to save it.

Disposition. Susan was sent home with a lab slip for a β-HCG determination to be performed in 48 hours and was given an appointment for the afternoon of the day of the β-HCG determination to follow up with the results.

FIRST FOLLOW-UP VISIT

SUBJECTIVE

Susan returns in 48 hours after having the β-HCG determination done that morning and says that she is still bleeding and cramping but has not seen any tissue. She denies any of the ectopic symptoms she was told about.

OBJECTIVE

Susan's vital signs are unchanged, as is her examination. Follow-up β-HCG results show a level of 780 mIU, a distinct fall from her previous level of 926 mIU.

ASSESSMENT

This is clearly an abnormal pregnancy. It is either an incomplete spontaneous abortion, since Susan is still bleeding, or an ectopic pregnancy. Since Susan is clinically stable, the decision is made to first do a D&C, and if products of conception are identified, this will stop the bleeding and complete the spontaneous abortion. If no products of conception are identified, the patient will need laparoscopy.

PLAN

A gynecology consultant is called, who agrees with the plan. Susan is admitted to the hospital that evening and undergoes a D&C. Scant tissue is obtained that shows decidua only on frozen section. Laparoscopy is therefore performed, which shows an unruptured 2-cm left ampullary ectopic pregnancy. The gynecologist does a linear salpingotomy through the laparoscope because the ectopic pregnancy is unruptured and small and is therefore able to conserve the tube with minimal blood loss. Susan is discharged the next morning with serial β-HCG determinations to follow until they fall to zero. Since Susan is Rh negative, she also will receive RhoGam. She will be told that she has only a 60% chance of achieving any pregnancy in the future, and if she does, she will be at increased risk of another ectopic (approximately 10% to 15%). Susan also will be told that she needs to come in as early as possible after a missed period to make sure that she has an intrauterine pregnancy.

DISCUSSION

As this case illustrates, the early diagnosis of ectopic pregnancy has been revolutionized by β-HCG determinations and vaginal probe ultrasound. In the past, up to 80% of ectopic pregnancies were ruptured at diagnosis, with a resulting high maternal mortality and morbidity, but now, because of improved technology, well over

80% of ectopic pregnancies are diagnosed before they rupture, resulting in saved lives and preserved tubal fertility in many cases. Likewise, the ability to visualize positive cardiac motion on vaginal ultrasound examination as early as 6 to 7 weeks helps gives reassurance to patients with established intrauterine pregnancies who are worried about threatened abortion. Often the answer can be given on the same day of presentation with a stat β-HCG determination and vaginal ultrasound and in the remaining cases after a repeat β-HCG determination and/or ultrasound in a few days. Of course, some ectopic pregnancies will still rupture and present as an acute abdomen and be hemodynamically unstable. However, these patients pose no difficulties in diagnosis and usually go straight to the operating room from the emergency room. They are becoming increasingly rare with the advent of this new technology, however.

SUGGESTED READING

Ectopic pregnancy. In DeCherny AH (ed.): Obstetrics and Gynecology Clinics of North America. Philadelphia, W.B. Saunders, 1991.

Noller KL, Avant RF: Obstetrics. In Rakel RE (ed.): Textbook of Family Practice, 4th ed. Philadelphia, W.B. Saunders, 1990, pp. 605–606.

Sutherland J, Nichols-Johnson V. Office gynecology. In Rakel RE (ed.): Textbook of Family Practice, 4th ed. Philadelphia, W.B. Saunders, 1990, p. 812.

QUESTIONS

1. In a normally growing pregnancy, the β-HCG levels double every
   a. 12 to 24 hours.
   b. 24 to 48 hours.
   c. 48 to 72 hours.
   d. 72 to 96 hours.
   e. 7 days.

2. The "discriminatory zone" is that level of β-HCG above which
   a. An ectopic pregnancy will be able to be seen on ultrasound.
   b. Most ectopic pregnancies occur.
   c. An ectopic pregnancy is ruled out.
   d. A viable intrauterine pregnancy should be seen on ultrasound.
   e. There is no need to do further β-HCG determinations.

3. The most reliable finding that helps rule out an ectopic pregnancy is
   a. A closed os on pelvic examination.
   b. Uterine examination that is consistent with dates at 6 weeks' gestation.
   c. Intrauterine pregnancy seen on ultrasound.
   d. Extrauterine pregnancy not seen on ultrasound.
   e. Rising β-HCG levels.

4. An empty uterus on ultrasound and a single β-HCG above 1000 mIU in a patient who is actively bleeding and cramping is compatible with all the following diagnoses except
   a. Ectopic pregnancy.
   b. Complete spontaneous abortion.
   c. Incomplete spontaneous abortion.
   d. Normal intrauterine early pregnancy.
   e. Abdominal pregnancy.

Answers appear on page 450.

Contraception

JANET P. REALINI

INITIAL VISIT

SUBJECTIVE

Patient Identification and Presenting Problem. Beverly L. is a 32-year-old woman who comes in for her annual pelvic examination. She has been divorced for about a year, is beginning to date, and wants a reliable form of birth control.

Present Illness. Beverly has had two pregnancies; one pregnancy occurred at age 20 and was terminated by a therapeutic abortion. The second occurred 3 years ago and resulted in the delivery of a term infant—her son, who is now 2 years old. Beverly's first pregnancy occurred while she was relying on the "withdrawal technique," or "coitus interruptus," although she sometimes used condoms without spermicide. Following the abortion, she took oral contraceptives for 9 years. Beverly married at age 26 and discontinued oral contraceptives in order to get pregnant. After her son was born, she used a diaphragm to avoid pregnancy until she and her husband separated. She has not used any contraception for the past year because she has not been sexually active.

Beverly had no problems with the oral contraceptives other than spotting and bleeding between periods. This developed after years on the pill and resolved after she changed to another oral contraceptive formulation.

Beverly's periods are fairly regular, occurring every 24 to 30 days and lasting about 5 days. She has some premenstrual bloating and moderate cramps on the first day or two of her menses. The amount of bleeding seems more than before she had her son but is similar to the periods she had before she took birth control pills. Beverly's last menstrual period began 2 weeks ago and was normal for her.

Past Medical History. Beverly had asthma as a child, but she has had no asthma symptoms for many years. She has never had venous thrombosis, pulmonary embolism, or other cardiovascular problems. She had her appendix removed at age 8 and broke her right arm in a fall at age 10. She takes no medications and has no known drug allergies.

Family History. Beverly's parents are living and well, although her father had a heart attack several years ago at age 60. Beverly has two brothers, who are well. Her maternal grandparents died at advanced age of unknown causes; her paternal grandmother is 92 and has hypertension. Her paternal grandfather died in an automobile accident.

Health Habits. Beverly does not smoke cigarettes. She tried marijuana in high school but does not use it or any other recreational drugs now. She drinks alcohol only occasionally. She wears seat belts but does not exercise regularly. She tries to eat a balanced diet and avoids high-fat foods.

Social History. Beverly is an elementary school teacher and finds it stressful being a single parent. Her parents live in the same community and are supportive, often helping to care for her son when he is too ill to attend day care. She and her husband separated after years of an unhappy marriage, and he is planning to marry someone else.

Review of Systems. Beverly has some mild symptoms she attributes to anxiety, including worrying about her son's health and about finances. However, she is sleeping and eating well. She has occasional headaches, but they are not severe, nor are they preceded by auras. She has had several vaginal yeast infections in her life. She has some vaginal discharge now, but there is no foul odor or itching.

OBJECTIVE

Physical Examination. Beverly's vital signs are normal, with a blood pressure of 116/70. Beverly is mildly obese and in no distress. Her breast examination is negative for masses and discharge, and her axillae are free of nodes. Her pelvic examination reveals a normal marital introitus and a small amount of white vaginal discharge. The cervix has no lesions, appears parous, and is nontender on motion. The uterus is small, firm, mobile, anteverted, and nontender. The adnexae are without masses or tenderness, and a rectovaginal examination confirms the findings.

Laboratory Tests. Wet saline preparation of the vaginal discharge shows normal epithelial cells. No yeast cells are visible on potassium hydroxide preparation. A Pap smear is sent, as is a serum cholesterol.

ASSESSMENT

Working Diagnosis. Beverly is an essentially healthy woman in need of contraception. In addition, she should have a screening serum cholesterol determination as part of her health maintenance program. She appears to be coping well with recent stresses. The vaginal discharge appears to be normal: It is not symptomatic, and the microscopic findings are normal.

Differential "Diagnosis": Contraceptive Options. Many contraceptive options are available, each with its advantages and disadvantages, risks and benefits. The task of the family physician is to assist a woman (or couple) in making an informed choice from the options that are appropriate for her.

In Beverly's case, reversibility is probably a necessity, since she is recently divorced and may be interested in having more children in the future. High effectiveness is likely to be another of her requirements for her method of birth control because of her dating situation, although the level of effectiveness she will require to feel comfortable is not yet clear and should be explored. How high a failure rate would be acceptable to her? How big of a disaster would an accidental pregnancy be for her? How would she feel about abortion if an accidental pregnancy occurred? Table 20–15 summarizes the typical and lowest expected failure rates of birth control methods.

Because Beverly will be dating and not be in a stable, mutually monogamous relationship, at least at first, she may be at risk for exposure to sexually transmitted diseases (STDs). Some contraceptive methods have advantages for Beverly in that they offer some protection from these infections, and others are inappropriate for someone at some risk of STDs. No matter which contraceptive method she chooses, the family physician should discuss with her the risks of sexual activity and "safe sex" practices.

In addition, the family physician must be aware of the presence of contraindications to the various contraceptive methods (see Tables 20–16 and 20–17). "Absolute" contraindications proscribe use of the method under any circumstances. "Relative" contraindications are reasons to avoid a method, but individual considerations may override relative contraindications. When a relative contraindication is present, the task is to weigh the risks and benefits of each of the patient's options in coming to a decision. A woman who has many other sat-

TABLE 20–15. EFFECTIVENESS OF CONTRACEPTIVE METHODS

METHOD	FAILURE RATE*	
	Lowest Expected	Typical
Chance	86	86
Spermicides	3	21
Periodic abstinence:		20
Calendar	9	
Ovulation (cervical mucus) method	3	
Symptothermal†	2	
Postovulation (basal body termperature)	1	
Withdrawal (coitus interruptus)	4	18
Cap (with spermicide)	6	15
Sponge:		
Parous women	9	28
Nulliparous women	6	18
Diaphragm (with spermicide)	6	18
Condom (without spermicide)	2	12
Intrauterine device:		3
Progesterone T	2.0	
Copper T 380A	0.8	
Oral contraceptives:		3
Combination	0.1	
Progestin only	0.5	
Depot medroxyprogesterone acetate	0.3	0.3
Norplant implants	0.04	0.04
Female sterilization	0.2	0.4
Male sterilization	0.1	0.15

*Percentage of couples experiencing an accidental pregnancy during the first year of use.

†Cervical mucus (ovulation) method supplemented by calendar in the preovulatory and basal body temperature in the postovulatory phase.

Source: Adapted from Trussell J, Hatcher RA, Cates W, et al. Contraceptive failure in the United States: An update. Stud Fam Plann 1990; 21:51–4. (Used with permission from the Population Council.)

TABLE 20–16. ORAL CONTRACEPTIVES: CONTRAINDICATIONS

ABSOLUTE
Thromboembolism
Cerebrovascular disease
Coronary artery disease
Undiagnosed abnormal genital bleeding
Known or suspected pregnancy
Estrogen-dependent malignancy (including breast, endometrium, melanoma)
Benign or malignant liver tumor that developed during estrogen use

RELATIVE
Hypertension
Diabetes mellitus or history of gestational diabetes
Hyperlipidemia
Liver disease
Cholestatic jaundice of pregnancy
Smokers over 35 years old
Severe migraine
Age over 40 (unless at low cardiovascular risk)

isfactory contraceptive methods from which to choose may be able to avoid a method that is relatively contraindicated for her. On the other hand, a woman whose only alternatives are pregnancy or other, less acceptable methods may use a method that is relatively contraindi-

TABLE 20–17. INTRAUTERINE DEVICES: CONTRAINDICATIONS

ABSOLUTE
Pregnancy, known or suspected
Undiagnosed abnormal genital bleeding
Gynecologic malignancy, known or suspected (including unresolved abnormal Pap smear)
Acute cervicitis
Previous major pelvic surgery
Abnormalities of the uterus with a distorted uterine cavity
History of ectopic pregnancy
Presence or history of pelvic infection
Presence or history of sexually transmitted disease
Presence or history of postpartum endometritis or infected abortion

RELATIVE
Dysmenorrhea
Hypermenorrhea
Multiple sexual partners
Nulliparity
Anemia
Coagulopathy
Congenital or rheumatic heart disease
Corticosteroid therapy

cated for her—especially if pregnancy would be medically dangerous or psychologically disastrous for her.

The patient's preferences and those of her sexual partner are also important in the choice of a contraceptive method. Her previous experiences with methods may influence her choice. Her lifestyle and health concerns are also important. For example, some women prefer to avoid use of hormones; others find it distracting or embarrassing to use any device at the time of intercourse.

Combination estrogen–progestin oral contraceptives (OCs) are a definite possibility for Beverly. They have the advantage of being highly effective when taken properly and readily reversible if she decides to have a baby. She has had satisfactory previous experience with them and has no contraindications to them. However, they do have drawbacks as well. They require good compliance to be effective: She will have to remember to take her pill every day. They also have "minor" side effects, such as nausea and breakthrough bleeding, although these are generally mild and transient and are easily managed. OCs are associated with rare, serious cardiovascular thromboembolic events, including venous thromboembolism, myocardial infarction, and stroke, but the risk of these is minimal for young, nonsmoking women. OCs do not protect well against STDs, although they may reduce the risk of pelvic inflammatory disease. If STDs are a concern, Beverly may need to have her partner(s) use condoms, in addition to her use of OCs.

The "minipill" contains a small dose of progestin and no estrogen. Because of frequent bleeding abnormalities and the need for exact, unfailing compliance, minipills are seldom considered in women who are candidates for the more effective combination OCs.

Norplant, a system of six rods inserted under the skin on the inside of the arm, slowly releases a progestin. It is extremely effective for 5 years and is reversible with surgical removal. Norplant is an option that Beverly should consider because of its high effectiveness and reversibility. However, it does not protect against STDs, and it is relatively expensive if used for only short periods of time. Beverly may be unsure for how long she would want to use it. Other disadvantages include frequent irregular bleeding and, occasionally, weight gain. On the other hand, Norplant has the advantage of requiring little patient compliance. If Beverly would have trouble remembering to take a pill every day, Norplant may offer her freedom from worry about using her method correctly.

Depot medroxyprogesterone acetate injections are ordinarily considered only when contraceptive options are quite limited, since they are not approved by the FDA for contraception.

Intrauterine devices (IUDs) are not appropriate for Beverly at this stage of her life because she is not in a stable, mutually monogamous relationship. IUDs are very effective in preventing pregnancy and have the advantage of requiring little patient compliance once they are inserted. However, because of the increased risk of pelvic inflammatory disease and subsequent tubal infertility, IUDs are not appropriate for women at risk for STDs.

Several of the barrier methods of contraception are appropriate options for Beverly. Condoms, especially if used with spermicide, are the most effective of these methods both in preventing pregnancy and in reducing the risk of STDs. Vaginal spermicides, diaphragms, and cervical caps are slightly less effective for both contraception and STD prevention but are more convenient for some women because cooperation from her partner is not necessary. A diaphragm or cervical cap could be fitted at this visit if Beverly were interested. Fitting of cervical caps requires special training. The Today contraceptive sponge has a relatively high failure rate in parous women like Beverly and thus should not be as strongly considered.

Periodic abstinence methods are useful and helpful for many women. The "calendar method" proscribes intercourse on fertile days of a woman's cycle. The earliest fertile day is the length of her shortest cycle minus 18; the latest fertile day is the length of her longest cycle minus 11. The character of cervical mucus also may be followed to help determine the fertile period ("ovulation method"). "Postovulation" periodic abstinence is the most effective rhythm method: Intercourse is limited to days at least 3 days after the ovulatory basal body temperature rise.

Because of their relatively high failure rate in actual use, periodic abstinence methods are more likely to be attractive to women or couples with religious restrictions on their contraceptive choices and to those who feel the risk of pregnancy is acceptable. A stable and cooperative couple relationship is important for good compliance with these methods. Beverly may reject periodic abstinence because of its lower effectiveness or because of its limitations on when intercourse can occur safely. These methods also offer no protection against STDs.

"Withdrawal," or "coitus interruptus," means that the penis is withdrawn from the vagina prior to ejaculation. It is inexpensive but not highly effective. It may not be appropriate for Beverly because it requires cooperation from her partner, and her situation is unclear and changing. Withdrawal is unlikely to offer protection from STDs.

Abstinence from sexual activity and noncoital sex are contraceptive alternatives but usually have been rejected by the patient before seeking medical assistance. There are some people who may not have considered these possibilities, however.

When a couple has completed its family and desires no more children, sterilization becomes an option. Although progress has been made in reversal techniques, these procedures should be considered permanent and would thus be inappropriate for Beverly at this time of her life.

PLAN

Diagnostic. Pap smear and serum cholesterol were sent. No other laboratory tests or x-rays are indicated.

Therapeutic. Beverly's contraceptive options were reviewed with her, and her preferences and input were elicited. She thought about a Norplant implant but was concerned about the likelihood of menstrual irregularities. She considered several of the barrier methods but settled on combination oral contraceptives because of their high effectiveness and her previous satisfactory experience with them. Her plan was to get to know any potential sex partners well and to use condoms in addition to OCs if significant STD risk was possible.

A triphasic oral contraceptive was chosen because it minimizes both estrogen and progestin dose. A 28-day pack was prescribed so that she would only have to remember to take a pill every day and not have to remember when to start and when to stop her pills.

Patient Education. Use of the OCs was reviewed with Beverly. She was to start the pills on the first day of her period and take one pill every day at the same time of day. If she missed a pill, she was to take it as soon as she remembered; if 24 hours had passed since the missed pill, two pills were to be taken together. If two pills were missed in a cycle, she was instructed to use a backup barrier method of birth control until the end of the cycle. If three or more pills were missed, the pills should be discontinued, a barrier method used, and the pills restarted when her period began. She was encouraged to call the office with any questions she might have.

Beverly was told that spotting or bleeding in the first few cycles is common; she should not be alarmed if it happens to her. This breakthrough bleeding usually goes away within the first few months without specific intervention. If Beverly has bleeding, she should continue the pills; she was encouraged to call the office if she had questions or needed reassurance. Other potential "minor" side effects were reviewed with her, such as nausea, feeling bloated, and headache. Signs and symptoms of serious complications (leg pain or swelling, chest pain, shortness of breath, neurologic symptoms, and progressive headaches) were reviewed. Beverly was given a patient package insert to read.

Beverly also was instructed in the proper use of condoms. Latex condoms protect against STDs, whereas the expensive "skin" condoms do not prevent STD transmission reliably. Oil or petroleum-based lubricants destroy latex condoms rapidly and should not be used. After coitus, the penis must be removed from the vagina prior to loss of erection; the rim of the condom should be held at the base of the penis during removal. The condom should be inspected to make sure it is intact and then discarded.

Disposition. Beverly was given a 3-month supply of low-dose OCs, and a follow-up appointment was scheduled for 3 months.

FIRST FOLLOW-UP VISIT

SUBJECTIVE

Beverly reported that she had been taking one pill every day without fail and that her withdrawal bleeding during the 4th week of each pack had been lighter than her usual periods, with a lot fewer cramps than usual. During the 2nd pill pack, she had some spotting during the 2nd week of the cycle, but this resolved. She had not missed any pills. She had no complaints and was relieved to have a reliable form of contraception. She was sexually active with one partner, who, in turn, had no other partners. He had no known risk factors for HIV infection.

OBJECTIVE

Beverly's blood pressure remained essentially unchanged at 108/68. Her Pap smear had been reported as normal, and her total serum cholesterol was 180.

ASSESSMENT

Beverly seems to tolerate the OCs well. The early breakthrough bleeding appears to have resolved on its own and needs no further investigation or therapy.

Low-dose OCs such as the ones prescribed for Beverly often have associated breakthrough bleeding. When bleeding occurs during the first few months of OC use, it is generally self-limited and requires no intervention other than reassurance. With the low doses of estrogen and progestin in triphasic OCs, taking the pill at the same time every day may minimize breakthrough bleeding.

If breakthrough bleeding occurs after many months on the pill, it often resolves with switching to another low-dose pill. Alternatively, small doses of additional es-

trogen may be given until the bleeding stops for one or two cycles; this often allows the patient to continue the same OC preparation. Lack of withdrawal bleeding after months on a pill is another common problem. After pregnancy is excluded, switching to another pill may be necessary.

PLAN

Beverly was given a prescription for 10 packs of pills. She will need a Pap smear and pelvic examination once a year, and her blood pressure should be measured at least once a year. (Some physicians prefer to check the blood pressure of patients on OCs twice a year.) Beverly was again encouraged to call about any problems, and the protocols for missed pills were reviewed, as were the potentially serious symptoms previously discussed.

QUESTIONS

1. Of the following, the most effective method of contraception is
   a. Combination estrogen–progestin oral contraceptives.
   b. Condoms used with spermicide.
   c. The Today vaginal sponge.
   d. Periodic abstinence based on a calendar method.

2. Absolute contraindications to the use of oral contraceptives include
   a. Breast cancer.
   b. Moderate obesity.
   c. A history of postpartum thrombophlebitis.
   d. A history of preeclampsia.
   e. Fibrocystic breast disease.

3. Contraindications to the use of an intrauterine device include
   a. Trichomonal vaginitis.
   b. Multiparity.
   c. Irregular vaginal bleeding of uncertain etiology.
   d. Hypertension.
   e. Previous pelvic inflammatory disease.

4. When counseling patients about contraception, the family physician's task is best described as
   a. Choosing the method with the lowest health risk.
   b. Recommending the method with the highest possible effectiveness.
   c. Avoiding nonreversible methods.
   d. Assisting patients in reviewing their options.
   e. Explaining which method is the best choice.

Answers appear on page 450.

Shortness of Breath

ROLAND A. GOERTZ

INITIAL VISIT

SUBJECTIVE

Patient Identification. John H., a 53-year-old diesel mechanic, has worked for his company for over 15 years. He has progressed to the position of supervisor and presents to the doctor after no interim visits for over 10 years.

Presenting Problem. John states he has been healthy for most of his life. However, he details a troublesome episode of breathlessness while playing a backyard game of football with his sons 2 days earlier.

Present Illness. John describes feeling guilty about spending too little time with his family the last few months because of a heavy work schedule demanding much overtime. He was particularly sensitive that he had not participated in many activities with his two sons, one age 14 and the other age 12. The fall weather had lifted one of his all too frequent episodes of fatigue, and a game of backyard football seemed appropriate.

His sons were ecstatic, and they began a vigorous game. John began experiencing breathlessness soon after the game had begun. The breathlessness became worse and worse, and he would have had to stop, but his wife's call to dinner intervened. This episode frightened John, and he presented to his family physician as soon as he could arrange time off.

John revealed that he has felt fatigued for the past several months. He also noted his belt size seemed to be increasing and his ability to work long hours and lift heavy implements was decreasing. He attributes these problems to "getting older." He also described difficulty sleeping for a number of months. He would arrive home late, slip into bed quietly, and soon notice a "suffocating" feeling. Arising and "getting fresh air" would stop the sensation. Sleeping with his head raised on several pillows prevented the feeling. These night episodes were occasionally accompanied by a dry, "hacking" cough. John also noted three or four episodes of frightening nightmares that terminated with him awaking, feeling severely short of breath. Arising and walking around in his bedroom seemed to resolve these episodes also. He attributed the night-time episodes to his stressful role of supervisor, recently worsened by long hours and a heavy workload.

Past Medical History. John had an appendectomy at age 10 and has been healthy since then. He had no unusual childhood illnesses. He denied any serious accidents or injuries, despite his job risks. He had no known medication allergies, and he was taking no regular medication.

Family History. John's father died at age 67 of a cerebrovascular accident; he had a long history of hypertension. His mother died at age 74 from a myocardial infarction; she also had adult-onset diabetes. John's only brother is 49 years old and healthy, but he also has not had a medical evaluation for a number of years. John did not know how his grandparents had died and knew little about them.

Health Habits. John stopped smoking 3 years ago after a 30 pack-year history (one pack of cigarettes daily for 30 years). He states that the media and his family finally convinced him to stop. He drank heavily before the children were born. He now only occasionally drinks beer, and he never goes out with the "boys" anymore. He denies any illicit drug use. He almost never exercises, saying, "When do I have time?" He has been monogamous. He uses seat belts. He does not follow any particular diet and eats large amounts of red meat, fats, and simple carbohydrates.

Social History. John and his wife have been married 23 years. He voices a stable love for his wife that appears to have strengthened through the years. There have been some problems with his oldest son recently: He stays out late and has been drinking. John feels guilty about the little time he has spent with him. John completed high school and trade school. He has worked as a diesel mechanic all his adult life and with his current employer for over 15 years. His income provides all significant wants.

Review of Systems. John acknowledges periods of fatigue that have worsened recently. He recently bought larger pants and belts. He denies any gastrointestinal or genitourinary symptoms. He admits to feeling anxious and somewhat depressed.

OBJECTIVE

Physical Examination. John's vital signs are blood pressure 180/110, heart rate 88, weight 195 lb, and height 72 in. He appears in no distress but does seem nervous. Physical examination is normal, except for 2+ edema of the feet and mild tenderness with deep palpation over the liver area. Cardiac examination reveals no murmurs or extra sounds. The apical impulse is bounding and slightly laterally displaced. Pulmonary examination is negative.

Laboratory Tests. A multiple-panel blood analysis showed 24 normal values. The liver enzymes were high normal. Urinalysis was normal, except for a slightly increased specific gravity. CBC was normal. ECG demonstrated nonspecific T-wave changes but no signs of acute injury. Chest x-ray showed mild, but definite, generalized cardiomegaly.

ASSESSMENT

Working Diagnoses. *Congestive heart failure* and *pulmonary disease* are the most likely diagnoses that explain John's findings and symptoms.

1. *Congestive heart failure.* Clinically, "heart failure" can be described as a syndrome that causes limitation of a patient's activity because of the heart's inability to function successfully. Congestive heart failure is common and is frequently diagnosed and treated by family physicians. New treatment modalities and appropriate early diagnosis can significantly improve morbidity and mortality (see Rakel RE, *Textbook of Family Practice* for further explanation). The physician must thoroughly evaluate the patient for precipitating and/or underlying causes of congestive heart failure (see Tables 20–18 and 20–19).

Appropriate care includes treatment of any identifiable causes. Coronary artery disease and hypertension (present in John) are the most common causes. The common pathway of the multiple etiologies of heart failure is eventual heart muscle damage and subsequent failure of the heart to adequately pump blood. A combination of classic findings occurs as this process worsens: dyspnea on exertion, paroxysmal nocturnal dyspnea, orthopnea, fluid retention, unexplained weight gain, and easy fatigability. "Dyspnea" (breathlessness) on exertion is often the earliest symptom of heart failure. John's night episodes are classic descriptions of orthopnea and paroxysmal nocturnal dyspnea. "Orthopnea" is dyspnea occurring in the recumbent position. The postural change mentioned above is instrumental in causing this symptom. Sleeping on several pillows to elevate the upper body and relief by assuming the upright posture are often revealed in the patient's history. "Paroxysmal nocturnal dyspnea" is severe shortness of breath with feelings of suffocation that occurs several hours into the night and awakens the patient from sleep. Coughing and wheezing are common. The episodes are often frightening and accompanied by nightmares. Sitting upright or walking around for a period of time usually provides relief. Fluid shifts caused by the postural change from an upright to a recumbent position and a poorly performing heart are factors in producing this symptom.

Weight gain, anorexia, fatigue, and abdominal distension or discomfort are general systemic symptoms seen in congestive heart failure. Systemic venous congestion resulting in distension of the liver is the probable cause of John's right upper quadrant tenderness.

2. *Pulmonary disease.* John has symptoms involving lung function. His past smoking history and possible vapor exposure at work make consideration of other causes of dyspnea imperative. Asthma, pneumonitis, pulmonary fibrosis, chronic obstructive pulmonary disease (COPD), and carcinoma should be considered. These diagnoses became less likely with the finding of an enlarged heart and the absence of any lung lesions or findings of COPD on chest x-ray. The absence of a sudden acute process makes asthma or acute pneumonitis less likely possibilities.

Differential Diagnoses. Congestive heart failure is a "clinical syndrome." Therefore, it is defined by the presence of an array of symptoms and findings. As a clinical syndrome, it is not unto itself a diagnosis unless no underlying cause is identified. When evaluating a clinical syndrome, the physician is asked to pursue a slightly different thought process than when asked to evaluate a certain finding or symptom. Most findings or symptoms generate a list of possible diagnoses that can be ranked from most likely to least likely. For example, dyspnea (one of John's symptoms) has a lengthy list of potential causes, including COPD, asthma, pneumonitis, pleural effusion, pneumothorax, pulmonary embolism, atelectasis, and hyperventilation. The physician's responsibility in evaluating a clinical syndrome such as heart failure is to decide its presence or absence. An extensive search for the array of findings and symptoms is relied on. The list of differential diagnoses is entertained

TABLE 20–18. COMMON PRECIPITATING CAUSES OF HEART FAILURE

Medical noncompliance
Physical, dietary, or emotional excess
Infection
Anemia
Alcohol abuse
Myocardial infarction
Pulmonary embolism
Thyrotoxicosis
Infective endocarditis
Malignant hypertension
Myocarditis
Pregnancy
Arrhythmias

Source: From Rakel RE. Textbook of Family Practice, 4th ed. Philadelphia, W.B. Saunders, 1990, p. 917, with permission.

TABLE 20–19. COMMON CAUSES OF HEART FAILURE

Coronary artery disease:
  Left ventricular failure
  Mitral regurgitation
  Left ventricular aneurysm
  Ruptured ventricular septum
Hypertension
Valvular disease:
  Mitral stenosis
  Mitral regurgitation
  Aortic stenosis
  Aortic regurgitation
  Prosthetic valve malfunction
  Infective endocarditis
Cardiomyopathy:
  Dilated
  Restrictive
  Hypertrophic
Constrictive pericarditis

Source: From Rakel RE. Textbook of Family Practice, 4th ed. Philadelphia, W.B. Saunders, 1990, p. 917, with permission.

when the clinician is fairly certain the syndrome is present. In the case of heart failure, there are classic findings and symptoms. The differential involves multiple complex causes, simplified by the two previous tables. This discussion cannot do justice to all the different etiologies. Further investigation and study of comprehensive texts are required.

PLAN

Diagnostic. Laboratory findings in early congestive heart failure are minimal, and none is specific. The ECG may be normal or reflect evidence of underlying cardiac disease. Chest x-ray may show generalized cardiac enlargement or specific chamber enlargement indicative of a particular cardiac process. Evidence of pulmonary congestion, such as pulmonary artery enlargement, interstitial edema, Kerley's B lines, increased vascularity of the lung apices, or pulmonary effusions, may be seen. An echocardiogram revealing decreased cardiac function is especially useful if the symptom and findings are not sufficient to diagnose heart failure. Nuclear cardiac evaluations and cardiac catheterization may be necessary in a confusing or complicated case. Once the clinical syndrome of congestive heart failure is diagnosed, the goal is to identify underlying treatable disease using specific tests.

Therapeutic

1. Decrease dietary salt to 3 to 4 gm/day, maintain good nutrition and limit calories to prevent obesity, and limit saturated fats to prevent coronary heart disease. Coronary artery disease is the most common cause of congestive heart failure.
2. Physical activity should be restricted to a level below stimulation of symptoms. Adequate sleep and anxiety-relieving techniques are important.
3. Diuretics are a key first-line pharmacologic treatment for hypertension and congestive heart failure. Both these problems warrant treatment. A diuretic, hydrochlorothiazide 25 mg/day, was started. An angiotensin-converting enzyme (ACE) inhibitor such as enalapril (Vasotec), is also a good first-choice drug that may be used to treat both problems. Some studies suggest that the early use of an ACE inhibitor may reduce morbidity and mortality.

Patient Education

1. The patient was instructed to keep daily weight records in order to monitor the effectiveness of the diuretic and the salt-restricted diet.
2. A low-salt and "heart healthy" diet was extensively discussed.
3. Possible side effects of diuretic use should be explained. The likely need of medication "for the rest of his life" to treat hypertension and heart failure was introduced.
4. The mechanisms underlying congestive heart failure were explained. Appropriate reassurance that multiple treatments were available was given.

5. John was urged to openly discuss his situation with his wife and to bring her along at his next visit.

Disposition. John was asked to return in 1 week, but to return earlier if any worsening occurred.

FIRST FOLLOW-UP VISIT

SUBJECTIVE

One week later John was feeling better, with less fatigue, but he was still experiencing exertional dyspnea. He did not have any episodes of dyspnea during the night. He admitted to being anxious.

OBJECTIVE

John appeared in no distress but was obviously anxious. His blood pressure was 154/100. His weight was 190 lb. He no longer had right upper quadrant abdominal tenderness, and his feet had minimal edema. The rest of his examination was normal.

ASSESSMENT

1. *Congestive heart failure* due to years of untreated hypertension was the continuing diagnosis.
2. *Hypertension.*

PLAN

1. Enalapril 5 mg/day was added.
2. A referral to a cardiologist was arranged, with further evaluation to include an echocardiogram. John's presentation with congestive heart failure as the initial problem after years of good health and his continuing symptoms were felt to warrant a thorough evaluation by a cardiologist for any treatable causes. It was hoped that John's anxiety would be relieved by an early referral and later return to the family physician for follow-up.

SUGGESTED READING

Braunwald E (ed.). Heart Disease: A Textbook of Cardiovascular Medicine, 3rd ed. Philadelphia, W. B. Saunders, 1988.
Rakel RE. Textbook of Family Practice, 4th ed. Philadelphia, W. B. Saunders, 1990, pp. 916–922.

QUESTIONS

1. The most frequently noted early symptom of heart failure is
   a. Orthopnea.
   b. Fluid retention.
   c. Dyspnea on exertion.
   d. Paroxysmal nocturnal dyspnea.

2. Specific laboratory findings in early heart failure are
   a. Elevated blood urea nitrogen.

b. Decreased hemoglobin and hematocrit.
c. Hyperkalemia.
d. Elevated creatinine.
e. None of the above.

3. Identification of any precipitating causes of heart failure is important to appropriately treat the disease. Which of the following are possible precipitating causes?
a. Infection
b. Thyroid disease
c. Physical, dietary, or emotional stress
d. Anemia

4. The clinician must extensively evaluate a patient for cause when a clinical syndrome is identified. Congestive heart failure is a clinical syndrome. Common causes are
a. Coronary artery disease.
b. Hypertension.
c. Valvular heart disease.
d. Cardiomyopathy.

Answers appear on page 451.

Nosebleed

JANE E. CORBOY

INITIAL VISIT

SUBJECTIVE

Patient Identification and Presenting Problem. Edward is a 49-year-old white man who is seen for the first time 1 week after an emergency room visit for a nosebleed.

Present Illness. Edward developed epistaxis while making a presentation to the board of directors of the agency where he is an administrator. The bleeding was stopped by the application of direct pressure and ice to the nasal bridge, but it resumed more heavily about an hour later without provocation. He went to the local emergency room, where his blood pressure was found to be 200/120. The emergency room physician gave him a single dose of sublingual nifedipine, which brought Edward's blood pressure down to 160/94. The physician placed an anterior nasal pack, admonished Edward to seek follow-up care with his family physician the following day, and issued a prescription for furosemide (Lasix) 40 mg and labetalol (Normodyne) 200 mg. Edward had the prescriptions filled (at a cost of more than $50) and started taking the pills the following day. He had no further nasal bleeding. Three days later he mentioned the episode to a family physician friend and asked when he could stop taking "all these pills."

Past Medical History. Edward had never been diagnosed with hypertension, although he had several isolated readings of diastolic pressures over 95 mmHg over 5 years ago. He has not seen a primary care physician on a regular basis.

Edward reports frequent upper respiratory infections and bronchitis and one hospitalization for pneumonia. He does not regularly take decongestants, cold preparations, or asthma inhalers. In his early twenties, he was hospitalized for a syncopal episode and had an extensive workup without a definitive diagnosis. Since then, he has taken aspirin three or four times a day to "prevent headaches." He reports heavy alcohol use in his teens and twenties. He moderated his use after urinating blood and being told he would have kidney and liver failure if he continued to drink. He has had no treatment for alcohol-related illnesses. He has no known allergies; his only medications are aspirin and the medications prescribed in the emergency room.

Family History. Edward's mother died in her middle thirties of breast cancer after undergoing what Edward recalls as experimental cobalt treatments that caused extensive radiation damage to the chest wall. Edward's father remarried several times and was in chronically poor health related to alcoholism. He died in his middle fifties in the immediate postoperative period following surgery for kidney stones. He was not known to have hypertension or heart disease. Several paternal uncles also were treated for alcohol-related illnesses, but none was known to have hypertension or heart disease. Edward's paternal grandfather died of a "stroke" at age 70.

Social History. Edward is an administrator for a health services agency. His work involves both day-to-day "crisis management" and long-range program planning and development. He has worked in a variety of settings, including university-level teaching, research, and consulting. Most recently, he worked in a similar agency in another city more than 10 years before moving to his current position 6 months prior to the epistaxis incident.

He describes his reactions to stressful situations as intense, but he prides himself on appearing externally calm and controlled.

Edward has been married for nearly 30 years and has one daughter, age 20, who is away at college, and two stepdaughters in their thirties from his wife's first marriage. He reports no impairment in sexual functioning.

Health Habits. Edward smokes up to three packs of cigarettes a day and has smoked since he was 13 years old. His alcohol intake is less now than in his youth, but occasionally heavy. He has no regular exercise, but about once a month he plays racquetball with great intensity. He usually has only coffee for breakfast, skips lunch, and eats a large dinner, usually at a restaurant. He has not made any effort to modify fat intake. He drinks four to six cups of coffee a day. Several years ago he stopped adding salt to his food.

Review of Systems. Edward generally has been in good health. He reports a persistent nonproductive cough and somewhat decreased stamina over the past few years associated with a 15- to 20-lb weight gain.

OBJECTIVE

Physical Examination. Edward's vital signs in the office included a heart rate of 76 and a blood pressure of 170/114 in both arms while seated and without change on standing. His weight is 190 lb, and his height is 71 in. Head and neck examination was unremarkable, except for the funduscopic examination, which showed mild arteriolar narrowing without hemorrhage or papilledema. The thyroid gland was normal, and the neck was without venous distension or bruit. The heart examination showed a regular rhythm without murmurs, gallops, or rubs, and the peripheral pulses were 2+ throughout without bruits. Auscultation of the lungs revealed a prolonged expiratory phase with occasional wheezes that clear with coughing. Abdominal examination was without masses, bruits, tenderness, or striae.

Laboratory Tests. Edward brought results of laboratory tests obtained in the emergency room, including a normal CBC, clotting studies, and urinalysis. The chemistry profile showed normal electrolytes, glucose, uric acid, and renal and hepatic functions; a total serum cholesterol of 213; and nonfasting triglycerides of 220.

ECG showed a normal sinus rhythm, rate of 84, a QRS axis of 0 degrees, amplitude in lead I of 20 mm, and no ST depression, abnormal Q waves, or T-wave inversion.

ASSESSMENT

Working Diagnoses. The most likely diagnoses to explain Edward's findings are

1. *Essential hypertension.* With diastolic readings of 114 and 120, his hypertension is classified as "moderate" to "severe" (see Tables 20–20 and 20–21). Secondary causes, although unlikely, should be considered (see Differential Diagnoses).

TABLE 20–20. APPROPRIATE TECHNIQUES FOR MEASURING BLOOD PRESSURE

The patient should be seated with the arm bared and supported at heart level.

Measurement should begin after 5 minutes of rest.

The cuff size must be appropriate—the rubber bladder should encircle at least two-thirds of the arm circumference.

A mercury sphygmomanometer is most accurate, followed by a recently calibrated aneroid manometer and then a calibrated electronic device.

Systolic and diastolic readings should be recorded, and the disappearance of sound should be used for the diastolic value.

Two or more readings should be averaged. If the difference between the two is more than 5 mmHg, additional readings should be obtained.

TABLE 20–21. CLASSIFICATION OF BLOOD PRESSURE AND FOLLOW-UP CRITERIA FOR INITIAL BLOOD PRESSURE MEASUREMENT FOR ADULTS AGED 18 YEARS OR OLDER

RANGE, mmHg	CATEGORY*	RECOMMENDED FOLLOW-UP+
Diastolic:		
≤85	Normal blood pressure	Recheck within 2 years
85–89	High normal blood pressure	Recheck within 1 year
90–104	Mild hypertension	Confirm within 2 months
105–114	Moderate hypertension	Evaluate or refer promptly to source of care within 2 weeks
≥115	Severe hypertension	Evaluate or refer immediately
Systolic:		
<140	Normal blood pressure	Recheck within 2 years
140–159	Borderline isolated systolic hypertension	Confirm within 2 months
≥160	Isolated systolic hypertension	Evaluate or refer promptly to source of care within 2 weeks

Source: Adapted from Chobanian, A. The 1988 Report of the Joint National Committee on Detection, Evaluation, and Treatment of High Blood Pressure. Arch Intern Med 1988; 148(5):1023–1038, with permission.

*Classification based on the average of two or more readings on two or more occasions.

†A classification of borderline isolated systolic hypertension (SBP 140 to 159 mmHg) or isolated systolic hypertension (SBP ≥160 mmHg) takes precedence over high normal blood pressure (diastolic blood pressure 85 to 89 mmHg) when both occur in the same person. High normal blood pressure (DBP 85 to 89 mmHg) takes precedence over a classification of normal blood pressure (SBP > 140 mmHg) when both occur in the same person. If recommendations for follow-up of diastolic and systolic blood pressure are different, the shorter recommended time for recheck and referral should take precedence.

2. *Multiple cardiovascular risk factors,* including hypertension, smoking, borderline hypercholesterolemia, sedentary lifestyle, and (possibly) "type A" personality.

Differential Diagnoses

1. *Labile or "white coat" hypertension.* This is unlikely because of the presence of funduscopic and ECG

changes suggesting some degree of underlying sustained hypertension.

2. *Drug-induced hypertension.* Hypertension can be associated with the use of oral contraceptives (not likely here), anabolic steroids, thyroid hormones, appetite suppressants, over-the-counter decongestants, cold preparations, nonsteroidal anti-inflammatory drugs, and some antidepressant medications, especially monoamine oxidase inhibitors.

3. *Renovascular hypertension.* This would be suggested by a renal artery bruit, but one was not heard. A bruit is present in only 50% of patients with renovascular hypertension, and this condition is more likely when accelerated hypertension occurs in a younger person.

4. *Renal parenchymal disease.* This would be suggested by the presence of a history of renal infections, trauma or hematuria, family history of polycystic kidneys, a flank mass on physical examination, or laboratory abnormalities in the urinalysis and renal function.

5. *Pheochromocytoma.* Should be considered if there is a history of episodic palpitations, diaphoresis, weight loss, and headache. Physical findings are those of sympathetic overactivity, such as tachycardia, tremor, sweating, and orthostatic hypotension. Laboratory abnormalities include hyperglycemia, leukocytosis, and elevated hematocrit.

6. *Hyperaldosteronism.* This would be suggested by a history of muscle weakness, cramps, and polyuria and by hypokalemia on initial chemistry profile (before the administration of diuretics).

7. *Cushing's disease.* Suggested by a history of weight gain, physical findings of truncal obesity with striae, and glucose intolerance.

8. *Coarctation of the aorta.* This is associated with symptoms of leg claudication and physical findings of delayed or absent femoral pulses and large discrepancies between readings in the two arms.

PLAN

Diagnostic. The goal of the diagnostic plan is to ascertain the significance of the blood pressure elevation. The specific objectives are as follows:

1. *Confirm the presence of sustained blood pressure elevation.* Edward has had an elevated blood pressure reading twice in a 2-week period. He reports feeling anxious on both occasions and doubts the accuracy of the readings. Review of his records from a podiatrist visit 5 years ago showed a blood pressure of 150/100.

2. *Assess end-organ (heart, kidney, central nervous system, vascular system) damage.* Edward's chemistry profile included normal renal function and urinalysis without blood, protein, or casts, indicating lack of renal parenchymal damage. A normal neurologic examination and lack of history of transient ischemic attack (TIA) or stroke argues against CNS involvement. Funduscopic examination with arteriolar narrowing confirms preexisting hypertension but no retinal damage. ECG showed increased voltage and a borderline (leftward) axis, suggesting early left ventricular enlargement, but it did not meet the criteria for left ventricular

hypertrophy. There was no sign of ischemia or previous myocardial infarction.

3. *Identify other conditions that affect treatment choices (diabetes, asthma or COPD, hyperlipidemia, gout).* Edward's smoking history indicates possible reactive airways or COPD, but it does not suggest the presence of the other conditions. His physical examination suggests some degree of COPD as well. His chemistry profile shows a normal random glucose and uric acid and borderline lipids. A chest x-ray might be considered both to evaluate his lung disease and to confirm the presence or absence of cardiomegaly.

4. *Identify curable secondary causes of hypertension.* As discussed under Differential Diagnoses, Edward's history excludes drug-induced hypertension. He has no history of renal disease, symptoms of pheochromocytoma, hyperaldosteronism, or Cushing's disease. His physical examination displays no signs of coarctation or of the endocrine causes of hypertension. The normal electrolytes and renal function exclude most of the renal and endocrine causes as well.

5. *Evaluate overall cardiovascular risk status.* As noted under Working Diagnoses, Edward's risk factors include smoking, hypertension, hyperlipidemia, and a sedentary lifestyle. His family history is not known. He does not have diabetes mellitus.

All the preceding objectives may be met by a focused history and physical examination, limited laboratory testing (CBC, urinalysis, and serum potassium, glucose, uric acid, blood urea nitrogen, and cholesterol determinations), and an ECG. Patients with suspected secondary hypertension may require more specialized testing.

Therapeutic. The goal of treatment of hypertension is to prevent cardiovascular morbidity and mortality. The specific objectives are

1. To reduce and maintain blood pressure under 140/90.
2. To preserve or improve the patient's well-being.
3. To reduce other cardiovascular risk factors.

The methods include nonpharmacologic and pharmacologic therapy.

NONPHARMACOLOGIC. These modalities are the first line and cornerstone of all other treatments of hypertension.

1. *Weight reduction.* The goal is to achieve a body weight within 15% of ideal body weight by calorie and fat restriction and moderate exercise.

2. *Sodium restriction.* This includes refraining from adding salt to foods and observing sodium labeling on processed foods. Sodium intake should be limited to 1.5 to 2.5 gm/day.

3. *Limitation of alcohol intake.* Alcohol intake should be limited to 1 oz ethanol daily (the amount contained in 24 oz beer, 8 oz wine, or 2 oz 100-proof liquor).

4. *Smoking cessation.* Smoking cessation may have little impact on reduction of blood pressure, but it has a

significant effect on overall cardiac risk status. Smokers should be encouraged to quit and should be counseled on cessation strategies at every opportunity.

5. *Relaxation.* Only modest reductions of blood pressures have been demonstrated, but these techniques may aid patients in dealing with everyday stresses more effectively.

6. *Exercise.* Aerobic activity such as walking, swimming, bicycling, or running when done for 20 to 40 minutes three or four times weekly is helpful in reducing blood pressure and weight and in improving the patient's lipid profiles and general sense of well-being.

7. *Other dietary interventions.* Recent findings suggest that a high potassium intake and an increased intake of calcium and magnesium supplementation may have beneficial effects on blood pressure. In patients taking diuretics, supplementation of potassium may enhance blood pressure control. However, these data are too inconclusive to make recommendations at present. Similarly, while reduced intake of saturated fats and increased intake polyunsaturated fats are associated with lower blood pressure, modifications of dietary fats can be recommended only because of the beneficial effects on blood cholesterol level and reduction of overall cardiac risk factors.

PHARMACOLOGIC. Most patients with moderate to severe hypertension will require one or more antihypertensive medications (Table 20–22). The 1988 report of the Joint National Commission on Diagnosis, Evaluation, and Treatment of Hypertension recommends an "individualized step-care" approach to therapy, considering the patient's other medical conditions, lifestyle, and other characteristics that might affect the efficacy of treatment. The four drug categories considered appropriate first-step treatment include

1. *Diuretics.* Edward expressed concern about his history of renal compromise due to alcohol overuse.

2. *Beta-blockers.* Because of Edward's smoking history and already decreased exercise tolerance, both Edward and his physician felt that a beta-blocker might exacerbate bronchospasm.

3. *Angiotensin-converting enzyme inhibitors.* Because of Edward's preexisting cough, his physician felt that gauging the presence of this side effect would be difficult. Also, Edward again expressed reservations about the possible renal effects.

4. *Calcium-channel blockers.* Despite Edward's concerns about the possible side effect of headache, this category of drugs has the least troublesome side-effect profile and offers the advantage of a once-daily dosage regimen with the sustained-release formulations of nifedipine or verapamil. Edward agreed to try Procardia XL 30 mg daily for a 2-week period. He was given samples sufficient to last 20 days and asked to return for a follow-up visit to assess drug efficacy and adverse effects.

Patient Education. The goal of patient education is to increase adherence to the treatment plan (Table 20–23). The specific objectives include the following:

1. *Inform the patient of the significance of the disease.* Edward was given specific figures showing the increasing risk of heart disease with each additional cardiovascular risk factor. He was surprised and resistant to accepting that hypertension is asymptomatic and a lifelong condition.

2. *Assess patient motivation to adhere to treatment and possible barriers to compliance.* Edward was frightened by the bleeding episode and wanted to avert future episodes. He was not initially convinced of the validity of his blood pressure readings, so he was advised to monitor his blood pressure at home or work. He was resistant to the idea of lifelong medication and expressed numerous concerns about potential side effects or complications of treatment.

3. *Describe the nonpharmacologic methods of treatment.* Edward was given information on a prudent diet for weight reduction, sodium restriction, and limitation of caffeine and alcohol. He agreed to start a walking program and to consider relaxation techniques such as muscle relaxation, deep breathing, and visualization. He was not willing to stop smoking now.

4. *Educate the patient on the basic pathophysiology of hypertension, rationale for therapy, and treatment options.* Edward and his physician discussed each of the medication categories, including efficacy, potential side effects, and cost. They discussed a target blood pressure and agreed on a mutually acceptable treatment plan, including timing of follow-up visits, use of medication, and Edward's above-mentioned lifestyle changes.

FIRST FOLLOW-UP VISIT

SUBJECTIVE

Edward reports no nose bleeds. He has been checking his blood pressure at the neighborhood grocery store and getting readings in the 160 to 170/90 to 100 range. He has been walking occasionally. He has tried to reduce his fat and salt intake and is drinking slightly less coffee. He has not changed his smoking pattern. He has taken his medication faithfully and has not noticed any significant side effects. He is somewhat disappointed that his blood pressure is not any lower as a result of his efforts.

OBJECTIVE

Edward's blood pressure is 168/100 in the right arm, seated, without orthostatic change; his pulse is 78; and his weight is 189 lb. The remainder of his physical examination is unchanged.

ASSESSMENT

Although Edward's blood pressure is still elevated, it is now in the "mild" range. He has made significant efforts to modify his diet and exercise habits, which should result in weight loss and further reduction of his blood pressure.

TABLE 20–22. DRUGS AVAILABLE FOR TREATMENT OF HIGH BLOOD PRESSURE: THEIR POTENTIAL ADVERSE EFFECTS

DRUGS	SELECTED ADVERSE EFFECTS	PRECAUTIONS AND SPECIAL CONSIDERATIONS
FIRST-LINE DRUGS		
Diuretics		
Thiazides	Hypokalemia, hyperuricemia, glucose intolerance	May be ineffective in renal failure; hypokalemia increases digitalis toxicity; may precipitate acute gout; increases blood levels of lithium
Loop diuretics	Same as for thiazides	Effective in chronic renal failure
Potassium-Sparing Agents		
Amiloride		
Spironolactone		
Triamterene		
Beta-Adrenergic Blockers	Bronchospasm, peripheral arterial insufficiency, fatigue, insomnia, sexual dysfunction, exacerbation of congestive heart failure, masking of symptoms of hypoglycemia, hypertriglyceridemia, decreased high-density lipoprotein cholesterol (except for pindolol and acebutolol)	Should not be used in patients with asthma, chronic obstructive pulmonary disease, congestive heart failure, heart block and sick sinus syndrome; use cautiously in insulin-treated diabetics and patients with peripheral vascular disease; should not be discontinued abruptly in patients with IHD
Acebutolol		
Atenolol		
Betaxolol		
Carteolol		
Labetalol		
Metoprolol		
Nadolol		
Penbutolol sulfate		
Pindolol		
Propranolol hydrochloride		
Timolol		
ACE Inhibitors	Rash, cough, angioneurotic edema, hyperkalemia, dysgeusia	Can cause reversible acute renal failure in patients with bilateral renal arterial stenosis in a solitary kidney; proteinuria may occur; hyperkalemia can develop
Captopril		
Enalapril		
Fosinopril		
Lisinopril		
Ramipril		
Calcium Antagonists	Edema, headache, tachycardia (all patients); constipation, flushing	May cause liver dysfunction
Bepridil		
Diltiazem		
Felodipine		
Nicardipine		
Nifedipine		
Nitrendipine		
Verapamil		
Isradipine		
SECOND-LINE DRUGS		
Centrally Acting Adrenergic Inhibitors	Drowsiness, sedation, dry mouth, fatigue, sexual dysfunction	Rebound hypertension may occur with abrupt discontinuance, particularly with prior administration of high doses or with continuation of concomitant beta-blocker therapy; may cause liver damage, Coombs-positive hemolytic anemia, and orthostatic hypotension in elderly
Clonidine		
Guanabenz		
Guanfacine hydrochloride		
Methyldopa		
Clonidine patch (Catapres-TTS)		
Peripherally Acting Adrenergic Inhibitors (Alpha adrenergic blockers)	First-dose syncope, orthostatic hypotension weakness, palpitations	Orthostatic hypotension in elderly
Prazosin hydrochloride		
Terazosin hydrochloride		
Doxazosin mesylate		
Vasodilators	Headache, tachycardia, fluid retention; positive antinuclear antibody test; hypertrichosis	
Hydralazine		
Minoxidil		

Source: Adapted from Rakel RE. Textbook of Family Practice, 4th ed. Philadelphia, W.B. Saunders, 1990.

PLAN

Diagnostic. No further diagnostic testing is needed at this visit. It would be advisable to repeat the lipid profile after a 12-hour fast within the next 2 to 3 months to clarify Edward's coronary risk status related to hypercholesterolemia.

Therapeutic. Edward will continue Procardia XL 30 mg daily until his follow-up visit.

TABLE 20–23. DETERMINANTS OF ADHERENCE TO TREATMENT FOR CHRONIC DISEASE

The patient's perceived vulnerability to the disease
The patient's understanding and acceptance of treatment goals
The simplicity of the treatment
The least interference with the patient's lifestyle
The amount of social and family support

Patient Education

1. The physician commended Edward on his efforts and assured him that further improvement would likely occur if he persists. He was reminded that hypertension is a lifelong disease and that a "quick fix" is not a realistic goal.

2. Edward was encouraged to include his family members in his treatment program, and he stated that his wife accompanies him on his walks.

3. The physician discussed smoking cessation and explored Edward's readiness to consider quitting. Edward reiterated his unwillingness to quit now.

4. Edward expressed his satisfaction with his current medication regimen and agreed to continue for another month and then return for evaluation.

DISCUSSION

Hypertension is one of the most prevalent conditions seen by family physicians. Some 60 million Americans have elevated blood pressures or are taking antihypertensive medications, equivalent to one-quarter of the U.S. population. The prevalence is higher with increasing age and in certain ethnic and racial groups. In the past 20 years, public education, screening programs, and improved therapeutic options have enhanced the detection and treatment of this important risk factor for cardiovascular disease. In 1971, less than one in four of those suspected of having hypertension was aware of their condition and only one in four of those diagnosed was adequately treated. In 1972, the National High Blood Pressure Education Program began a massive public health effort targeting hypertension detection, evaluation, and treatment. These efforts have resulted in (1) a greater public awareness of the need for treatment of high blood pressure, (2) a greater rate of diagnosis and effective treatment of hypertension, and (3) significant decreases in mortality related to stroke and coronary artery disease in the past 20 years.

Most adults know their blood pressure reading and know the normal blood pressure range. Those with limited access to the health care system or those who have had only episodic care are the most likely to have undiagnosed or untreated hypertension. Edward's lack of attention to his condition seems unusual considering his employment in a health care setting and his expected awareness of the disease. However, his health care had been compromised by the lack of a personal primary care physician to inform him of his blood pressure readings and emphasize the importance of follow-up and his lack of confidence in physicians in general. Every patient contact is an opportunity to initiate hypertension control by detecting high blood pressure, informing the patient of the significance of high blood pressure, and arranging for definite follow-up care.

Hypertension should not be diagnosed on a single reading. At least two subsequent measurements with average diastolic pressures of over 90 mmHg or systolic pressures of over 140 mmHg are required for the diagnosis. The intervening time may be used for starting dietary modifications, assessing other cardiac risk factors, and developing rapport with the patient and an understanding of his or her lifestyle.

In 1984, the Joint National Committee on Detection, Evaluation, and Treatment of High Blood Pressure recommended a step-care approach using thiazide-type diuretics and beta-blockers as initial therapy. Since then, two other drug classes (calcium antagonists and ACE inhibitors) have been added as first-line drugs. There has been a proliferation of antihypertensive drugs in each of these classes as well as in the other classes (α_1-blockers, centrally acting α_2-agonists, peripherally acting adrenergic inhibitors, and vasodilators) that may be added as second-step agents. Examples of drugs in each category are listed in Table 20–23.

When selecting initial therapy, the following factors should be considered:

1. *Demographics.* Older patients may respond better to diuretics and calcium antagonists, as do blacks and Hispanics. Younger, white patients may respond better to beta-blockers or ACE inhibitors.

2. *Lifestyle.* Many of the drugs have troublesome adverse effects. For example, beta-blockers may reduce exercise tolerance or performance in an active person. Diuretics may be undesirable for a person with a physically demanding occupation if dehydration from sweating is not considered. Many of the drugs, especially diuretics, beta-blockers, central α_2-agonists, and peripheral adrenergic inhibitors, may cause male sexual dysfunction. There is increasing awareness of their effects on female sexual function as well.

3. *Coexisting conditions.* Some conditions may be worsened by antihypertensive drugs, and others may improve as a beneficial side effect of the medication. For example, beta-blockers may worsen asthma, peripheral vascular disease, and hyperlipidemia; may block symptoms of hypoglycemia in an insulin-requiring diabetic; and may impair glucose control in type II (non-insulin-dependent) diabetics. On the other hand, beta-blockers are an excellent choice in a patient with concomitant angina pectoris, migraine headache, or performance anxiety. Similarly, ACE inhibitors have been shown to improve renal hemodynamics in diabetics and may be the drug of choice in this group. ACE inhibitors may cause hyperkalemia in diabetics with nephropathy and hyporeninemic hypoaldosteronism and acute, reversible renal insufficiency in patients with bilateral renal artery stenosis.

4. *Economic considerations.* The cost of some of the newer, safer medications may be a significant barrier to compliance. The least expensive drugs are the thiazide

diuretics, averaging 20 cents per day or less for the drug, but many patients require a potassium supplement or a potassium-sparing agent, at a cost of about 40 cents per day. Beta-blockers cost around 50 cents per day, with a lower cost for generic propranolol. ACE inhibitors average around $1 per day, whereas calcium antagonists may be as high as $2 daily.

If initial therapy is not successful in attaining blood pressure control within 1 to 3 months, the physician should consider possible causes of refractory hypertension, including

1. Nonadherence to therapy
2. Drug-related—doses too low, interactions with other drugs, inappropriate combinations
3. Associated conditions—weight gain, excessive alcohol intake, renal insufficiency, other causes of hypertension
4. Volume overload—excess sodium intake, fluid retention from antihypertensive drug, renal damage

If none of these conditions exists, the physician may either increase the dose of the original drug, add a second drug (usually a diuretic if not the initial drug), or change to a drug in a different class. Occasionally, several such modifications are necessary before good blood pressure control is attained. The physician should be aware of the sense of frustration some patients will experience in this situation and must continue to include the patient in discussions of the therapeutic plan. In patients who achieve blood pressure control for at least 1 year, the physician may attempt to reduce drug dosages and even discontinue some, if not all, drugs while continuing nonpharmacologic methods. Regular follow-up must be maintained, since hypertension may recur.

SUGGESTED READING

Castle H. Cardiovascular disease (hypertension). In Rakel RE (ed.): Textbook of Family Practice, 4th ed. Philadelphia, W. B. Saunders, 1990, pp. 870–874.
Chobanian A (Committee Chair). The 1988 Report on the Joint National Committee on Detection, Evaluation, and Treatment of High Blood Pressure. Arch Intern Med 1988; 148(5):1023–1038.
Kozeny GA, Afable RF. Hypertension, refractory. In Taylor RB (ed.): Difficult Medical Management. Philadelphia, W. B. Saunders, 1991, pp. 325–332.

QUESTIONS

1. Match the blood pressure reading with the appropriate follow-up. Each option may be used once, more than once, or not at all.
   a. 150/95 in a 40-year-old man
   b. 170/85 in a 72-year-old woman
   c. 180/108 in a 35-year-old woman
   d. 110/88 in a 28-year-old man
      (1) Recheck within 2 years
      (2) Recheck within 1 year
      (3) Confirm within 2 months
      (4) Evaluate or refer to source of care within 2 weeks
      (5) Evaluate or refer immediately to source of care

2. Which of the following tests is *not* included in the routine evaluation of hypertension?
   a. Serum potassium
   b. Urinalysis
   c. Electrocardiogram
   d. Liver function tests
   e. Complete blood count

3. Sexual dysfunction is a frequent side effect of
   a. Diuretics.
   b. Beta-blockers.
   c. ACE inhibitors.
   d. Calcium antagonists.
   e. Central α_1-agonists.

4. Appropriate first-line drug treatment for moderate hypertension includes
   a. Propranolol.
   b. Hydrochlorothiazide.
   c. Hydralazine.
   d. Captopril.
   e. Verapamil.

Answers appear on page 451.

JANE E. CORBOY

INITIAL VISIT

SUBJECTIVE

Patient Identification and Presenting Problem. Jim W. is a 61-year-old white accountant who has had chest pains for the past month.

Present Illness. Jim first noticed the pain when he was cleaning the apartment of his younger sister, who had committed suicide the previous week by jumping from the window of her third-floor apartment. Jim and his oldest daughter drove 700 miles to his sister's home the day after learning of the suicide. They started packing and cleaning the apartment the following day. Jim noticed an aching tightness in his throat and midchest while carrying boxes up and down stairs, scrubbing, and vacuuming floors. The pain did not radiate or change location. He had no nausea, diaphoresis, or shortness of breath with the pain. The discomfort lasted for 2 to 5 minutes after he reached the top of the stairs. He took Tums without relief or prevention of the pain.

Since he returned home, Jim has noticed the pain less frequently. He has had one or two episodes a week that have occurred with the moderate exertion of lifting and unpacking boxes. He had not had similar pain in the past, but he admits that his activity level had been quite low for several years. He has never had chest pain lasting more than 30 minutes.

Past Medical History. Jim has had a hiatal hernia and reflux esophagitis for several years. He regularly takes an antacid/antigas medication after meals and at bedtime. He has no history of hypertension, diabetes, previously known heart disease, asthma, or psychiatric disease.

Family History. Jim's father died at age 32 of peritonitis due to appendicitis. His father's two brothers died suddenly in their sixties of uncertain causes. His mother is 89 years old and has hypertension and osteoarthritis. Besides his deceased sister Jim has no other siblings. There is no family history of premature heart disease, diabetes, hyperlipidemia, or stroke.

Social History. Jim is the plant accountant for the local factory of a national manufacturing company. He has worked for the same company since his teens with time off for military service during World War II. He describes his work as stressful because of his management responsibilities. Jim completed high school and some college. He has been married for 35 years. He and his wife have three daughters, ages 19, 28, and 29, all living away from home. Since his sister's death, Jim's mother has moved in with Jim and his wife.

Health Habits. Jim has never smoked. His alcohol intake is less than one drink per week. Jim usually eats three meals a day with moderately high fat intake and enjoys a late-night snack of ice cream or cheese and crackers. He drinks one or two cups of coffee daily. Jim occasionally plays tennis or golf but has no regular exercise routine.

Review of Systems. Positive only as in the history of present illness. His esophageal reflux symptoms had been somewhat worse over the past several months associated with increased weight.

OBJECTIVE

Physical Examination. Jim is a moderately obese white man in no acute distress. His vital signs are blood pressure 160/102, pulse 82, height 5 ft 8 in, weight 180 lb. Significant physical findings involving the cardiovascular system include mild arteriovenous narrowing on funduscopic examination, no carotid bruits, cardiac examination normal except for distant heart sounds, and peripheral pulses mildly decreased in the lower extremities. Abdominal examination showed slight epigastric tenderness. The remainder of the examination, including neurologic examination, is normal. Jim does not want to discuss his feelings about his sister's death.

Laboratory Tests. A fasting multitest chemistry panel was notable for a total cholesterol of 266. His HDL cholesterol was 42, triglycerides 175, and the calculated LDL cholesterol 189.

ASSESSMENT

Working Diagnoses. The most likely diagnoses to explain Jim's symptoms are as follows:

1. *Angina pectoris.* Jim gives a classic description of chest tightness or pain brought on by exertion and emotional stress and relieved by rest. In a man with cardiovascular risk factors of hypertension, sedentary lifestyle, and elevated cholesterol level, angina pectoris is the most likely, as well as the most critical, diagnosis to consider.

2. *Grief reaction, unresolved.* Jim's unwillingness to discuss his feelings about his sister's recent, unexpected, and violent death may be due to his immediate concerns about his own health. It would be useful to know if he had discussed his reactions to the event with his family or church pastor, since unresolved grief may negatively affect his physical well-being.

3. *Hypercholesterolemia.* With total cholesterol over 240, LDL cholesterol over 160, and a total to HDL cholesterol ratio of 6.4, Jim's cholesterol profile places him in high risk for atherosclerotic heart disease.

Differential Diagnoses

1. *Musculoskeletal chest pain.* Chest pain arising from the chest wall, ribs, and costochondral joints is usually sharp in nature. It may worsen with moving the arms or a severe cough. Physical examination shows tenderness on palpation of the chest wall. Movement of the arms often reproduces the patient's pain. With Jim's history of lifting heavy boxes at the time the pain started, this diagnosis is possible. Without the chest-wall tenderness, it must be a diagnosis of exclusion.

2. *Esophageal disease.* Esophageal pain may be from reflux or spasm. Reflux pain is classically burning in nature and occurs shortly after meals. It may worsen with activities that increase reflux, such as reclining or straining, and thereby increasing intraabdominal pressure. Antacids usually provide rapid relief. Esophageal spasm causes a substernal pressure-type pain, which may last 2 to 5 minutes, similar to angina. It usually radiates to the back rather than to the arms. The pain is more likely to occur after meals and usually is not associated with exertion. Antacids provide variable relief of the pain of esophageal spasm. Jim's history of hiatal hernia makes esophageal disease a reasonable inclusion in the differential diagnosis.

3. *Pericarditis or pleuritis.* Chest pain from inflammation of the pleura or pericardium is sharp and is worsened by a deep breath or cough. It is usually associated with other symptoms reflecting the primary disease or condition, such as fever and cough with pneumonia, dyspnea with a pulmonary embolism, and positional pain and fever with pericarditis. Physical examination reveals friction rubs over the inflamed pleura or pericardium.

4. *Anxiety.* Either situational anxiety or a primary anxiety disorder may cause chest pain, discomfort, or palpitations. Usually, situational anxiety occurs in association with stressful life events and the symptoms are transitory. With generalized anxiety disorder, the patient may have unrealistic worries about several life events. Physical symptoms reflect muscle tension, autonomic hyperactivity, and excessive CNS arousal. Panic attacks may cause intense discomfort and multiple symptoms, including dyspnea, dizziness, trembling, sweating, nausea, chills, fear of dying or of losing control, along with chest pain or palpitations. Jim certainly has undergone a stressful event and may have worries and concerns, but his symptoms are not consistent with a true anxiety disorder.

PLAN

Diagnostic. The goal of the diagnostic plan for angina is to establish the significance of the patient's symptoms. The specific objectives are as follows:

1. *Evaluate risk factors for accelerated atherosclerosis.* The history will reveal smoking, poor exercise habits, and a family history of heart disease. Physical examination may reveal hypertension, xanthomas, or xanthelasmas. Abnormal measurements of cholesterol, creatinine, and glucose may suggest hyperlipoproteinemia, renal insufficiency, or diabetes. Jim has two major cardiac risk factors: hypertension and hypercholesterolemia. His family history is unclear but suspicious for heart disease.

2. *Identify conditions that may exacerbate or trigger angina symptoms.* Conditions that increase myocardial oxygen demand, such as thyrotoxicosis or fever, are detectible on history and physical examination. The history and physical examination may suggest certain conditions that decrease oxygen supply, such as anemia and hypoxemia. Laboratory tests, including hemoglobin or hematocrit and arterial blood gases, provide confirmation.

3. *Determine the presence and extent of coronary artery disease.* Jim's *resting ECG* was normal, and he did not have pain during the examination. An *exercise ECG* or treadmill stress test may elicit ECG changes with exercise. Jim's physician scheduled him for an exercise ECG to be done before his next visit in 1 week. *Coronary angiography* to define the coronary artery anatomy and left ventricular function is important in determining the patient's prognosis. The risks and indications for angiography are discussed below.

Therapeutic. The goal of therapy of angina is to reduce mortality from coronary artery disease. The specific objectives are as follows:

1. Reduction of cardiovascular risk factors, as discussed under Patient Education.

2. Treatment of coexisting conditions that aggravate angina.

3. Amelioration of the fundamental disparity between myocardial oxygen supply and demand.

The methods include pharmacologic (medical) therapy and "invasive" therapy, which will be discussed at greater length in the Discussion section. Jim's physician prescribed propranolol 40 mg four times daily.

Patient Education. The goal of patient education in angina is to enable the patient to reduce his or her morbidity and mortality from cardiovascular disease. The specific objectives are as follows:

1. *Inform the patient of the meaning of his or her chest pain symptoms.* Jim's physician advised him that his chest discomfort is likely to represent an imbalance of the heart muscle's oxygen supply and demand. It therefore signifies a threat to the health of the heart. Jim and his physician discussed that he should stop and rest immediately at the onset of pain to avoid prolonging the precarious situation.

2. *Recommend lifestyle modifications to reduce further cardiovascular risk.* Jim and his physician discussed a low-fat, low-cholesterol, reduced-caffeine diet. Because of the mild hypertension, Jim also received instructions on reducing his salt intake.

3. *Educate the patient on basic pathophysiology of angina, rationale for therapy, and treatment options available.* Jim received information on basic coronary artery anatomy. He learned that treatment aims to increase blood flow to the heart, either with medications or by mechanical means. He received 0.4-mg nitroglyc-

erin sublingual tablets with instructions to carry them with him at work and at home. He understood that he should use one under his tongue at the onset of pain and a second tablet if his pain does not disappear after about 5 minutes. Jim and his physician also briefly discussed the treatment plan of medical versus surgical management depending on the outcome of his treadmill test.

FIRST FOLLOW-UP VISIT

SUBJECTIVE

Jim had only one episode of chest pain in the preceding week. The pain occurred while he was climbing stairs at work and was promptly relieved with the nitroglycerin. He and his family have sorted his sister's belongings and have given away or discarded most of the household goods and clothing. He reports that he read some of her letters and diaries in an attempt to understand her suicide. He has begun to discuss the event with his wife.

OBJECTIVE

Jim has no significant changes in his physical examination, including vital signs. His exercise ECG showed downsloping ST-segment depression in leads I, II, aVF, and V_3–V_6 that occurred 5 minutes into the exercise portion of the test at a heart rate of 120 (75% of predicted maximum heart rate). Jim reported chest tightness at the time of the ECG changes, and the examination was stopped. There was no fall in blood pressure, and the ECG changes and pain resolved approximately 5 minutes after stopping exercise.

ASSESSMENT

1. *Coronary artery disease.* With Jim's symptoms, cardiac risk factors, and a positive stress test, the diagnosis of atherosclerotic cardiovascular disease is almost certain. The diffuse ST-segment depression indicates that a large portion of the myocardium is at risk.
2. *Grief reaction.* Jim has begun to address his questions and come to terms with his sister's death.

PLAN

Jim was referred to a cardiologist for a coronary angiogram and left ventriculogram. The angiogram showed 90% occlusion of the left main coronary artery, 95% occlusion of the left anterior descending artery proximal to the obtuse marginal branch, and 95% blockage of a dominant right coronary artery in its midportion. Left ventricular function was good, with a 60% ejection fraction and no discrete areas of hypokinesis. Jim was referred to a cardiovascular surgeon for coronary artery bypass surgery.

DISCUSSION

Angina pectoris is one of the four cardinal manifestations of ischemic heart disease. The other three are myocardial infarction, congestive heart failure, and arrhythmia. The major determinants of myocardial oxygen consumption are listed in Table 20–24. Since angina usually represents a *transient* imbalance in myocardial oxygen supply and demand, patients may present with angina before the myocardium is permanently damaged. Because patients with angina pectoris have a better prognosis than those with silent ischemia or prolonged ischemia, the physician must recognize classic angina symptoms and diagnose and treat the condition accurately and promptly.

The resting ECG may show an old myocardial infarction, but it may be completely normal if the patient does not have pain. An ECG done while the patient has pain may show transient ST-segment depression or T-wave inversion in the leads that correlate with the location of the ischemic segment (see Table 20–25). This finding helps to predict the coronary artery obstruction as well as establish that the pain is indeed angina.

Patients who have classic angina and numerous risk

TABLE 20–24. DETERMINANTS OF MYOCARDIAL OXYGEN CONSUMPTION

DETERMINANTS OF OXYGEN DEMAND
Heart rate
Wall tension
  Blood pressure
  Ventricular size
  Ventricular wall tension
Contractility
Metabolic rate

DETERMINANTS OF OXYGEN SUPPLY
Coronary artery patency
  Spasm
  Fixed obstruction
  Platelet aggregation
Blood oxygen-carrying capacity
  Hemoglobin content
  Oxygen saturation

TABLE 20–25. CORRELATION BETWEEN ECG CHANGES, LOCATION OF ISCHEMIA AND CORONARY ARTERY INVOLVED

ECG LEADS WITH ST = SEGMENT DEPRESSION	AREA OF ISCHEMIC MYOCARDIUM	CORONARY ARTERY
II, III, aVF	Inferior	Right coronary artery
V_1, V_2 (elevation)	Posterior	Right coronary artery
V_2–V_4	Anteroseptal	Left anterior descending branch
V_3–V_5	Anterior	Left anterior descending branch
I, aVL	High lateral	Circumflex or Diagonal branch
V_5, V_6	Apical	Left anterior descending branch, or posterior descending of right coronary artery

Source: Adapted from Scientific American Medicine. Ischemic Heart Disease: Angina Pectoris. New York, Scientific American, 1991, sec. 1, chap. 9, pp. 1–20, with permission.

factors for heart disease may not need an exercise ECG, since the outcome of this test should not dissuade the physician from suspecting heart disease in these patients. However, if the diagnosis is uncertain, an exercise ECG may assist the diagnosis. Exercise-induced ECG changes associated with typical angina pain, fatigue, or a fall in blood pressure are strongly predictive of the presence of coronary artery disease. The exercise ECG is also useful in detecting exercise-induced ECG changes or arrhythmias that have not caused angina pain. These changes represent "silent ischemia." Table 20–26 lists the criteria for ECG changes that most reliably indicate the presence of myocardial ischemia. False-negative tests (a negative test in a person with coronary artery disease) occur about a third of the time, and false-positive tests occur in about 10% of people who do not have coronary artery disease. Because of the imperfect sensitivity and specificity of the test, the physician should consider the likelihood of the disease before performing the test. A negative test does not rule out angina in a person with numerous risk factors and a high likelihood of disease.

Other noninvasive diagnostic studies include the thallium stress test, which combines ECG measurements with a radioisotope uptake scan. It provides increased sensitivity and specificity over the standard exercise ECG but is more expensive. Other imaging techniques are available, including gated wall-motion studies of left ventricular function, magnetic resonance imaging (MRI) of the heart, and others.

Coronary angiography provides the most accurate information about the status of the coronary arteries and left ventricular function. Because of its invasive nature, it also has greater risks than the previously discussed examinations. These risks include myocardial infarction, stroke, and death. The physician must balance these risks against the value of the information gained by the procedure and recommend the procedure only for those patients for whom the benefits outweigh the risks. Table 20–27 lists the indications for angiography.

The rationale for medical therapy is to reduce the discrepancy between myocardial oxygen demand and oxygen supply to the heart. Oxygen demand is reduced by reducing heart rate at rest and with exercise, decreasing blood pressure, reducing left ventricular volume, and decreasing contractility. The oxygen supply may be enhanced by increasing coronary artery patency by preventing spasm, dilating fixed obstructions, or preventing platelet clumping. Each of the major categories of antianginal medications acts on one or more of these mechanisms. Some classes of drugs complement or are

TABLE 20–26. EXERCISE ECG CRITERIA FOR ISCHEMIA

ST-segment depression that:

1. Is over 1 mm in amplitude.
2. Is horizontal or of downsloping contour.
3. Occurs early in exercise.
4. Persists for a few minutes after exercise.

TABLE 20–27. INDICATIONS FOR CORONARY ANGIOGRAPHY

Incapacitating angina in patients on maximal medical therapy
Young or vigorous patients who have a large area of cardiac muscle at risk
Patients who are incapacitated by atypical chest pain, to exclude the diagnosis of coronary artery disease
Patients undergoing cardiac surgery for valvular heart disease, to assess the presence or extent of coronary artery disease

synergistic with others. Some target different mechanisms; others interfere with the compensatory responses that limit the effectiveness of the other agent.

Beta-blockers act on the demand side of the myocardial oxygen equation by reducing heart rate, blood pressure, and myocardial contractility. Beta-blockers are effective in the treatment of angina. They may reduce the risk of myocardial infarction and ischemia-related arrhythmia. Side effects include worsening or provocation of congestive heart failure or asthma. Other adverse effects include impotence, decreased exercise tolerance, and lethargy. They may block the hypoglycemic symptoms in patients with insulin-dependent diabetes mellitus. Beta-blockers are classified as "nonselective" or "cardioselective." Those which are cardioselective have less risk of inducing bronchospasm at standard therapeutic doses. Other characteristics that distinguish the different beta-blockers include duration of action, degree of lipid solubility, and the presence of intrinsic sympathomimetic activity. Each of these characteristics affects the agent's side-effect profile or dosing frequency. These qualities may affect the patient's acceptance of and adherence to therapy.

Nitrates primarily affect ventricular volume by reducing left ventricular filling pressure. The mechanism of action is venous dilatation and some arteriolar dilatation. A secondary effect of nitrates is to dilate coronary arteries, relieve coronary artery spasm, and improve collateral flow. Side effects of nitrates relate to their vasodilating effects. Reflex tachycardia results from the decreased blood pressure. Headache and flushing resulting from vasodilation may discourage the patient from using these effective drugs. Beta-blockers counter the tachycardia of nitrates and also may decrease the headache. Nitrates may be taken sublingually, like nitroglycerin, with rapid onset and short duration. Other dosing routes for angina are oral and transdermal. Patients on maintenance nitrates develop tolerance and loss of efficacy if the drugs are used continually. The patient should omit the bedtime dose of oral nitrates or remove the nitroglycerin patch at bedtime to prevent tolerance to the drug.

The *calcium antagonists* each have different effects on the myocardial oxygen demand–supply ratio. Verapamil and bepridil decrease heart rate, blood pressure, and contractility. The effects are similar to those of the beta-blockers, but they do not precipitate asthma. Nifedipine, felodipine, nicardipine, and israpidine have a greater effect on peripheral and coronary dilatation. In this way, they behave similarly to the nitrates. Diltiazem's effects are between those of the other two groups. The different calcium antagonists have different side effects as well. The most common side effects with verapamil are constipation, bradycardia, and fatigue. Nifedipine most commonly causes headache, dizziness, and flushing. Calcium antagonists are useful additions to the standard beta-blocker and nitrate combination in patients who have not responded to maximal therapy. Another use is in patients who cannot tolerate beta-blockers because of lung disease, diabetes, or other conditions.

Other components of medical management include treating hypertension, congestive heart failure, and other underlying medical conditions. In addition, 325 mg aspirin daily may prevent myocardial infarction by reducing platelet aggregation.

Surgical therapy or angioplasty is recommended for patients who have certain conditions. Each of these groups has a large amount of myocardium at risk from myocardial infarction. First, those with left main coronary artery disease have better survival with surgery than with medical therapy. Patients with three-vessel disease and decreased left ventricular function also have improved survival rates with surgery. Two-vessel disease is also an indication for surgery, if one of the vessels is the proximal left anterior descending artery. Finally, those with intractable angina or silent ischemia on maximal medical management may benefit from surgery.

The indications for percutaneous transluminal coronary angioplasty (PTCA) are similar to those for coronary artery bypass grafting. However, because the procedure is less invasive, it may be appropriate to use angioplasty on single-vessel lesions as well.

SUGGESTED READING

Hennekens CH, Buring JE, Sandercock P, et al. Aspirin and other antiplatelet agents in the secondary and primary prevention of cardiovascular disease. Circulation 1989; 80:749.

Rakel RE. Textbook of Family Practice, 4th ed. Philadelphia, W. B. Saunders, 1990.

Scientific American Medicine. Ischemic Heart Disease: Angina Pectoris. New York, Scientific American, 1991, sec. 1, chap. 9, pp. 1–20.

Varnauskas E. The European Coronary Surgery Study Group: Twelve-year follow-up of survival in the randomized European Coronary Surgery Study. N Engl J Med 1988; 319:332.

QUESTIONS

1. Major risk factors for atherosclerotic heart disease include which of the following?
   a. Smoking
   b. Hypertension
   c. Diabetes mellitus
   d. Hypertriglyceridemia
   e. Family history of heart disease

2. Match each of the following types of chest pain with the associated conditions.
   a. Sharp, over costochondral joints
   b. Squeezing, radiates to back, worse after meals
   c. Sharp, worse with deep breath or cough
   d. Dull, heavy, occurs with exertion
      (1) Angina pectoris
      (2) Esophageal spasm
      (3) Pleurisy
      (4) Musculoskeletal pain

3. Which of the following antianginal drug classes causes venous pooling, decreased ventricular filling pressure, coronary artery dilatation, and tachycardia?
   a. Beta-blockers
   b. Calcium antagonists
   c. Platelet inhibitors
   d. Nitrates

Answers appear on page 451.

Preschool Physical Examination

MICHAEL A. CROUCH

INITIAL VISIT

SUBJECTIVE

Patient Identification. Gary A. is a 24-year-old Caucasian freshman medical student being seen for a preschool physical examination.

Presenting Problems. Although his general health has been quite good in the past, Gary has been experiencing abdominal pain, loose bowel movements, chest discomfort, and palpitations intermittently for about 2 weeks.

Present Illness. Gary began experiencing cramping periumbilical pain and loose bowel movements following a farewell weekend with college friends, just prior to moving to University City to begin medical school. The abdominal pain originally began while he was packing his belongings in his car. The most severe episode occurred midway through the first day of orientation week and was quite uncomfortable (8 on a scale of 10). Each episode has lasted from 30 to 45 minutes. The pain has occurred at all different times of the day but has not awakened him from sleep. The pain is unrelated to mealtime or physical activity. Neither antacids nor bismuth subsalicylate (PeptoBismol) has produced prompt pain relief, but a dose of bismuth subsalicylate seemed to normalize his bowel movements for about 12 hours. His bowel movements have been a normal brown color, with a quite loose but not liquid consistency. The stool has contained small amounts of mucus at times, without visible blood.

Gary began experiencing bilateral chest discomfort and palpitations some time after the onset of the abdominal pain. He has had episodes lasting 5 to 10 minutes, occurring two to three times a week, associated with unusually forceful and rapid heartbeat. The episodes typically occurred at rest, after he had been experiencing abdominal pain for an hour or more. The symptoms were relieved by his getting up and moving around restlessly.

Past Medical History. Gary has had no surgery, accidents, or serious injuries and has never been hospitalized. He has no known medication allergies. He takes no medications on a regular basis and denies using cathartic laxatives or stool softeners.

Family History. Gary's father, a dairy farmer, died suddenly at age 48, presumably from a heart attack. His mother is in good health at age 58. His only brother has hypercholesterolemia. His only sister has had no serious health problems. His paternal grandfather died from colon cancer at age 75. His other three grandparents died from unknown causes past the age of 80. He admits to worrying quite a bit about the possibility of his having inherited a predisposition to heart disease from his father. He is also worried about getting colon cancer like his grandfather did.

Health Habits. Gary does not smoke. He drinks small amounts of alcohol on rare occasions and denies using any illicit drugs. He always wears seat belts when driving his car. For the past 5 years he has always used latex condoms when having intercourse. He exercises regularly, usually running about 3 to 4 miles at least three times a week. He has avoided eating red meat, pork, and whole-milk dairy products for 2 years, after reading that they could increase one's risk of heart disease and cancer.

Social History. Gary is single. He has been seeing one girlfriend regularly for 2 years and is sexually active exclusively with her. They are planning to marry following his first year in medical school. He describes his relationships with his girlfriend, mother, and siblings as close and supportive. He is unsure that he will be able to compete well academically in medical school and is concerned about how he will handle the heavy academic load and mental stress he has heard about. He made excellent grades in college while being active in intramural sports and social life with friends.

Review of Systems. Gary has had no change in his appetite, weight, energy, or general mood. He has experienced no nausea or vomiting. He has felt somewhat jittery and restless while sitting in lectures for the past few days. He has also had uncharacteristic difficulty getting to sleep recently. He denies having thoughts of imminent life-threatening illness or death.

OBJECTIVE

Physical Examination. Gary's vital signs are all within normal limits, including blood pressure of 110/70, heart rate of 92, weight of 160 lb, and height of 70 in. His affect is normal, except for looking mildly nervous. His physical examination is notable only for cool clammy hands, moist axillae, mild diffuse tenderness of the abdomen, and questionably diminished deep tendon reflexes and slow recovery. His thyroid gland and Achilles tendons are normal to inspection and palpation. His peripheral pulses are all normal.

Laboratory Tests. A multitest "executive profile" drawn 2 days prior to Gary's office visit is notable only for a total cholesterol level of 300 mg/dl (7.7 mmol/liter). The panel did not include cholesterol subfractions or triglycerides, but it did include normal liver and renal function tests.

ASSESSMENT

Working Diagnoses. Two likely diagnoses best explain the patient's symptoms and findings:

1. *Adjustment disorder with anxious mood.* This is expressed as situational anxiety, mild sleep disorder, symptoms of autonomic overactivity, and irritable bowel syndrome.

2. *Familial heterozygous hypercholesterolemia* (type IIa in the Frederickson classification). This based on the suggestive family history and the very high total cholesterol value despite a "heart healthy" lifestyle. Even this severe form of hypercholesterolemia is asymptomatic until atherosclerotic lesions progress to a critical extent, usually after age 30. Although the likelihood of Gary's having symptomatic coronary artery disease now is quite low, he most likely has some degree of coronary atherosclerosis already. His concern about developing early heart disease in his thirties or forties is well founded. The severity of cholesterol elevation might be exacerbated by the stress of beginning medical school and his ambivalence about his ability to succeed academically and cope well with the demands of his chosen profession. Although unlikely, secondary causes of hypercholesterolemia should be kept in mind (see Differential Diagnoses).

Differential Diagnoses. Gary's symptoms and findings suggest several other possibilities, including

1. *Hypothyroidism.* This is unlikely because of the mild tachycardia, but it is a cause of secondary hypercholesterolemia worth keeping in mind. It usually presents with considerable fatigue in younger patients.

2. *Generalized anxiety disorder.* This is not an appropriate diagnosis at this point because of the short duration of symptoms.

3. *Somatization disorder.* This is not an appropriate diagnosis at this point because of the relatively limited scope and duration of somatic symptoms. If this episode is not handled well, however, the patient might gradually become more preoccupied with somatic symptoms.

4. *Panic disorder.* This is unlikely because of the lack of intense acute fear of imminent personal catastrophe. If the patient is biologically predisposed despite a lack of suggestive family history, his concerns could eventually be expressed as panic attacks or agoraphobia.

5. *Hypochondriasis with cardiac and cancer neuroses.* This should be kept in mind as a plausible possibility given the patient's family history and current symptoms. The patient would be vulnerable to developing an exaggerated fear of heart disease in his forties as he approaches and reaches the age at which his father died. Such fear would be rational to some extent, given his lipid disorder.

Several less likely diseases also must be considered because of their seriousness and potentially grave consequences if not diagnosed promptly:

1. *Acute pancreatitis secondary to severe hypertriglyceridemia.* This is unlikely because of the relatively brief duration of the pain episodes and the patient's slender physique, regular aerobic exercise, low alcohol intake, and nondiabetic status.

2. *Hyperalphalipoproteinemia.* This is unlikely, especially in a male. Patients with this condition have a very high level of HDL cholesterol. High levels of HDL cholesterol are usually associated with low risk for atherosclerosis. In rare cases, however, the HDL cholesterol does not function normally in transporting peripheral cholesterol to the liver, and the patient is at risk for coronary disease despite the high HDL cholesterol level.

3. *Angina pectoris caused by atherosclerotic coronary artery disease.* This is highly unlikely in such a young adult. Patients with *homozygous* familial hypercholesterolemia develop heart disease early in life, but if Gary had the homozygous form, he would have already experienced severe atherosclerotic consequences (stroke or myocardial infarction) by adolescence.

4. *Coronary vasospasm causing atypical angina.* This is rare in Gary's age group and less likely in men than in women.

PLAN
Diagnostic

1. Fasting lipoprotein analysis (lipid profile) is the most appropriate initial test. Measurement of total cholesterol, HDL cholesterol, and triglycerides and a calculated estimate of LDL cholesterol will allow verification and categorization of common lipid disorders.

2. Thyroid-stimulating hormone (TSH) level. This is a reasonable test to obtain to exclude hypothyroidism, a treatable secondary cause of high cholesterol.

3. Electrocardiogram (ECG). Although very unlikely to show abnormalities, a normal ECG may provide useful reassurance to some patients. Neither the patient nor the physician thought an ECG was necessary.

Therapeutic

1. Diet low in saturated fat and cholesterol. It is recommended to continue following step 1 of the American Heart Association (AHA) guidelines until the lipid profile results are obtained. Given the level of total cholesterol, a step 2 AHA diet will be necessary for dietary modification to have a chance to significantly lower the severe LDL cholesterol elevation. A high water-soluble fiber intake (e.g., oat bran) is recommended.

2. Aerobic exercise. Gary is advised to continue his current routine throughout medical school and residency training as much as possible. Exercise increases lipoprotein lipase activity, sometimes lowers LDL cholesterol somewhat, raises HDL cholesterol 5 to 15 mg/dl, and has a relaxing effect.

3. Lipid-altering medication. This is probably advisable if the lipid profile results show the anticipated severe LDL cholesterol elevation. Discussion of pros and cons and specific alternatives was deferred until the second visit.

4. Relaxation techniques. Gary was introduced to options of deep breathing, progressive muscle relaxation, and visual imagery to help reduce effects of stress and deal with acute and chronic anxiety.

Patient Education

1. The cholesterol elevation was provisionally characterized as severe pending two repeat measurements to confirm persistence of the elevation.

2. The strong role of cholesterol elevation as a risk factor in heart disease was explained. The physician gave Gary a pamphlet with answers to common questions about cholesterol to read and discuss during the return visit.

3. The importance of rechecking the cholesterol level and obtaining a fractionated fasting lipid profile to look at LDL and HDL cholesterol levels was stressed.

4. Gary was urged to encourage his sister and fiancée to have their cholesterol checked if they had not already done so.

5. Gary was asked to keep a 3-day food diary, recording everything he ate and drank for 72 hours, noting serving sizes and method of preparation.

6. Gary's anxiety as an entering medical student was normalized, and a likely good adjustment was predicted. Anxiety was reconnoted as a useful signal of stress and as an energy-mobilizing catalyst.

Disposition. Gary was asked to return in 1 week for follow-up of his cholesterol and anxiety problems. Referral was not thought to be indicated for either problem at this point.

FIRST FOLLOW-UP VISIT

SUBJECTIVE

Gary returned for follow-up 1 week after his initial visit. He was feeling much better. He attributed his improvement mainly to relief from worry about his symptoms indicating some serious underlying illness such as heart disease or cancer. His abdominal pain, chest discomfort, and palpitations had resolved. He was still having occasional loose bowel movements, but he was not bothered by them.

Gary was anxious to discuss his lipid profile results. In the intervening week he had discovered that a paternal aunt and a paternal uncle both developed heart disease in their fifties and that both had high cholesterol levels. He had already encouraged his sister and fiancée to undergo cholesterol screening, and they expressed an intention to do so soon. He expressed curiosity about the wisdom of taking fish oil capsules.

OBJECTIVE

Gary looked less nervous than on the first visit. His heart rate was 72 (compared with 90 the previous week). His 3-day food diary showed a low intake of foods high in saturated fat and cholesterol, congruent with the step 1 American Heart Association dietary guidelines. He also showed an increase in water-soluble fiber intake, with oatmeal for breakfasts and oat bran muffins for lunches. The fasting lipoprotein analysis showed a total cholesterol of 310 mg/dl (8.0 mmol/liter), HDL cholesterol of 40 mg/dl (1.0 mmol/liter), triglycerides of 100, and an estimated LDL cholesterol of 250 mg/dl (6.5 mmol/liter). The TSH result was 2.0, well within normal limits.

ASSESSMENT

1. *Familial heterozygous hypercholesterolemia* (FHC) with severely elevated total and LDL cholesterol (see Tables 20–28 and 20–29). Below average HDL cholesterol. The average for males is 45 mg/dl (1.15 mmol/liter). FHC is a very strong risk factor for early coronary artery disease, with clinical heart disease occurring in males at an average age of 42. Aggressive medical treatment to lower LDL cholesterol as much as possible, ideally to <130 mg/dl (3.4 mmol/liter), should be established and maintained lifelong.

2. *Adjustment disorder with anxious mood.* This is mild and is responding well to reassurance and education about stress coping strategies.

PLAN
Diagnostic

1. Repeat fasting lipid profile. It is advisable to examine short-term variations and establish pretreatment baseline for LDL cholesterol. This repeat analysis ide-

TABLE 20–28. DIETARY AND DRUG TREATMENT BASED ON LDL CHOLESTEROL

LDL CHOLESTEROL LEVEL	PATIENT DESCRIPTION CLASSIFICATION
<130 mg/dl	Desirable LDL cholesterol
130–159 mg/dl	Borderline high-risk LDL cholesterol
≥160 mg./dl.	High-risk LDL cholesterol

LDL CHOLESTEROL LEVEL TO INITIATE DIET THERAPY TO LOWER CHOLESTEROL

Risk Factor Status	Initiation Level	Goal
No CHD or less than two other risk factors	≥160 mg/dl	<160 mg/dl
With CHD or two other risk factors	≥130 mg/dl	<130 mg/dl

DRUG TREATMENT PLUS DIETARY TREATMENT

No CHD or less than two other risk factors	≥190 mg/dl	<160 mg/dl
With CHD or two other risk factors	≥160 mg/dl	<130 mg/dl

Source: Fram Rakel RE. Textbook of Family Practice, 4th ed. Philadelphia, W.B. Saunders, 1990, with permission.
Note: Risk factors include family history, cigarette smoking, HDL-C<35 mg/dl, hypertension, diabetes, and male sex.

TABLE 20–29. LDL CHOLESTEROL CUTPOINTS BASED ON PRESENCE OF RISK FACTORS FOR CORONARY HEART DISEASE

LDL cholesterol > 160 in any patient
Low-density lipoprotein (LDL) cholesterol > 130 in any patient with two or more of the following:
    Prior history of coronary heart disease
    Male sex
    Family history of premature coronary heart disease (less than 55 years of age)
    Cigarette smoker (greater than 10 per day)
    Hypertension
    High-density lipoprotein (HDL) cholesterol level less than 35
    History of any occlusive vascular disease
    Severe obesity (more than 30% overweight)
Other risk factors:
    High stress personality profile (probable)
    Inactivity (probable)
    Oral contraceptive use in smokers over 35 years of age

Source: Fram Rakel RE. Textbook of Family Practice, 4th ed. Philadelphia, W.B. Saunders, 1990, with permission.

ally should be done several weeks later. Once treatment is started, a lipid profile should be repeated about 4 weeks after each change in the regimen. Once a regimen has achieved satisfactory results, a lipid profile should be repeated every 3 to 6 months to monitor the ongoing response.

2. Soft-tissue roentgenograms of the Achilles tendons. Xanthomas show up as tendon thickening. Re-

measurement after a year of treatment can be used as an index of therapeutic response to lipid-altering medications. Although this is not done routinely in clinical practice, it is reasonable to provide tangible evidence of benefit for the patient.

3. Apolipoprotein B determination. Elevation indicates higher risk for atherosclerosis. It is unclear how much this measurement adds to risk assessment.

4. Lipoprotein (a) [Lp(a)] determination. Elevation indicates higher risk for atherosclerosis. It is also unclear how much this measurement adds to risk assessment.

Therapeutic

1. Step 2 AHA diet. Further restriction of foods high in saturated fat and cholesterol is recommended, and this is to be continued lifelong to help reduce LDL cholesterol elevation. The physician recommended use of nonhydrogenated corn, safflower, soybean, and olive oil in cooking and avoidance of oils high in saturated fat, including coconut and palm oil (see Table 20–30). Gary was encouraged to bring his fiancée along to the next visit for a more detailed discussion of food selection and preparation.

2. Lipid-altering medication. The general pros and cons of this were discussed. Lovastatin was presented as the medication most likely to produce satisfactory results with monotherapy. Its high cost, uncertain long-term safety, and lack of directly proven benefit for heart disease prevention were presented as potential disadvantages. Psyllium hydrophilic mucilloid and niacin were presented as inexpensive over-the-counter choices for initial or adjunctive treatment. Sustained-release niacin alone might give good results at 2 to 3 gm/day, but liver toxicity should be watched for during the first few months. Cholestyramine was presented as a costly adjunctive treatment for use at a low to medium dose to avoid the constipation caused by a high dose. Probucol was discussed as a costly potential adjunctive treatment

to prevent the development and progression of atherosclerotic lesions. Plans were made to initiate drug therapy after obtaining the results of the second lipid profile. Some experts advocate withholding medical treatment until three lipid profiles have been obtained over a several-month period to observe variations over a longer time interval (see Tables 20–31 and 20–32).

3. Relaxation techniques. The physician explained deep breathing, progressive muscle relaxation, and visual imagery in more detail, encouraged Gary to try them, and loaned Gary an audiotape with relaxation instructions.

Patient Education

1. The physician discussed the general pros and cons of the over-the-counter and prescription medications for lowering LDL cholesterol.

2. The genetic inheritance pattern of familial hypercholesterolemia and the reproductive implications of Gary's marrying someone who also has familial hypercholesterolemia were discussed.

3. The heart disease risk factor pamphlet was discussed, and Gary's questions were answered.

4. The physician told Gary that while one or two capsules of fish oil high in eicosopentanoic acid (EPA) would not be harmful, it would probably not be helpful either. Higher doses affect blood lipids but entail high amounts of fat-soluble vitamins that could be toxic, as well as a substantial caloric intake. Intake of fish high in EPA (e.g., halibut, sardines) was encouraged in lieu of beef and pork.

Disposition. Gary was asked to return in 4 weeks for a repeat fasting lipid profile. An office visit was scheduled in 5 weeks to discuss the lipid results and tentatively to initiate lipid-altering medical treatment with lovastatin (Mevacor).

DISCUSSION

Gary's symptoms are quite common expressions of anxiety related to difficulty coping with stress at home, school, or work. Most patients in this situation respond well to simple reassurance, normalization, and empathic support, coupled with developing an effective repertoire of strategies for preventing and coping with stress and anxiety. This patient's anxiety appears to stem partly from irrational fear about acute heart disease and a more rational fear of eventually having heart disease. Discussing and treating Gary's major risk factor could greatly reduce his anxiety if the treatment is successful and well tolerated. If treatment does not go well, however, Gary's anxiety could escalate. It would be important to clarify that Gary's long-term LDL cholesterol range is the important determinant of prognosis, not any particular LDL cholesterol level.

Familial heterozygous (type IIa) hypercholesterolemia is relatively uncommon, with an incidence of about 1 in 400 in the general population. Mild and moderate hypercholesterolemia, however, is extremely common.

TABLE 20–30. FOODS DIVIDED INTO FATTY ACID COMPOSITION GROUPS

MORE THAN 30% SATURATED FATTY ACIDS	20% TO 30% SATURATED FATTY ACIDS	LESS THAN 20% SATURATED FATTY ACIDS
Butterfat	Poultry	Fish
Beef, lamb, pork, veal	Margarine*	Margarine*
Butter	Shortening	Oils, including peanut, corn, olive, safflower, sesame
Margarine* Shortening Coconut, palm oils	Cottonseed oil	Nuts

Source: From Gallagher-Allred CR, Townley NA. Dietary management in hyperlipidemia. In Nutrition and Health Promotion in Primary Care Series. Columbus, Department of Family Medicine, The Ohio State University, 1980, p. 10, with permission.

*The kind of fat and composition of fat in margarine vary considerably.

TABLE 20–31. DRUGS USED IN THE TREATMENT OF HYPERCHOLESTEROLEMIA

	DRUGS OF FIRST CHOICE			OTHER DRUGS	
	Bile Acid Binders	*Nicotinic Acid*	*HMG CoA Reductase Inhibitors (Lovastatin, Pravastatin, Simvastatin)*	*Gemfibrozil*	*Probucol*
Average effect					
LDL-C	↓	↓	↓	↔ ⇕	↓
HDL-C	↔ (or slight ↑)	↑	↑ ↔	↑ (slight)	↓
Triglycerides	↔ ↑	↓	↓ ↔	↓	↔
CHD risk reduction	Proven	Proven	Not proven, new drug	Proven	Not proven
Side effects	GI effects; constipation; malabsorption of digitalis, thyroid, and vitamins	Flushing, LFT* ↑, arrhythmia, gout, glucose intolerance, GI effects	Minimal side effects LFT ↑, fatigue, headaches, myopathy (rare)	Increased gallstones, LFT ↑, myopathy (rare)	GI effects, mild diarrhea, possible heart conduction disturbances
Contraindications	GI disease, peptic ulcer disease, severe hemorrhoids	Peptic ulcer disease, liver disease, gout, cardiac arrhythmias, bundle-branch block	Liver disease	Biliary obstruction, gallstones, liver disease	Ventricular irritability, prolonged QT interval
Dosage	Cholestyramine: 8 to 24 gm per day; Colestipol: 10 to 30 gm per day; taper on slowly	500 mg to 2 gm t.i.d.; taper on slowly and take with food	Lovastatin, 20 to 80 mg daily; pravastatin, 10 to 80 mg daily; simvastatin, 5 to 40 mg daily Take with evening meal Use a lower dose in the elderly	300 to 600 mg b.i.d.	250 to 500 mg b.i.d.

Source: Fram Rakel RE. Textbook of Family Practice, 4th ed. Philadelphia, W.B. Saunders, 1990, with permission.
*LFT = liver function tests

Over 50% of American adults have levels of LDL cholesterol high enough to promote coronary atherosclerosis, even in the absence of other risk factors. Over half the patients who experience myocardial infarctions have total cholesterol values between 200 and 240 mg/dl (5.2–6.1 mmol/liter) and LDL cholesterol levels below 160 mg/dl (4.1 mmol/liter). Individuals with diabetes or hypertension and cigarette smokers are at especially high risk if their LDL cholesterol levels are even mildly elevated and/or their HDL cholesterol levels are below average. After menopause, women rapidly catch up to men with respect to their risk for heart disease unless they receive estrogen replacement therapy.

When starting a program of dietary change to lower LDL cholesterol, it can be very helpful to ask patients to bring in their spouse, children, and other key family members for a family conference to discuss the rationale and details of a heart-healthy diet. Teaching patients and spouses how to interpret the information on food labels is an important component of patient education. Figuring out ways to deal with ethnic food preferences and customs is an important need for some families.

The main dietary changes for lowering elevated LDL cholesterol entail reducing the intake of foods high in saturated fat—fatty cuts of beef and pork and whole milk dairy products. Healthier replacements for these foods include chicken, fish, low-fat or nonfat dairy products or substitutes (not those with coconut or palm oil), and complex carbohydrates (starches such as breads, rice, and potatoes and water-soluble fiber such

as oat bran). The best oils for cooking include monounsaturated olive oil and polyunsaturated corn, safflower, and soybean oils. Olive oil has recently gained favor because it lowers LDL cholesterol as much as polyunsaturated oils, and it does not have the HDL cholesterol–lowering effect seen with the polyunsaturated oils.

Patients who have an average American intake of saturated fat and cholesterol usually respond to dietary modification by lowering their total and LDL cholesterol levels by about 10% to 15% of the baseline value. Patients who already have a low intake of saturated fat seldom respond well to dietary modification because they have so little room for change. Increased intake of water-soluble fiber often lowers LDL cholesterol by 5% to 15%. Cholesterol-lowering medication usually lowers the LDL cholesterol an additional 10% to 40% below the level achieved by dietary modification.

Although the cost-effectiveness of treating patients with borderline high LDL cholesterol is controversial, several prospective studies have established that lowering high LDL cholesterol with medication reduces the risk of coronary heart disease greatly during the ensuing 5 to 10 years in men. Patients with severe LDL elevation and/or very low HDL cholesterol levels are most likely to benefit from treatment.

Guidelines for the diagnosis and management of hypercholesterolemia in children are being developed. Dietary prevention ideally should begin early in life to minimize or postpone the development of atherosclerosis in

TABLE 20–32. HOW TO RECOMMEND AND WRITE PRESCRIPTIONS FOR CHOLESTEROL-LOWERING MEDICATIONS

MEDICATION	COMMENTS
OVER-THE-COUNTER	
Psyllium hydrophilic mucilloid/PHM:	Costs patient $7–11/mo for regular plain no-name PHM or Metamucil with sugar
Metamucil or no-name equivalent 1 heaping teaspoonful (tablespoonful of sugared/flavored form) in 8 oz of water/liquid, t.i.d. with meals	Costs $15–21/month for sugarfree form Costs $11–21/month for orange or lemon-lime flavor Costs $25/month for Instant Mix Metamucil
Fiberall Fruit and Nut Fiber Wafer, 3.4 gm 1 to 2 t.i.d. with 8 oz or more of liquid	Costs $35–40/month if sole PHM source Convenient lunchtime substitute for liquid dose
Nicotinic acid/niacin, 500 mg SR tab. #100	See nicotinic acid below for comments
Initial dose 1 tab., b.i.d.	Costs patient $8–10 for a bottle of 100
Increase to 2 tabs., b.i.d. 2nd week	Maximum dose 3 gm/day; little side effects with SR form except occasional hepatitis ts $10–12/month for 2 gm/day, $15–20/month for 3 gm/day
PRESCRIPTION MEDICATIONS	
Cholestyramine (Questran), powder	Proven preventive benefit; inconvenient; constipating; more than 15-year safety record
Disp.: 3 cans (378 gm/can)	Will cost patient $60–70 for 3 cans
Sig.: 1 scoop, b.i.d.(starting dose)	Will last 2 months ($30–35/month)
2 scoops, b.i.d. (usual maintenance dose)	Will last 1 month($60–70/month)
2 scoops, t.i.d. (max. maintenance dose)	Will last 3 weeks ($90–105/month) if patient takes it all
Probucol (Lorelco), 500-mg tab (new size)	Well tolerated; convenient; regresses xanthomas; Inhibits foam-cell formation; reverses cholesterol transport; LDL catabolism; antioxidant effect 10-year safety record; HDL lowering probably benign
#100	Will cost patient $60–80 for 100
Sig.: 1 tab. b.i.d. with meals	Will last 7 weeks ($45/month)
Nicotinic acid/niacin	Lowers LDL and VLDL; raises HDL; 20-year safety record
Nicolar, 500-mg tab.	Intense flushing/itching (can block with 1 ASA tab.) Well tolerated after initial adjustment period Hepatitis occasionally; arrhythmia/hyperglycemia rare
#200	Will cost patient $70 for 200
Sig.: 2 tabs. b.i.d. with meals	Will last 7 weeks ($45/month)
Nicobid, 500-mg SR cap	Less flushing/itching than Nicolar
#200	Will cost patient $90–110
Sig.: 2 tabs. b.i.d with meals	Will last 7 weeks ($50–65/month)
Gemfibrozil (Lopid), 300/600-mg tab	Short safety record; erratic LDL effect; raises HDL Beneficial in Helsinki study
#100	Will cost patient $75 for #100 300-mg or 50 600-mg
Sig.: 1 or 2 tabs. b.i.d. with meals	Will last 7 weeks ($45/month)
Lovastatin (Mevacor), 20-mg tab	Highly effective LDL lowering; ? long-term safety
#60	Will cost patient $85 for 60
Sig.: 1 tab. q.d. with evening meal (initial)	Will last 2 months ($45/month)
1 tab. b.i.d.or 2 tabs. q.d. (medium)	Will last 1 month ($85/month)
1 tab. t.i.d. (high)	Will last 3 weeks ($135/month)
Pravastatin (Pravachol), 20 mg tab	Highly effective; ? long term safety
#60	Will cost patient $75 for 60
	Will last 2 mos. ($40/mo)
Sig: 1 tab, q.d. with evening meal	Will last 1 month ($80/mo)
2 tabs, q.d.	Will last 3 wks ($120/mo)
3 tabs, q.d.	
Simvastatin (Zocor), 10 mg tab	Same as Pravastatin
Same regimens as pravastatin and lovastatin	

adulthood. Although most clinicians are reluctant to use lipid-altering drugs in children, medication should be considered if a child's severely elevated LDL cholesterol does not respond well to dietary modification.

The benefit of medical management has not been studied in females. Women will probably benefit about as much as men with similarly elevated LDL cholesterol levels and comparable risk factors. Postmenopausal estrogen replacement may have more powerful preventive potential than LDL cholesterol–lowering medications, especially for women with low HDL cholesterol levels.

Treatment of high LDL cholesterol in the elderly is even more controversial. The estimated potential benefit of treatment (enhanced quality of life for more of the remaining lifespan) must be weighed carefully against the expense and possible adverse effects of medications being considered for each elderly patient.

The importance of triglyceride elevations as a heart disease risk factor continues to be controversial. Severe elevation above 400 mg/dl appears to increase the risk for heart disease in female patients, especially those with diabetes, and should be treated with niacin or gemfibrozil. It is unclear whether lesser elevations of triglycerides should be treated medically if weight loss, exercise, alcohol abstinence, and improved control of diabetes do not satisfactorily lower the fasting level of triglycerides.

Mounting evidence has established low HDL cholesterol as a powerful independent risk factor, even if LDL cholesterol is only mildly elevated (130–159 mg/dl) or in the high range of normal (100–129 mg/dl). Although the initial National Cholesterol Education Program (NCEP) guidelines do not recommend medical management for low HDL cholesterol per se, the results of the Helsinki study suggest that treating low HDL cholesterol is at least as beneficial as lowering elevated LDL cholesterol levels. Hygienic approaches, including regular aerobic exercise, weight loss, and smoking cessation, tend to raise HDL cholesterol by 5 to 15 mg/dl, as does treatment with niacin or gemfibrozil. Lovastatin and cholestyramine sometimes elevate HDL cholesterol slightly. Although probucol lowers HDL cholesterol, this is probably not an adverse effect, since HDL cholesterol lowering correlates even better than LDL cholesterol lowering for atheroma regression in probucol-treated patients. Apparently, the smaller HDL particles in probucol-treated patients carry less total cholesterol at any given point in time but are more efficient in moving excess LDL cholesterol from peripheral storage areas back to the liver.

SUGGESTED READING

Rakel RE. Textbook of Family Practice, 4th ed. Philadelphia, W. B. Saunders, 1990, pp. 227–229, 866–867, 870, 1226–1228.

Report of the Expert Panel on Detection, Evaluation, and Treatment of High Blood Cholesterol in Adults. Arch Intern Med. 1988; 148:36–69.

Recommendations for treatment of hyperlipidemia in adults (Joint Statement of the Nutrition Committee and the Council on Atherosclerosis). Circulation 1984; 69:1067A–1090A.

Snyder S. Comparison of cholesterol-lowering regimens. Am Fam Physician 1990; 42:761–768.

QUESTIONS

1. High LDL cholesterol is defined by the National Cholesterol Education Program guidelines as an LDL cholesterol level of
    a. 130 mg/dl (3.4 mmol/liter) or higher.
    b. 160 mg/dl (4.1 mmol/liter) or higher.
    c. 190 mg/dl (4.9 mmol/liter) or higher.
    d. 200 mg/dl (5.2 mmol/liter) or higher.
    e. 240 mg/dl (6.1 mmol/liter) or higher.

2. Which of the following foods contain the *least* saturated fat and cholesterol when eaten in average serving amounts?
    a. Eggs and liver
    b. Beef and pork
    c. Olive and safflower oil
    d. Whole milk and butter
    e. Coconut oil and palm oil

3. Among the following over-the-counter and prescription medications, which one lowers LDL cholesterol the most effectively?
    a. Cholestyramine
    b. Gemfibrozil
    c. Lovastatin
    d. Niacin
    e. Probucol

Answers appear on page 451.

Severe Lethargy

STEVEN D. MORSE

INITIAL VISIT

SUBJECTIVE

Patient Identification and Presenting Problem. Karen is a 25-year-old Caucasion female who lives with her spouse. On a cold December evening just after Christmas, she is brought to the emergency department (at 10 p.m.) because of severe lethargy. Her husband Doug is present and assists in providing clinical data.

Present Illness. Karen moved to this area 6 months ago so her spouse could pursue a promising career opportunity. This move forced her to leave behind an extended family to whom she feels quite close. Owing to the demands of his new job, Doug is away from home for prolonged periods, and Karen has been tearful and easily angered recently in interactions with him. On the evening of admission, a sudden alteration of weekend plans caused them to argue. Doug left the house at about 6 p.m. to "take a walk and clear my head." When he returned at about 9 p.m., he found Karen in the bedroom extremely lethargic and surrounded by empty pill vials and a nearly empty bottle of Scotch. After several unsuccessful attempts to awaken her, he summoned an ambulance and had her transported to the hospital. He has also had the presence of mind to bring the pill bottles for review; Tylenol 3 tablets are noted (prescribed for him for a severe ankle sprain; 20 tablets are unaccounted for) and Valium 5 mg tablets are noted as well (originally prescribed for him as an adjunct for a low back strain; an unknown number of these are unaccounted for).

Past Medical History. Karen has no past history (per her spouse) of any medical or surgical illness and has never been hospitalized. She has no known allergies and has apparently never before sought or needed psychiatric help.

Family History. Karen's parents and multiple siblings are alive and well. Her grandparents are likewise alive and in good health. There is no known history of familial disease, either medical or psychiatric. Karen and Doug have been married for 4 years and have had no past problems; he appears very concerned and supportive.

Health Habits and Social History. Doug states that Karen is a nonsmoker who drinks only socially and does not use recreational drugs. She is, to his knowledge, sexually active only with him, and she uses oral contraceptives for birth control. Karen does not exercise regularly; she has no dietary restrictions.

Review of Systems. This is currently unobtainable; Karen's husband states she has volunteered no physical complaints recently.

OBJECTIVE

Physical Examination. Physical examination reveals a well-nourished and well-developed white female. Her blood pressure is 110/70; heart rate is 96; respiratory rate is 14; and rectal temperature is 97°F. She is somnolent and resposive only to painful stimuli, with feeble but somewhat purposeful symmetrical responses. The examination is of note for pinpoint pupils, alcohol on the breath, a feeble to absent gag reflex, and mild acrocyanosis.

Laboratory Tests. Appropriately in this case, diagnostic and therapeutic efforts are carried out in tandem. Multiple studies were obtained rapidly (Table 20–33). These revealed a combined metabolic and respiratory acidosis, an elevated alveolar–arterial oxygen gradient,

TABLE 20–33. KAREN'S LABORATORY DATA

CBC: Normal
Electrolytes: Na 141, K 4.1, Cl 103, HCO$_3$ 19
BUN/Creatinine: Normal
Blood glucose: 131 mg%
Arterial blood gases (room air): pH 7.28, pO$_2$ 62, pCO$_2$ 48, carboxyHgb 5.0%
Portable AP CXR: "Possible infiltrate right lower lobe"
12-lead ECG: Normal
Serum ethanol level: 321 mg%
Serum acetaminophen level: 300 μ/ml
Serum drug screen: Sent out; available in 5 to 6 hours
Urinalysis (by Foley catheter): pH 6.0, spec. grav. 1028, dipstick 1+ ketones, 2+ glucose, sediment: none
Cultures obtained and pending: Blood (two), urine, sputum
Serum pregnancy test (screen): Negative

a possible right lower lobe aspiration pneumonia, and potentially dangerous serum levels of ethanol and acetaminophen.

ASSESSMENT

Working Diagnosis. Karen appears to have depression of her mental status due to a polypharmacy drug ingestion. The majority of intentional drug ingestions are polypharmacy, and most such ingestions include ethanol. The patient's small pupils suggest that narcotics are a contributor to her mental status, and the measured high ethanol level (available later) proves its role as well. While the elevated acetaminophen level recorded acutely is not a factor in her mental state, it is a dangerous level based on estimated time of ingestion (Fig. 20–8) and will require antidotal therapy once the

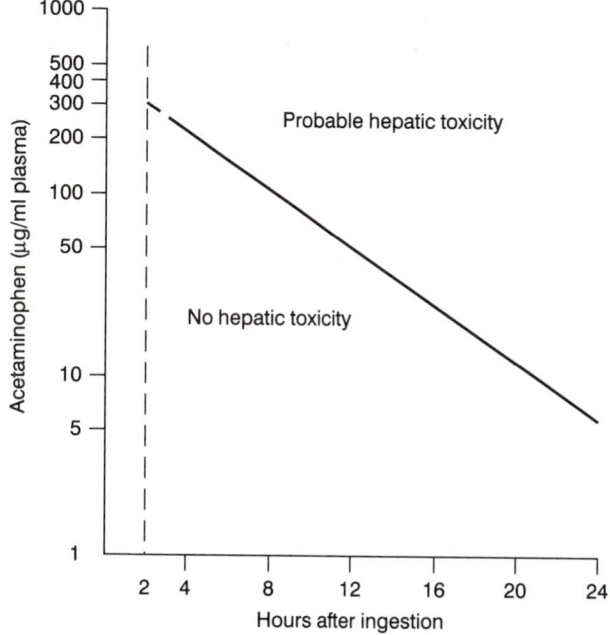

Figure 20–8. Semilogarithmic plot of plasma acetaminophen levels versus time. (From Rumack, B. H., and Matthew, H.: Pediatrics, 55:871, 1975, with permission.)

patient has been acutely stabilized. Any contribution of other (as yet unsuspected) drugs to her status will be more apparent upon return of her drug screen, but acute management will not be altered.

Secondary diagnoses, such as depression or other psychiatric illness, can only be adequately assessed and managed once stabilization and resumption of prior mental status have been achieved. However, these issues must not be forgotten.

Differential Diagnosis. Other explanations for Karen's clinical presentation are not likely given the scenario and the (rapidly) available data. However, one consideration that must be included is that of *CNS injury due to occult trauma* (including spouse abuse). Should the rapid resumption of normal mental status not occur with supportive and antidotal therapies, CT scanning of the brain should be carried out as rapidly as possible.

PLAN

The first step in stabilization of this obtunded patient should involve airway access and control. A cuffed endotracheal tube of appropriate size should be placed orally or nasally as atraumatically as possible. This will afford protection from further aspiration and allow maintenance of stable gas exchange and good pulmonary toilet.

Once the patient has been intubated, a large-bore orogastric or nasogastric tube should be placed to permit removal of the gastric contents, including pill fragments, by saline lavage. Once this has been accomplished, instillation of activated charcoal and a cathartic such as sorbitol should be considered. Activated charcoal is a nonspecific adsorbent of small organic molecules. A cathartic will decrease GI transit time for any unabsorbed drug, thus improving its excretion from the gut. One may wish to delay this instillation for a brief period, however, to permit the unencumbered instillation of *N*-acetylcysteine (Mucomyst) into the stomach via gastric tube to begin the antidotal regimen for acetaminophen overdose (loading dose 140 mg/kg, followed by 70 mg/kg every 4 hours for 17 doses). This agent blunts or aborts the delayed hepatotoxicity of acetaminophen ingestion, which occurs due to reduced glutathione depletion and the buildup of toxic metabolic intermediates in hepatocytes.

Once airway protection is achieved and the patient is appropriately ventilated, in addition to gastric decontamination, intravenous access should be accomplished, and coincident with this, blood (if not previously obtained) should be sent to the laboratory for studies for guidelines in further management (see Table 20–34).

It is appropriate in the management of the obtunded patient to empirically provide several intravenous agents: One ampule (25 gm) of 50% dextrose, 0.8 to 2.0 mg naloxone (Narcan), and 100 mg thiamine should be given in the adult, in addition to some degree of supplemental oxygen. In known or suspected benzodiazepine ingestion it is appropriate to administer a test dose of flumazenil (Mazicon), a benzodiazepine antagonist, as

well. Dextrose provides a substrate for cerebral metabolism and combats hypoglycemia due to insulin, malnutrition, or the toxic effects of drugs, including ethanol and narcotics in overdoses. The morbidity of its administration is extremely low, even in patients with preexisting hyperglycemia. Naxolone, a narcotic antagonist without agonist properties, is a useful antidotal agent in cases of overdose with opiates and associated agents (such as propoxyphene); in chronically narcotic-dependent individuals, the drug may precipitate a withdrawal syndrome (short-lived but sometimes severe) requiring acute symptom management. In addition, if a patient awakens after use of this short-lived agent, combativeness may occur, and prophylactic placement of soft restraints should be considered in selected patients to avoid damage to the patient or staff, extubation, or abrupt exit from the emergency department by the patient. If a gratifying response to initial naloxone is achieved, the initial bolus may be supplemented both with intramuscular naloxone and possibly a continuous infusion of the drug titrated to the patient's mental status (often 0.4–0.8 mg/h is sufficient to prevent profound depression of mental and respiratory status). If it is expected that a dramatic response to naloxone will occur, carry out any other needed maneuvers first (once the airway is stabilized) to avoid the added difficulties inherent in a combative or violent patient.

The use of thiamine will prevent cerebral damage due to glucose loading in the face of preexisting thiamine depletion. While this is more often a problem in the chronic malnourished patient, the agent should be given liberally because of its extremely low morbidity and cost.

In appropriately selected cases, the use of intravenous flumazenil (Mazicon), a benzodiazepine receptor antagonist, may reverse obtundation from benzodiazepine ingestion. Careful observation is required, however, to avoid resedation and seizures (especially in patients with chronic benzodiazepine dependence or those who also take tricyclic antidepressants).

Once the preceding maneuvers have been carried out, the patient should receive a careful "secondary survey" or more detailed examination, assessing response to initial maneuvers, seeking occult trauma or medical disease states, and ensuring that there have been "fingers and tubes in every orifice." Further studies (such as CT scanning of the head or other cavities) can now be rationally considered.

A catheter should now have been placed to follow urinary output; urine should always be dipsticked in the emergency department to provide a clue to additional disease. The urine and gastric contents should supplement serum samples for drug screening. An ECG should be obtained to screen for occult ischemia or myocardial infarction (MI), and the patient should be monitored (even the young patient may have MI in the face of cocaine or amphetamine use). The additional value of the ECG is in screening for an unsuspected cardiotoxin in the overdose (such as tricyclic antidepressants; look for QTc prolongation or QRS widening).

In obtunded females who are of childbearing age,

who may require multiple studies, procedures, and drugs, it is prudent to routinely obtain a pregnancy test early in evaluation to allow for rational modifications of therapy and reduce possible subsequent risks of medicolegal liability. A positive test may even provide a clue to psychological stress leading to the ingestion and allow for appropriate discussion and planning later in the hospital course.

Response to Treatment and Disposition. After the modalities discussed above were instituted, Karen became much more responsive; her pupils became dilated and briskly reactive to light. While still sleepy, she followed simple motor commands appropriately and symmetrically. She was admitted to the intensive care unit and was rapidly weaned from ventilator support. A full antidotal course of *N*-acetylcysteine therapy was carried out, with no apparent elevation of transaminases on serial study. She recovered normal mental status, and restraints were removed. Upon interviewing her, she relates her progressive feelings of isolation, hopelessness, and helplessness brought on by her husband's career change and their move. She has no close friends locally. Her feelings culminated in the impulsive ingestion. A psychiatric consultant sees her, and he finds her free of any active suicidal ideation or thought disorder and recommends outpatient treatment but no pharmacotherapy. Goal-directed counseling is begun.

Karen's inpatient course is only complicated by fever on the second hospital day and a cough productive of yellow sputum. She is treated for aspiration pneumonitis with parenteral antibiotics and rapidly improves.

The only drugs detected in Karen's full drug screen, which returns on the second hospital day, are acetaminophen, codeine, diazepam, ethanol, and various metabolites. She is discharged from the hospital after several days, in good health, for planned office follow-up.

DISCUSSION

Karen's case illustrates the acute approach to a common emergency situation, the obtunded drug-overdosed patient. Assessment and management of such a patient must proceed simultaneously. The sequence of events must include attention to airway access and protection, ventilation and maintenance of circulation, gastrointestinal tract decontamination, antidotal therapy as appropriate, and then secondary evaluation and differential diagnostic assessment. GI tract decontamination may be accomplished in the alert patient (with an intact gag reflex and no contraindications) with ipecac and then charcoal/sorbitol if the ingestion is recent. If patients are poor risks for emesis but decontamination is required, gastric intubation and lavage with a large-bore tube are appropriate, after the airway is secure.

Most overdoses are polypharmacy in the adult, and the patient's history is often incomplete, inaccurate as to dose and/or timing, or grossly in error or incomplete as to agents taken. This may be due to obtundation, fear, or sociopathy. The overdosed patient must be approached with this in mind, and a wide diagnostic approach must be taken to rule out unsuspected toxins. However, while medical and laboratory assessment should be aggressive, interpersonal interaction in these cases, even in difficult situations, should be nonjudgmental and supportive, even if the patient simultaneously requires restraints. This will minimize patient combativeness and attendant risks to staff, maximize the chances for later compliance, and minimize later medicolegal risk.

It is important to keep in mind that due to invasive procedures, patient combativeness, and other factors (such as intravenous drug use), emergency department staff may be exposed to blood or bodily fluids with little advance warning. Precautions should always be taken to minimize the chance of such exposures with their attendant risks of hepatitis or HIV transmission.

Should the patient with putative drug overdose and altered mental status refuse treatment, it is important to remain supportive but to reinforce to the patient and family/friends the need for treatment and the potentially self-destructive nature of the actions that have been performed by the patient. If necessary, psychiatric colleagues can be utilized to secure involuntary commitment for required medical treatments in the case of suicidal and ill or dangerous but resistant patients.

Fortunately, while useful antidotal therapies (such as those used in this case) are not common, most overdoses are well managed with aggressive supportive therapy as reviewed. Exotic modalities such as dialysis are useful only for a few drugs with specific characteristics regarding protein binding and volume of distribution.

Vigorous supportive therapy must continue for these patients after discharge from the acute hospital stay to prevent a recurrence of the overdose due to unresolved stressful situations in the environment or unaddressed and untreated psychopathology. It is an unfortunate fact that despite our best efforts, many overdose patients will repeat their behavior and present again for care.

QUESTIONS

1. The most common drug in polypharmacy drug overdose cases is
   a. Aspirin.
   b. Ethanol.
   c. Heroin.
   d. Cocaine.

2. The proper priority sequence in the obtunded overdose patient is
   a. Circulation, airway, gastric decontamination, secondary survey.
   b. Gastric decontamination, airway, circulation, secondary survey.
   c. Airway, circulation, gastric decontamination, secondary survey.
   d. Airway, circulation, secondary survey, gastric decontamination.

3. All the following have specific and available anti-dotal therapy *except*
   a. Acetaminophen.
   b. Cocaine.
   c. Carbon monoxide.
   d. Insulin.
   e. Diazepam.

4. Activated charcoal is of use in all the following ingestions *except*
   a. Digoxin.
   b. Aspirin.
   c. Lithium.
   d. Theophylline.
   e. Acetaminophen.

Answers appear on page 451.

Confusion with Lethargy

STEVEN D. MORSE

INITIAL VISIT

SUBJECTIVE

Patient Identification and Presenting Problem. Joseph K. is a 65-year-old white man who lives alone in a boarding house. When money is available, he tends to drink heavily. He has sporadically attended the family practice center. An ambulance has been summoned to his room on this February evening because his landlord found him sitting in a chair, confused and lethargic. The landlord had come to his room to argue with him about the overdue rent. He arrives at the emergency department just after the ambulance and admits that in retribution for his tenant's tardiness he had "turned the heat down a little" in the building recently.

Present Illness. Joseph's past medical history is significant to his current state. His office records reveal a prior history of episodic congestive heart failure, for which he has been maintained on furosemide (40 mg/day) in the past. In addition, he has a history of chronic ethanol abuse and a paranoid personality disorder treated with chlorpromazine (50 mg/day). His last recorded visit to the office setting was 7 months ago.

Because of his current mental status, and because he is reclusive and lives alone, little information is available regarding recent symptoms. Joseph is somewhat confused and lethargic but can slowly answer very simple questions and follow some simple commands. He states he has not had alcohol in "days" and has obtained his nourishment at the local Salvation Army soup kitchen in the last week. He denies any focal complaints and says he has been taking his medications regularly. However, although he is aware that he is at the hospital, he states the year is 1974 and Richard Nixon is the president.

Past Medical History. Aside from his recorded psychiatric and cardiac histories, neither Joseph nor his records reveal any other medical problems. Nor can his landlord suggest any other difficulties. Joseph was last hospitalized 18 months ago for dehydration due to overdiuresis and self-neglect. He has not been hospitalized for congestive failure in over 3 years. An inpatient psychiatric stay has not occurred in 6 years. He has no known allergies.

Family History. Joseph is single, reclusive, and reticent to any discussion about family. He appears to be childless and to have no close relatives.

Health Habits and Social History. Joseph's drinking history is well-documented in the available medical records; there is no documentation of alcohol withdrawal syndrome, seizures, or any acute or chronic visceral complications of ethanol abuse. The landlord states that Joseph smokes heavily, but there is no history of drug abuse. Joseph has lived in his current boarding house for 2 years, is unemployed, and obtains most meals through social service agencies. To Joseph's credit, although the rent is often late, the landlord says that the patient makes a point of getting and taking his prescibed medication; it seems to be a point of pride for him. Sexual history is not obtainable.

Review of Systems. This is entirely negative when presented to the patient, except for the statements that he feels thirsty and cold; he repeatedly asks for water and blankets.

OBJECTIVE

Physical Examination. Physical examination reveals a disheveled and confused elderly white man who appears poorly nourished and whose hands and nails are heavily nicotine stained. There is no odor of alcohol on his breath. Mental status review reveals moderate disorientation, as noted above; the patient is very slow to converse but attempts to do so intermittently. He slowly follows simple one-step commands.

The blood pressure is 80/40; pulse is 50 and regular; respiratory rate is 14; and oral temperature by electronic probe is 31°C (89°F); a rectal temperature is taken and is found to be 31.5°C (90°F).

The examination is otherwise of note for anicteric sclerae, dry mucous membranes and poor skin turgor, clear lungs, a benign cardiac examination, and an absence of organomegaly on abdominal examination. The stool is hemoccult negative. The neurological examination is grossly nonfocal; the reflexes are questionably "hung up." There is no asterixis. The skin reveals spider angiomata and palmar erythema. The extremities, while quite cool, have good capillary refill and are free of edema, bullae, or anesthesia.

Laboratory Data. Multiple laboratory studies were obtained; they are listed in Table 20–34. Initial patient management in this case, however, should not await their return. The patient's cardiac rhythm was monitored (Fig. 20–9).

Laboratory studies revealed a leukocytosis and a slight macrocytic anemia (probably blunted due to hemoconcentration). A metabolic acidosis is present, as is dehydration given the high sodium and BUN and elevated BUN/creatinine ratio. Mild to moderate hyperglycemia is present. Arterial blood gases (measured and reported at 37°C) suggest an additional respiratory acidosis and rule out carbon monoxide as an agent causing confusion. Note, however, that the arterial blood gas values as reported are inaccurate and must be corrected

back to reflect the patient's true core temperature (Table 20–35). Such a correction reveals that acidosis in the patient is not profound and that pO_2 and pCO_2 are actually lower than reported.

Urinalysis corroborates dehydration. There is no ethanol present. The ECG and rhythm strip demonstrate J or Osborne waves, characteristic of systemic hypothermia, and would point to the diagnosis even if the core temperature had not as yet been measured.

ASSESSMENT

Working Diagnosis. Joseph appears to be suffering from *systemic hypothermia* brought on by relatively slow exposure to low environmental temperatures and exacerbated by his preexisting medical and psychiatric difficulties and his medical regimen.

"Systemic hypothermia" is defined as a core (usually rectal) temperature of less than 95°F (35°C). Metabolic heat production rises in response to cold stress until this core temperature is reached. At even lower core temperatures, metabolic heat production declines and leads to progressive cooling and multisystem dysfunction.

A wide range of settings and situations can predispose to hypothermia (Table 20–36). The elderly, neonates, the intoxicated, those who are obtunded or psychiatrically deranged, those with diseases or on drugs that impair heat generation or conservation, and those who become glycogen-depleted and exhausted in the cold are all at increased risk.

Joseph is not currently intoxicated. However, if alcohol were present, it could exacerbate his syndrome. It is a vasodilator and a sedative, and it can induce hypoglycemia. Phenothiazines, which the patient uses, also vasodilate via alpha-blocking effects and further impair heat conservation. They also may sedate a patient and impair appropriate behavioral responses to cold stress.

TABLE 20–34.   JOSEPH'S LABORATORY DATA

CBC: Hgb 12.5, Hct 37, (MCV 103) WBC count 14.3, polys 89, bands 4, lymphs 7
Electrolytes: Na 149, K 3.1, Cl 105, HCO_3 20
BUN 68, creatinine 1.8, PT 12.1, PTT 29.2
Blood glucose, 280 mg%
Arterial blood gases (room air, reported at 37°C):   pH 7.21, pO_2 90, pCO_2 52, carboxyhemoglobin 7.0%
Portable CXR: No infiltrates or CHF; cardiomegaly noted
ECG: Sinus bradycardia and diffuse Osborne waves noted
Serum ethanol level: <10 mg/dl
Serum drug screen: Positive only for chlorpromazine (returns on day 2)
Urinalysis (catheterized specimen):   pH 5.0, spec. grav. 1.035, dipstick positive for glucose only, sediment: none
Cultures obtained and sent: Blood (two), urine
Serum ammonia: Normal
Liver function tests: Normal
Serum ketones: Negative
Thyroid function tests: Sent
Serum cortisol: Sent

TABLE 20–35.   VARIANCE OF BLOOD GASES WITH BODY TEMPERATURE*

	↑ 1°C	↓ 1°C
pH	↓ .015	↑ .015
pCO_2 (mmHg)	↑ 4.4%	↓ 4.4%
pO_2 (mmHg)	↑ 7.2%	↓ 7.2%

Source: From Rakel RE. Textbook of Family Practice, 4th ed. Philadelphia, W.B. Saunders, 1990, with permission.
   *Departures from values at 37°C.

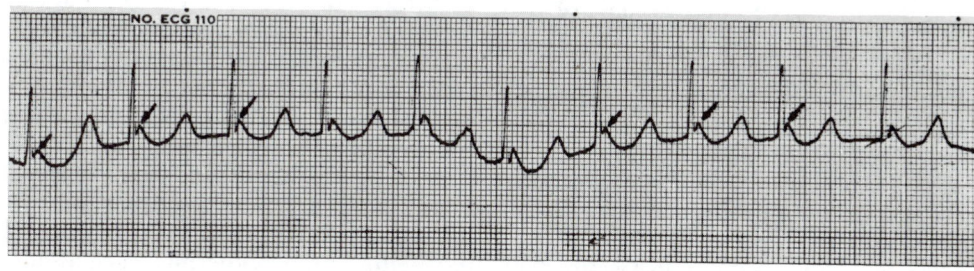

Figure 20–9. Osborne waves (←) in this hypothermic patient. These waves disappeared with rewarming.

TABLE 20–36. CLINICAL SETTINGS FOR HYPOTHERMIA

Exposure
Drugs
   Alcohol
   Barbiturates
   Phenothiazines
Endocrinopathies:
   Hypoglycemia
   Diabetic ketoacidosis
   Myxedema
   Hypoadrenalism
   Panhypopituitarism
Central nervous system dysfunction:
   Wernicke's encephalopathy
   Anorexia nervosa
   Cerebrovascular disease
   Head trauma
   Spinal cord transection
Sepsis
Malnutrition
Skin dysfunction—burns, erythrodermas

Source: Fram Rakel RE. Textbook of Family Practice, 4th ed. Philadelphia, W.B. Saunders, 1990, with permission.

While it is more conjectural, they also may inhibit hypothalamic response to temperature stress.

Joseph is also dehydrated and volume-contracted, as demonstrated by hemoconcentration and other laboratory data. This is due to his continued diuretic use, fluid compartment shifts due to hypothermia, and renal tubular dysfunction leading to inappropriate salt and water loss in chronic cold stress ("cold-induced diuresis").

Differential Diagnoses. Other entities deserve consideration in this hypothermic patient. It is reasonable to consider the possibility of *undiagnosed endocrinopathy* and screen for this. *Hypoglycemia* should be empirically reversed early on (see below), and any other disease states should be managed as they become manifest. *Masked narcotic overdose* should be considered and empiric naloxone therapy given. In this patient as well, *Wernicke's encephalopathy* should be treated/avoided with empiric thiamine treatment on presentation. *Sepsis* should be sought and managed if documented or if suspicion is high.

Careful secondary survey should be carried out, with consideration given to possible *occult head trauma, spinal axis trauma,* or *stroke.* The physician should not miss clues that this syndrome is related to *hepatic failure* or *myxedema* and should take care not to miss signs of *frostbite* in more severe exposures on secondary survey (not likely in this slow-onset scenario) and screen for associated "silent" diseases in the elderly (such as *myocardial infarction* on ECG).

PLAN

Mortality in hypothermia is dictated mainly by the presence and severity of other disease states, and rates of mortality vary widely in reported series. The only entity in which depression of core temperature is directly related to mortality is myxedema coma.

Cardiovascular and neurologic changes in hypothermic patients are often profound. Bradycardia, lengthening of ECG intervals, and T-wave inversions may be seen. Atrial arrhythmias may occur due to chamber distension. Muscular tremors may be seen on ECG, even at temperatures so low that gross shivering has ceased. Of all ECG changes, the Osborne wave is most characteristic. In severe cases, one may see ventricular fibrillation and, at lower temperatures, asystole.

Mentation progressively deteriorates in hypothermia as cerebral blood flow decreases in parallel with temperature. Coma eventually supervenes, and the EEG becomes flat at severe levels of core temperature depression (at or below 68°F).

Profound hypothermia may simulate death, with fixed and dilated pupils, asystole, apnea, and coma. However, severely hypothermic patients can tolerate prolonged hypoxia, hypotension, and circulatory arrest and still undergo complete medical and neurologic recovery, especially if previously well. An important dictum of environmental medicine is that "no one is dead until they are warm and dead."

Many other organ systems become dysfunctional in the hypothermic patient. Tracheobronchial secretions increase in volume and become viscid ("cold-induced bronchorrhea"); aspiration may further complicate matters. Hemoconcentration, due to fluid shifts, occurs. Ileus and diminished hepatic enzyme function both gradually develop. Pancreatitis is uncommon clinically but can occur.

As core temperature drops, renal blood flow falls and with it glomerular filtration rate. However, in patients in whom hypothermia develops over days (like Joseph), volume depletion can occur on a renal basis due to cold-related distal tubular dysfunction with excess salt and water loss ("cold-induced diuresis").

Glucose utilization is impaired in hypothermia as metabolic demands fall. Hyperglycemia, while common, does not accurately reflect the presence of diabetes mellitus. Only extreme hyperglycemia or documented ketoacidosis should be actively treated, since any insulin given may become extremely potent in the face of diminished hepatic degradation. Also, fluid shifts precipitated by insulin due to glucose movement may exacerbate hypovolemia.

A variety of therapeutic approaches can be taken to the patient with systemic hypothermia (Table 20–37). Passive rewarming by removal from cold stress and use of blankets is safe and effective if patients are mildly hypothermic. In extreme cases, active core rewarming may be needed, such as GI irrigation with heated fluids, dialysis, extracorporeal blood rewarming, and even more extreme methods. Two means of providing some degree of active core rewarming that are of low morbidity and that can be used on most patients include warming intravenous fluids ("room temperature" fluids add to cold stress in a cold patient) and giving heated humidified air or oxygen by nebulizer for inhalation.

Controversy exists regarding active external rewarming methods in hypothermia (such as hot water immersion, electric blanket use, etc.). These methods are safest

TABLE 20–37.   THERAPY IN HYPOTHERMIA

Don't miss head trauma, frostbite, injection sites (e.g., insulin, opiates, and so on)
Hospitalize and monitor if temperature is less than 91°F (33°C)
Use glass thermometer that reads into *low* range or electronic probe
Usual ABCs of CPR; handle cautiously to avoid cardiac arrest
Minimize drug use; avoid insulin when possible
Atrial arrhythmias revert with rewarming
PVCs—check pO_2, check pH, use lidocaine if needed, check electrolytes
Warm intravenous fluids with blood coils to 99°F to 112°F (37–43°C)
Heated oxygen, good pulmonary toilet
Thyroxine (400 μg) and steroids (300 mg hydrocortisone) for myxedema coma
Warm oral fluids if awake
Rewarming—active or passive
Prolong CPR—no one is dead until warm and dead

Source: From Rakel RE. Textbook of Family Practice, 4th ed. Philadelphia, W.B. Saunders, 1990, with permission.

where least needed, in young and mild cases. In severe cases, they inhibit access to patients for resuscitative efforts, cause vasodilation and shock in volume-depleted patients, may cause burns, and can in theory even suppress endogenous heat production by abolishing core-to-surface temperature gradients. In theory, vasodilation induced by active external rewarming can shunt cold peripheral pooled blood back to the body's core and produce "core temperature afterdrop," which may worsen visceral dysfunction. Careful thought should be given to any active external rewarming method before use to assess risk on an individual basis owing to the theoretical risks. Most active core rewarming methods (except as described above) should be reserved for severe cases because of the morbidity associated with these complex invasive maneuvers.

In Joseph's case, blankets were placed. Intravenous fluids were heated using blood-warming coils, and heated nebulized oxygen (30% FiO_2) was given via mask. Joseph was empirically given one ampule 50% dextrose, 0.8 mg naloxone, and 100 mg thiamine intravenously for his confusional state.

Intravenous fluids (5% dextrose in normal saline) with multivitamins and supplemental magnesium were given liberally; potassium supplementation also was provided in the intravenous fluid. The blood pressure rapidly improved with volume challenge and rewarming, and within 2 hours of arrival, the rectal temperature (continuously monitored) was 95°F and the patient was shivering and fully alert and oriented (although actively paranoid) with a blood pressure of 120/80 mmHg. Joseph's Osborne waves resolved, and his cardiac rate accelerated. He was fully cultured, and tests of endocrine function were sent, but antibiotics, steroids, and thyroxine were not empirically used owing to his rapid improve-

ment (Some or all of these agents might well be utilized in more severe and refractory cases in an empiric fashion pending results of studies.)

Disposition.   Joseph was discharged from the hospital on the third day of his stay. He returned in 1 week to the office. He had no complaints and appeared reasonably well. Meals-on-wheels services, arranged via social service, are now attempting to ensure his adequate nutrition. It will be important to reinforce to him the need to decrease ethanol use, avoid environmental cold stress, and liberalize fluid and electrolyte intake at this time of year. His landlord has been counseled about his responsibility to help the patient avoid undue environmental cold stress (a call to the city licensing and inspection board proved most persuasive in this regard) and heat stress for that matter; he now appears willing to be a kinder and gentler individual in this regard. Only time will tell.

QUESTIONS

1. The major determinant of mortality in systemic hypothermia is
   a. Patient age.
   b. Core temperature depression.
   c. Associated diseases.
   d. Presence of frostbite.
   e. Speed of rewarming.

2. The most characteristic ECG change in systemic hypothermia is
   a. T-wave inversion.
   b. Delta waves.
   c. Osborne waves.
   d. Bradycardia.
   e. Long intervals.

3. Hypothermic patients usually should not receive
   a. Dextrose.
   b. Naloxone.
   c. Oxygen.
   d. Insulin.
   e. Thiamine.

4. Risks of active external rewarming include all the following *except*
   a. Shock due to vasodilation.
   b. Burns due to contact.
   c. Core temperature afterdrop.
   d. Introduction of infection.
   e. Poor patient accessibility.

Answers appear on page 451.

Leg Pain

DAVID GONZALEZ, WILLIAM L. FRANZEN, Jr., and DAVID C. CAMPBELL

INITIAL VISIT

SUBJECTIVE

Patient Identification and Presenting Problem. Sarah L., a 43-year-old female recreational runner, presents with a lengthy history of pain on the distal lateral aspect of her right leg. Sarah began running at a recreational level (3–20 miles/week at a 9–12-minute/mile pace) 18 months prior to the evaluation. After 2 months of running, her total was 10 to 15 miles (3 miles per workout, three to four times per week). At this level of running, Sarah did not experience any problems. She increased her workout intensity to a total of 18 to 24 miles per week in preparation for a competitive race. At this level of running, she started complaining of pain on the distal lateral aspect of her right leg. She described this pain initially as dull, aching, but well circumscribed. The pain would begin after 3 to 4 miles of running and persisted until she stopped running. Her initial assessment was "no pain, no gain," so she ran through the pain. Her pain became more disabling, and at the time of her initial presentation, Sarah described the pain as throbbing and "like a rubber band getting tighter with more and more running." Sarah also related that pain was present when walking. At this stage there was no difference in the nature or the quality of the pain with variations of running distance, course, intensity, or running surface. Sarah then requested medical evaluation.

OBJECTIVE

Physical Examination. A general physical examination revealed a well-nourished and healthy 43-year-old white female. The focus of the musculoskeletal examination was limited to the right distal lower extremity. The patient entered the office ambulating independently without an antalgic gait. Visually, there was no evidence of soft-tissue swelling or muscle atrophy. Digital palpation of the right distal lower extremity elicited marked tenderness at the musculotendinous junction of the peroneus muscle group, particularly posterolaterally. Mild tenderness also was noted throughout the peroneus muscle belly. Biomechanical evaluation of the right ankle and foot was unremarkable. Range of motion was found to be within normal limits throughout the gastrocnemius–soleus complex and peroneal muscle group (tested with the foot in inversion). When isolating the peroneal muscle group for flexibility, moderate discomfort was elicited near the musculotendinous junction. Manual muscle testing of the right extrinsic foot musculature demonstrated weakness (3/5) in the peroneus longus and brevis (positioning of the foot in plantar flexion and eversion prior to testing are imperative for isolating this muscle group). The distal lower extremity pain was elicited with contraction of this muscle group.

ASSESSMENT

Diagnostic Tests. Plain radiographs obtained at the time of the initial evaluation were negative. A bone scan was performed and revealed accumulation of tracer on the lateral aspect of the distal fibula of the right leg. This finding was consistent with a possible stress fracture. At this point, the patient's leg was immobilized.

A second plain radiograph was obtained after 4 weeks of immobilization and again failed to show radiologic evidence of a distal fibula stress fracture. In view of this, an MRI scan was ordered.

The MRI scan revealed mild fluid accumulation around the flexor hallucis longus, suggestive of tendinitis. There were no radiographic findings suggestive of a stress fracture or any soft-tissue pathology on the lateral aspect of the right lower extremity.

Differential Diagnosis. The differential diagnosis of anterior distal leg pain includes "*shin splint*," *stress fractures, compartment syndrome,* and *chronic tendinitis.* There is, however, considerable overlap in the clinical findings for each of these entities. Therefore, the diagnosis must be based on the history and on a few differentiating clinical findings common to each of the clinical entities.

This is a case of a recreational runner who develops distal lateral leg pain after increasing her weekly mileage to a level II intensity (that is, 20–40 miles/week) in a short period of time. The cause of most runners' injuries are multifactorial, including training errors, biomechanical conditions, environmental conditions, the surface of running, personality traits, and even preexisting medical conditions. Most of the injuries are related to training errors in combination with biomechanical deficiencies. Training errors commonly cited include excessive or rapid increases in mileage, intensive interval training, inadequate warmup and stretching, improper shoes, and inappropriate running surface.

When examining the dynamics involved in running, one must review the running gait. Running is a repetitive, cycled motion that consists of a nonsupported or airborne phase which includes a follow-through, forward swing, and foot descent and a supported phase which includes heel strike, midstance, and toe-off. This motion results in a force of two to three times the body weight (5000 times per mile per foot) exerted through the calcaneus and distributed to the lower extremity, predisposing the musculoskeletal structure to injury. The presence of minor anatomic or biomechanical abnormalities can significantly increase the likelihood of an injury-related event.

SHIN SPLINTS. Traditionally, the term "shin splints" has been described as pain appearing below the knee to the ankle and aggravated with running. The anatomic location, its etiology, and its clinical course have been the subject of different interpretations.

This term has been used as a "waste basket" to include the diagnoses of (1) strain of the musculotendinous areas, (2) stress bone reactions, (3) stress fractures of the tibia and distal fibula, (4) periostitis, (5) compartment syndromes, (6) and chronic tendinitis. It is important from a treatment point of view to be more specific in the diagnosis.

The location of the pain may assist on the further characterization of this entity. The diagnosis of "anterior shin splints" is related to the muscle–tendon group involved in a specific phase of the running gate, including the tibialis anterior, the extensor hallucis brevis and longus, and the extensor digitorium longus (decelerators of the leg). "Anterior shin splints" is typically described as pain over the lateral border of the distal third of the tibia that increases with active dorsiflexion and passive plantar flexion. This finding distinguishes anterior shin splints from anterior compartment syndrome, periostitis, peroneal tendinitis, and stress fracture of the distal fibula.

The syndrome of "posterior shin splints" involves pain localized to the posteromedial border of the distal two-thirds of the tibia, over the posterior tibialis longus, flexor digitalis longus, and flexor hallucis longus (primarily invertors and supinators of the foot). This entity has been described in runners with excessive femoral anteversion and hyperpronation. Also, running on a banked track and running on the shoulder of a road have been described as precipitators of this condition.

Both anterior and posterior syndromes are the result of overuse of the musculotendinous structures, which have been subject to repetitive loading and stretching. These excessive forces induce multiple microtears with subsequent inflammation and decrease of tensile force, resulting in weakness of the involved muscle group.

The diagnosis of these conditions is based on the history of overuse, the nature of the pain, the resulting limitations of activity, reproducibility of the symptoms, findings of associated weakness, and evaluation of the biomechanical factors involved. The differential diagnosis, again, includes the continuum of tendinitis–periostitis–stress fractures and compartment syndrome. The use of diagnostic testing is limited. Plain radiographs are usually negative unless the extent of the injury suggests stress bone reaction with periostitis (in which case, hypertrophy of the cortex and subperiosteal bone formation can be found). The bone scan will give the classic "streaking phenomena," indicating bone activity in cases of severe tendinitis or periostitis. The usefulness of MRI for evaluation of this entity is still under investigation.

BONE STRESS REACTIONS AND STRESS FRACTURES. The next diagnostic consideration in the evaluation of distal leg pain is bone stress reactions and stress fractures. When the bone is exposed to applied stress, remodeling occurs, which consists of bone resorption followed by new bone formation. Abnormal stress to a bone with normal elastic resistance may produce a variety of bone abnormalities, reflecting the physiologic adaptations of the bone. Changes in the magnitude or frequency of the stress leads to remodeling with the production of new bone. If there is an imbalance in this remodeling process (that is, the osteoclast activity is greater than the bone deposition), then a structural defect or fatigue stress fracture develops. If there is no actual structural defect, then this process is referred to as "bone stress reaction."

Bone stress reaction has been classified by a grading system that takes into consideration (1) physical findings, (2) imaging examinations, and (3) risk of structural failure. The radiographic diagnosis of bone stress reaction has in the past been limited to plain films and bone scans. The sensitivity for detecting bone stress reactions on plain films is poor (20%–25%). If radiographs are taken within 3 to 4 weeks after the onset of the bone stress, the results are almost always negative. When present, the changes seen on plain films are subperiosteal bone formation or cortical thickening, giving evidence of the healing reaction. The differential diagnosis of these radiographic findings include osteoid osteoma, osteomyelitis, osteogenic sarcoma, Paget's disease, exostoses, and tumors that result in new bone formation.

The bone scan has been the preferred imaging technique for diagnosing stress fracture. The bone scan also may be positive in cases of grade 0 and grade 1 bone stress reactions (see Table 20–38), which clinically are referred to as "periostitis" and "shin splints." Bone scans are read in three phases: (1) the dynamic or angiographic phase, (2) the blood pooling or tissue phase, and (3) the metabolic or delayed phase. The bone scan of a stress fracture will be abnormal in all three phases, giving a focal area of activity. In periostitis and shin splints, the angiographic and blood pool images will be normal and the so-called streaking phenomena will give a longitudinal increase in trace over the anterior cortex of the tibia.

Recently, the use of other imaging techniques, such as the MRI, has provided the clinician with an additional diagnostic tool. MRI is very sensitive to changes in soft-tissue and skeletal structures. Research is presently under way that in the future may allow clinicians to utilize the MRI scan for assessing the severity of the insult and to predict the risk of structural failure.

The classical symptoms of a stress fracture include the early onset of pain with running, pain on walking, erythema over the affected area, and exquisite pain on percussion of the bone. The pain starts early during exercise and later becomes more intense, to the extent of limiting daily activities. The differential diagnoses of stress fracture include osteoid osteoma, Brodie's abscess, osteomyelitis, and eosinophilic granuloma.

CHRONIC COMPARTMENT SYNDROME. The next diagnostic challenge to be considered is chronic compartment syndrome. Although symptoms could develop in any of the four compartments, the runner usually suffers from exertional anterior compartment syndrome. The classical presentation of symptoms alerts the phy-

TABLE 20–38. CLASSIFICATION OF BONES STRESS REACTIONS

GRADE 0: *Characterizes the physiologic response of bone to a change in mechanical environment, either load or repetitions of loads.*

Bone scan positive
Not symptomatic
No risk of bone failure
X-rays negative

GRADE 1: *Describes clinically significant stress reaction.*

Bone scan positive
Symptoms: local pain exacerbated by activity and a history of increase activity or onset of a new activity
No risk of bone failure
X-rays negative

GRADE 2: *Characterizes clinically significant stress reaction.*

Bone scan positive
Symptoms: localized pain with mild tenderness to palpation but no palpable mass
X-rays positive; barely detectable changes

GRADE 3: *Stress reaction with potential structural damage.*

Bone scan positive
Symptoms: localized pain not completely abated with rest; marked local tenderness with palpable fullness or mass; increase in discomfort if activities were not stopped.

GRADE 4: *Clinically significant stress reaction of bone that has failed structurally, a frank fracture.*

X-rays shows evidence of frank fracture and evidence of chronic process or remodeling.

sician to consider this diagnosis. The runner describes pain in the lower leg precipitated by exercise, with associated paresthesia, and a sensation of fullness and pressure in the anterior leg. Physical examination often reveals weakness in the affected anterior compartment musculature.

The diagnosis of this entity requires a thorough history and physical examination, radiographic evaluation, EMG studies, and intramuscular pressure recordings at rest and during exercise. The slit-catheter method is used to determine the intramuscular pressure. A resting pressure in the compartment of more than 12 mmHg, pain elicited during exercise, and a failure of the pressure to return to preexercise levels within 5 minutes confirms the diagnosis.

CHRONICALLY INFLAMED MUSCULOTENDINOUS JUNCTION. The final consideration for the differential diagnosis is the chronically inflamed musculotendinous junction. In overuse injuries, repetitive and additive forces produce an area of microtrauma that triggers the inflammatory response. This physiologic response has the responsibility of bringing into action vasoactive substances, chemotactic factors, and agents responsible for the healing process. A prolonged response, however, will lead to chronic inflammation and destruction of the surrounding tissues. This prolonged healing phase will bring dysfunctional consequences. Resting a chronically inflamed musculotendinous junction will lead to a vicious cycle of injury, weakness, imbalance, inflexibility,

and ultimately, functional adaptations with overloading of the tissues and further aggravation of the injury. The diagnosis of a chronically inflamed musculotendinous group is made after clearly excluding the other entities previously discussed.

PLAN

Therapeutic

1. *Shin Splints.* The treatment of shin splints is based on a dynamic protocol that addresses the following: decrease of the pain and inflammation, improvement of the biomechanical deficiencies, and prevention of future development. The approach to management of this overuse syndrome must be coordinated by the family physician with the physical therapist or the athletic trainer. Interventions to decrease the pain and inflammation include the use of the concept of "relative rest"; that is, rest from activities that aggravate the pain but continue other activities to prevent further weakness and stiffness. The use of ice to decrease the inflammation and pain is recommended. The use of medications to decrease the inflammatory response in the acute phase should not interrupt the normal physiologic healing response.

A thorough biomechanical evaluation must be part of the treatment. This is geared toward avoiding training errors, assessing weak links in the biomechanical function, designing a flexibility and strengthening program, and evaluating the running gait, including the foot–shoe binomial. Lastly, a well-designed strategy toward prevention should be delineated. This should include learning good techniques of warming-up and cooling-down, continued emphasis on flexibility programs, and a sound plan to gradually return to activity and progress symptom free.

2. *Stress fractures.* The management of stress fractures is determined by the risk of structural failure. Stress fractures of the tibia are considered high risk, whereas those of the distal fibula, which are more prevalent, are considered low risk. After confirmation of a tibial stress fracture by bone scan, running should be avoided for 3 weeks. Bicycling, walking, and swimming are prescribed for maintaining the cardiovascular level. If simple weight-bearing ambulation is painful, cast immobilization, "air cast" immobilization, or partial weight bearing on a walking surgical shoe are alternatives. This treatment should last 2 to 3 weeks, until the inflammation resolves. The rehabilitation protocol should include appropriate heel cord stretching, ankle stretching, and strengthening exercises to avoid postinjury weakness and stiffness. In a small number of cases, a nonunion fracture develops, and surgical consultation is recommended.

3. *Chronic compartment syndrome.* The treatment includes a progressive rehabilitation effort directed toward breaking the injury cycle and returning the injured athlete to his or her preinjury level. The use of physical modalities (ice, ultrasound, electric stimulation) in the early phases of treatment is encouraged. The early use

of therapeutic exercise strategies will shorten the treatment time. Isokinetic exercise (both concentric and eccentric) has been shown to increase the tensile properties of the affected tissues, breaking the injury cycle by creating a balance between demands and performance.

DISCUSSION

Sarah was properly diagnosed as having chronic peroneal tendonitis. Clinical findings that supported the diagnosis were threefold:

1. Focal tenderness with palpation to the peroneal muscolotendinous structures
2. Reproduction of symptoms when isolating the peroneal muscle group during manual muscle testing
3. Reproduction of symptoms with passive stretching of the peroneal muscle group

A major factor that contributed to Sarah's developing a chronic soft tissue lesion was overtraining during the early stage of symptoms. The philosophy "no pain—no gain" was adopted as a training principle. This training error led to repetitive active loading of the musculotendinous unit resulting in soft tissue fatigue and subsequent failure.

Sarah was placed on an aggressive rehabilitation protocol designed to improve strength and extensibility in the peroneal musculature. Progressive resisted exercise and electrical muscle stimulation were incorporated to address the strength deficiencies in the peroneal group. The stretching program was aimed at restoring normal length in the gastroc-soleus and peroneal muscle groups. Piroxicam 20 mg daily was prescribed. Sarah was placed on a walking program and after 2 weeks of treatment no symptoms were reported. Physical examination after the 2-week period revealed good strength and length to the peroneals wihout any symptom reproduction during muscle contraction or stretching. Sarah was then allowed to start a progressive running program.

SUGGESTED READING

Andrish J, Work J. How I manage shin splints. Physician Sports Med 1990; 18(12):113–114.

Apple D. End-stage running problems. Clin Sports Med 1985; 4(4):657–670.

Becker E, Griffith H. Radiologic diagnosis of pain in the athlete. Clin Sports Med 1987; 6(4):699–711.

Brown, D. Ankle and leg injuries. In Team Physician Handbook. Philadelphia, Hanley and Belfus, 1990.

Campbell DC, Yetter JT. Sports medicine. In Rakel RE (ed.): Textbook of Family Practice, 4th ed. Philadelphia, W. B. Saunders, 1990.

Cavanagh PR. The Running Shoe Book. Mountain View, Calif., Anderson World, Inc., 1980.

Hunther-Griffin L. Overuse injuries. Clin Sports Med 1987; 6(2):225–258, 273–320, 371–388, 405–468.

Jackson DW. Shin splint: An update. Physician Sports Med 1978; 10(6):51–64.

Jones DC, James SL. Overuse injuries of the lower extremity. Clin Sports Med 1987; 6(2):273–290.

Kaplan P. Imaging stress injuries of bone. Study under development.

Kibler W. Clinical aspects of muscle injury. Med Sci Sports Exerc 1990; 22(4):450–452.

Markey KL. Stress fractures. Clin Sports Med 1987; 6(2):405–425.

Matire J. The role of nuclear medicine bone scans in evaluating pain in athletic injuries. Clin Sports Med 1987; 6(4):713–737.

McBryde AM. Stress fractures in runners. Clin Sports Med 1985; 4(4):737–751.

McKeag DB. The concept of overuse: The primary care aspects of overuse of syndromes in sports. Primary Care 1984; 11(1):43–59.

McKeag DB, Dolan C. Overuse syndrome of the lower extremity. Physician Sports Med 1989; 17(7):108–123.

Mellion MB. Office Management of Sports Injuries and Athletic Problems. Philadelphia, Hanley and Belfus, 1988.

Rorabeck CH, Bourne RB, Fowler PJ. The role of tissue pressure measurement in diagnosing chronic anterior compartment syndrome. Am J Sports Med 1988; 16:143–146.

Stafford S, Rosenthal D, Gebhardt M. MRI in stress fracture. AJR 1986; 147:553–556.

Stanish WD, Curwin S, Rubinovich M. Tendinitis: The analysis and treatment for running. Clin Sports Med 1985; 4(4):593–609.

Sutton J, Nilson K. Repeated stress fractures in an amenorrheic runner. Physician Sports Med 1989; 17(4):65–71.

Torg J, Vegso J, Torg E. Rehabilitation of Athletic Injuries. Chicago, Year Book, 1987.

Yao L, Lee J. Occult intraosseous fracture: Detection with MRI. Radiology 1988; 167:749–751.

QUESTIONS

1. Which of the following are true regarding stress fracture?
    a. Plain radiographs are usually diagnostic in the early stages of this condition.
    b. Results from abnormal stress to the bone and an imbalance in the remodeling process.
    c. The bone scan of a stress fracture is typically abnormal in all three phases of the scan.
    d. The differential diagnosis includes osteoid osteoma.
    e. Stress fractures of the distal fibula are more common and more serious than stress fractures of the tibia.

2. Which of the following are true regarding chronic compartment syndrome?
    a. The anterior compartment is the most commonly involved in runners.
    b. Classic symptoms include pain, even at rest, but without associated paresthesia.
    c. Using a slit-catheter method to determine intramuscular pressure, the resting pressure is elevated, rises with exercise, and is slow to recover.
    d. Weakness in the affected musculature may be found on physical examination.

3. Which of the following are true in a chronically inflamed musculotendinous junction?
    a. Microtrauma and a resulting inflammatory response are typical.

b. The athlete should rest the involved area for at least 10 days prior to initiation of therapy.

c. Isokinetic exercises are contraindicated in the treatment of this problem.

d. Physical modalities such as ultrasound and electrical stimulation are of very limited use in this condition.

4. Which of the following are true regarding the management of stress fractures?

a. It is the same regardless of location.

b. The athlete's running program may continue during treatment.

c. Bicycling and swimming must be avoided because of the unusual stresses they place on the lower extremities.

d. Immobilization is not indicated because of the atrophy that may result.

e. Once healed, stress fractures seldom recur, so specific rehabilitation is not needed.

Answers appear on page 451.

Knee Injury

WALTER L. CALMBACH

INITIAL VISIT

SUBJECTIVE

Patient Identification. Mike is a 17-year-old Caucasian high school junior who presents with right knee pain.

Presenting Problems. Mike reports recurrent right knee pain for 6 months. He first injured his knee playing football. He recalls planting his right foot firmly and then turning sharply to the left. He heard a distinct "pop" and felt excruciating pain. He was taken to the sidelines and examined by a trainer, who applied an Ace wrap and an ice pack. He remembers that the knee began swelling fairly quickly during the first hour after injury. The pain subsided over the next day or two, and although the swelling decreased more slowly, Mike declined seeing a physician at that time. However, since then he has had recurrent problems with his knee. Occasionally, his knee will "give out" on him, especially when climbing stairs. Sometimes his knee will "lock" in one position, and it takes some time to resume normal motion. Occasionally, the knee will "pop" and will become swollen with even slight trauma.

Past Medical History. Mike has no serious medical illnesses, takes no medications, and has no other history of trauma. He was hospitalized for an appendectomy at age 6; otherwise, he has no history of hospitalization or surgery. Mike has no medication allergies, but gives a vague history of "seasonal allergies."

Family History. Mike's father is alive and well, age 48, and has no medical illnesses. His mother is 47 and has mild hypertension, for which she is taking medication. Mike has one brother and two sisters, all of whom are without medical problems.

Social History. Mike has no history of smoking, and he drinks alcohol (beer) "occasionally." He denies any history of illicit drug use or experimentation.

Review of Systems. Review of systems is negative, except for occasional "seasonal allergies."

OBJECTIVE

Physical Examination. On physical examination, with the patient seated and the knees flexed at 90 degrees, there is slight swelling of the right knee joint compared with the left. A small amount of joint fluid is ballotable medial and lateral to the patella. There is no warmth or redness and no tenderness of the tibial tuberosity. Putting the knee through a short arc of range of motion, there is no joint-line tenderness.

With the patient supine and the knee extended to zero degrees, ballottement again produces a small amount of joint fluid medial and lateral to the patella. The patient gives no reaction when the patella is displaced slightly laterally (negative patellar apprehension test). When the patient contracts the quadriceps, the patella fits snugly into the patellofemoral joint without tenderness or crepitus.

While supporting the patient's leg, the passive range of motion is found to be normal: 0 degrees extension to 135 degrees flexion.

With the patient supine, the knee is flexed to 90 degrees. After stabilizing the patient in this position by sitting on the lateral aspect of the foot (Fig. 20–10), anterior and posterior distracting forces are applied to the proximal tibia. The tibia seems to sublux slightly anteriorly (positive anterior drawer sign) but has a definite end point posteriorly (negative posterior drawer sign).

To confirm these findings, Lachman's maneuver is applied. With the patient supine, the knee is flexed to approximately 25 to 30 degrees. The examiner grasps

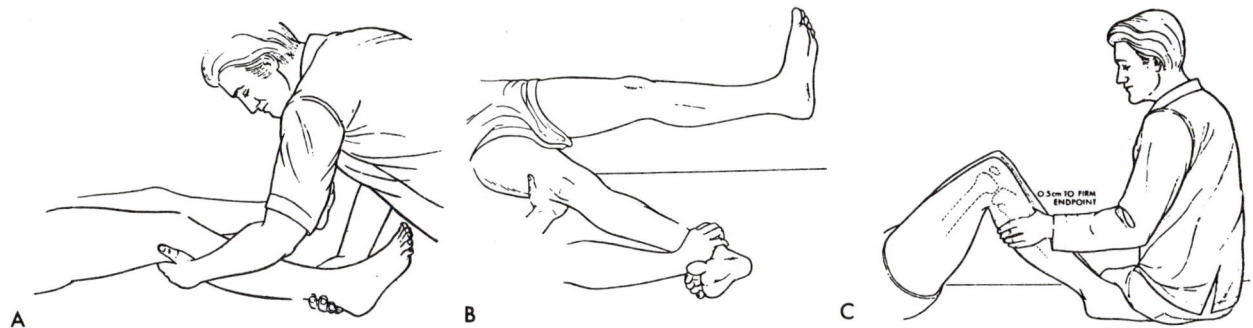

Figure 20–10. A, Abduction-adduction stress test of knee ligaments. The patient must lie on the examining table with the hip extended over the edge to relax the hamstrings. The examiner places one hand on the lateral side of the thigh and one hand above the ankle. Test the uninjured side first. B, The test should be done on the injured side with the knee in 30 degrees of flexion and in full extension. Instability of the knee in full extension is indicative of a serious ligamentous disruption (Grade III injury). C, Anterior-posterior drawer testing for cruciate ligament injury. The patient lies with the hips flexed 45 degrees and the knees flexed 90 degrees. The examiner rests gently on the patient's feet and checks the uninjured side first. The tibia is drawn forward in external rotation, neutral rotation, and internal rotation. Forward displacement of 0.5 cm. more than on the uninjured side and without a firm endpoint is a positive result. (From Connolly, J. F.: DePalma's The Management of Fractures and Dislocations: An Atlas. 3rd ed. Philadelphia, W. B. Saunders Co., 1981 with permission.)

the distal femur with one hand and the proximal tibia with the other hand. The examiner now applies anterior and posterior distracting forces. The anterior subluxation of the tibia is confirmed.

While supporting the leg, the knee is extended to 0 degrees, and varus and valgus stresses are applied. On valgus stress, widening at the medial aspect of the joint is noted (positive valgus laxity). Varus stress does not produce any widening.

While alternately internally and externally rotating the distal tibia, the knee is repeatedly flexed and extended (McMurray's test). No "locking" of the knee is reproduced.

ASSESSMENT

Working Diagnoses. There are three injuries of the right knee that can explain Mike's symptoms and findings:

1. *Anterior cruciate ligament (ACL) tear.* The history of a planted foot with a sharp turn in the opposite direction, hearing a "pop," swelling of the knee within 1 or 2 hours after the injury (suggesting hemarthrosis), and the knee "giving way" are all consistent with a tear of the anterior cruciate ligament.

2. *Medial collateral ligament (MCL) tear.* The MCL is often injured when the ACL is torn. The same valgus stress is responsible for both. On physical examination, valgus stress with the knee extended 0 degrees demonstrates motion at the medial aspect of the knee. The fact that there is no tenderness with this maneuver, as well as no joint-line tenderness, is consistent with the history of injury 6 months ago.

3. *Meniscal injury.* Either the lateral or medial meniscus can be injured when valgus stress is sufficient to tear the ACL and/or the MCL. Of the two, the medial meniscus is more often injured. When the meniscus is torn, a "flap" of cartilage can prevent normal motion and can sometimes cause the "locking" that the patient

reports. The "shock absorber" function of the menisci also can be disturbed, contributing to the joint effusion with even minimal trauma. The outer one-quarter to one-third of the meniscus is innervated, and a tear in this area can cause joint-line pain, which the patient does not have.

Differential Diagnoses. Mike's history and physical examination suggest several other possibilities, including

1. *Posterior cruciate ligament (PCL) tear.* Occasionally, the physical examination can seem to demonstrate anterior subluxation when the real injury is a PCL tear that allows the tibia to sublux posteriorly. With a PCL tear, though, there is a definite end point when anterior force is applied. Another way to assess the PCL is to place the knee at 90 degrees with the patient supine and observe the knee from a lateral position. If the PCL is torn, the proximal tibia will "sag" posteriorly and be seen easily from a lateral viewpoint.

2. *Ligamentous laxity.* While it seems unlikely that laxity alone could explain the patient's findings, it must be remembered that ligamentous laxity does occur, and both knees should be examined. Patients with lax knee ligaments are more likely to sustain knee injuries.

3. *Patellar subluxation.* In some patients, the patella can sublux (slip) laterally, causing chronic and recurrent anterior knee pain. This is usually found in adolescent females, in whom ligamentous laxity and relative genu valgum ("knock kneed") combine to facilitate lateral subluxation. This is relatively unlikely in this adolescent male who demonstrates a negative patellar apprehension test.

4. *Periostitis of the tibial Tubercle (Osgood–Schlatter's disease).* Repetitive strain at the developing epiphysis of the tibial tubercle can cause chronic irritation and inflammation of the periostium and tenderness at the tibial tubercle. This too is a common cause of anterior knee

pain in children and adolescents, whose ossification centers have not yet fused. It is more commonly found in males than in females and is slightly more common in the left knee. This patient, however, showed no tenderness of the tibial tuberosity.

A less likely diagnosis that must be considered due to its seriousness and the potential for long-term disability is *hip pain referred to the knee*. In particular, avascular necrosis of the femoral head should be kept in mind, particularly in a young athlete, who may be at risk for steroid use; the glucocorticoid side effects of some anabolic steroids may promote the development of avascular necrosis of the femoral head. Avascular necrosis eventually leads to severe arthritis of the joint. While no treatment is currently available, prompt diagnosis may prevent the same problem from affecting the contralateral hip.

PLAN

Diagnostic. In the acute phase, at the time of the injury, knee arthrocentesis could have been done, to demonstrate hemarthrosis consistent with a tear of the anterior cruciate ligament. At this point, however, the best way to assess the ACL is through physical examination, or even examination under general anesthesia. Arthrography can sometimes be used to confirm an ACL tear, as well as injury to the menisci. Similarly, arthroscopy can demonstrate cruciate injury and meniscal injury. Magnetic resonance imaging (MRI) is an excellent non-invasive procedure. MRI is useful in determining the extent of injury prior to examination under general anesthesia and therapeutic arthroscopy.

Therapeutic. Many factors must be weighed in determining a treatment plan for a patient such as Mike, a young athlete with several injuries, apparently incurred 6 months prior to presentation. First and foremost, the patient's performance level and degree of dysfunction must be considered in tandem. For example, if the patient wishes to pursue competitive-level sports requiring sharp pivoting, he will need surgical repair and augmentation of the ACL, surgical repair of the MCL, and partial or total meniscectomy, followed by approximately 1 year of intense rehabilitation.

Primary repair of the torn ACL should be supplemented by an augmentation procedure that strengthens the repaired ACL by augmenting it with an autograft (usually taken from the middle third of the patellar ligament). Autografts also can be taken from the semitendinosus, gracilis, iliotibial band, or fasciae latae.

The combination of ACL tear with a MCL tear also argues in favor of surgical therapy. A torn meniscus may be repaired, or perhaps a partial meniscectomy will be adequate (e.g., a "parrot-beak" or "bucket-handle" tear). Complex tears of a meniscus require total meniscectomy.

Conversely, if the patient plans a more sedentary lifestyle or wishes to pursue sports that do not require sharp pivoting (e.g., swimming, cycling), a more conservative approach may be warranted. After an acute injury, the knee is splinted, allowing a small range of motion. The patient ambulates with the aid of crutches until the effusion is resolved and painless range of motion is restored. If a conservative approach is planned, some basic principles of ACL rehabilitation must be kept in mind. The goal is to restore range of motion, strength, ligamentous stability, and functional capabilities.

Rehabilitation is extremely important. Immobilization should be avoided or at least kept to a minimum. Emphasis should be placed on restoring range of motion and muscle strength. An initial rehabilitation program should include

1. Patellar mobilization: passive range of motion exercises
2. Hamstring stretching exercises
3. Hamstring strengthening exercises: for example, stationary bicycle with toe clips, swimming, "running water" in a life vest
4. Quadriceps strengthening exercises: for example, straight-leg raises
5. Partial weight bearing, progressive ambulation, controlled stress, progressive resistive exercises (e.g., ankle weights, exercise benches, weight boots)

Patient Education

1. Mike is counseled regarding his options: surgery versus conservative therapy. The risks and benefits of both are explained.
2. The rehabilitation program is outlined in detail, particularly the importance of muscle-strengthening exercises. The patient is told why straight-leg raises are the preferred way to begin quadriceps strengthening and is warned about the subluxation caused by active extension between 45 degrees of flexion and full extension.

Disposition. Mike was asked to consider his future plans and decide whether surgical intervention or conservative management was preferable. A physical therapy program was agreed on, and referral was postponed until the patient had made his decision.

FIRST FOLLOW-UP VISIT

Mike returned 1 week later, saying that he had thought it over, discussed it with his parents and his coach, and decided that he would prefer to try the conservative, nonsurgical approach for now. He had some questions about the effectiveness of delayed reconstructive surgery if that should become necessary, but otherwise he seemed comfortable with his decision. It was emphasized that his physical activities would have to be modified and that competitive-level sports requiring sharp turns on a planted foot (e.g., football, basketball, baseball) should not be considered. However, after proper conditioning, recreational sports, such as swimming, cycling, and jogging, should pose no problem for him. Mike reported that his knee continued to be mildly painful, but that the physical therapy program was progressing very well. He could not yet see the benefit of the straight-leg raising exercises, and he had some questions about resistive knee extension exercises. The importance of not extending the knee from 45 to 0 degrees while performing resisted extension was emphasized.

OBJECTIVE

Mike's physical examination is unchanged.

ASSESSMENT

Mike has a history and physical examination consistent with both ligamentous and cartilaginous injuries. The ACL and MCL injuries are largely defined by physical examination. Since the patient prefers a conservative approach, physical therapy and rehabilitation measures will be attempted. A meniscal tear is suspected owing to the history of occasional "locking" of the knee, although physical examination was unable to reproduce this abnormality and confirm the diagnosis.

PLAN

Diagnostic

1. Since the patient does not want surgical repair at this time, there will be no opportunity for physical examination of the knee under anesthesia. This is an important adjunct to routine physical examination because the patient is obviously totally relaxed and the type and degree of ligamentous injuries can be assessed.

2. The question of meniscal injury remains. If no surgery is contemplated, invasive diagnostic procedures such as arthroscopy or arthrography are probably not indicated. MRI can detect meniscal tears quite well and spare the patient an invasive procedure.

The frequency of "locking" and the degree to which "locking" interferes with normal daily activities should be assessed. Although the patient might wish to avoid surgery, he may require meniscal repair, a partial meniscectomy, or even complete meniscectomy.

Therapeutic

1. Hamstring stretching exercises
2. Hamstring strengthening exercises
3. Quadriceps strengthening exercises (e.g., straight-leg raises, resisted extension, 90 to 20 degrees, *not* between 20 and 0 degrees)
4. Elastic knee support (Taping the knee or using an elastic knee support may prevent reinjury by increasing the patient's proprioceptive input from the knee.)
5. Progress to running: one-mile jog at a slow pace, in a straight line, on a flat surface. Once this has been established, the patient can try 80-yard dashes: half speed, then three-quarters speed, finally full speed.

Patient Education

1. Quadriceps strengthening and hamstring strengthening and stretching exercises are important in maximizing protection of the knee from further injury.
2. Activities such as running downhill or actively extending the knee from 20 degrees flexion to 0 degrees full extension, especially with weights, will tend to cause anterior subluxation of the tibia. These activities are to be avoided.
3. As rehabilitation proceeds, an elastic knee brace should be worn. Such a brace is no substitute for intact ligaments, but it will increase proprioceptive feedback to the patient, allowing the quadriceps and hamstring muscles to adjust.
4. Sports requiring pivoting on a planted foot can reproduce the injury. Sports such as jogging, cycling, and swimming are to be preferred.

Disposition. Mike is instructed to follow the rehabilitation program outlined and return to clinic in 1 month for evaluation of progress and management of any problems that might arise.

DISCUSSION

Anterior knee pain is a common presenting complaint, especially among young patients. Although the differential diagnosis is broad, a few elements are fairly common.

Periostitis of the tibial tubercle (Osgood–Schlatter's lesion) is a common cause of anterior knee pain in young patients in whom ossification centers have not yet fused. A combination of repetitive trauma and/or overuse can result in the slow onset of vague symptoms with intermittent pain and swelling at the tibial tubercle.

Patients are usually 11 to 15 years old (age range 9 to 15 years), males are slightly more commonly affected than females, and the left knee is more commonly affected than the right. Symptoms have usually been present for months before the patient seeks medical attention and are aggravated by running, jumping, kneeling, squatting, or climbing stairs. Symptoms are relieved by rest and restriction of activities.

On physical examination there is localized tenderness and swelling at the tibial tubercle and the insertion of the patellar ligament. There is no joint effusion. Painful symptoms can be reproduced if the patient tries to extend the knee against resistance or with forced passive flexion of the knee.

Treatment requires rest and restriction of activities. The knee is immobilized in extension for 3 or 4 weeks, during which period the patient continues hamstring stretching and strengthening exercises. After the period of immobilization, quadriceps strengthening exercises are added. Activities requiring jumping (e.g., basketball, hurdles) or repetitive knee flexion and extension (e.g., bicycling) are modified or restricted.

Prognosis is excellent, and the patient usually returns to full activity, although with residual prominence of the tibial tubercle.

Patellar subluxation is another common cause of anterior knee pain, especially among teenage females. In these patients, the vastus medialis of the quadriceps muscle is relatively weak, and the alignment of the quadriceps muscle, the patella, and the insertion of the patellar ligament is such that the patella is pulled laterally (the so-called Q-angle). The patient reports a sensation of "giving way," of lateral slippage, or of hypermobility of the patella.

On physical examination the patellar apprehension test is positive: If the examiner gently subluxes the patella laterally, the sensation of discomfort is reproduced. It is important to recognize patellar subluxation, if only to prevent patellar dislocation, which can result in an osteochondral fracture. It must be differentiated from chondromalacia patella (a degeneration of the patellar cartilaginous surface that produces crepitus on physical examination) and patellar tendonitis.

Treatment consists of an elastic sleeve around the knee, usually with a crescent-shaped pad laterally to prevent subluxation of the patella. The key to therapy is to strengthen the quadriceps, first with straight-leg raising exercises, progressing to flexion-to-extension exercises. Hamstring stretching exercises and use of the stationary cycle are also useful.

Anterior cruciate ligament (ACL) injuries are usually the result of noncontact deceleration; that is, the foot is planted and there is a quick pivot in the opposite direction. The patient often hears a "pop," and there is usually rapid joint swelling caused by hemarthrosis due to a torn ACL. An ACL injury is often associated with other injuries as well, especially medial collateral ligament (MCL) injuries and meniscal injuries.

If the injury has been present for some time, the patient may report that the knee "gives way" from time to time, especially when climbing stairs. In the acute phase, pain and hemarthrosis may make physical diagnosis difficult. If the mechanism of injury and history are typical for an ACL injury, the patient may benefit from an examination under anesthesia.

In the postacute phase, physical findings are more straightforward. A small effusion is usually present, the anterior drawer test is usually positive, as is Lachman's maneuver; that is, the proximal tibia subluxes anteriorly when anterior distracting forces are applied.

Surgery in the acute phase is usually reserved for young patients with marked anterior tibial subluxation who wish to continue competitive-level sports, especially those requiring jumping or pivoting. Patients who also sustain MCL or meniscal injuries and those who possess general joint laxity are also candidates for surgical intervention.

Conservative therapy is usually more appropriate for patients over age 30 or those with only mild anterior tibial subluxation (i.e., grade II sprain of ACL rather than complete rupture). Conservative management is probably indicated in patients who can modify their activities or who have relatively "tight joints" (i.e., no joint laxity). Finally, conservative therapy is appropriate for patients with isolated ACL injuries (e.g., intact MCL and meniscus).

Primary surgical repair of a torn ACL should be augmented with an autogenous graft; the central third of the patellar ligament is often used, as are the semitendinosus tendon, the gracilis tendon, or the iliotibial band. If conservative therapy fails, reconstructive surgery is available.

Medial collateral ligament (MCL) injuries often can be treated without surgery. Injuries that do not produce instability should be treated conservatively. A mild sprain (grade I) can be treated simply with ice, compression, and activity as tolerated. Quadriceps strengthening exercises can be initiated when pain subsides.

Moderate to severe sprains (grade II) require immobilization in a cast or splint with the knee in extension. A cast brace can sometimes be used to allow limited-arc motion (e.g., 40 to 70 degrees) in the early healing phase. This brace can provide varus/valgus stability, and range of motion can be increased to full arc as healing progresses.

Complete MCL tears can produce an unstable knee; these patients benefit from primary surgical repair. Patient age and activity may suggest conservative therapy rather than surgery. Also, if the ligament is avulsed at the femur rather than being ruptured at midsubstance, patients do well with conservative therapy.

Meniscal injuries occur as a result of a combination of compressive and rotatory forces (e.g., sharp pivoting on a planted foot). Most commonly, this causes a "bucket-handle" tear of the meniscus. The central portion of the meniscus is displaced to the center of the joint and causes occasional "locking" of the knee or limited extension. The patient will report locking, popping, or catching. In true locking, full extension is blocked and can be relieved by rotation and passive extension.

Physical examination reveals joint-line tenderness (pain from a torn meniscus is referred to the joint line) and joint effusion. If the injury is of long standing, the patient may show quadriceps atrophy. McMurray's test is positive, as is Apley's test (with the patient prone and the knee flexed to 90 degrees, an axial load is applied to the distal extremity with slight internal and external rotation). Having the patient squat, first with the feet in external rotation and then with the feet in internal rotation, also can demonstrate a torn meniscus. Arthrography, arthroscopy, and MRI can confirm the diagnosis.

A simple tear in the outer one-quarter to one-third of the meniscus can be repaired primarily. Symptomatic "bucket-handle" or flap tears may require partial meniscectomy. Total meniscectomy is needed in cases of complex tears or extensive meniscal degeneration.

Operative therapy is indicated for these types of tears, for patients with pain during activities of daily living, or when a locked knee is not reducible by conservative means. After meniscectomy, the joint space may be narrowed, changes in the femoral condyles are accelerated, and early degenerative changes in the joint can be seen. Therefore, the indications for surgery must be weighed carefully against the consequences of surgery.

SUGGESTED READING

American Academy of Pediatrics Committee on Sports Medicine. Knee brace use by athletes. Pediatrics 1990; 85(2):228.

Andersson C, Odensten M, Good L, Gillquist J. Surgical or nonsurgical treatment of acute rupture of the anterior cruciate ligament: A randomized study with long-term follow-up. J Bone Joint Surg 1989; 71A(7):965–974.

Berg E, Henderson JM, Simon RR. Office diagnosis of knee pain. Patient Care 1990; 24:48–78.

Casteleyn PP, Handelberg F, Opdecam P. Traumatic haemarthrosis of the knee. J Bone Joint Surg 1988; 70B(3):404–406.

Cowart VS. Several choices availabe for repair of ligamental tears in the knee. JAMA 1990; 263(2):197, 201.

DeHaven KE. Decision-making factors in the treatment of meniscus lesions. Clin Orthop 1990; 252:49–54.

Indelicato PA, Hermansdorfer J, Huegel M. Nonoperative management of complete tears of the medial collateral ligament of the knee in intercollegiate football players. Clin Orthop 1990; 256:174–177.

Insall J. "Chondromalacia patellae": Patellar malalignment syndrome. Orthop Clin North Am 1979; 1(1):117–127.

Insall J, Falvo KA, Wise DW. Chondromalacia patellae: A prospective study. J Bone Joint Surg 1976; 58A(1):1–8.

Kannus P. Long-term results of conservatively treated medial collateral ligament injuries of the knee joint. Clin Orthop 1988; 226:103–112.

Kannus P, Jarvinen M. Conservatively treated tears of the anterior cruciate ligament: Long-term results. J Bone Joint Surg 1987; 69A(7):1007–1012.

McInerney VK, Mailly KH, Paonessa KJ. Rehabilitation of the sports-injured patient. Orthop Clin North Am 1988; 19(4):725–735.

Polisson RP. Sports medicine for the internist. Med Clin North Am 1986; 70(2):469–489.

Swenson EJ Jr, Hough DO, McKeag DB. Patellofemoral dysfunction. Postgrad Med 1987; 82(6):125–146.

Terry GC. Office evaluation and management of the symptomatic knee. Orthop Clin North Am 1988; 19(4):699–713.

Zarins B, Adams M. Knee injuries in sports. N Engl J Med 1988; 318(15):950–961.

QUESTIONS

1. On physical examination of the knee, which one of the following assesses the anterior cruciate ligament?
   a. Patellar apprehension test
   b. Posterior drawer sign
   c. Lachman's maneuver
   d. Varus or valgus stress
   e. McMurray's test

2. Conservative therapy for acute knee injuries is recommended in which of the following cases?
   a. A young athlete
   b. A patient over age 30
   c. An isolated ACL tear
   d. Multiple injuries: ACL tear, MCL tear, and medial meniscus injury
   e. Sedentary lifestyle

3. Match each of the following major clinical manifestations with the knee disorders listed.
   a. Foot planted, sharp pivot, rapid hemarthrosis
   b. Teenage female, weak vastus medialis of quadriceps
   c. History of "locking" of knee
   d. Teenage male, associate with repetitive trauma or overuse, treated by rest
      (1) Patellar subluxation
      (2) Tibial tubercle periostitis (Osgood–Schlatter's lesion)
      (3) Anterior cruciate ligament tear
      (4) Medial collateral ligament tear
      (5) Meniscal injury

4. Total meniscectomy is required in which one of the following situations?
   a. History of occasional locking of knee
   b. "Bucket-handle" tear of meniscus
   c. Positive joint effusion
   d. Complex tear of meniscus
   e. Associated joint-line tenderness

5. Anterior subluxation of the tibia can be expected in which of the following activities?
   a. Climbing stairs
   b. Straight-leg raising exercises
   c. Extending the knee betwee 20 degrees of flexion and full extension
   d. Running downhill
   e. Swimming

Answers appear on page 451.

Low Back Pain

WALTER L. CALMBACH

INITIAL VISIT

SUBJECTIVE

Patient Identification and Presenting Problem. Tomas is a 42-year-old Hispanic construction worker who presents with a 2-day history of sudden-onset low back pain.

Present Illness. Tomas is a slightly obese Hispanic male who developed sharp, right-sided low back pain that has worsened over the last 2 days. The pain began immediately after Tomas tried to lift a 50-lb bag of cement. He is not experiencing any paresthesias in his legs, nor any leg weakness. He has no bowel or bladder incontinence.

Past Medical History. Tomas has no previous history of back injury or back surgery and no previous motor vehicle accident (MVA). There is no history of surgery or hospitalizations, and he has no allergies. He is taking no medications, except for occasional Tylenol or aspirin for relief of his back pain.

Family History. Tomas's father is 62 years old and has a history of recent-onset hypertension, for which he takes no medication. Tomas's mother is 60 years old and has mild hypertension, type II diabetes mellitus, and a history of cholecystectomy for cholelithiasis "years ago." Tomas has two older brothers and two younger sisters and is unaware of any medical problems they may have. There is no family history of stroke, myocardial infarction, liver disease, renal disease, tuberculosis, or bleeding disorders. Tomas is unaware of the cholesterol status of any of his family members.

Health Habits. Tomas drinks about 2 beers each night, slightly more on weekends. He has never missed work or had medical problems related to alcohol abuse. He smoked about 2 packs of cigarettes per day for about 9 years, but he stopped smoking at age 25. He does not use any illicit drugs.

Social History. Tomas has been married for 22 years and lives in a rented home with his wife and three of their four children.

Review of Systems. Essentially negative. In particular, Tomas has no history of polyuria, polyphagia, or polydipsia; no headaches or epistaxis; and no urinary frequency or hesitancy.

OBJECTIVE

Physical Examination. Tomas's blood pressure is 136/84; his pulse rate is 68; his respiration rate is 12; and his temperature is 98.6°F. *Head:* Normocephalic, atraumatic. *Eyes:* Extraocular muscles intact; pupils equal, round, and reactive to light and accomodation. Funduscopic examination shows sharp disc margins with mild "copper-wiring" of arterioles without A-V nicking, retinal hemorrhages, or exudates. ENT examination is normal. Neck examination shows full range of motion without tenderness, full carotid pulses without bruit, nonpalpable thyroid, trachea in the midline, and no adenopathy. Lungs are clear with normal breath sounds. Heart examination shows normal S_1 and S_2 sounds without murmur, rub, or gallop rhythm; there is no lift or leave, and PMI is not palpable. His abdomen is flat, without scar; bowel sounds are normal. There is no tenderness or guarding, no organomegaly, and no bruits. Liver span is approximately 8 cm.

BACK EXAMINATION. On standing, Tomas shows splinting to the right side. There is mild right paravertebral muscle tenderness in the lumbar area without midline tenderness. Tomas is able to flex the spine to approximately 70 degrees; lateral bending and rotation are limited by pain in the right paravertebral lumbar area. Tomas is able to toe-walk and heel-walk, although this increases his right-sided pain.

In the seated position with hips and knees flexed at 90 degrees, the knees are gently extended. Tomas is able to extend the left knee to 0 degrees without difficulty; however, extending the right knee to 20 degrees causes a sharp "electrical" pain to "shoot" from the right lumbar area through the back of the leg to the dorsum of the right foot.

Sensation to light touch and pinprick is equal bilaterally. Deep tendon reflexes are normal at the knee and ankle, but dorsiflexion of the right first toe is slightly weak compared with the left.

Rectal examination shows normal sphincter tone, no masses, normal prostate without tenderness or nodularity, and heme-negative stool. The cremasteric reflex is intact bilaterally.

Laboratory Tests. Lumbosacral films are ordered (five views: AP, lateral, two obliques, and a "spot" or close-up film of the L5–S1 interspace). These show normal alignment of the vertebral bodies, no spondylolysis (i.e., the pars interarticularis is intact), and no spondylolisthesis (i.e., the posterior aspect of the vertebral bodies are well aligned and do not encroach on the spinal canal). The pedicles are intact and show no sign of infectious or metastatic disease. There is no vertebral body collapse or "wedging" of a vertebra, and there are no osteophytes or other signs of degenerative changes. There is slight narrowing of the L5–S1 interspace compared with other disc spaces, but this may be due to the relative angle at which this interspace is filmed.

ASSESSMENT

Working Diagnosis. At this point, the most likely diagnosis is *lumbar disc herniation impinging on the L5 nerve root.* Disc herniation in a patient of this age after heavy lifting is fairly common. Over time, there is degeneration of the intervertebral disc, leading first to protrusion of the disc into the spinal canal and sometimes progressing to extrusion and sequestration of disc material (Figs. 20–11 to 20–13). The two most common sites for disc herniation are at the L4–L5 interspace and the L5–S1 interspace. The patient's description of paresthesias radiating from the back through the posterior thigh and to the dorsum of the foot are consistent with some irritation of the L5 nerve root (Table 20–39).

Differential Diagnoses (Table 20–40)

1. *Muscle strain, ligamentous strain.* There are many muscles and ligaments that support the spine, and these can be injured through the same mechanism of heavy lifting. Such patients also will demonstrate splinting to one side and paravertebral muscle tenderness. However, paresthesias consistent with dermatomal distribution of the lumbar nerves are not found in patients with musculoskeletal strain; motor function and deep tendon reflexes are intact.

2. *Posterior facet syndrome.* The posterior facet joints are often overlooked in the evaluation of back

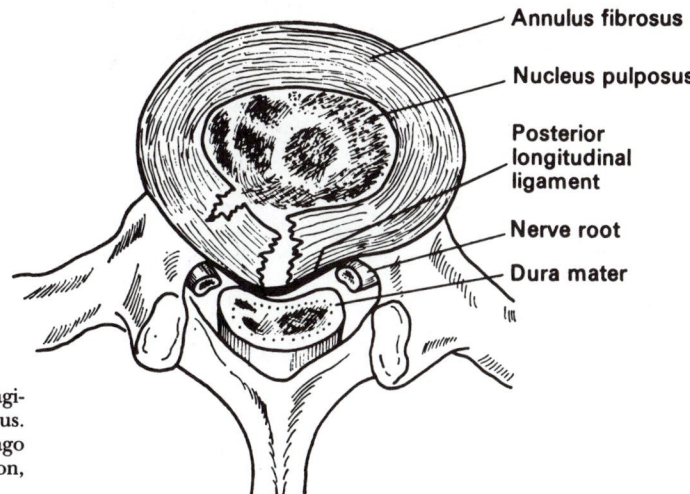

Figure 20–11. The disc structure includes an outer fibrocartilaginours annulus fibrosus and an inner, more fluid nucleus pulposus. Either of these structures may rupture and produce either lumbago sclatica. (From Cyriax, J.: Orthopaedic Medicine. Vol. 1. London, Cassell Ltd., 1978 with permisssion.)

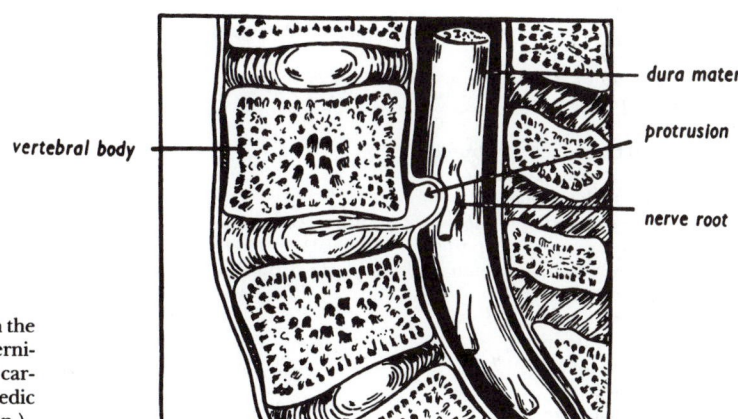

Figure 20–12. Herniation of the nucleus pulposus through the tear in the annulus produces a collar stud abscess type of herniation that does not reduce spontaneously the way a moveable cartilaginous displacement reduces. (From Cyriax, J.: Orthopaedic Medicine. Vol. 1. London, Cassell Ltd., 1978 with permission.)

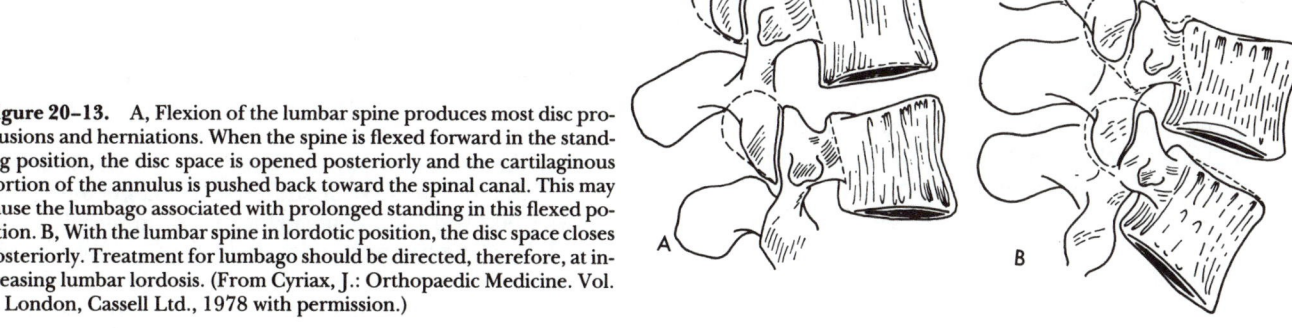

Figure 20–13. A, Flexion of the lumbar spine produces most disc protrusions and herniations. When the spine is flexed forward in the standing position, the disc space is opened posteriorly and the cartilaginous portion of the annulus is pushed back toward the spinal canal. This may cause the lumbago associated with prolonged standing in this flexed position. B, With the lumbar spine in lordotic position, the disc space closes posteriorly. Treatment for lumbago should be directed, therefore, at increasing lumbar lordosis. (From Cyriax, J.: Orthopaedic Medicine. Vol. 1. London, Cassell Ltd., 1978 with permission.)

pain, but they share the load of supporting the spine with the vertebral bodies and the intervertebral discs. The facets are posterolateral zygapophyseal joints; the joint capsule is innervated by the posterior primary ramus of the dorsal nerve root. A tear in the capsule causes referred pain to the buttocks and posterior thigh. Treatment involves moist heat, nonnarcotic analgesics, muscle relaxants, and facet nerve blocks. If conservative measures fail, spinal fusion or facet arthrodesis may be required.

3. *Degenerative joint disease (DJD) or osteoarthritis (OA).* DJD of the lumbar spine is common, especially among elderly patients, those with a history of back trauma, or patients with abnormalities of the spine (e.g., spondylolysis). In such cases, plain films of the lumbar spine are helpful in diagnosing DJD. However, care must be taken to avoid ascribing pain to osteoarthritic changes when the pain may in fact be due to another cause.

4. *Spinal stenosis.* This degenerative process can

TABLE 20–39. LEVELS OF INNERVATION FOR MOTOR FUNCTION IN LOWER LIMBS

NERVE LEVEL	MOTOR FUNCTION
L2,3	Hip flexion
L4,5	Hip extension
L3,4	Knee extension
L3–S1	Knee flexion
L4,5	Ankle dorsiflexion
S1–S2	Ankle plantar flexion
L4	Foot inversion
L5–S1	Foot eversion

Source: From Rakel RE. Textbook of Family Practice, 4th ed. Philadelphia, W.B. Saunders, 1990, with permission.

TABLE 20–40. DIFFERENTIAL OF ETIOLOGIC FACTORS IN BACK PAIN

Tumors:
  Benign (such as meningiomas, neuromas, osteoid osteomas, Paget's disease)
  Malignant—primary bone or neural tumors and metastatic
Trauma:
  Acute sprain or strain
  Chronic sprain or strain
  Fractures
  Subluxed facet (facet syndrome)
  Spondylolisthesis with strain
Toxicities from heavy metals
Congenital asymmetries of facets or transitional vertebrae
Metabolic disorders—osteoporosis or osteomalacia
Inflammatory arthritis—rheumatoid and Marie–Strümpell's disease
Infections, acute and chronic
Degenerative disc or facet disease
Mechanical disturbance:
  Poor muscle tone
  Poor posture
  Unstable vertebrae
  Scoliosis (severe)
Extrinsic disease such as aortic aneurysm, uterine fibroids, prostate disease, hip disease, etc.
Psychologic to include hysteria, malingering, and acute remunerative spinal pain (Green–Poultice disease)

Source: From Rakel RE. Textbook of Family Practice, 4th ed. Philadelphia, W.B. Saunders, 1990, with permission.

mimic vascular claudication symptoms. Patients report dull achy back pain and posterior thigh pain with standing or walking, relieved by rest or sitting down. This problem can be differentiated from vascular claudication by the lack of ischemic changes and the presence of full pulses. Also, symptoms of vascular insufficiency are more quickly brought on by activity and more quickly relieved by rest than are symptoms of spinal stenosis.

Several less likely diagnoses also must be considered (Table 20–40):

1. *Multiple myeloma.* This disease will affect the vertebral bodies, predisposing the patient to pathologic fractures of the spine. The diagnosis can be confirmed by bone biopsy or by serum and/or urine protein electrophoresis.

2. *Carcinomatous metastases to the spine.* This is especially true for cancers of the lung, breast, kidney, thyroid, and prostate. On plain films of the spine, the ped-

icles are often obscured, and the vertebral bodies may show osteolytic or osteoblastic lesions.

3. *Osteomyelitis.* Hematogenous spread of bacteria to the vertebral body is not uncommon, and osteomyelitis can be overlooked as a cause of back pain. Many patients can initially present without fever or leukocytosis, and as many as 50% will have their diagnosis delayed 3 months. Tuberculosis, diabetes mellitus, IV drug abuse, alcohol abuse, steroid use, and disseminated malignancy are associated with an increased risk of osteomyelitis. Fever is usually present but may be absent in debilitated patients whose immune systems are impaired. An elevated erythrocyte sedimentation rate (ESR) is a nonspecific but confirmatory finding. Blood culture can define the pathogenic organism, and bone scan or MRI can localize the lesion.

4. *Spinal cord tumors.* Spinal cord tumors and nerve root tumors (neurofibroma, neurilemmoma) are rare causes of back pain, and diagnosis requires a high index of suspicion. These lesions are best confirmed by MRI.

5. *Psychogenic causes.* It would be a mistake to assume that most patients with back pain have a psychogenic cause for their pain, but it does occur in some patients. In some cases the pain is psychosomatic in origin, and treatment is aimed at the underlying cause of anxiety.

PLAN

Diagnostic. While the differential diagnoses outlined must be kept in mind, the patient's presentation is fairly typical for L5 nerve root irritation due to a herniated intervertebral disc. Further characterization of the lesion is not necessary at this point, and the patient warrants a course of conservative therapy. If the patient's symptoms do not resolve with conservative therapy, or if they worsen, reevaluation is required in order to direct further investigative studies (Table 20–41).

Therapeutic. Tomas's symptoms are of recent onset, and he demonstrates no muscle weakness or loss of bowel or bladder control. Therefore, an attempt at conservative management is warranted.

In the acute phase, the patient will benefit from a combination of physical and pharmacologic modalities. Strict bed rest on a firm surface is recommended for 3 to 7 days (some experts suggest 14 days), combined with nonnarcotic analgesics, such as nonsteroidal anti-inflammatory agents. There is some question as to the efficacy of muscle relaxants (e.g., Valium, Flexeril), but these are often used. Physical modalities such as moist heat, massage, and manipulation are also helpful.

Once the acute pain has resolved, the patient can begin work on abdominal strengthening exercises and weight loss. These will decrease the amount of strain placed on the lumbar spine and help prevent reinjury. In the same way, sending the patient to "back school," where he can learn simple measures to prevent reinjury, is an important adjunct to education provided by the physician.

TABLE 20–41. POSSIBLE DIAGNOSTIC TESTS FOR LOW BACK PAIN

BLOOD

Hgb
Hct
WBC
Differential
ESR
Blood culture
Serum protein electrophoresis
Acid phosphatase
Alkaline phosphatase
Fasting blood sugar
Liver function tests

URINE

Urinalysis
Urine culture
Bence–Jones protein
Urine protein electrophoresis

RADIOLOGY

Plain films, lumbar spine
CT scan
Myelogram
MRI

NUCLEAR MEDICINE

Bone scan
Gallium scan

PATHOLOGY

Needle biopsy/open biopsy
Culture
Gram stain
Histology

PHYSICAL MEDICINE

Electromyography/nerve conduction
Velocity (EMG-NCV)

PSYCHIATRIC

Psychiatric evaluation
Psychometric testing

Patient Education. At this point, Tomas is very concerned about his back pain, and care should be taken to explain to him how this occurred, what he can expect, what the treatment plan is, and a rough idea on when he might return to work. In particular, Tomas should be instructed on the importance of strict bed rest on a firm surface for approximately 3 to 7 days. He should understand the usefulness of moist heat and its proper application, as well as how and when to use prescribed medications. He should not attempt abdominal strenthening exercises until the acute episode has resolved.

Tomas also should be told about possible surgical alternatives. In most cases, conservative therapy is sufficient, but if his symptoms do not resolve, or if they get worse, he may require referral to an orthopedist for possible chemonucleolysis, discectomy, or laminectomy.

Disposition. Tomas is sent home to strict bed rest for 3 to 7 days, with instructions to apply moist heat to his back for about 30 minutes approximately four to six times a day. He is given a nonsteroidal anti-inflammatory agent and a muscle relaxant and is told to return in 1 week, or earlier if symptoms worsen.

FIRST FOLLOW-UP VISIT

SUBJECTIVE

Tomas returns 1 week later feeling much better. He still reports occasional "electrical pains" that radiate from his back through the posterior thigh to the dorsum of the foot, but he denies any leg weakness or bowel or bladder incontinence. He says his back pain is much decreased.

OBJECTIVE

On physical examination, Tomas still has right-sided paravertebral muscle tenderness in the lumbar area, but no midline tenderness and no tenderness in the obturator foramen area of the buttock. Heel-walking and toe-walking are intact, as are motor strength and deep tendon reflexes. In particular, dorsiflexion of the foot and first toe are intact. Straight-leg raising is still limited on the right side, but Tomas says the pain is less severe than a week ago. The cremasteric reflex and rectal sphincter tone are intact.

ASSESSMENT

Tomas's symptoms seem to be decreasing while his physical examination is stable or improving. He probably has a small degree of disc herniation impinging on the right L5 nerve root and causing his current symptoms. The protruding disc material will probably degenerate further and cease to cause impingment and symptoms.

PLAN

Diagnostic. Many tests are available, but they are probably not indicated at the moment, since Tomas is improving (see Table 20–42). These tests must be used selectively and judiciously and are required in only a subset of patients with back pain. If his symptoms should worsen, several options may be considered:

1. *Myelogram.* Myelogram using the water-soluble dye metrizimide is especially useful in diagnosing intradural and extradural masses and is indicated when tumor is suspected, when symptoms are referable to several different lumbar areas, when the cauda equina syndrome is present, when spinal stenosis is considered, and when the diagnosis is not clear or disc herniation is not suspected. Its diagnostic accuracy is in the range of 75% to 80%, although the false-positive rate is about 10% and the false-negative rate is about 16%.

2. *Computed tomography (CT).* CT scan is especially useful in lesions involving the bone (e.g., spinal stenosis, facet joint disease, and bony lesions such as metastases or osteophytes). In particular, CT scanning is 72% to

100% effective in detecting disc herniation. Although it has the benefit of being a noninvasive test, it does expose the patient to a fair dose of ionizing radiation, is usually restricted to the axial plane, and is not useful for intrathecal pathology or for differentiating scar tissue due to previous back surgery from disc herniation.

3. *Magnetic resonance imaging (MRI).* MRI is a noninvasive technique to examine soft tissues in multiple planes without the drawback of exposing the patient to radiation. It has replaced CT as the "gold standard" for noninvasive examination of lumbar spine injuries and offers excellent differentiation among the several soft tissues of the spine.

4. *Electromyography and nerve conduction velocity (EMG-NCV) tests.* Some authors feel this test adds little to physical examination, but others find it helpful in differentiating the radiculopathy of nerve root impingement from peripheral neuropathy (e.g., irritation of the sciatic nerve in the obturator foramen or the peripheral neuropathy of diabetes or heavy metal exposure).

Theraupeutic

1. Continue nonsteroidal anti-inflammatory agents.
2. Discontinue muscle relaxants.
3. Continue moist heat therapy, and refer Tomas to physical therapy for additional modalities (e.g., ultrasound, diathermy, massage).
4. If available in the community, send Tomas to "back school" to learn simple ways to avoid undue stress on the lumbar spine.

Patient Education

1. Instruct Tomas on the importance of good "back hygiene": how to lift properly with the back straight and the knees bent, how to relieve back strain during prolonged standing by placing one foot on a 6-in footstool, and so on.
2. Review abdominal strengthening exercises with Tomas: In the supine position, bring the knee toward the chest by flexing the knee and hip; bent-knee "sit-ups" or "head-lifts"; and pelvic-tilt exercises. It should be emphasized that these exercises are not to be started until the acute episode has resolved.
3. A diet and weight-loss program should be started. Tomas should understand that maintenance of ideal body weight will decrease the strain placed on the lumbar spine.
4. Tomas should be encouraged to view back pain as a chronic problem that can be managed by close cooperation between him and the physician. A "cure," that is, a totally pain-free spine, may not be possible and should not be an expectation. All attempts should be made to prevent Tomas from becoming an "invalid" due to back pain. Patient education and active patient involvement in management of this chronic problem can greatly reduce the morbidity of back injury.

Disposition. Tomas will implement the diet, weight-loss, and exercise regimens discussed and return to clinic in 4 weeks to check on progress. He is told to return sooner if problems develop, such as worsening of back pain or appearance of new symptoms.

DISCUSSION

Tomas's presentation is fairly typical for lumbar disc herniation: acute onset of back pain, usually associated with trauma, paresthesias consistent with nerve root irritation, and resolution of symptoms with conservative management. However, it must be remembered that most patients with low back pain do not present with sciatica.

When abnormal compression or strain is applied to the intervertebral space, the annulus fibrosus may tear, allowing herniation of part or all of the nucleus pulposus. This degeneration can lead to protrusion of disc material, extrusion into the spinal canal, or even sequestration of disc material within the spinal canal.

Most patients with disc herniation enjoy resolution of symptoms spontaneously with conservative management. This consists of bed rest on a firm surface, use of nonnarcotic analgesics, moist heat to help minimize muscle spasm, and physical therapy modalities such as ultrasound, diathermy, and massage. Although muscle relaxants are often prescribed, their effectiveness is not clear.

In the subacute phase, the patient can be counseled regarding weight loss and abdominal strengthening exercises, both of which will decrease the amount of compression and strain forces applied to the lumbar spine. If a "back school" is available in the community, the patient will benefit from group discussion of back anatomy and causation of symptoms, as well as instruction on good "back hygiene": proper techniques for sitting, standing, and lifting to help protect the back from further injury. Finally, the "back school" can reinforce weight-loss counseling and the proper way to perform abdominal strengthening exercises.

If symptoms do not resolve, or worsen, or if motor weakness or bowel or bladder incontinence are present, special diagnostic tests may be required to elucidate the pathogenic mechanism. Myelogram, CT scan, and MRI all have their place in diagnosis. If available, MRI of the lumbar spine is the single test that can provide the most information about the spinal canal, the spinal cord, the intervertebral discs, and any soft-tissue masses.

Some cases of disc protrusion or extrusion can be treated by "chemonucleolysis," or dissolution of disc material by chymopapain injected into the intervertebral disc space. Such therapy is successful in approximately 70% of selected patients, but it will not be effective if disc material is sequestered within the spinal canal. Chemonucleolysis is not without risks; anaphylaxis occurs in 0.5% to 1.0% of patients, paraplegia occurs in about 1 in every 3500 patients, and subarachnoid hemorrhage occurs in about 1 in every 7000 patients.

Surgical discectomy can have up to a 95% success rate in carefully selected patients. This procedure is not a therapy for low back pain alone but is appropriate for symptoms of radiculopathy unresponsive to conservative management.

Spinal fusion may be necessary for patients with unrelenting chronic low back pain, usually due to degenerative changes at the intervertebral or facet joints. Decompressive laminectomy is reserved for patients with acute motor weakness or bowel/bladder dysfunction caused by disc material or other mass.

SUGGESTED READING

Bassam BA: Low back syndromes. Postgrad Med 1990; 87(4):209–216.

Connally JF, Jardon OM. Orthopedics In Rakel RE (ed.): Textbook of Family Practice, 4th ed. Philadelphia, W. B. Saunders, 1990.

Deyo RA, Loeser JD, Bigos SJ. Herniated lumbar intervertebral disc. Ann Intern Med 1990; 112(8):598–603.

Frymoyer JW. Back pain and sciatica. N Engl J Med 1988; 318(5):291–300.

Keim HA, Kirkaldy-Willis WH. Low back pain. Clin Symp 1980; 32(6):1–35.

Kirkaldy-Willis WH. Managing Low Back Pain, 2nd ed. New York: Churchill-Livingstone, 1983.

Macnab I. Disc degeneration and low back pain. Clin Orthop 1986; 208:3–14.

Mandel P, Lipton MH, Bernstein J, et al. Low Back Pain. Thorofare, N.J., SLACK, 1989.

Mooney V. The syndromes of low back disease. Orthop Clin North Am 1983; 14(3):505–515.

Shields CB, Williams PE Jr. Low back pain. Am Fam Physician 1986; 33(3):173–182.

Yon-Hing K, Kirkaldy-Willis WH. The pathophysiology of degenerative disease of the lumbar spine. Orthop Clin North Am 1983; 14(3):491–504.

QUESTIONS

1. Disc herniation occurs most frequently at which of the following intervertebral spaces?
   a. L1–L2, L2–L3
   b. L2–L3, L3–L4
   c. L3–L4, L4–L5
   d. L4–L5, L5–S1
   e. L5–S1, S1–S2

2. What motor function is impaired by nerve root injury at the L5 level?
   a. Hip flexion
   b. Knee flexion
   c. Knee extension
   d. Foot dorsiflexion
   e. Foot plantar flexion

3. In treating acute lumbar disc herniation, what are the main elements of conservative management?
   a. Bed rest
   b. Analgesics
   c. Steroids
   d. Moist heat
   e. Tylenol with codeine

4. What are the indications for surgical discectomy?
   a. Low back pain
   b. Acute lumbar disc herniation
   c. Disc herniation with paresthesias
   d. Disc herniation with paresthesias unresponsive to conservative therapy
   e. Spinal stenosis

5. What is the single best diagnostic test in evaluating a patient with probable acute lumbar disc herniation?
   a. Plain films, lumbar spine
   b. EMG-NCV
   c. Myelogram
   d. CT scan
   e. MRI

Answers appear on page 451.

Stiffness in Fingers

CHARLES M. PLOTZ

INITIAL VISIT

SUBJECTIVE

Patient Identification and Presenting Problem. Ann B. is a 57-year-old housewife who complains of low back pain and stiffness of her fingers.

Present Illness. Ann's complaints had a gradual onset about 4 years previously, but there was an episode of severe low back pain requiring a few days of bed rest about 2 years before. The back pain is aggravated by lifting, bed-making, and prolonged activity and is somewhat relieved by rest and simple analgesics. The finger stiffness is somewhat worse in the morning and is relieved by running her hands under warm water. There is a little pain, but Ann is mainly disturbed by "the knobby appearance" of her hands. There are no other significant joint complaints.

Family History. Ann's mother had similar complaints, but she has been dead for over 30 years and little is known of her medical history.

Social History. Ann has been married happily for 35 years and has two grown children, also married. She has never worked, and the only medication she takes is occasional aspirin or ibuprofen for the pain and a multivitamin pill most mornings.

Review of Systems. Unremarkable. Ann is 5 years postmenopausal and had a negative Pap smear and mammography within the past year.

OBJECTIVE

Physical Examination. On physical examination Ann is a slightly obese, pleasant middle-aged woman appearing about her stated age. She maintains a certain postural rigidity and complains of low back pain when getting on the examination table.

Ann's height is 64 in; weight is 144 lb; blood pressure is 128/76. EENT is normal, except for presbyopia consistent with her age. Her neck is supple and unremarkable. Heart, lungs, and abdomen are unrevealing, as are rectal and pelvic examinations. Skin is negative.

Hands reveal nodule formation and deformity at proximal and distal interphalangeal joints with no synovial fluid excess. Wrists are normal, as are the other peripheral joints. Straight-leg raising is to 90 degrees, with some complaint of low back pain. There is tenderness to percussion over the lower lumbar spine. Neurologic examination is entirely negative.

Laboratory Evaluation. Initial laboratory tests reveal a normal CBC and urine. ESR (Westergren) is 27 (normal 0–20 for women). Further tests were done, and a treatment plan was outlined.

ASSESSMENT

This is a reasonably common presentation to the family physician. Musculoskeletal complaints rank high on the list of symptoms that cause patients to consult the physician.

Differential Diagnoses

1. *Rheumatoid arthritis (RA).* In favor of rheumatoid arthritis we have the involvement of proximal interphalangeal (PIP) joints of the fingers, the morning stiffness, the mild elevation of ESR, and the patient's sex. Opposed to this diagnosis is the involvement of the distal interphalangeal joints, the lack of evidence of synovitis, the absence of wrist involvement, and the minimal elevation of ESR and only transitory morning stiffness.

2. *Osteoarthritis (OA).* In favor of this diagnosis are the *nodular* involvement of distal interphalangeal joints (Heberden's nodes) and of PIP joints (Bouchard's nodes), the chronic low back pain (although the acute episode 2 years previously is not common in osteoarthritis), the patient's age, and the minimal morning stiffness and mild elevation of ESR. Against the diagnosis are the lack of evidence of osteoarthritis in other weight-bearing joints.

3. *Gout.* This is an episodic disease with intermittent severe attacks associated with elevated uric acid. The nodules sometimes associates with it, called "tophi," collect around cartilage, particularly that of the ear, and only in severe advanced tophaceous gout would there be nodules over all the fingers. Chondrocalcinosis, or "pseudogout," is often seen in association with osteoarthritis but usually involves larger joints and again leads to a chronic course with acute flare-ups. Gout is unlikely here in either form.

4. *Sciatica.* In favor of sciatica is the low back pain and somewhat positive straight-leg raising test. The acute episode 2 years previously could have been a herniated disc, although there is no history of any episode that might have caused this. There is no neurologic involvement, and disc herniation leading to sciatica often causes unilateral depression of deep tendon reflexes and some sensory change. It is unusual for a sciatic syndrome to affect both sides. Finally, of course, the sciatic syndrome would in no way cause the involvement of hands.

Working Diagnosis. On balance, then, both gout and sciatica can be discarded out of hand. The evidence so far presented is largely in favor of osteoarthritis (Table 20–42).

PLAN

Diagnostic. In general, rheumatic disease can be divided into inflammatory conditions (e.g., rheumatoid arthritis, infectious arthritis, systemic lupus, etc.) and those which are noninflammatory (e.g., osteoarthritis, posttraumatic syndromes, etc.). The best quick way to decide whether or not inflammation is present is the ESR, preferably done by the Westergren method, which allows for a wider range. If the ESR is normal—and in the absence of such mitigating factors as polycythemia, sickle-cell disease, and severe dehydration—it is unlikely that an inflammatory process is present. If the ESR is elevated, it is possible that there is inflammatory arthritis, but be aware that many other conditions (e.g.,

TABLE 20–42. BASIC DIFFERENTIAL DIAGNOSIS OF RHEUMATOID ARTHRITIS (RA) AND OSTEOARTHRITIS (OA)

	RA	OA
Sex difference	F >M 2:1	None
Age	Younger more common	Older more common
Involvement of DIP joints	Uncommon	Common
Involvement of PIP joints	Common	Uncommon
Involvement of wrists	Common	Uncommon
Symmetrical involvement	Common	Less common
Evidence of synovitis	Common	Only acute episodes
Morning stiffness	Considerable	Minimal
Systemic manifestations	Common	Uncommon

neoplastic disease, any infectious process, anemia, etc.) can cause elevations of ESR. Marked elevation of the ESR—over 100 (Westergren)—should alert one to the possible presence of multiple myeloma or polymyalgia rheumatica.

X-rays are helpful because inflammatory disease is often associated with bone erosion and osteoarthritis is associated with hypertropic changes. The two can coexist. Chondrocalcinosis is revealed by the thin line of calcification seen within the joint. Gout is associated with "punched out" lesions, which represent tophaceous deposits in the periarticular bone. Spine x-rays can reveal, in addition to arthritis, destructive lesions associated with neoplasia or infection and osteoporosis, a common affliction in postmenopausal women.

Rheumatoid factor is present in about 60% of patients with rheumatoid arthritis, and the simplest way of detecting it is with the latex fixation test of Singer and Plotz. There are numerous false-positive results, however, and a positive latex test should be considered confirmatory rather than diagnostic.

Let us now add to our knowledge of the patient. A repeat ESR was 12, and on closer questioning Ann reports that she had had a mild respiratory infection at the time of the initial test. This indicates that Ann does not have an inflammatory disease. X-rays of the hands show productive lesions at all the IP joints, with some distortion and bone rather than soft-tissue swelling. This is characteristic of the presence of both Heberden's and Bouchard's nodes and is diagnostic of osteoarthritis. X-rays of the lumbosacral spine again reveal the hypertrophic changes of osteoarthritis but here also show considerable osteoporosis and wedging of L4 consistent with an old compression fracture. This most likely was the result of the acute episode reported 2 years previously. The remainder of the laboratory and x-ray data are not contributory.

Therapeutic. After 4 years of symptoms, it is worthwhile to talk with Ann and her husband and learn a little more about what has motivated her to seek help now. Two things are significant. A maternal aunt had "crippling arthritis," and this has haunted Ann since childhood. Second, a close friend of Ann's recently consulted a physician because of back pain and was found to have metastatic breast carcinoma.

Before anything else then, Ann needs the reassurance, which can now be given, that she does not have any form of crippling arthritis and that tests and x-rays have revealed no evidence of any kind of cancer. It is conceivable that this is the only thing that needs to be done for Ann, since her tension and anxiety will be relieved and her symptoms may become much more bearable.

A major tenet of treatment is that "less is more." Every therapeutic intervention carries with it its own risk, and the physician must always weigh the risk–benefit ratio. It is clear that there is no evidence for rheu-

matoid arthritis, and therefore, the use of major second-line drugs is contraindicated. Even if rheumatoid arthritis is suspected, it would almost certainly be wrong to start with these agents. In non-life-threatening diseases, it is usually better to use the safest procedures before proceeding to those which are more dangerous.

The local injection of corticosteroids is often useful in localized painful conditions that have an inflammatory component. In osteoarthritis, for instance, when a knee develops synovitis and is painful, it is sometimes a good idea, once you are sure that the inflammation is not secondary to infection, to remove fluid and inject a long-acting corticosteroid. In general, such injections, into weight-bearing joints, should not be given more often than every 4 to 6 months for fear of inducing a Charcot joint. In this patient there is really no localized area of great pain or inflammation. The spine pain is secondary to osteoporosis and compression fracture. There is therefore no indication for steroid injection.

Simple home physiotherapeutic measures are always useful. Warmth and range-of-motion exercises are soothing and preserve mobility. Furthermore, when generalized osteoporosis is present, as in Ann, it is advisable for the patient to keep as active as possible, since rest promotes bone loss. Thus, when vertebral compression occurs due to osteoporosis, rest may be necessary during the acute fracture stage, but as soon as possible, exercise and general activity should be encouraged.

QUESTIONS

1. Which of the following are typical of osteoarthritis?
   a. Involvement of the PIP joints
   b. Involvement of the DIP joints
   c. Ear nodules
   d. Involvement of the wrists
   e. Most common in older persons

2. When compared with patients with osteomyelites, those with rheumatoid arthritis
   a. Are younger.
   b. Have symmetrical joint involvement.
   c. Have involvement of DIP joints.
   d. Have systemic manifestations.
   e. Have evidence of synovitis.

3. If in the differential diagnosis of arthritis you are confined to a single laboratory determination, which of the following would be most useful?
   a. Latex fixation
   b. X-ray of spine
   c. Erythrocyte sedimentation rate
   d. Antinuclear antibody
   e. Serum uric acid

Answers appear on page 451.

Skin Irritation

SHELLEY P. ROATEN, Jr.

INITIAL VISIT

SUBJECTIVE

Patient Identification. Marla A. is a 48-year-old Caucasian homemaker who complains of a skin condition.

Presenting Problems. Although her health has generally been good in the past, Marla has noticed rough areas of her skin for several months, areas that are sometimes slightly tender to touch. During a vacation to a beach resort on the Atlantic coast last month, she also noticed a growth on her right hand after it bled briefly following a minor injury. Two weeks ago, she applied hydrocortisone cream to the lesion for several days, with no apparent response. In retrospect, Marla also recalls that she changed to a mild soap for bathing several weeks ago because of "skin irritation."

Past Medical History. Marla has had no surgery or serious illnesses and takes no medications routinely. She suffered a fibular fracture in adolescence, which healed without sequelae, and she had a facial laceration repaired after a sailing accident.

Family History. Marla's father was a cattle rancher and real estate broker who died of injuries resulting from a tractor accident at age 63. Marla recalls that her father was treated for "skin cancers" several times prior to his death. Her mother is in good health at age 69. Her brother is an investment banker in good health at age 51, and he has no history of skin problems. Marla has two healthy children in college.

Health Habits. Marla does not smoke, and she drinks small amounts of alcoholic beverages on occasion. Two years ago, Marla and her husband began walking 2 miles each day and reduced dietary fat and cholesterol. Marla sometimes remembers to use a sunscreen during her summer vacation trips, but she rarely wears a hat or gloves. Her last Pap smear and breast examination were performed 8 months ago.

Social History. Marla and her husband both enjoy outdoor activities, including gardening and fishing. For many years they have met another couple for an annual summer vacation at the same beach resort, and they usually have a skiing trip to Colorado or Utah. They also play tennis and bridge with friends.

Review of Systems. Marla can recall no recent changes in the use of skin or hair products other than changing her bath soap. She has a tendency to develop dry skin, particularly in the winter months, and she uses a moisturizing cream as needed. She reports no changes in activities, appetite, weight, or sleep patterns.

OBJECTIVE

Physical Examination. Marla's vital signs are within normal limits, including a blood pressure of 134/80, a heart rate of 64, weight of 118 lb, and height of 64 in. Marla is neatly dressed; has light brown short hair, hazel eyes, little or no makeup; and has tan skin. There are scattered, ill-defined, light brown, slightly scaly macules on her forehead and the dorsal surfaces of both hands. Some are slightly erythematous. On her right hand there is a solitary, firm, erythematous, nontender nodule with a slightly scaly surface and a diameter of about 6 mm. There are a few seborrheic keratoses on her abdomen and upper back. There are no palpable lymph nodes in any location, and the remainder of the examination is normal.

Laboratory Tests. None were done at this visit. A chemistry profile obtained at the previous visit 8 months ago was entirely normal.

ASSESSMENT

Working Diagnoses. There are three likely diagnoses that explain Marla's skin lesions:

1. *Actinic keratoses.* The scattered scaly macules in sun-exposed areas are characteristic of actinic (solar) keratoses, a reaction to cumulative overexposure to ultraviolet light.
2. *Squamous cell carcinoma.* A firm, discrete nodule arising within a field of actinic keratoses is highly suggestive of squamous cell carcinoma. The margins of the tumor are usually indistinct, and the surface is smooth or slightly scaly. Fast-growing squamous cell carcinomas may exhibit central ulceration.
3. *Seborrheic keratoses.* These common, benign tumors are usually brown or black in color, with a soft, pitted and furrowed surface. There are often multiple lesions spread over the face, neck, back, chest, abdomen, and extremities, particularly the backs of the hands.

Differential Diagnoses. Seborrheic keratoses are so common and of such typical appearance that it is unlikely that any further diagnostic testing would be necessary after examination. Occasionally, unusual color, size, shape, or location may prompt a biopsy, especially if the patient reports any concerns about growth or other recent changes in the lesion. A variety of methods can be used to remove them for cosmetic reasons.

Marla's actinic keratoses are also fairly characteristic in appearance and location, particularly in view of her history of significant sunlight exposure. The appearance of slightly scaly, erythematous areas on the forehead might suggest *seborrheic dermatitis,* but there are no signs of this condition in other areas, and the presence of similar scaly lesions on the hands supports the primary diagnosis. Although biopsy would offer additional confirmation, it is rarely necessary.

The solitary nodule on Marla's right hand could be any of several *neoplasms,* either malignant or benign. One might consider *Bowen's disease, keratoacanthoma, basal cell carcinoma, a wart,* or possibly some other lesions. Bowen's disease on glabrous skin is probably best thought of as "squamous cell carcinoma in situ" and is thus distinguished histologically. A keratoacanthoma is a benign (though ugly and fast growing) tumor that may occur in this location but is typically bud-shaped or dome-shaped with a central keratinaceous plug, occasionally with ulceration. Basal cell carcinoma is a neoplasm that can occur in this setting, induced by prolonged exposure to sunlight. Most basal cell carcinomas exhibit central ulceration and a distinct pearl-colored, translucent border with telangiectasia.

PLAN

Diagnostic. If a solitary skin tumor is not recognized as a benign lesion with absolute certainty, the only prudent response is complete removal and histologic examination. Complete excision, followed by suture removal in about 7 days for this location, is the most desirable method for use by a family physician, who typically has little training and experience with the alternatives. Properly done, excisional biopsy provides an excellent specimen for the pathologist and an acceptable cosmetic result.

No additional diagnostic testing is necessary at this time. Squamous cell carcinomas have the potential for local and distant metastasis, so the presence of any palpable lymph nodes in the region of the tumor would indicate the need for additional lymph node biopsy and possibly more extensive surgery.

Patient Education. At least the following issues should be discussed:

1. General wound care and suture removal, and discussion of the pending histologic examination.
2. Brief outline of the subsequent treatment plan for actinic keratoses.
3. Protection from sunlight and attention to any new lesions.

Marla received instructions for wound care and suture removal. She also was informed about the significance of the biopsy, which was expected to confirm the tentative diagnosis of squamous cell carcinoma and confirm that all the lesion was excised. Since actinic keratoses are precursors of squamous cell carcinoma, Marla was given an outline of subsequent treatment alternatives and a pamphlet that explains the relationship of these lesions to sunlight exposure. The use of 5-fluorouracil cream was recommended at a later visit. The advice included information about avoidance of peak times of the day for sun damage and alternatives for protection, emphasizing choice of clothing and sunscreen preparations.

Disposition. Marla was asked to return in 1 week for suture removal and biopsy result and then in 1 month to begin treatment for the actinic keratoses. Sutures were removed 1 week later from a wound that appeared to be healing well, and the biopsy confirmed the diagnosis of squamous cell carcinoma and the absence of tumor cells at the margins of the specimen.

FOLLOW-UP VISIT, 1 MONTH

SUBJECTIVE

Marla returned 1 month later, and her wound was healing well. With her usual enthusiasm, she was eager to discuss the pamphlet and options for protection from further sun damage. She expressed some embarrassment that this problem had never occurred to her in view of her other efforts to maintain good health habits. Since her usual outdoor activities were important to her and her husband, both have already begun using protective clothing and a topical sunscreen labeled with a sun protective factor (SPF) of 15.

OBJECTIVE

Wound healing was nearly complete, and there were no changes in the other skin lesions.

ASSESSMENT

1. Squamous cell carcinoma, probably cured by excision
2. Multiple actinic keratoses requiring treatment
3. Multiple seborrheic keratoses for which no further treatment is planned

PLAN

Diagnostic. No further diagnostic testing was required or planned at this visit.

Therapeutic. A topical preparation of 5% 5-fluorouracil cream (Efudex) was the treatment option selected for Marla's actinic keratoses. She was instructed to apply a thin film twice daily in the areas affected by scaly lesions.

Patient Education

1. The anticipated brisk inflammatory response to treatment was discussed, as well as the other potential side effects that should prompt Marla to call for additional advice.
2. The physician answered questions prompted by the pamphlet that was provided at a previous visit, and other issues related to sunlight and sunscreen protection were discussed.

During the 3- to 4-week course of treatment, Marla understood that she should temporarily discontinue the sunscreen but should limit sun exposure to brief periods.

Disposition. A follow-up visit was scheduled in 2 weeks, with tentative plans for one additional visit 2 weeks later.

DISCUSSION

This patient's skin lesions are often seen in primary care practice. In Marla's case, the seborrheic keratoses can be regarded as an incidental finding that does not mandate any particular treatment. Because of its destructive potential, the squamous cell carcinoma requires relatively prompt attention, after which treatment of the premalignant actinic keratoses can be addressed.

Seborrheic keratoses rarely pose any diagnostic dilemma for the experienced clinician. These slow-growing, benign lesions gradually increase in size and number after middle age. They are typically brown, but they range in color from flesh-colored to black and have a sharply circumscribed border and usually a characteristic pitted and furrowed surface texture. Except for irritation by clothing or cosmetic considerations, they pose no significant threat to health. Dermatologist Walter B. Shelly has dubbed them the "barnacles of old age." If necessary, they can usually be removed by freezing with liquid nitrogen or by dermal curettage after local anesthesia. Those lesions with unusual features or rapid growth should prompt excision and pathologic examination to differentiate them from other lesions of greater significance.

Actinic keratoses (solar keratoses) eventually affect nearly all of the elderly light-skinned population and may be found in much younger adults who have significant exposure to sunlight. Increased incidence in males compared with females probably reflects greater likelihood of excessive sunlight. Lesions are often multiple, a fact clearly confirmed by 5-fluorouracil treatment, which inflames even keratoses that are clinically inapparent.

Under the microscope, there is a very thin superficial layer of atypical epidermal cells, and there may be areas of squamous cell carcinoma in situ. Given time, a few of these actinic keratoses will evolve into squamous cell carcinoma. Some keratoses also may result in the exuberant hyperkeratosis that produces a projection called a "cutaneous horn," which may conceal a carcinoma at its base.

Treatment is indicated to halt the potential progression to carcinoma. The most common therapeutic options for actinic keratoses are cryotherapy with liquid nitrogen and chemotherapy with topical preparations of 5-fluorouracil. Other cryotherapeutic agents probably should not be used for this indication, since they fail to quickly achieve the low temperature and "quick-freeze" destructive capacity of liquid nitrogen on glabrous skin. The nitrogen can be applied with a large cotton-tipped applicator (twice for 10 to 15 seconds) or with a spraying device. The patient should expect some stinging upon application and some erythema or blistering to follow.

If there are larger areas or large numbers of actinic keratoses, topical application of 5-fluorouracil is usually a more reasonable choice, at least in part due to the time and effort that would be required with liquid nitrogen. Clinically, 5-fluorouracil has little visible effect on normal skin, but it causes a prompt inflammatory response at the sites of actinic lesions, even some that may not have been recognized by inspection. The patient should be forewarned of these reactions, which progress from erythema to erosion to ulceration during the first 1 or 2 weeks. Areas with poor cutaneous penetration, such as the dorsal aspect of the hand, may benefit from occlusion with plastic wrap after application. This is not generally done, however, because of the brisk eczematous reaction that ensues. Sunlight enhances the cutaneous reaction and should ordinarily be minimized. Patients with many lesions may prefer to treat areas sequentially to reduce the discomfort and cosmetic problems. Some physicians also prescribe concomitant use of topical steroids to reduce the irritation, which does not appear to interfere with the ultimate results. Treatment continues for about 3 weeks, or until the peak of the reaction appears to be past. Complete healing may require several weeks.

Any clinical lesion that survives the attack with liquid nitrogen or 5-fluorouracil deserves biopsy. Therapeutic alternatives under investigation include immunotherapeutic agents and retinoids.

Squamous cell carcinoma (SCC) of the skin may arise de novo or in response to a variety of precipitating factors, of which the most common is exposure to the ultraviolet component of sunlight. Other associated exposures include arsenic, coal tar, radiation, and several oils. People with light skin, regardless of race, are more susceptible to this sun damage. SCC that arises from an actinic keratosis is considered to have a relatively low risk of metastasis (probably less than 5%), but it can be locally destructive. Risk of metastasis is higher for carcinomas that arise de novo and those on the lip.

Because of its capacity for local destruction and metastasis, SCC of the skin must be treated with some respect and reasonable assurance of complete removal. Common methods of therapy include excision, electrocoagulation, irradiation, and Mohs' technique for chemosurgery. Excision is the method most often employed by family physicians, and it is suitable for most lesions. Electrosurgery can be employed for small carcinomas (less than 10 mm) and is useful for multiple small SCCs that may arise within an area of radiation dermatitis. Radiation treatment is usually reserved for large lesions, especially for those for which other methods would result in significant disfigurement. Mohs' technique is desirable when peripheral extensions of the tumor may be present, since the method is performed in multiple steps under microscopic control, and is useful when bone or cartilage may be involved.

Any patient who has had SCC or actinic keratoses needs to be aware of the need for both protection from sunlight and long-term surveillance for new or recurrent lesions.

SUGGESTED READING

Arnold HL, Odom RB, James WD. Andrew's Diseases of the Skin, 8th ed. Philadelphia, W. B. Saunders, 1990, pp. 749–751, 754–756, 777–782.

Fitzpatrick TB, et al. (eds.). Dermatology in General Medicine, 3rd ed. New York, McGraw-Hill, 1987, pp. 746–758, 733–739.

Roaten S Jr, Lea WA. Dermatology. In Rakel RE (ed.): Textbook of Family Practice, 4th ed. Philadelphia, W. B. Saunders, 1990, pp. 1130–1131.

QUESTIONS

1. Predisposing factors associated with the development of squamous cell carcinoma include which of the following?
   a. Ultraviolet irradiation
   b. Fair skin
   c. Coal tar
   d. X-ray irradiation
   e. Topical corticosteroids

2. Proper treatment will reduce the risk of subsequent squamous cell carcinoma of the skin arising from which of the following?
   a. Seborrheic keratoses
   b. Seborrheic dermatitis
   c. Actinic keratoses
   d. Keratoacanthomas
   e. Junctional nevi

3. A 64-year-old man has several small, scattered, well-circumscribed, brown or black nodules on his forearms and abdomen. The individual lesions have a soft, pitted, and furrowed surface. One of them has the same general appearance but has a diameter of 2.5 cm. This description is most characteristic of
   a. Cherry angiomata.
   b. Lentigo maligna.
   c. Superficial spreading melanoma.
   d. Seborrheic keratoses.
   e. Actinic keratoses.

4. Acceptable treatments of actinic keratoses include which of the following?
   a. Freezing with liquid nitrogen
   b. Topical application of 5-fluorouracil
   c. Topical application of methotrexate
   d. Freezing with ethyl chloride
   e. Photochemotherapy with psoralens

Answers appear on page 451.

Recurring Rash

SHELLEY P. ROATEN, Jr.

INITIAL VISIT

SUBJECTIVE

Patient Identification. Rebecca D. is a 29-year-old Caucasian homemaker and vocational nurse scheduled for a Pap smear and routine examination. She has been divorced and she remarried 2 years ago; she has children ages 7 and 5 years; and she has worked part time for the past year in a clinic for sexually transmitted diseases.

Presenting Problem. Rebecca called about 1 month ago to schedule an appointment for her regular Pap smear. She also wants advice about a rash that has appeared since the appointment was made.

Present Illness. Rebecca first noticed a few spots on the upper part of her chest 2 or 3 weeks ago, but on closer inspection she found other lesions on her back and shoulders. They seem to be getting lighter in color. There has been no itching or other associated symptoms, and Rebecca does not recall any single lesion that appeared before the others. In retrospect, she remembers a similar rash several months ago during the winter. At that time, she believes that the spots were darker than the surrounding skin; this time the small patches appear lighter. During the winter she used a skin moisturizing lotion, and the initial rash seemed to fade gradually in early spring. She sought no medical attention for the first rash, but now she would like to improve the appearance of her skin.

Rebecca's pelvic examinations and Pap smears have been normal in the past, and she has had regular menstrual cycles. She stopped taking oral contraceptives 2 years ago at the time of her marriage, since her husband had a previous vasectomy. Rebecca takes no other medications regularly, but she does report occasional use of acetaminophen for headaches and Ex-Lax or another laxative tablet for constipation. She takes a laxative when she fails to have a daily bowel movement, but she denies discomfort and has not noticed any abnormality of the stools. She last took an Ex-Lax tablet about 2 weeks ago.

Past Medical History. Rebecca had an appendectomy at 10 years of age and otherwise was hospitalized only for normal childbirth. She has had no other surgery or serious injuries. An accidental needle puncture at work 6 months ago caused some anxiety but no other apparent sequelae.

Family History. Rebecca's father and mother are in good health at ages 55 and 54, respectively. Her husband is 35 years of age, enjoys good health, and works as a laboratory technician in the hospital. Their children are also well, and no other person in the family has a rash. Rebecca's sister is in good health at age 31.

Health Habits. Rebecca does not smoke, and she drinks alcoholic beverages only occasionally. Other than some experimentation with marijuana during her college years, there is no history of illicit drug use. Rebecca sometimes does aerobic exercises with a videotape and has recently started to "watch calories" in an annual effort to lose weight before summertime activities begin. She has no particular diet plan and is not fond of most vegetables or fruits. She has not attempted any dietary modification in response to the bowel irregularity, which has occurred about every month or two since her first pregnancy.

Her husband plays tennis about once per week in a doubles league. Although his cholesterol levels have been normal, his father and uncle both take medications for elevated cholesterol. He mentioned recently to Rebecca that they should give some thought to cholesterol reduction, but they have made no specific plans.

Social History. Rebecca and her husband moved from Cincinnati to Austin, Texas, after their marriage 2 years ago. They have dinner and go to movies with friends, and the family enjoys camping and backpacking trips. They are active in school and church activities with their children. Rebecca's husband is her only sexual partner, and she had one other relationship between her divorce and second marriage.

Review of Systems. Rebecca feels well and reports no changes in activity, energy, or mood. There has been a weight loss of 4 lb since she started to reduce calories, but she still feels hungry most of the day. She has moderate menstrual flow every 30 days, the last beginning 10 days ago. There is no history of vaginal discharge or lesions now or in the past, except for one episode of monilial vaginitis during her second pregnancy.

OBJECTIVE

Physical Examination. Rebecca's vital signs are all within normal limits, including blood pressure of 122/78, heart rate of 72, weight of 138 lb, and height of 63 in. General examination is unremarkable, including breasts, pelvis, and rectum. Inspection of the skin reveals multiple ovoid, slightly hypopigmented macules and small patches scattered randomly on her upper chest over the sternum, upper back, and shoulders. Most of the lesions have tiny dry scales, exhibited particularly well when scratched gently with a fingernail.

Laboratory Tests. Stool examination for occult blood is negative. Appropriate slides were made for the Pap smear with cytobrush and spatula. A chemistry profile, CBC, and urinalysis obtained prior to her current employment were all within normal limits, and repeat testing is not thought to be necessary at this time.

ASSESSMENT

Working Diagnoses

1. *Tinea versicolor* is the most likely explanation for the rash. Despite some other distracting clues, both the history and appearance of the skin lesions are practically diagnostic in this case. In view of the medications taken and the small risk of syphilis exposure, some additional confirmation of the diagnosis is probably justified.

2. Rebecca's health habits are less than ideal, especially her dietary patterns and relative lack of exercise. Rather than using appropriate dietary modifications to promote bowel regularity, she has resorted to medications as an expedient, but less desirable, remedy. Since she has not experienced discomfort or observed dry, hard stools, she probably also has unrealistic expectations about bowel regularity.

Differential Diagnoses. Although the cause of Rebecca's rash is probably established on clinical evidence, other possibilities traditionally considered in the differential diagnosis of tinea versicolor include leprosy, syphilis, pityriasis rosea, pityriasis alba, seborrheic dermatitis, drug eruptions, and vitiligo.

1. *Leprosy.* Although no exposure to the disease is evident in this patient, leprosy occurs in southern states, including Florida, Louisiana, and Texas. The macular cutaneous lesions of leprosy are frequently the first visible expression of the disease, and they may resemble tinea versicolor. Most patients, however, report regional numbness prior to the onset of skin lesions, and there is localized loss of cold and light touch sensation.

2. *Syphilis.* Secondary syphilis may have a variety of cutaneous manifestations that mimic other disorders, including multiple pink, slightly scaly macules or papules. There is often generalized adenopathy. Unlike tinea versicolor, the "syphilid" rash is prone to involve the face, palms and soles, and anal or genital areas. Although the risk seems fairly remote in Rebecca's case, changes in sexual partners and the possibility of occupational exposure require some consideration. Since serologic tests are positive in essentially all cases of syphilis, a simple blood test could resolve the uncertainty, if needed.

3. *Pityriasis rosea.* Pityriasis rosea is a mild inflammatory rash of unknown etiology characterized by multiple scaly, salmon-colored macules or papules with a distribution similar to tinea versicolor. The individual lesions are usually ovoid, with their long axes parallel to the skin's lines of cleavage. Many patients will recognize a large, single "herald patch" preceding the other lesions.

4. *Pityriasis alba.* Pityriasis alba usually occurs in children and adolescents, who exhibit oval, hypopig-

mented, scaling macules and patches on the face, neck, shoulders, and upper arms. The etiology is unknown, and the lesions gradually resolve over months or years.

5. *Seborrheic dermatitis.* In patients with seborrheic dermatitis, the skin patches are erythematous with a faint yellowish hue, and the scales are rather large and have an oily texture, instead of the fine "dusty" scales of tinea versicolor. Although seborrheic dermatitis is found on the chest and back, the absence of facial or scalp involvement would be relatively unusual.

6. *Drug eruption.* There are a variety of drugs, among them the phenolphthalein in some laxatives, that can cause a "fixed drug eruption" characterized by abnormally pigmented or erythematous macules and patches. The lesions tend to appear recurrently in the same locations after each ingestion of the offending agent and then recede gradually. In this case, the timing and persistence of the patient's eruptions make a drug reaction unlikely.

7. *Vitiligo.* Patches of vitiligo can occur almost anywhere on the skin regardless of age or race. The hypopigmentation is usually more pronounced than in tinea versicolor, and scaling is not a common feature unless the areas have been sunburned.

PLAN

Diagnostic. A preparation of scales from the skin lesions with 10% potassium hydroxide solution revealed characteristic hyphae and clusters of spores commonly referred to as "spaghetti and meatballs."

Therapeutic

1. After a brief review of options, Rebecca elected to begin treatment of the rash with selenium sulfide 2.5% lotion (Selsun), to be followed later by use of similar lotion/shampoo (Selsun Blue) available without a doctor's prescription.

2. Rebecca also received printed copies of balanced diets of 1000 and 1200 calories and an American Heart Association booklet containing advice about dietary fats and cholesterol. She was advised about the use of dietary modifications to reduce constipation, in preference to laxative use.

Patient Education

1. The use of selenium sulfide lotion was explained, beginning with daily applications to scalp and affected areas of skin during a shower for 1 week; the lotion or lather is left on the skin for about 10 minutes and then rinsed. An alternative initial regimen is one or two applications left on overnight.

2. Rebecca understood that even after successful treatment, repigmentation of the areas to blend with normal surrounding skin takes time, and recurrences are likely. Following the first course of treatment, she decided to try a preventive application of Selsun Blue or a similar lotion/shampoo about once each month.

3. The relationship between bowel patterns and specific foods was discussed, emphasizing the role of dietary fiber, fresh fruits and vegetables, and adequate liquid intake. There was also a brief discussion of the difference between constipation and absolute adherence to a daily schedule.

Disposition. No specific date was set for a return visit other than for routine health maintenance. When the physician telephoned 1 week later to report normal results from the Pap smear, Rebecca reported no problems with use of the lotion, and she had lost another 2 lb. She and her husband have begun walking each evening for about a mile, and they bought a copy of the *Low-Fat, Low-Cholesterol Cookbook* (American Heart Association/Time Books). It was agreed that Rebecca would make another appointment if the constipation continued or if she had any difficulty with treatment.

DISCUSSION

Rebecca's presentation is typical, in that patients often use routine visits to mention minor complaints, including mild "irregularity" and rashes that do not itch. Rebecca was concerned only about the appearance of the rash, which would soon be more evident in summer clothing.

Her history of "constipation" certainly sounds benign, with further assurance from the negative test for stool blood. Dietary advice and encouragement are a reasonable first approach, with further attention to the problem if it persists.

Observant patients with tinea versicolor may note that the rash appears to change color or even seems to come and go with the seasons, and such observations strongly support the diagnosis. Tinea versicolor is caused by the fungus *Malassezia furfur,* the yeast phase of which is named *Pityrosporum orbiculare.* The organism apparently interferes with the transfer of melanin pigment to the keratinocytes so that the rate of change in pigmentation within lesions is noticeably delayed in comparison with surrounding skin. While normal skin tans, the lesions lag behind and appear relatively light in color. Conversely, as normal skin areas lose the tan, the lesions may appear darker (and hence the name "versicolor").

The diagnosis of tinea versicolor is ordinarily made by history and examination. The diagnosis also can be supported, when necessary, by the observation of yellowish fluorescence under Wood's light or by microscopic examination of scales to identify fungal elements. Scales can be scraped gently onto a microscope slide, to which one adds 10% to 20% potassium hydroxide solution and a cover slip. The slender hyphae and clusters of small, round spores are said to resemble "spaghetti and meatballs." In addition to use of the Wood's light for diagnosis, it is also sometimes used to monitor progress during treatment if the patient's degree of concern justifies close observation.

Malassezia furfur has some properties that distinguish it from the common dermatophytes that cause tinea corporis, tinea cruris, and other common fungal infections of the skin. Although this organism can be treated with many of the topical medications for fungi, it is not re-

TABLE 20–43. REPRESENTATIVE MEDICATION PRICES, RETAIL

Clotrimazole cream (Lotrimin), 30 gm	$21.10
Ketoconazole tablets 200 mg (Nizoral), #14	38.50
Selenium sulfide lotion 2.5% (Selsun), 120 ml	16.20
Selenium sulfide shampoo (Selsun Blue), 120 ml	3.60
Sodium thiosulfate solution (Tinver), 120 ml	21.30
Tolnaftate cream (Tinactin), 15 gm	5.63

sponsive to griseofulvin. If mistakenly identified as tinea corporis and treated with griseofulvin, the patient wastes time and money.

Another problem with planning treatment is that the organism is commonly found on individuals with no skin lesions and on normal skin areas of people with the rash. The cause of variation in susceptibility to the rash is unknown, and recolonization after treatment is the rule rather than the exception. "Cure" is a hazardous term to use with reference to tinea versicolor. Although some patients prefer to attempt treatment for cosmetic reasons, they must understand that resolution of the rash is gradual and recurrence is likely unless preventive medication is used periodically. There is no generally accepted regimen for prevention of recurrence.

Successful treatments have been reported with a variety of topical preparations, including clotrimazole (Lotrimin), tolnaftate (Tinactin), sodium thiosulfate solution (Tinver), selenium sulfide lotions (Selsun, Exsel, Selsun Blue), 2% benzoyl peroxide, and 50% propylene glycol in water. More recently, success has been demonstrated with various oral dosage regimens of ketoconazole (Nizoral). Suggested dosages of ketoconazole include 200 mg daily for 2 to 4 weeks or 400 mg as a single dose. Some representative retail costs of these medications at a local pharmacy are shown in Table 20–43.

Because of safety and low cost, many physicians still favor use of the time-tested selenium sulfide preparations; the 2.5% lotion is available by prescription, and the lower strength is available as Selsun Blue without prescription. Although several treatment schemes have been used, the package insert with Selsun lotion suggests daily use for 1 week, rinsed off 10 minutes after each application. Others report good response to a single application left on the affected areas overnight. Shampooing the hair at the same time is recommended, since organisms are harbored in the scalp. Although no proven regimen exists for prevention, it seems reasonable to recommend an application every few weeks, or the patient could just resume treatment at the earliest sign of recurrence.

In summary, Rebecca visited her physician for a Pap smear and routine examination, but the visit revealed other health matters that deserved attention. Most patients are likely to be receptive to general advice and encouragement related to proper diet and exercise, with more detailed management plans in response to specific problems, such as hypercholesterolemia. Tinea versicolor is a common, benign rash often mentioned by the patient as an afterthought or detected as an incidental finding during examination. When treatment is desired, the physician needs to share some key information with the patient to arrive at a treatment plan with reasonable expectations.

SUGGESTED READING

Arnold HL, Odom RB, James WD (eds.). Andrews' Diseases of the Skin, 8th ed. Philadelphia, W. B. Saunders, 1990, pp. 347–350.
Braunwald E, et al. (eds.). Harrison's Principles of Internal Medicine, 11th ed. New York, McGraw-Hill, 1987, p. 179.
Fitzpatric TB, et al. (eds.). Dermatology in General Medicine, 3rd ed. New York, McGraw-Hill, 1987, pp. 2197–2200.
Roaten S Jr, Lea WA. Dermatology. In Rakel RE (ed.): Textbook of Family Practice, 4th ed. Philadelphia, W. B. Saunders, 1990, pp. 1133–1134

QUESTIONS

1. The causative organism of tinea versicolor is
   a. *Microsporum audouinii.*
   b. *Trichophyton tonsurans.*
   c. *Tinea corporis.*
   d. *Malassezia furfur.*
   e. *Tinea versicolor.*

2. Appropriate treatment alternatives for tinea versicolor include which of the following?
   a. Topical clotrimazole (Lotrimin)
   b. Topical selenium sulfide (Selsun)
   c. Oral griseofulvin (Grifulvin, Fulvicin)
   d. Topical nystatin (Mycostatin)
   e. Oral ketoconazole (Nizoral)

3. Changes in pigmentation within lesions of tinea versicolor are due to
   a. Increased production of melanin.
   b. Abnormal transportation of melanin.
   c. Deposition of dark fungal spores in scales.
   d. Decreased production of melanin.
   e. Reduced penetration of ultraviolet light.

Answers appear on page 451.

Diabetes Mellitus

KAY F. McFARLAND and JAN C. UPDIKE

INITIAL VISIT

SUBJECTIVE

Patient Identification and Present Illness. Karen, a 19-year-old college student with insulin-dependent diabetes, presented to the emergency room at 11:00 a.m. with a history of vomiting four times and not being able to keep fluids down for 12 hours. Because of the nausea and vomiting, she omitted her insulin before breakfast. She had not been measuring her blood sugars on a regular basis at school; the last glucose determination, done several days before, was 180 mg/dl at bedtime. She denied fever, chills, cough, dysuria, or muscle aches.

Past Medical History. Karen had been hospitalized two times for diabetes, 10 years ago at the time of diagnosis and 6 months ago for an episode of ketoacidosis. Her present medications are insulin, NPH 10 units, regular 2 units before breakfast, and NPH 4 units and regular 2 units before supper and aspirin three to four tablets per week for headaches. She has no allergies to medications.

Family History. Karen's maternal grandmother died from renal failure secondary to diabetes. She has no other family history of diabetes. Her mother, father, brother, and sister are all living and well.

Health Habits. Although Karen does not follow a calorically measured diet, she avoids foods high in fat and sugar primarily for the purpose of weight control. She does not drink alcohol and has never smoked. She has not ever used illegal drugs. She is quite active and runs at least 1 mile or more five times per week.

Social History. Karen is in her second year of college, majoring in history. She has to study hard to make slightly above average grades and has not had time to participate in any organized school social groups. She broke up with her boyfriend about 7 months ago and had not had sex or even dated since then. Her mother is a school teacher with whom she is quite close. Her father is a lawyer who has always worked long hours.

Review of Systems. Karen has had some blurring of vision for several days and has noticed this in the past when her blood sugar level was elevated. Following her last ophthalmology appointment 3 months ago she was told that she had mild eye changes of diabetes. Other positive findings include a history of frequent headaches, particularly in the last year, which she describes as "tension related," a weight loss of about 20 lb over the past 8 months from dieting, and constipation intermittently, for which she uses milk of magnesia. Her last menstrual period was 5 months ago. Her periods have been a little irregular since their onset at age 13, but she had never skipped more than 2 months in the past.

OBJECTIVE

Physical Examination. On examination, her temperature is 97.1°F; her heart rate is 124; her respirations are 26; her blood pressure is 80/62; and her weight is 105 lb. She is alert and oriented, but she appears acutely ill. Her skin is warm and without rashes. Her pupils are equal, round, and reactive to light and accommodation. On funduscopic examination, she is noted to have scattered microaneurysms and several blot hemorrhages, but no exudates. Her throat is clear, without erythema, and her mucous membranes are dry. Her lungs are clear to auscultation and percussion. The heart is regular, without murmurs, rubs, or gallops. The abdomen is tender and firm with guarding, but there is no rebound tenderness. The liver percusses to 8 cm. The spleen is not palpable; bowel sounds are active. She has normal female genitalia, and pelvic examination is within normal limits. Cranial nerves II through X are normal. Knee and ankle reflexes are present and equal bilaterally.

Laboratory Tests. On admission, her glucose is 493 mg/dl, BUN 24 mg/dl, potassium 5.4 mEq/liter, chloride 97 mEq/liter, bicarbonate 12 mEq/liter, and sodium 140 mEq/liter. Her WBC count is 11,800, with 79% neutrophils, 4% bands, 15% lymphocytes, and 2% monocytes. Urine specific gravity is 1.035, pH 6; glucose and ketones are positive. Protein, nitrites, and microscopic examination are negative. Her urine pregnancy test is negative.

ASSESSMENT

Working Diagnosis. Karen is felt on admission to have (1) *diabetic ketoacidosis,* (2) *diabetic retinopathy* (background), (3) *amenorrhea,* and (4) *leukocytosis.*

The diagnosis of diabetic ketoacidosis was based on the elevated serum glucose (>300 mg/dl), a low serum bicarbonate (<17 mEq/liter), and urine ketones that were strongly positive. There was no obvious precipitating cause of the ketoacidosis. Karen did not have a fever, respiratory symptoms, or dysuria. She did have a leukocytosis, which might have been a sign of infection, but ketoacidosis in the absence of infection may cause leukocytosis. Karen was not taking any medications such as steroids that would have caused an increase in insulin need.

Because no obvious cause of ketoacidosis could be found, the history was reviewed with Karen again. The interviewer mentioned that some diabetic women decrease their insulin dose or even sometimes omit their afternoon dose to help lose weight. Karen, then, indicated that she had done this frequently in the past few months. She was quite concerned about getting fat, since she had gained weight rapidly when her insulin dose was increased 8 months previously.

Karen has background diabetic retinopathy, diagnosed by the presence of the microaneurysms (minute aneurysmal dilatations of retinal capillaries) and blot hemorrhages. She has blurred vision related to changes in the lens due to hyperglycemia. This bears no relationship to the retinopathy. She does not have any changes of proliferative retinopathy, which is characterized by the appearance of a network of small vessels that are friable and bleed easily.

Karen also has amenorrhea with a normal pelvic examination and negative pregnancy test. Although she has a history of irregular menses, she has not had more than an interval of 2 months between periods until the past few months. The weight loss is felt to be a factor or the primary cause of the amenorrhea, although a more extensive evaluation is felt to be warranted.

Differential Diagnoses. Metabolic acidosis with an increased anion gap may be due to the *failure of secretion of inorganic acids,* as in renal failure. It also may be due to the presence of *excess organic acids* caused by increased production of lactate; ingestion of alcohol, salicylates, paraldehyde, methanol, and ethylene glycol; or starvation. *Alcoholic ketoacidosis* generally occurs in patients with a long history of excessive alcohol use, a recent history of binge drinking with little or no food intake, and recurrent vomiting. *Lactic acidosis* is suspected when there is evidence of decreased tissue perfusion and no other obvious cause of acidosis. Lactic acidosis is verified by finding a plasma lactate level of >4 m mol/liter.

The most common causes of secondary amenorrhea are physiologic (pregnancy, menopause, or lactation). Since none of these applied to Karen, other causes were considered, such as *drug use.* She is not taking oral contraceptives or phenothiazines, which may cause amenorrhea. She has no clinical signs of *hypothyroidism* and had normal thyroid function tests a few months earlier. *Polycystic ovarian disease* is a possibility, since Karen has irregular menses, but she has no evidence of hirsutism. Karen has no history of galactorrhea, sarcoidosis, or other findings such as a visual-field loss to suggest a *pituitary tumor.* Weight loss seems to be the most likely possibility.

PLAN

Therapeutic. In the emergency room, a presumptive diagnosis of diabetic ketoacidosis was made on the basis of the history and the finding of an elevated fingerstick blood sugar and dipstick urine strongly positive for ketones. Normal saline was started at 300 cc/hour, and regular insulin 10 units was given intravenously prior to the return of the chemistry panel, which confirmed the diagnosis. Potassium was added to the fluids as soon as it was known that her serum potassium level was normal. The scheme for management of diabetic ketoacidosis is shown in Table 20–44, and this plan was followed.

TABLE 20–44. TREATMENT OF DIABETIC KETOACIDOSIS

Insulin⟶Fluids⟶Potassium⟶Close follow-up

INSULIN
10 units regular insulin bolus IV, **then**
　　10 units/hour regular insulin continuously IV
Decrease amount IV insulin when blood sugar < 250 mg/dl
Start NPH insulin before breakfast or supper when CO_2 > 18 mEq/liter and patient is eating
Initial NPH dose = preketoacidosis dose or 0.7 units/kg/day.

FLUID AND ELECTROLYTES
0.9% NaCl IV:
　　300 cc/hour initially
　　Switch to D_5W when blood sugar < 250 mg/dl
KCl—up to 20 mEq/h, begin when serum K normal/low
Glucose:
　　Begin D_5W 150–300 cc/h when blood sugar < 250 mg/dl
　　Discontinue when patient is alert and eating/drinking
Phosphate—indicated if phosphorus < 1 mg/dl
HCO_3—do not give unless pH < 6.9

LABORATORY TESTS
Glucose—hourly (by fingerstick) until < 250 mg/dl; **then** q3–4h until ketoacidosis is resolved
CO_2, K—every 3–4 hours until CO_2 > 18 mEq/dl
Urine ketones—every voided specimen until negative

A CT scan of the sella turcica and a prolactin determination obtained to evaluate amenorrhea were both normal, and Karen was reassured in this regard. Weight loss was felt to be the cause of the amenorrhea, and Karen was encouraged to gain weight slowly. The possibility of an eating disorder was not completely dismissed, and Karen's change in weight over the next few weeks was to be closely monitored.

Patient Education. A diabetes educator was asked to review the basic principles of diabetes care with Karen even though she already knew how to give herself insulin, was aware of the need to give insulin on a regular basis before meals, and also understood the value of monitoring her glucose at home in order to make logical decisions regarding needed changes in her insulin dose. She had a meter to evaluate her own blood sugar levels, and it was documented that her values agreed very closely with those obtained in the laboratory. Karen agreed to monitor her blood sugars before meals and at bedtime and to call if her glucose levels were over 250 mg/dl or if she had insulin reactions prior to her scheduled follow-up visit.

FIRST FOLLOW-UP VISIT

On the first follow-up visit 1 week after hospitalization, Karen expressed concern about having gained 3 lb and was worried that she would "balloon up" like a "blimp" if this pattern continued. She had checked her blood sugar two or three times a day, but she admitted that she just could not check it four times because of her schedule. She commented that her fingers felt like "pin cushions."

A finger stick blood sugar in the office was 142 mg/dl, and the urine was negative for ketones. Karen's blood pressure was on the low side at 92/68, and her heart rate was 64 beats/minute. She brought her record of glucose measurements, with fasting blood sugars ranging between 70 and 174 mg/dl, those before lunch ranging between 160 and 243 mg/dl, before supper between 103 and 155 mg/dl, and at bedtime between 76 and 198 mg/dl.

It was felt that her glucose levels generally had been within a satisfactory range, although the noontime levels were slightly higher than the rest. Therefore, she was advised to increase her regular insulin 2 units before breakfast. When additional insulin was recommended, she again commented on her fear of gaining weight. The rest of the visit was spent with her talking about these concerns. She was reassured that if her weight increased to near her ideal body weight, adjustments could be made in her insulin as well as in her diet to help prevent further weight gain. She agreed that it would be wise for her to gain about 10 lb, but she became very anxious when she was told that her ideal weight would be around 120 to 125 lb based on a height of 65 in and medium frame. It was felt that this needed to be discussed further both with a psychologist and on a return visit. Karen was given an appointment to return in 3 weeks.

Frequent appointments for support were considered to be an important part of Karen's management in order to encourage her to continue taking her insulin on a regular basis and to work with her regarding her eating. The emphasis was on trying to find common ground between her goal for weight control and those of her physician, who felt that the primary goal was to prevent ketoacidosis and hypoglycemic reactions. Rather than insisting on a preset number of calories, it was decided that her weight would be used as the indicator of her caloric need, and Karen felt relieved that a rigid, unbending program was not going to be insisted on.

Karen also voiced some concern that the high blood sugars might cause her to have further changes in her eyes. It was agreed that she would add 2 units of regular insulin before meals if her blood sugars were elevated, but the baseline insulin would not be changed unless she called to discuss this change.

DISCUSSION

Diabetes is a common metabolic disorder that is easy to diagnose because its primary manifestation is hyperglycemia. Table 20–45 outlines the methods used for diagnosis. Eventually, diabetes affects most organ systems, the most significant changes taking place in the eyes, kidneys, blood vessels, and nerves. There is an unresolved controversy as to whether the pathologic changes seen in diabetes are primarily due to abnormally high glucose levels or other factors are more important in the development of long-term complications.

Diabetes can be divided into at least three categories that differ in both etiology and pathogenesis. A distinction is made between "type I diabetes," which is char-

TABLE 20–45. DIAGNOSIS OF DIABETES MELLITUS

1. Random blood sugar > 200 mg/dl with classic symptoms (polyruia, polydipsia, weight loss)
2. Fasting blood sugar > 140 mg/dl × 2
3. Two values on glucose tolerance test > 200 mg/dl by 2 hours
4. During pregnancy: FBS > 105 mg/dl × 2 or after 100 mg oral glucose; two values > 190 mg/dl (1 h), 165 mg/dl (2 h), 145 mg/dl (3 h)

acterized by absolute insulin deficiency and dependence on injected insulin to prevent ketosis and sustain life; "type II diabetes," which is non-ketosis-prone diabetes in which the abnormality is an ineffectiveness of insulin action rather than a total lack of insulin; and "other types of diabetes," previously known as "secondary diabetes," which include cases of pancreatic disease, hormonal disorders, and drug-induced glucose intolerance.

Type I diabetes may begin at any age, although the onset is usually before age 40. These patients present with the classic symptoms of hyperglycemia, including polyuria, polydipsia, and recent weight loss despite increased food intake. There also may be complaints of recent onset of blurred vision, vaginal itching, and fatigue. Signs of recent weight loss and hepatomegaly frequently are the only significant physical findings. Type II non-insulin-dependent diabetes mellitus, on the other hand, frequently is insidious in onset. Many of these patients are obese and have a strong family history of diabetes. They may present with blurred vision, perineal pruritis, impotence, or paresthesias. Rapid weight loss is uncommon. The most frequent physical findings are retinopathy (microaneurysm, hemorrhages, exudates, proliferation of new vessels), neuromuscular changes (absent ankle reflexes, loss of vibratory sensation), and peripheral vascular disease (rubor on dependency, pallor on elevation, absent pedal pulses, gangrene).

The treatment plan for diabetes must be adapted to the needs and lifestyle of each individual in order to minimize the impact of the disease. Listening to the patient's concern is a starting point, and a great deal of flexibility is necessary in planning a treatment regimen that is practical. In the absence of complications, emphasis is placed on achieving the best possible glucose levels with the least possible change in the patient's lifestyle. With these factors in mind, the objectives of therapy in the rough order of their importance are (1) prevention of ketosis, (2) avoidance of severe hypoglycemic reactions, and (3) normal growth and development in children and maintenance of optimal body weight in adults.

The purpose of diabetes education is to encourage each patient to assume primary responsibility in the management of the disease, with the physician being a supportive consultant and supervisor. Patients must understand the basic principles of a healthy diet, the rational use of insulin or oral hypoglycemic agents, the effects of exercising and illness on glucose levels, home monitoring of blood sugar and urine ketone levels, and appropriate foot care. They must be able to recognize the symptoms and appropriate treatment of hyperglycemia and hypoglycemia. Smoking and excessive use of alcohol should be discouraged. These basic principles of diabetic care need to be explained in detail at the time of diagnosis and reviewed regularly thereafter. It is important that the recommended regimen be individually tailored to each patients' specific needs, since this is essential to promote optimal psychologic and social adaption.

The goals of the diabetic diet can best be achieved by making the dietary prescription as simple as possible. Emphasis should be placed on achieving and maintaining normal weight, regular timing of meals, avoidance of refined carbohydrates and saturated fats, and relative consistency of meal portions from day to day. The total caloric intake need not be specified unless weight gain or reduction is desired. To avoid hypoglycemic episodes, the patient with insulin-dependent diabetes normally should eat his or her meals within a half hour of the same time each day. Midafternoon and bedtime snacks also may need to be added. The actual content of the meal is not as important as its timing in patients with widely fluctuating blood sugars. Patients should avoid foods that are high in sugar content, such as candy, cake, cookies, and pie. In addition, foods high in saturated fats, such as red meat, eggs, and fried foods, should be limited, but the emphasis should be directed toward nutritionally balanced meals rather than a restrictive diet.

Oral hypoglycemic agents should be reserved for patients who are not ketosis prone and in whom dietary management fails to control symptoms related to hyperglycemia. The most commonly used oral agents are the sulfonylureas—tolbutamide, chlorpropamide, acetohexamide, tolazamide, glyburide, and glipizide. Since these drugs are metabolized and/or excreted by the liver or kidneys, their use is contraindicated in patients with liver disease, renal impairment, and erratic or inadequate caloric intake. Serious prolonged hypoglycemia can occur with any of these agents and is particularly threatening in the elderly. Other side effects of the sulfonylurea drugs are uncommon but include gastrointestinal symptoms, skin eruptions, cholestatic jaundice, hematologic reactions, and a disulfiram-like reaction. Periodic monitoring of the blood sugar in all patients on oral hypoglycemic agents is necessary in order to modify the dose or switch to insulin treatment when glucose levels cannot be maintained within an acceptable range.

The goal of insulin therapy is to normalize blood sugars with the simplest possible regimen while avoiding the complications of therapy. If normal blood sugar levels cannot be achieved with diet alone, the use of the insulin is indicated in patients who (1) have symptomatic hyperglycemia, (2) develop hyperglycemia due to infection, trauma, surgery, or the use of medications such as steroids, (3) become pregnant, or (4) have ever had ketoacidosis. A reasonable starting dose is a single NPH dose before breakfast—0.5 units per kilogram of body weight for children or 20 to 30 units for adults. Since most patients with type I diabetes will require at least two injections daily, some physicians initiate therapy with divided doses to avoid having patients feel that they

are getting worse if a second dose is added later. Except in adolescents and during pregnancy, the total insulin requirement rarely exceeds 1 unit/kg per day. Doses in excess of this amount may actually lead to wider glucose fluctuations in type I diabetic patients and steady gain in weight in those with type II diabetes.

The goal is to keep fasting blood sugar levels below 140 mg/dl and postprandial levels below 200 mg/dl while avoiding hypoglycemia. Changes in the doses of intermediate-acting insulin generally are not made more than once or twice weekly and then in increments of about 10%. The major objective is to prevent hyperglycemia from occurring rather than to treat an already elevated blood sugar level. Adding or subtracting 2 to 4 units of regular insulin before meals often is beneficial in modifying the effect of stress and dietary changes on glucose levels. A plan for modifying insulin doses may be found in Table 20–46.

Hypoglycemia is a major complication of treatment with insulin, as well as with oral hypoglycemic agents. The most common causes of hypoglycemia are omission or delay of meals and unusually heavy exercise; other common causes are chronic insulin overdose and errors in measuring injected insulin. Insulin-dependent diabetic patients should be instructed always to have immediate access to sugar in some form and wear a bracelet or necklace identifying them as having diabetes. They should be taught the symptoms of hypoglycemia and instructed to eat immediately if there is any possibility that they may be having an insulin reaction. The patient's family and friends also should be instructed regarding the symptoms that may occur during hypoglycemia, such as sweating, tremulousness, abnormal behavior, and impaired thinking.

Blood sugar testing methods applicable to home use now offer the most accurate means of monitoring diabetic control. A number of reflectance meters for home glucose monitoring are available for less than $150 and are quite accurate when proper technique is used. Insulin-treated diabetic patients should be encouraged to measure and record their blood sugar levels several times per week and more frequently during times of stress, such as during an illness or a change in daily routine.

Glycohemoglobin, also called "hemoglobin A1C" and "glycosylated hemoglobin," is used as a measure of long-term control. The test is most valuable in insulin-dependent patients who have wide daily changes in glucose levels.

The physician's records should include periodic measurement of weight, blood pressure, insulin dose, other medications taken, number and percent of high and low blood home glucose values reported, frequency and timing of hypoglycemic reactions as well as office glucose results, dipstick urine protein measurements, and glycohemoglobin levels. Patients who are monitoring their own blood sugar at home should bring their instrument to the office at each visit in order to check their meter results against those obtained in the physician's office. Also, periodic recording of the funduscopic examination, peripheral pulses, and vibratory sensation in

TABLE 20–46. GUIDELINES FOR INSULIN USE

TIME OF HYPERGLYCEMIA	ONE DOSE DAILY, MORNING	TWO DOSES DAILY, MORNING AND EVENING
Fasting	Increase morning NPH* **Alternatives** 1. Split dose to b.i.d. 2. Change to ultralente	Increase evening NPH
Between breakfast and lunch	Increase morning regular	Increase morning regular
Between lunch and supper	Increase NPH	Increase morning NPH or add regular before lunch
After supper or at bedtime	Increase dose of NPH **Alternative** Add regular before supper	Increase regular in evening

*May use lente instead of NPH.

Note: Average dose 0.7 units/kg/day; type I: two or more doses/day; type II: one or more doses/day. Adolescents and pregnant women may need higher insulin doses. Regulate insulin dose based on pattern of glucose levels; alter by 10% every 3 to 4 days for outpatients. Decrease insulin dose for repeated or unexplained hypoglycemia.

lower extremities should be made. Patients may need to be seen weekly or biweekly until blood sugar levels are stable, and then the intervals between visits may be extended. Periodic creatinine levels should be determined in those who have had diabetes for more than 10 years because of the increased frequency of renal impairment in these patients.

SUGGESTED READING

American Diabetes Association. Physician's Guide to Insulin-Dependent (Type I) Diabetes: Diagnosis and Treatment. American Diabetes Association, Inc., 1988.

Baker C, McFarland KF. Endocrinology. In Rakel RE (ed.): Textbook of Family Practice, 4th ed. Philadelphia, W. B. Saunders, 1990, pp. 1149–1163, 1194–1195.

McFarland KF. Diabetes mellitus type I. In Taylor RE (ed.): Difficult Medical Management. Philadephia, W. B. Saunders, 1990, p. 209.

QUESTIONS

1. Two common serious complications of insulin-dependent diabetes mellitus are hypoglycemia and diabetic ketoacidosis. Match the signs and symptoms listed below with the complication they describe.
   a. Sweating
   b. Hunger
   c. Tremors
   d. Rapid onset of weakness
   e. Dehydration
      (1) Diabetic ketoacidosis
      (2) Hypoglycemia

2. The classic patient with type I diabetes is
   a. Hyperinsulinemic.
   b. Not ketosis prone.
   c. Insulin dependent for survival.
   d. Under 40 years old.
   e. 25% or more overweight.

3. New-onset symptomatic insulin-dependent diabetes patients with *no* ketoacidosis present with
   a. Polydipsia.
   b. Polyuria.
   c. Low CO_2.
   d. Blood sugar above 200 mg/dl.
   e. Tachypnea.

4. The classic patient with type I diabetes is
   a. Hyperinsulinemic.
   b. Not ketosis prone.
   c. Insulin dependent for survival.
   d. Under 40 years old.
   e. 25% or more overweight.

Answers appear on page 451.

Intermittent Tachycardia

KAY F. McFARLAND and JAN C. UPDIKE

INITIAL VISIT

SUBJECTIVE

Patient Identification and Presenting Problem. Mary N., a 45-year-old teacher, was seen for evaluation of intermittent tachycardia. At first she attributed the episodes of fast heart beat to stress, but when the palpitations continued into the summer months, she became concerned. During the past 2 months she also has had extreme mood variability, tremulousness, difficulty getting to sleep, and a 10-lb weight loss despite an increased appetite. She feels warm most of the time and wonders if she is having postmenopausal hot flashes. She has no history of heart disease.

Past Medical History. Mary's only hospitalizations were for delivery of her three children, ages 14, 16, and 19. She developed a rash after receiving penicillin as a teenager.

Family History. Mary's mother and father, ages 69 and 66, are living and well. She has three brothers, one of whom has a seizure disorder.

Health Habits. Mary has no history of tobacco use. She drinks alcohol socially, averaging less than two drinks per week. Mary does little vigorous exercise, but she does walk three to five times per week about 2 miles at a time.

Social History. Mary taught high school algebra for several years before her children were born and returned to teaching about 7 years ago. She has been married 23 years and feels that she has a strong marriage. Her primary stress is from discipline problems at school.

Review of Systems. Mary has had burning, tearing, and itching of her eyes for several weeks. She also has noticed that her eyes are prominent in a recent family photograph. She has not had any chest pain but has had shortness of breath intermittently for several weeks. The only other positive finding on the review of systems is increased fatigue, especially late in the day.

OBJECTIVE

Physical Examination. On physical examination, Mary's blood pressure is 150/70; her heart rate is 120; her height is 63 in; and her weight is 115 lb. She appears restless, moves constantly, and her speech is rapid. On eye examination her pupils are equal, round, and react to light. Extraocular movements are normal. She also has bilateral lid retraction and lid lag. Funduscopic examination is normal. She has bilateral proptosis, 17 mm on the right and 18 mm on the left. Her thyroid is diffusely enlarged and estimated to be two to three times

normal size. Her heart rate is regular, with a grade II scratchy systolic murmur heard in the pulmonic area. Her skin is fine, warm, and moist. Her liver is percussed to 8 cm.; the spleen is not palpable. Bowel sounds are normal. There are small inguinal nodes palpable bilaterally. Pelvic examination is normal. Knee and ankle reflexes are brisk bilaterally.

Laboratory Tests. The initial dipstick urine is negative. No other laboratory tests were available when she was first seen.

ASSESSMENT

Diagnoses

1. *Tachycardia secondary to Graves' disease with hyperthyroidism.* Painless thyroiditis, which frequently occurs postpartum, also would be a consideration, since it is associated with a diffuse goiter, but not with eye signs. A multinodular goiter may cause hyperthyroidism and needs to be considered, but by examination the gland is diffuse, which is evidence enough to exclude this. Finally, it was considered that Mary could be taking exogenous thyroid medication to cause the symptoms, but this seemed unlikely, since she has never been on any such medication in the past. The presence of a diffuse goiter and exophthalmos with the symptoms of hyperthyroidism at age 45 makes Graves' disease the most likely possibility.
2. *Graves' ophthalmopathy.*
3. *History of penicillin allergy.*

PLAN

Diagnostic. T_4, T_3 uptake, free thyroxine index (FTI), T_3 RIA, CBC, and liver enzymes were ordered.

Therapeutic. Mary was started on a beta-blocker, propranolol 20 mg b.i.d. The day after Mary was seen, the following test results were reported: T_4 21 μg/dl, T_3 uptake 36%, WBC 5000, with 61% neutrophils, 35% lymphocytes, 2% monocytes, and 2% eosinophils. Mary was started on propylthiouracil (PTU) 150 mg b.i.d., and the side effects of the medication were discussed, including possible development of rash, sore throat, fever, fever blisters, or muscle aches. Mary was instructed to stop the PTU and call if any of these symptoms occurred.

FIRST FOLLOW-UP VISIT

SUBJECTIVE

Mary returned for her first follow-up visit 2 weeks later. After starting the beta-blocker, she had not had any more episodes of the tachycardia and had felt well until a couple of days before her return. Her only specific complaint was related to a sore throat that she had developed that morning. On examination, her throat appeared normal.

OBJECTIVE

Because of the sore throat, a repeat CBC count was ordered, and Mary was told to omit the propylthiouracil that night and the next morning until the laboratory test results were known. Later that afternoon her WBC count was found to be 3100, with 30% neutrophils, 10% monocytes, 8% eosinophils, and 52% lymphocytes. It was felt that Mary had granulocytopenia from the PTU. Mary was called and told to discard the PTU and never to take the medication again. She was seen the next day and started on lithium carbonate 300 mg b.i.d. Future treatment with radioactive iodine was discussed. Mary was warned about being around anyone with an infectious disease. A repeat WBC count was ordered.

DISCUSSION

Graves' disease is the most common cause of hyperthyroidism in the third and fourth decades of life. The diagnosis is based on finding a diffuse goiter with hyperthyroidism and either proptosis or pretibial myxedema. However, classic eye signs are present in only 50% of patients, and pretibial myxedema is rare. In the absence of eye signs or pretibial myxedema, the diagnosis is based on finding hyperthyroidism in patients with a diffuse goiter and an elevated radioactive iodine uptake. Other causes of hyperthyroidism are listed in Table 20–47.

The gland in Graves' disease is normal to soft in consistency and symmetrically enlarged, usually two to four times normal in size. The eye signs are characterized by lid lag, stare (widened pupil fissure), injection of the conjunctiva, and periorbital edema. With more advanced disease, ophthalmoplegia (extraocular muscle weakness) producing diplopia may occur. The ophthalmopathy and hyperthyroidism of Graves' disease may follow entirely independent courses.

Many patients with hyperthyroidism present with an

TABLE 20–47. ETIOLOGY OF HYPERTHYROIDISM

DISORDER	CONDITION OF GLAND
Graves' disease	Diffusely enlarged
Toxic multinodular	Nodular enlargement
Hyperfunctioning adenoma	Solitary nodule
Subacute thyroiditis	Tender enlargement
Autoimmune thyroiditis	Normal size or enlarged
Exogenous thyroid	Normal or small
Rare causes:	
Radiation thyroiditis	Normal
Thyroid carcinoma	Solitary nodule
Excessive TSH stimulation	Diffusely enlarged
Excessive iodine intake	Normal or enlarged
Struma ovarii	Normal or small
Trophoblastic disease	Normal or enlarged

TABLE 20–48. SIGNS AND SYMPTOMS OF HYPERTHYROIDISM*

SUBJECTIVE FINDINGS	OBJECTIVE FINDINGS
Nervousness	Goiter
Heat intolerance	Tachycardia
Palpitation	Tremor
Dyspnea	Hyperkinesis
Fatigue/weakness	Warm, moist hands
Weight loss	Thyroid bruit
Eye symptoms	Lid lag

*In relative order of frequency.

unmistakable constellation of symptoms, such as fullness in the throat, heat intolerance, increased sweating, and weight loss despite a good appetite. Other common complaints include tremulousness, insomnia, headache, palpitations, and eye symptoms of itching, burning, and tearing. Careful questioning may reveal other symptoms, such as emotional lability, dyspnea on exertion, or muscle weakness. For example, some patients may have difficulty walking up stairs and use a handrail to pull themselves up because of the weakness of the quadraceps muscles. Their inability to concentrate and lability in mood may negatively effect their job performance and interpersonal relationships and may interfere with their taking medications regularly. The symptoms and signs associated with hyperthyroidism are listed in relative order of frequency in Table 20–48.

The most characteristic physical findings of hyperthyroidism are thyroid enlargement and tachycardia. A tremor may be striking or detectable only when the hands are outstretched. Lid lag and retraction, with a crescent of sclera visible over the iris, may be present in patients with hyperthyroidism of any etiology, whereas the classic eye signs of Graves' disease—periorbital edema, exophthalmos, conjunctivitis with tearing, and ocular muscle palsies—may occur with or without hyperthyroidism. The skin has a silky quality, and the hair is fine and brittle. Thinning of the hair, especially in the temporal regions, is common. Typical nail changes involve separation of the distal nail from its bed, making it difficult to keep the fingernails clean. The change, called "onycholysis" or "plummer's nails," is most commonly found on the fourth digit. The palms may be red, warm, and moist. Cardiac manifestations include a third heart sound, edema, and atrial fibrillation. As a result of the elevated cardiac output, the arterial pulses are bounding, and the difference between the systolic and diastolic blood pressures may be greater than 70 mmHg. A fine tremor may be striking. Atrial fibrillation and congestive heart failure are more commonly seen in older patients, in contrast with mood lability and hyperkinesis in younger patients.

T_4 and T_3 uptake and the free thyroxine index may be the only tests needed in most cases to establish the diagnosis of hyperthyroidism. If the clinical impression is not substantiated by these tests, they may be repeated and a serum T_3 by radioimmunoassay may be ordered. About 10% of cases of hyperthyroidism are associated with T_3 toxicosis and a T_4 at the upper level of normal. Thyroid-stimulating hormone (TSH) measured by ultrasensitive measures also may be used to confirm the diagnosis and now is being used more frequently as a screening test for both hypothyroidism and hyperthyroidism. The radioactive iodine uptake and thyroglobulin level may be helpful at times in differentiating Graves' disease from painless thyroiditis and excess thyroid hormone administration. In hyperthyroidism associated with painless thyroiditis and with exogenous thyroid hormone administration, the ^{123}I uptake is suppressed, whereas the uptake is high in Graves' disease. Serum thyroglobulin is decreased with exogenous thyroid hormone administration and high in other forms of hyperthyroidism.

Antithyroid drugs, ^{131}I ablation, and subtotal thyroidectomy are all effective in treating the hyperthyroidism due to Graves' disease. The chief advantage of antithyroid drug therapy is that it does not cause permanent thyroid damage and some patients experience permanent remission of hyperthyroidism following several months of treatment. As many as 10% of patients, however, have reactions to the medication or require some other form of therapy.

Propylthiouracil and methimazole are the two most widely used drugs that inhibit thyroid hormone synthesis. The choice between these drugs is largely a matter of individual choice. Propylthiouracil inhibits extrathyroidal T_4 conversion to T_3 and because of this action may be preferred when a rapid response to therapy is desired. Methimazole, on the other hand, has the advantage of coming in two dosage strengths and may be given once daily, whereas propylthiouracil comes in only one strength and is given twice daily. Methimazole requires fewer tablets and is taken less frequently than PTU, which may lead to better patient compliance.

The usual beginning dose of propylthiouracil is 150 to 200 mg b.i.d.; the beginning dose for methimazole is 30 mg daily. If there is an adverse reaction to an antithyroid drug, or if the patient finds that taking the medication on a regular basis is unacceptable, the drug should be stopped and another treatment modality chosen. Clinical improvement may be evident in 1 or 2 weeks, and usually the patient becomes euthyroid between 2 and 3 months after initiation of therapy. If the antithyroid drugs fail to control the hyperthyroidism, one should suspect inadequate dose or noncompliance. Once the patient is euthyroid, the dose of the antithyroid medication may be decreased by a third every couple of months as long as the hyperthyroidism is controlled. There is no clear indication how long the drug should be continued after the patient has been rendered completely euthyroid, but commonly, the drugs are continued for 6 months to a year.

Side effects of the antithyroid drugs are not uncommon, but fortunately, most are mild and reversible. Serious reactions include agranulocytosis, thrombocytopenia, anemia, hepatitis, arthritis, and fever. Usually, a WBC and liver enzymes are obtained at the start of therapy. Continued periodic monitoring of the WBC count and liver function is not helpful, because adverse reactions may occur rapidly, even when these tests are normal. Therefore, the tests are repeated only if the patient develops symptoms or signs suggestive of a toxic reaction. Patients should be instructed to contact their physician if they develop any new symptoms, particularly fever or sores on their lips or in their mouth, while on these drugs. When a severe reaction occurs, the medication should be stopped. It is usually wise to give ^{131}I rather than to change to another antithyroid drug.

Inorganic iodine is rapidly effective in controlling hyperthyroidism, for it not only inhibits thyroid hormone synthesis but also prevents the release of thyroid hormone from the gland. Very small doses are needed, and two drops of saturated solution of potassium iodine mixed in juice once daily is more than adequate, except during "thyroid storm," when a larger dose is given.

Lithium carbonate acts like iodine, inhibiting thyroid synthesis and release, but because of its narrow therapeutic range, it should not be used routinely. However, if ^{131}I therapy is anticipated in a patient with hyperthyroidism and the patient has a reaction to the other antithyroid drugs, lithium is a good choice until the patient becomes euthyroid.

The most common use of iodine is a 7- to 10-day course prior to surgery to decrease the vascularity of the gland and in the treatment of thyroid storm. Iodine should not be used as a sole form of therapy for hyperthyroidism, however, because a week or two after the initiation of therapy with iodine alone there may be escape from the beneficial effects of the medication. This is usually not true after ^{131}I therapy, when the thyroid is very sensitive to the effects of iodine. Iodine, however, should not be given for at least 3 days after ^{131}I therapy to ensure maximum effect of the radioactive isotope.

Beta-blockers have been used widely in the treatment of hyperthyroidism and are effective in reducing associated tachycardia, palpitations, heat intolerance, and nervousness. The drugs do not normalize metabolic rate and should not be used alone, except in cases of transient hyperthyroidism due to autoimmune thyroiditis. Beta-blockers are contraindicated in patients with asthma and normally should not be used in those with congestive heart failure.

The major advantage of ^{131}I therapy is that it is simple and effective. Antithyroid therapy often is used prior to and following ^{131}I treatment in severely symptomatic patients, because weeks may elapse before the patient becomes euthyroid after treatment with the isotope. ^{131}I permanently damages the thyroid, eventually causing hypothyroidism in most cases. Past concerns regarding a high risk of carcinoma of the thyroid, leukemia, or genetic damage to the offspring of women treated with ^{131}I in the childbearing years has not been substantiated by more than 30 years of follow-up of treated patients. The amount of radiation to the ovaries from a therapeutic dose of ^{131}I is about the same or less than the radiation associated with an intravenous pyelogram or barium enema.

Allergy to iodine does not preclude the use of ^{131}I because the amount of iodine used is very small. Pregnancy, however, is an absolute contraindication to ^{131}I therapy. Therefore, all women in the reproductive age group should be questioned about pregnancy and/or a pregnancy test should be done prior to ^{131}I therapy.

The risk and expense of subtotal thyroidectomy are greater than those of ^{131}I and antithyroid drugs, and this method generally should be reserved for those patients who are noncompliant, for those in whom other methods are unacceptable, and for children. Surgery is also suitable for patients who insist on a rapid cure, because there is a lag of several weeks between treatment with ^{131}I and restoration of the euthyroid state. If hyperthyroidism recurs after surgery, ^{131}I should be recommended because the incidence of complications after a second operation is greatly increased. Subtotal thyroidectomy may be the treatment of choice in patients with very large multinodular goiters, particularly those whose iodine uptake is low. The advantage of surgery is that it is a definitive form of therapy that renders a patient euthyroid quickly. On the other hand, possible adverse effects are numerous, including the risk of general anesthesia, injury to the recurrent laryngeal nerve with vocal cord paralysis, and permanent hypothyroidism or hypoparathyroidism.

Patients who undergo thyroidectomy should first be rendered euthyroid with antithyroid medications and should receive a 7- to 10-day course of iodine preoperatively. In addition to the patients who are rendered hypothyroid immediately following surgery, 1% to 2% will become hypothyroid each succeeding year and will require thyroid replacement therapy.

"Thyroid storm," a severe form of hyperthyroidism, is life-threatening and requires aggressive management even prior to confirmation of the diagnosis by thyroid function tests. The condition is usually precipitated by trauma or medical illness in a patient who has had hyperthyroidism for some time. It may occur spontaneously in those who have discontinued antithyroid medication. The most common sign is the presence of fever and tachycardia in a patient with known hyperthyroidism. Other striking features include marked agitation, mental confusion even to the point of coma, jaundice, and psychosis.

Treatment should begin with propylthiouracil 200 mg every 4 hours. If the patient is unable to swallow the tablets, they may be crushed and put down a nasogastric tube; a parenteral form of the medication is not available. Iodine is subsequently given, preferably orally, but intravenously if necessary. Five drops of saturated solution of potassium iodine is given orally four times daily. Propranolol 20 to 40 mg every 4 hours also may be given orally.

SUGGESTED READING

Baker C, McFarland KF. Endocrinology. In Rakel RE (ed.): Textbook of Family Practice, 4th ed. Philadelphia, W. B. Saunders, 1990, pp. 1163–1172.

Hashizume K, Ichikawa K, Sakurai A, et al. Administration of thyroxine in treated Graves' disease. N Engl J Med 1991; 324(14):947–953.

McFarland KF, Saleeby G. Graves' disease: Manifestations and therapeutic options. Postgrad Med 1988; 83:275–282.

QUESTIONS

1. ^{131}I is widely prescribed as definitive therapy for hyperthyroidism. Absolute contraindications for its use are
   a. Pregnancy.
   b. Atrial fibrillation.
   c. Desire for future pregnancy.
   d. Diabetes mellitus.

2. What clinical signs help distinguish Graves' disease from other causes of hyperthyroidism? One or more of these must be present in addition to the hyperthyroid state to establish the diagnosis.
   a. Pretibial myxedema
   b. Fine tremors
   c. Proptosis and ophthalmoplegia
   d. Eye stare and lid lag
   e. Weight loss
   f. Heat intolerance (sweating)

3. Elevated levels of all the following support the diagnosis of Graves' disease except
   a. Ultrasensitive TSH.
   b. Free T_4 index (FTI).
   c. Serum free T_4.
   d. T_3 RIA.
   e. ^{131}I uptake.

4. Match the potential complications of drug therapy with the drug most likely responsible.
   a. Agranulocytosis
   b. Congestive heart failure
   c. Asthma
   d. Hepatitis
   e. Nephrotoxicity
      (1) Lithium
      (2) Propranolol
      (3) Propylthiouracil

5. Which test may be used to differentiate Graves' disease from thyroiditis and the ingestion of excess exogenous thyroid hormone?
   a. Free T_4 index
   b. Ultrasensitive TSH
   c. RAIU (thyroid radioiodide uptake)
   d. Serum free T_4
   e. Thyroglobulin level

Answers appear on page 451.

Nutritional Problems in the Elderly

PATRICK J. FAHEY and CHARLETTE GALLAGHER-ALLRED

INITIAL VISIT

SUBJECTIVE

Patient Identification and Presenting Problem. Mrs. A. is a 76-year-old Caucasian woman who has suffered a stroke recently and is being admitted to a nursing home temporarily for rehabilitation. She has lost weight and has poor nutritional intake. For many years she has been a pillar in school and church activities in a rural community.

Present Illness. Mrs. A. is admitted to the local nursing home following a cerebrovascular accident 2 weeks ago that caused her to be hospitalized. This event has left her with some residual right-sided weakness but no aphasia. She has decreased strength of both the upper and lower extremities on the right side and needs help with eating, walking, and getting out of a chair. At this time she is unable to care for herself at home or to be cared for by her 84-year-old husband who is in frail health. She expresses a sense of futility and anger at her present condition, and she is admitted to the nursing home for comprehensive rehabilitation therapy before discharge to home.

In obtaining her gastrointestinal and nutritional history, Mrs. A. complains of abdominal pain with several loose bowel movements throughout the day, starting shortly before her father's death. She is frequently nauseated and has occasional vomiting. Her dentures do not fit properly since she has lost weight, and she has trouble chewing some foods. She refuses to be evaluated for new dentures.

Past Medical History. Mrs. A. has had Parkinson's disease for a few years. The disease process has actually been fairly stable; she takes one Sinemet 25-100 tablet three times daily and has taken hydrochlorothiazide 25 mg daily for hypertension for years. She denies any drug allergies or major operations. She denies diabetes, cancer, and known heart disease.

Family History. Mrs. A.'s mother died of arteriosclerotic heart disease at age 64, and her father died 2 months ago of Alzheimer's disease at the age of 96. Mrs. A. and her husband, with the help of a hired homemaker, cared for Mrs. A.'s father in their home until his death. Mrs. A. has no brothers or sisters. She and her husband have one daughter who does not live nearby and is not involved in the care of her mother or father.

Health Habits. Mrs. A. denies smoking cigarettes or abusing alcohol. She is socially active and has engaged in regular physical exercise. Until recent months, she had eaten three well-balanced meals daily.

Social History. Mrs. A. is a retired third-grade school teacher and an artist who has many sculptured art objects displayed locally. While caring for her father, Mrs. A. continued to be involved in the school's tutoring program. Her church work is extensive, and she and her husband are large financial contributors to the maintenance of their local church. Mr. A. is a successful retired farmer.

Review of Systems. Mrs. A. experienced a significant change in appetite, weight, energy, and sleep patterns during the last 4 months of her father's life, which she attributes to her compulsion to care for her father and her dedication to school and church activities. Following her father's death, however, Mrs. A. experienced a general decline in her mood and seemed to enjoy her volunteer work less.

OBJECTIVE

Physical Examination. Mrs. A.'s blood pressure is elevated at 160/100. She is afebrile, and her pulse is regular, rate 72. Respirations are normal. Her weight upon admission to the nursing home is 115 lb, and her height is 66 in. Her usual adult weight is 140 to 145 lb. *Anthropometric measures:* Height is 95th percentile, triceps skinfold thickness is 40th percentile, and midarm muscle circumference is only 20th percentile.

Mrs. A. appears thin, pale, and weak, and her affect is nonexpressive, very different from the bounciness that is characteristic of Mrs. A. Her head, neck, and cardiorespiratory systems are normal. She has significant parkinsonian tremors and some upper and lower extremity weakness on the right side but no major problem with head and body positioning. She has no drooling and does not choke or cough when eating. When attempting to feed herself, however, she spills a large amount of food, becomes agitated, and frequently will not allow nursing assistance in feeding. She exhibits cogwheeling and a shuffling gate, and she needs assistance in walking due primarily to the weak right leg.

Laboratory Tests. Hemoglobin 12.7 gm/dl, hematocrit 37.5%, albumin 3.5 gm/dl, fasting glucose 120 mg/dl, and cholesterol 160 mg/dl; normal liver and renal function tests; urine analysis normal.

ASSESSMENT

Working Diagnoses

1. *Right-sided hemiparesis,* secondary to a recent *cerebrovascular accident,* recovering gradually.
2. *Significant recent weight loss.* Perhaps this is secondary to poor nutrient intake.

Mrs. A.'s usual weight (140–145 lb) is a reasonable

and desirable weight for Mrs. A. [To calculate reasonable body weight for a medium-frame adult female, use the Hamwi formula for women: 100 lb for the first 5 ft in height and add 5 lb for each inch over 5 ft, putting the resulting figure in a range of plus or minus 10%; therefore, for Mrs. A. at 5 ft 6 in, her reasonable body weight is $100 + (5 \times 6) = 130 \pm 13$ pounds.] Mrs. A.'s weight loss over the past 6 months of 20 to 25 lb represents a weight loss of 16%, which places her at risk for several nutrition-related disorders, including pressure sores, increased infections, and other complications. A typical dietary history elicited by the home's registered dietitian from Mrs. A. and her husband shows approximately 1100 kcal/day intake, with 10% from one alcoholic beverage consumed each evening. Mrs. A. consumes a high-fiber diet consisting of many home-grown vegetables and fruits; her typical breakfast has included bran and prune juice to "keep regular." She rarely experiences hunger between meals. Energy requirements for weight maintenance and weight gain are calculated using the Harris–Benedict equation with adjustment for mobility as follows:

Energy needs for weight maintenance for female
$$= [655 + (9.56 \times \text{weight}) + (1.85 \times \text{height})$$
$$- (4.68 \times \text{age})] \times \text{activity factor}$$
where weight $= 115$ lb $\div 2.2$ lb/kg $= 52.3$ kg
      height $= 66$ in $\times 2.54$ cm/in $= 167.6$ cm
      age $= 76$ years

Activity factor for ambulatory resident $= 1.3$
$$655 + 500 + 310 - 356 = 1109 \times 1.3$$
$$= 1442 \text{ kcal/day}$$

Energy needs for weight gain
(of 1 lb/week)
    $1442 + 500$ extra kcal/day $= 1950$ kcal/day

3. *Depression.* Reasons for depression include apathy over her apparent losses caused by her stroke, decreased independence, decreased mobility, and concern for her future. Mrs. A. is likely experiencing significant grief following the death of her father, which may enhance her depression.

Depression may be hard to identify and may be overlooked because of the masked facies with Parkinson's disease. Such patients may not be sad but will appear sad because of their inability to smile; on the other hand, they may be sad and the face may not reflect that appearance. Depression is supported by the fact that Mrs. A. speaks only when spoken to, despite her lack of aphasia.

4. *Abdominal pain with diarrhea and nausea.* A high probability for the cause here is irritable bowel syndrome, probably the result of stress, anxiety, depression, and unresolved grief. A high-fiber diet may be a contributor to frequent stools.

5. *Hypertension, chronic.* Risk factor for stroke.

6. *Feeding difficulties* caused in part by her neurologic problems, denture problems, and abdominal problems.

7. *Parkinson's disease.*

Differential Diagnoses

1. *Right-sided hemiparesis secondary to cerebrovascular accident.* Unilateral hemiparesis is confirmed; there is thus a fairly limited differential diagnosis. However, it would be important to have distinguished during the hospitalization the differential diagnoses as to the etiology of the cerebrovascular accident, such as ruling out a brain tumor and evaluating for cerebrovascular hemorrhage.

2. *Significant recent weight loss.* Considerations besides a poor nutrient intake include *hyperthyroidism* and *malignancy.* Hyperthyroidism would be less likely with a normal pulse rate and the fact that the patient is so withdrawn, although in older patients there is an entity called "apathetic hyperthyroidism," which could be considered. However, during Mrs. A.'s recent hospitalization, screening evaluations for a major malignancy such as a chest x-ray and abdominal and gynecologic examination did not reveal a malignancy that would tend to be more obvious by the time such a weight loss would be so profound. Consideration might be given to a pancreatic cancer, which can cause fairly significant weight loss before being discovered.

3. *Depression.* Other considerations besides depression include *hypothyroidism* and *anxiety disorder.* Hypothyroidism is unlikely due to the fact that Mrs. A. has actually lost a lot of weight, which would be more characteristic of hyperthyroidism, and the fact that Mrs. A. has been suffering from increased loose bowel movements, which is more characteristic of hyperthyroidism than hypothyroidism. Although Mrs. A. may have anxiety as a component of her depression, the total passivity that she expresses would be more consistent with a depressive disorder. Also, her profound lack of nutritional intake would be more consistent with a major depressive disorder than for the usual anxiety syndrome.

4. *Abdominal pain with diarrhea and nausea.* Other considerations besides irritable bowel syndrome include the following:

    a. *Pancreatic carcinoma.* As noted above, an undiagnosed pancreatic carcinoma can cause weight loss. In addition, it can cause diarrhea and nausea.

    b. *Carcinoma of the stomach or carcinoma of the colon.*

    c. *Lactose intolerance,* which may lead to diarrhea and abdominal discomfort.

    d. A *malabsorption syndrome,* which would lead to diarrhea and possibly abdominal pain. This would be unlikely, since the bowel movements would have such specific characteristics as being extremely foul-smelling if there were a problem with fat malabsorption, and this was not noted. The high amount of fiber intake may be worsening the loose stools, since fiber is nonabsorbed complex carbohydrate.

    e. *Diarrhea* and *cramping.* Perhaps the abdominal pain is secondary to this diarrhea, and the diarrhea itself is secondary to a metabolic problem such as *hyperthyroidism.*

    f. *Parasitic infection* giving pain, diarrhea, and weight loss. *Giardia* would be such an example; however, this kind of infection would be less likely without some sort of travel history or other exposure to such a disorder.

    5. *Hypertension, chronic.* The presence of this disorder is certainly a risk factor for stroke. Once the diagnosis is well established, there is little need to go through the differential diagnoses.

    6. *Feeding difficulties* have been observed by the staff. In terms of the possible etiology of Mrs. A.'s feeding difficulty, it is most likely related to her neurologic and denture problems.

    7. *Parkinson's disease.* The differential diagnosis does not need elaboration due to her classic features.

PLAN

Diagnostic

    1. Evaluate depression. Encourage Mrs. A. to discuss her personal losses, including the death of father, the poor health of her husband, and her own mortality and morbidity from recent stroke. Consult a psychologist or psychiatrist as needed. Order electrolytes, calcium, and TSH determinations, since depression may be secondary to a metabolic disorder.

    2. GI workup to rule out cancer as a cause of weight loss and abdominal problems. Could include digoxin levels, upper GI series, barium enema, possible CT scan, or endoscopies. Other tests for loose stools and weight loss include stool tests for ova and parasites, TSH determination to rule out hyperthyroidism (already ordered above), and a malabsorption screening test.

Dietary

    1. Stop weight loss within the first 2 weeks of admission to the nursing home. Place the patient on a no-added-salt diet (4-gm sodium) for hypertension and modify the texture of foods as appropriate. Provide her with her food preferences, and substitute menu items as needed based on her individual tolerances and preferences. If the salt restriction causes Mrs. A. to not enjoy her meals and therefore to eat less than is needed to promote weight gain, consider liberalizing the salt restriction in order to increase calorie consumption.

    2. Promote weight gain of 1 lb per week thereafter by encouraging foods high in caloric content. If Mrs. A. does not consume greater than 75% of her meals, request a commercial medical nutritional supplement with each meal. If weight gain does not occur, consider tube feedings as appropriate.

    3. The feeding goal for Mrs. A. is to self-feed with dignity. Encourage her to eat her meals where, when, and with whom she desires. Provide feeding devises as necessary, such as a hand brace, plate guard or grip, etc.

    4. Provide adequate fluid to prevent dehydration with frequent loose stools.

Nursing

    1. Prevent pressure sores with appropriate mattresses, skin care, changes of her position in the bed, and physical mobility.

    2. Monitor for drooling, cheeking, trouble swallowing, and speech dysfunction, which places her at risk for aspiration; maintain head and body position to prevent swallowing problems.

    3. Set up dental consult.

Physical Therapy

    1. Improve muscle strength with range-of-motion activities; lift self out of chair several times hourly to prevent pressure sores.

    2. Walking between parallel bars to increase activity, restore dignity, and prevent pressure sores.

Patient Education

    1. Discuss the importance of regaining lost weight and attaining her usual, reasonable weight. Teach Mrs. A. how to increase caloric intake (see Table 20–49).

    2. Instruct Mrs. A. on the importance of a mild salt restriction to augment antihypertensive medications and the need to avoid dehydration and hypokalemia with diuretic use. Instruct her to include two foods high in potassium at each meal (all fruits and vegetables are high in potassium).

    3. Discuss techniques to aid swallowing and prevent choking and aspiration secondary to stroke.

    4. Discuss the possible relationship between a high-fiber intake and frequent loose stools. Instruct Mrs. A. on the need to consume plenty of fluids to prevent dehydration with loose stools; with diarrhea, daily fluid needs are 30 to 40 cc/kg body weight at this point. Instruct Mrs. A. on foods high in water-soluble fiber (fruits, legumes, oats, barley) that may alleviate watery diarrhea. (Water-insoluble fiber foods include vegetables and whole-grain breads and cereals, and these, on the other hand, are efficacious in preventing/treating constipation.)

TABLE 20–49. SUGGESTIONS FOR INCREASING CALORIE INTAKE

Increase portion sizes
Eat more frequently, especially before bedtime
Choose high-calorie foods such as peanut butter, cream cheese, nuts, cheese cake, ice cream, milkshakes, eggnog, pie, cake, cookies, fudge, salad dressings
Choose higher-fat dairy products
Fortify casseroles, soups, or meat dishes with cheese, nonfat dry milk, cream, or half-and-half
Add margarine to hot vegetables
Add sauces or gravies to vegetables or meats
Fry foods instead of baking or broiling
Select higher calorie fruit juices instead of coffee or tea
Add sugar or syrup to fruits or juices
Supplement meals and evening snacks with commercial medical nutritional products

---

Source: Adapted from Rakel RE. Textbook of Family Practice, 4th ed. Philadelphia, W. B. Saunders, 1990, p. 1209, with permission.

5. Involve Mrs. A. and her husband in decision making about Mrs. A.'s rights, for example, in terms of life-sustaining measures, including resuscitation, hospitalization, tube feeding, and medications. Promote the understanding that the wishes of the patient and her husband will be respected, that they have the right to refuse treatment, and that they can expect and have a right to know the care planned and why.

6. Upon discharge, the nursing home staff, including the dietitian, social worker, and physical therapist, will provide a home visit to help the family rearrange the home so that the Mr. and Mrs. A. can get around with as little problem as possible. Alternative meal programs in the community will be contacted, and Mr. and Mrs. A. may then be added to the list of recipients for such services should such services be needed in the future.

Disposition. Mrs. A. was discharged to her home after 4 weeks in the nursing home following successful reversal of her weight loss and indeed an 8-lb weight gain, lessening of loose bowels, and a return to near-normal physical abilities. Mrs. A. was asked to make monthly follow-up appointments with her family physician.

FIRST FOLLOW-UP VISIT WITH FAMILY PHYSICIAN

SUBJECTIVE

During the month after discharge, Mrs. A. and her husband continued to live at home and do well. Mrs. A. even began to return to a few selected community activities. With her family physician's understanding, she is now beginning to work through her grief over her father's death. Her bowel problems seem to be improving. She is adhering to a no-added-salt diet for her blood pressure. She is quite pleased that her weight has improved nicely. She advises her physician that if she were in a situation where she could no longer have a meaningful existence, she would not wish to have life-sustaining measures in the future, including nutrition support.

OBJECTIVE

Mrs. A.'s blood pressure is 140/85; her weight is now 132 lb; her facial expression, although "masked," is definitely more vital than when she was admitted to the nursing home. She is alert and is speaking freely. Neurologically, although her Parkinson's disease remains the same, she clearly seems to be regaining some strength in her extremities that were weakened by the stroke.

ASSESSMENT

Mrs. A. is markedly improved in many respects. The most significant improvement is her weight gain, because of her increased caloric intake and reduced loose stools. Importantly, she is also doing much better regarding her depression.

PLAN

Arrangements are made for Mrs. A. to visit a dietitian next month to reevaluate her caloric and other dietary needs because as she gets back to her old weight, her needs will be less. A return appointment is scheduled in 1 month.

DISCUSSION

Poor calorie intake is the major cause of weight loss. In the elderly, it is often due to reversible causes. In Mrs. A.'s case, weight loss was primarily the result of depression associated with her father's death. Parkinson's disease, malabsorption, drug interactions, and poor-fitting dentures that resulted when significant weight loss occurred also were likely contributors to her weight loss. When the depression was resolved, Mrs. A.'s irritable bowel symptoms subsided, her appetite and intake improved, and weight gain occurred. Mrs. A.'s behavior surrounding her dentures is an indication of embarrassment (caused by loss of dignity) and depression. Parkinsonian tremors contribute to the embarrassment of spilled food and also increase daily calorie needs. Sinemet and digoxin are appetite suppressants. Alcohol also may dull the appetite. Upon admission to the nursing home, Mrs. A. appeared wasted but lacked the textbook characteristics of malnutrition. Her weight loss of 16% in 6 months was severe (see Table 20–50) and a major trigger for nutritional status workup. Her weight loss was largely due to loss of lean muscle mass (as evidenced by a midarm muscle circumference at the 20th percentile) with a lesser loss of adipose tissue (triceps skinfold at the 40th percentile). Normal serum albumin is not uncommon with recent weight loss resulting from inadequate caloric intake.

The goal of nursing home nutrition care was to reverse Mrs. A.'s weight loss and prevent complications associated with malnutrition. The diet was liberalized as much as possible to encourage enjoyment in eating. Foods high in calories were served, and tools were considered that would allow her dignity to be maintained with self-feeding. Physical therapy and psychosocial counseling to improve her mental outlook added to Mrs. A.'s appetite. Nutrition's contribution to improved

TABLE 20–50. EVALUATING THE SIGNIFICANCE OF WEIGHT LOSS*

TIME INTERVAL	SIGNIFICANT WEIGHT LOSS (%)	SEVERE WEIGHT LOSS (%)
1 week	1.0–2.0	>2.0
1 month	5.0	>5.0
3 months	7.5	>7.5
6 months	10.0	>10.0

Source: Adapted from Blackburn GL, et al. Nutritional and metabolic assessment of the hospitalized patient. JPEN 1977; 1:11, with permission.

*Percent weight change = $\dfrac{\text{(usual weight} - \text{actual weight)}}{\text{usual weight}} \times 100$

muscle strength was primarily through added calorie intake. Protein, vitamin, and mineral needs to rebuild tissue were significant, but since calorie needs were met for weight gain and a variety of foods were consumed, the increased needs for protein, vitamins, and minerals also were met.

If Mrs. A. had not been able to consume adequate calories in the nursing home through regular food alone, commercial medical nutritional supplements would have been an appropriate consideration. Such products are usually best taken with meals instead of between meals, but the decision should be left to the patient. These products can add significantly to the overall nutrient intake and are appropriate for tube feedings, if necessary. Tube feedings should be considered for Mrs. A. only if regular food and supplemented intake cannot meet her needs for weight gain. If tube feedings are necessary for an extended period, a percutaneous gastrostomy tube (PEG) is an appropriate consideration. Nasogastric tubes are uncomfortable and irritating and would have been demeaning to Mrs. A. A PEG tube is associated with few side effects and is less costly than surgically placed gastrostomy tubes.

QUESTIONS

1. What diet order is the most reasonable for the salt intake in the hypertensive patient?
   a. 1-gm sodium diet
   b. 6-gm sodium diet
   c. No-added-salt diet.

2. What is the Hamwi formula for calculating ideal body weight for adult females?
   a. 100 lb plus 1 lb per year lived
   b. 90 lb plus 7 lb for each inch over 5 ft
   c. 100 lb plus 5 lb for each inch over 5 ft

3. A recent significant weight loss in the elderly
   a. Should be assessed immediately for reversible causes.
   b. Should be treated with as liberal a diet as medically tolerated.
   c. Is characterized by loss of lean muscle mass more than loss of adipose tissue.
   d. Is accompanied by a significant reduction in serum albumin.

4. A high-fiber diet consisting primarily of water-insoluble fiber
   a. Is contraindicated in elderly patients without teeth or with ill-fitting dentures.
   b. May be helpful in alleviating watery diarrhea.
   c. Increases the need for fluid.
   d. May decrease the laxative cost for nursing home residents.

Answers appear on page 451.

Fatigue

Wm. MacMILLAN RODNEY

INITIAL VISIT

SUBJECTIVE

Patient Identification and Presenting Problem. Mrs. C. is a 70-year-old white widow who lives alone with two cats for whom she cares faithfully. She takes the bus to scheduled visits with the doctor, and she is a reliable historian. While she values the doctor's advice, she does not always follow it. For example, she has chosen not to accept referral for mammography. Recently, she has noted a decrease in her energy. She feels it is increasingly difficult to maintain her one-story, well-lit, one-bedroom bungalow. She fears that she may have to give up her home and independence.

Past Medical History. Mrs. C. has been well without hospitalization during the 10 years she has been in the practice. She has no allergies. She underwent hysterec-

tomy 25 years ago for unknown reasons, and old records are not available. She believes her ovaries and appendix were removed at the same time. Her gallbladder was removed 5 years ago for symptomatic cholelithiasis. Illnesses include mild osteoarthritis, for which she receives a nonsteroidal anti-inflammatory medication (Naprosyn 375 mg PO b.i.d.), and idiopathic essential hypertension, which has responded to 40 mg propranolol b.i.d. She has coronary artery disease, having sustained a silent inferior wall myocardial infarction of indeterminate age. This was noted on her first ECG 10 years ago. She carries sublingual nitroglycerin 0.3 mg in her purse as a prophylactic measure. She receives estrogen replacement therapy, and she suffers from hemorrhoids.

Family History. As an adoptee, Mrs. C.'s biologic parents are unknown. She has a 30-pack-year smoking history, but she quit 25 years ago. She watches her diet but acknowledges being 30 lb over her "ideal weight." Before delivering her three children, she weighed 137 lb. She does not drink alcohol. She is gravida 4, para 3, with one miscarriage. Her three living children have moved to a neighboring state. Whenever possible, she visits at Christmas or Thanksgiving by bus travel. She worries that this may no longer be possible.

Social History. Mrs. C.'s husband died 10 years ago, leaving her with a modest pension and Social Security. She has Medicare health insurance without supplementation. She has a tenth-grade education and remains an avid reader of mystery novels.

Review of Systems. Review of systems is negative for a new headache, change in vision, localized weakness, paresthesias, fainting, cough, dyspnea, palpitations, dysuria, frequency, change in bowel habit, and bright red blood per rectum. Mrs. C. states that she has experienced some mild, intermittent, poorly localized cramping and abdominal pains that have not been associated with meals. There is no memorable pattern, and these pains do not awaken her from sleep. She feels that her appetite is coming under control and acknowledges a 10-lb weight loss since a visit 3 months ago. She reports "watching what I eat." This week she has felt lightheaded when she gets up. She denies melena but on closer questioning comments on the unaesthetic nature of examining one's own bowel movement. She has been unwilling to retrieve stool specimens from the toilet bowl for fecal occult blood testing (FOBT). She agrees to attempt a bowel movement at the office today. If successful, nursing staff will obtain a specimen for FOBT.

OBJECTIVE

Physical Examination. On physical examination, Mrs. C. is a well-developed, well-nourished, cooperative, white female who appears slightly younger than her stated age. Vital signs include blood pressure 145/88, pulse 92 and regular, respiratory rate 16, and oral temperature of 37.4°C. On further examination, pertinent positive findings include mild A-V nicking, dentures, and diffusely scattered 2- to 4-mm nonpigmented skin tags on the upper torso and neck. Rales that clear upon deep inspiration occur at both posterior lung bases. There is a 2/6 midsystolic murmur at the left sternal border. The point of maximal impulse is localized to the 4th intercostal space in the midclavicular line. The abdomen is normal to inspection and auscultation. Deep palpation produces slight discomfort, more on the left than the right. Nonpulsatile masses are not felt, but the aorta is palpable midline above the umbilicus. Pelvic examination is normal, and the digital rectal examination is normal. Inspection reveals a left lateral skin tag near the anus. There are no fissures, fistulas, sinus tracts, or external hemorrhoids.

Laboratory Tests. A chest x-ray reveals no evidence of acute heart failure, although cardiomegaly is noted. Blood is drawn for thyroid, renal, and liver function studies. Electrolytes, glucose, urinalysis, and a hemogram are ordered. Serendipitously, Mrs. C. successfully creates an inhouse natural bowel movement that tests positive for occult blood (FOBT).

ASSESSMENT

Working Diagnosis. In this age group, a positive FOBT suggests the possibility of (but it is not pathognomonic of) *colorectal cancer.* Based on prevalence alone, secondary cancer prevention programs target breast, colorectal, and cervix/uterine cancers for these patients. Lung cancer is a primary prevention project through smoking cessation. Because of signs and symptoms noted above, further investigation will proceed. However, since it relates to colorectal cancer, this process is literally defined as a "case-finding" investigation (fully covered by Medicare) as contrasted with "asymptomatic screening" (not always covered by Medicare).

Differential Diagnoses

1. *Drug effect—NSAID-induced GI bleeding.* Since NSAIDs are well known causes of gastric irritation and subclinical bleeding, it would be tempting to attribute the positive FOBT to drug effect. Do not send these patients home with additional FOBT cards, because a positive result is likely to be a true positive. While it is recommended to discontinue NSAIDs 7 days prior to FOBT, this is not always possible. Furthermore, in a study of FOBT among rheumatoid arthritis patients, true positives outnumbered false positives 7 to 1. A positive FOBT requires further investigation.

2. *Hemorrhoids.* Hemorrhoids are present in over 70% of women this age. Most of these are subclinical and are only seen on retroversion (the J-maneuver, the turn-around maneuver) of the flexible sigmoidoscope or colonoscope. Instrumentation of the anus by digital examination or endoscopy can produce a false-positive FOBT. However, this patient has mild abdominal pain, a 10-lb weight loss, and recent lightheadedness. If the patient could not have produced a natural bowel movement, digital examination for FOBT would have been indicated. The presence of hemorrhoids is not sufficient to explain the signs and symptoms of Mrs. C.

3. *Acute GI bleeding.* Specifically, acute bleeding is a possibility. Orthostatic measurements are taken (supine blood pressure is 143/88, pulse 92; standing after 2 minutes blood pressure is 130/80, pulse 98). An in-the-office hematocrit is obtained (value of Hct = 40). These values must be normal to continue the workup as an outpatient. For acute gastrointestinal bleeding of unknown etiology, hospitalization is recommended when the patient is hemodynamically unstable.

4. *Diverticulitis.* Bleeding diverticulosis, also known as "diverticulitis," can cause brisk and/or chronic lower GI bleeding. These patients usually present with lower left quadrant abdominal pain, low-grade fever, and leukocytosis. Abdominal guarding occurs,

and in severe cases, perforation can lead to peritonitis. These patients should be hospitalized. Mrs. C. does not fit this picture. Based on age and prevalence, it is likely that Mrs. C. has diverticulosis unrelated to her major problem.

5. *Angiodysplasia.* During the 1980s, angiodysplasia emerged as a frequent cause of painless lower GI bleeding among seniors. Mrs. C. did not have the anemia or aortic stenosis associated with angiodysplasia. Nevertheless, these ectatic vessels of the bowel wall remain a possibility. Only colonoscopy will detect these lesions, unless bleeding is so brisk that they can be detected angiographically. Angiodysplasia is not highly probable as the cause, but it is possible.

6. *Thyroid.* The loss of energy remains unexplained, although it could be related to the working diagnosis of occult colorectal cancer. Thryoid dysfunction should be considered.

7. *Cardiac failure.* Based on the physical findings and the chest x-ray, cardiac failure is unlikely, although the cardiomegaly and previous myocardial infarction are ongoing separate problems.

8. *Miscellaneous and rare possibilities.* Follow-up on the hemogram and other tests would be mandatory to exclude rarer disease such as leukemia, diabetes, polymyalgia rheumatica, coagulopathy, and others.

9. *Abdominal aneurysm.* An in-the-office ultrasound is immediately performed, revealing a 4 × 3.5 cm aneurysm. While this is of importance, it does not explain all the signs and symptoms. At this size, outpatient management and further imaging studies of the aneurysm can proceed once a definitive diagnosis of the major problem is found. This aneurysm is not a contraindication for colonoscopy or air contrast barium enema.

10. *Upper GI tract disease.* If examination of the lower GI tract is negative, upper GI tract disease may be sought. The weight loss and abdominal pain could be early indicators for esophageal, gastric, or pancreatic disease. In this patient, the uterus, ovaries, appendix, and gallbladder have been surgically removed, but not all the old records are available. Organs mistakenly retained and/or poorly remembered should be kept in mind when the workup does not proceed to a logical conclusion.

11. *Colitis.* Colitis does occur among seniors, although Mrs. C. does not relate the more severe abdominal pain and markedly abnormal bowel movements consistent with infectious colitis. Idiopathic inflammatory bowel disease (ulcerative colitis or Crohn's) would be a rare possibility. Radiation colitis can affect patients who have received radiation therapy for pelvic tumors. This would not apply to Mrs. C. A normal colonoscopy will exclude these possibilities in over 90% of cases. Finally, ischemic colitis can be as difficult a diagnosis of exclusion among the elderly as irritable bowel syndrome (IBS) is among the young and middle-age adults. The patient has no abdominal angina related to meals. Even though it is likely Mrs. C. suffers from widespread atherosclerotic cardiovascular disease, it is not a likely cause of her pain, weight loss, and positive FOBT.

PLAN

Diagnostic. Given the possibilities and probabilities, a plan for the detection of colorectal cancer is suggested. Many possible permutations and combinations of flexible sigmoidoscopy, air contrast barium enema, and/or colonoscopy exist. There are several valid investigative pathways that have different strengths and weaknesses. Endoscopy techniques and barium enema techniques are both operator-dependent, with varying degrees of sensitivity and specificity. Under ideal conditions, false-negative rates can be minimized to 5% to 10% for either. In some cases, both techniques are required when the first technique is inconclusive.

All things being equal, patient access to the technique should be considered. If colonoscopy is unavailable, flexible sigmoidoscopy (FS) may be synergistic with air contrast barium enema (ACBE). This approach is frequent in Great Britain and some American communities. When available, colonoscopy offers the advantage of high specificity (almost zero false-positive results) and the ability to obtain tissue through biopsy. Polypectomy at the time of colonoscopy can be curative, although some lesions are not resectable by endoscopy.

On the other hand, colonoscopy is more expensive ($500 versus $250 for ACBE). Perforation of the intestine can require immediate surgery, although some perforations can be managed conservatively by IV antibiotics and close observation. Perforation occurs more frequently (1 in 500 to 1 in 1000) with colonoscopy than it does with ACBE. Complications are rare with both techniques.

Patient comfort is operator-dependent. Controlled studies suggest a patient preference for colonoscopy over barium enema. Probably this is due to the use of intravenous sedation and analgesia for colonoscopy. Meperidine (25–125 mg) and/or diazepam (1–12 mg) are slowly administered under controlled conditions to produce twilight sedation and analgesia. Therefore, informed consent must include the possibilities of drug reaction and phlebitis. These are rare. With ACBE, phlebitis risk is nonexistent. The bowel preparation is critical to the success of both techniques (see Table 20–51).

In the case of Mrs. C., the family physician performed colonoscopy in the office. Mrs. C. received a 24-hour clear-liquid diet and a mixed electrolyte purge solution (Golytely, Colyte, others) as her bowel prep. Multiple lesions were detected. At 15 cm of insertion depth, a pale, sessile, hemispheric, nonfriable lesion 5 mm in diameter was biopsied and sent to pathology. These pathology reports normally return 2 to 5 working days later.

At 35 cm, a pedunculated polyp (measuring 12–15 mm across its head) was found. This was left undisturbed while examination proceeded to the cecum. The bowel prep was excellent, and 97% of the mucosal surface was visualized directly. Haustrae, sharp turns, and isolated fecal debris make 100% visualization a conceptual "ideal" that is rarely attained. Therefore, a negative examination can never be viewed as a "guaranteed clean bill of health."

TABLE 20–51. COMPARISON OF DIAGNOSTIC METHODS FOR COLORECTAL CANCER*

VARIABLE	FLEXIBLE SIGMOIDOSCOPY, 35 cm	SHORT COLONOSCOPY, 65 cm	FULL COLONOSCOPY, 180 cm	AIR CONTRAST BARIUM ENEMA
Operator dependent?	Yes	Yes	Yes	Yes
Average patient charge	$90–$140	$90–$200	$250–$750	$150–$250
Doable in the office?	Yes	Yes	Yes	No
Continuity of care possible?	Yes	Yes	By family practitioner: Yes / By GI consult: No	No
Biopsy possible on same visit?	Yes	Yes	Yes	No
Equipment cost (avg.)	$4000–$7000	$4000–$7000	$10,000–$20,000	None
IV sedation used?	No	No	Yes	No
Hard-copy of diagnostic images routinely retained?	No	No	Video: Yes / Fiberoptic: No	Yes
Sensitivity under ideal conditions	40%–50%	60%–65%	90%–95%	90%–95%

*These are the most commonly used and most diagnostically powerful methods currently available for the early detection of colorectal cancer. Accessibility and community standards vary. It is not uncommon for physicians to utilize more than one technique in pursuit of diagnostic certainty.

At the hepatic flexure, an irregularly contoured, friable, asymmetrical, sessile lesion consuming 120 degrees of arc was found. Two biopsies were taken with minimal bleeding. The scope was withdrawn atraumatically. On withdrawal, multiple sigmoid diverticuli were noted. The turn-around maneuver examined the pectinate line. Mild internal hemorrhoids with no active bleeding were seen.

The patient tolerated the procedure well. Vital signs were observed until stable and the patient was alert. Mrs. C. was driven home by a friend from church, with a return appointment scheduled for 1 week.

Therapeutic. Prior to leaving, Mrs. C. was told of the findings and the probable need for removal of the polyp in the hospital. The lesion at the hepatic flexure would require surgical consultation. A videotape of the lesion would be shared with the surgeon when the pathology reports are returned.

The next day, the pathologist called with a preliminary report. The lesion at 15 cm was a hyperplastic polyp. The hepatic flexure lesion was "moderately well differentiated adenocarcinoma." In consultation with a surgeon, hospitalization was scheduled for the next day. A metastatic survey was negative. At laparotomy 2 days later, a Dukes B colonic adenocarcinoma was resected. Nodes were negative, and a primary reanastomosis of the remaining bowel segment was successful. Mrs. C. was discharged 10 days later. Removal of the remaining polyps by the family physician was accomplished 2 months later.

Patient Education. During the hospitalization, Mrs. C. was visited daily. During that time, she received information regarding the high likelihood of a "cure." Nevertheless, the need for surveillance was explained. The pedunculated polyp was felt to be a benign risk, with good surgical margins possible on endoscopic removal. Although data are limited regarding the safest time for subsequent removal following open laparotomy, a 1- to 2-month interval was felt to be safe. Once

removed, the colon was felt to have been cleared of pathology. A surveillance protocol was established. Mrs. C. underwent colonoscopy 1 year later. At that time, no additional lesions were found. Mrs. C. understands that she is at "above average" risk for additional lesions. She agreed to report any additional new symptoms and to follow up on a 3-year colonoscopy surveillance protocol as long as she is asymptomatic.

Disposition. Mrs. C. remains under the care of her family physician for her other illnesses and continuing support.

SUGGESTED READING

Blackstone MO. Endoscopic Interpretation: Normal and Pathologic Appearances of the Gastrointestinal Tract. New York, Raven Press, 1984, pp. 1–575.

Rodney WM (ed.). Flexible Sigmoidoscopy for the Family Physician. Kansas City, Mo., American Academy of Family Physicians, 1988.

Rodney WM, Felmar E. Why flexible sigmoidoscopy instead of rigid sigmoidoscopy? J Fam Pract 1984; 19:471–476.

Rodney WM, Derezin M. Gastroenterology. In Rakel RE (ed.): Textbook of Family Practice, 4th ed. Philadelphia, W. B. Saunders, 1990.

Smith CW (ed.). Gastrointestinal disease in primary care. Clin Office Pract 1988; 15(1):1–204.

QUESTIONS

1. A 63-year-old man presents with hemorrhoidal bleeding and a hematocrit of 36. Anoscopy examination confirms the presence of mild internal hemorrhoids. No bleeding is seen. Colonoscopy is not available. You would recommend

   a. Air contrast barium enema (ACBE).
   b. Flexible sigmoidoscopy and ACBE.
   c. Referral for hemorrhoidal surgery.
   d. Iron replacement therapy, Preparation H, and warm sitz baths.
   e. None of the above.

2. Which of the following is not associated with lower gastrointestinal bleeding?
   a. Ischemic colitis
   b. Cancer
   c. Hemorrhoids
   d. Diverticulosis
   e. Pancreatitis

3. Regarding the relative advantages and disadvantages of colonoscopy versus air contrast barium enema, which of the following statements is/are true?
   a. Colonoscopy is always the preferred method.
   b. Air contrast barium enema is less painful to patients and therefore preferred by them.
   c. Both have 5% to 10% false-negative rate under ideal conditions.
   d. All of the above
   e. None of the above

4. Regarding fecal occult blood testing, which of the following statements is/are true?
   a. A positive test in a patient taking nonsteroidal anti-inflammatory drugs can be disregarded.
   b. Screening FOBT can be performed by digital rectal examination.
   c. Under screening conditions described by most medical societies, fecal occult blood testing is appropriately performed on stools specimens that result from a natural bowel movement.
   d. All of the above
   e. None of the above

Answers appear on page 451.

Heartburn

Wm. MacMILLAN RODNEY

INITIAL VISIT

SUBJECTIVE

Patient Identification and Presenting Problem. Mr. W. is a married, 35-year-old white father of two. He is a registered nurse who works rotating shifts in the hospital. He is a reliable historian and a compliant patient who has been in the practice for 5 years. His index complaint is continuing epigastric and substernal pain over the past 3 months.

Present Illness. Mr. W. has experienced mild "heartburn" related to large meals sporadically over the past few years. He has self-medicated with over-the-counter (OTC) products, and these episodes were self-limited. Three months ago, after an "all-you-can-eat-night" at the hospital cafeteria, the gradual onset of a severe burning discomfort extending from the xiphoid to the jaw kept Mr. W. awake for 15 to 30 minutes past his normal sleep time. Although not as severe, these attacks have persisted at the rate of three to four times per week since then. By reading in his nursing textbooks he has implemented several clinical strategies that include (1) no meals after 8:00 p.m. and (2) raising his head by using two extra pillows. This seemed to help a little.

Two weeks ago he noted the gradual onset of diffuse upper abdominal pain during the day in contrast to his other pain, which had occurred in the evening and at bedtime. Although the pain occurred 1 to 2 hours after meals, it also came at other times. He started a regular antacid routine of 1 tablespoon with each meal. His pain continues. One week ago it radiated to his back, but not to his shoulders or jaw.

Two days ago, Mr. W. was awakened by his worst pain ever. He was going to come to the office as an emergency, but by morning the pain was gone. Analysis of this symptom: $(P^2Q^2R^2ST^3)$:

Provoked:	By going to bed (supine or prone posture), but the pain is not pleuritic.
Palliated:	By getting up and swallowing some antacids. The pain seems to go away with time.
Quality:	Sharp, burning
Quantity:	At its worst, it was 9 on a scale of 10. Now it is 0 to 1.
Region:	Diffuse upper abdomen and midchest
Radiation:	Radiation to the shoulders or jaw, but Mr. W. stated that the pain has radiated through to his back on several occasions.
Severity:	By morning, he felt well enough to go to work. He worked the full day without further problems.
Temporal factors:	1. Previous *onsets* were gradual; this one was sudden.
	2. Pains are *constant,* lasting 30 to 120 minutes.
	3. Pains have been *recurrent* over months, but this was *the first time* he was awakened.

Past Medical History. *Surgeries:* None. *Allergies:* None. *Hospitalizations:* None. *Illnesses:* Early morning insomnia and dysphoria diagnosed as depression 4 months ago. *Medications:* Prescription medications: Nortriptyline, 75 mg q.h.s. Over-the-counter medications: Tums, Alka-Seltzer tablets p.r.n., average consumption of two tablets after a meal once in a while; and a generic antacid (Maalox, Mylanta, Gelusil, and others) taken 1 tablespoon before each meal during the past week; this has not relieved his worsening pain.

Family and Social History. Mr. W. grew up as the only child of a divorced registered nurse who raised him lovingly. His father died at age 60 of a sudden "heart attack." Among bloodline relatives, there is no report of diabetes, high blood pressure, or tuberculosis. A maternal aunt has had breast cancer but is still alive. The father's side of the family is known for "bad nerves," including a "nervous stomach."

Mr. W. was a corpsman in the army for 4 years after high school. By working shifts in a nursing home, he was able to put himself through college, obtaining the nursing degree at age 28. His wife works as an accountant, and they have two healthy children, ages 7 and 5. He does not smoke. He drinks alcohol rarely. He jogs on weekends whenever he can.

Review of Systems. Mr. W. denies any new headaches, change in vision, dyspnea, wheezing, exercise-related chest pain, diaphoresis, night sweats, cough, syncope, palpitations, numbness, tingling, arthralgia, myalgia, weakness, or rash. He has experienced some nausea, but no actual vomiting. In particular, there has been no hematemesis, melena, diarrhea, or constipation. His appetite is good, but recently there has been some pain associated with eating. He has lost 5 lb. Mr. W. is sexually active with his wife. He denies dysuria and penile discharge.

OBJECTIVE

Physical Examination. Mr. W.'s height is 70 in; his weight is 235 lb; and he has the following vital signs: blood pressure 140/88, pulse 80 regular, respirations 14, temperature 37.0°C by mouth. Mr. W. is alert, cooperative, and overweight. *Integument:* Normal distribution and quality. *HEENT:* Unremarkable. *Chest:* Mild pectus excavatum; no point tenderness; lungs are clear. Bowel sounds can be heard on the left anteroinferior chest wall. *Heart:* The point of maximal impulse is localized to the 4th intercostal space within the left midclavicular line. There are no heaves, gallops, or murmurs. Pulses are appropriately strong and equal (carotid, brachial, femoral, and dorsalis pedis). *Abdomen:* The abdomen is convex, and bowel sounds are present. No bruits are heard. Although the abdomen is soft, examination is suboptimal secondary to the patient's increased girth. No masses are palpated. The liver percusses to a vertical span of 12 cm in the right midclavicular line. Moderate palpation creates reproducible discomfort in the upper abdomen, generally most prominent in the midline. Murphy's sign (simultaneous

palpation to the right costal margin in the midclavicular line while the patient takes a deep breath) is positive. Abdominal and inguinal hernias are absent. Testicles are normal in size, shape, and consistency. Mild external hemorrhoids are present without fissures, fistulas, or sinus tracts. Sphincter tone is normal, and the digital examination produces soft, dark brown stool that tests "trace" positive for occult blood. The musculoskeletal and neurologic examinations are normal. The patient appears appropriately concerned regarding his condition. He responds in a guarded but appropriate fashion to humor. He feels that his family is supportive. His job is difficult but fulfilling. He is hopeful regarding his illness and optimistic regarding his future.

Follow-Up Examination and Laboratory Tests. Blood pressure and pulse are remeasured in the supine and standing positions. Supine blood pressure is 140/90; pulse is 82; blood pressure standing after 2 minutes is 126/80; pulse is 92. The results of tests in the office laboratory are as follows: Hgb 14.1 (normal 14–18), WBC 8.0 (normal 4.2–10.0), aspartate aminotransferase (SGOT) 31 (normal 20–48), alanine aminotransferase (SGPT) 47 (normal 22–46), bilirubin total 0.9 (normal 0.5–1.1), amylase 44 (normal 30–55), lipase 62 (normal 28–60), lactate dehydrogenase (LDH) 224 (normal 100–250), cholesterol 360 (normal <240), and PT, APTT, and creatine phosphokinase (CPK) all normal. Urinalysis reveals a pH of 5.0 and a specific gravity of 1.014. The dipstick chemistries and the microscopic examination are normal.

The ECG reveals a normal sinus rhythm of 84 with an axis of −30 degrees. The intervals are measured as follows: PR 200 ms, QRS 110 ms, and QT 340 ms. There are no signs of enlargement or ischemia. The PA and lateral chest films are negative for effusions, infiltrates, and cardiomegaly. There is no air under the diaphragm.

ASSESSMENT

Working Diagnosis. The working diagnosis is *undifferentiated peptic disease* of the upper gastrointestinal system. This category of diseases include ulcer, gastritis, duodenitis, and esophagitis. Each of these distinct entities exists on a continuum that ranges from mild to severe.

Interpretation of the medical literature requires a common definition of terms. "Peptic ulcer disease" is a traditional catch-all phase, however, "peptic disease syndrome" more accurately describes the variety of these conditions. In one series from the offices of family physicians, less than 10% of dyspeptic patients actually had ulcers (Rodney et al.).

"Dyspepsia" is the preferred general term that encompasses all others (i.e., heartburn, indigestion, reflux, upper abdominal pain, meal-related epigastric pain). Patients may describe it partially or totally with such terms as "gas," "bloating," or even "food allergy."

Dyspepsia can reflect a single peptic disease or the concurrent existence of several. For example, a duodenal ulcer and esophagitis can exist simultaneously. Dyspepsia can occur in nonpeptic conditions such as cancer, cholelithiasis, pancreatitis, pneumonia, depression, and more. Commonly prescribed drugs such as erythromycin, NSAIDs, ampicillin, theophylline, and others can cause dyspepsia.

Describing the diagnostic dilemma that faces the clinician of first contact, a widely respected gastroenterologist has said, "It has been taught that there are classic symptoms which differentiate types of peptic ulcer diseases with regard to meals, types of pain, and other symptoms. With endoscopy, all of these concepts have been dramatically revised. We have detected patients with large ulcers who had minimal, if any, symptoms. Other patients have had disabling symptoms with a totally normal endoscopic examination" (Rogers).

Differential Diagnoses

1. *Gastric or duodenal ulcer.* These can perforate requiring immediate hospitalization. These patients usually present with unrelenting abdominal pain that can radiate to the back and/or shoulder. When the condition advances to generalized peritonitis, the abdomen becomes rigid and bowel sounds usually disappear. Less advanced cases may be detectable only by the appearance of free air under the diaphragm. A chest x-ray was ordered to rule out this possibility of silent perforation.

2. *Bleeding secondary to peptic disease.* This can range from subclinical to life-threatening. A positive fecal occult blood test (FOBT) is consistent with peptic disease, colorectal cancer, intestinal A-V malformations, coagulopathy, hemorrhoids, and others. Normal coagulation chemistries are reassuring, but these laboratory tests are not mandatory when the patient does not bleed excessively with normal activities (e.g., brushing of teeth).

Although the age of 35 does not exclude colorectal cancer, it is reasonable to pursue the more probable diagnosis of peptic disease. This decision is based on the strong history. Similarly, the finding of hemorrhoids is not sufficient to explain and dismiss a positive FOBT in this setting.

Immediate analysis of the FOBT includes a hematocrit or hemoglobin (Hgb) along with orthostatic measurements. A Hgb of less than 10 and/or significant orthostatic changes require close observation in the hospital.

3. *Upper GI neoplasia.* Cancer is always a consideration; however, Mr. W. exemplifies the clinical situation where a thoughtful analysis and empirical therapy precede full-scale technologic investigations designed to "rule out cancer." Immediate endoscopy, CT scans, and upper GI x-rays are not indicated at this time. Consider other possibilities and return to this one if the patient becomes increasingly ill or unstable.

4. *Emotional disorder.* Depression and/or anxiety can be expressed as a chronic nervous, painful stomach. Severe depression may include anorexia, weight loss, and insomnia. Mr. W. has been recently diagnosed with this depression. His appetite has been unchanged, although some episodes of eating have become more painful.

The awakening with severe pain is not characteristic of depression. Depression may exhibit early morning insomnia with difficulty getting back to sleep. Anxiety may lead to difficulty initiating sleep. Neither is usually associated with severe, burning, substernal pain. This pattern is consistent with severe esophagitis. Furthermore, sitting up, swallowing, and antacid ingestion can palliate a severe attack in 30 to 120 minutes. Pain at bedtime is common among patients with gastroesophageal reflux disease (GERD). These patients may have difficulty initiating sleep. In contrast to the poorly defined symptoms of anxiety-related insomnias, GERD patients know exactly why they cannot sleep. It is because of epigastric-substernal pain. Ironically, strong sedatives can produce sleep which overrides the symptom while the underlying esophageal pathology continues unabated. These symptoms of Mr. X are *not* characteristic of depression or anxiety.

5. *Side effects from drugs.* Dyspepsia can be initiated or exacerbated by a variety of widely prescribed medications. Mr. W. does not take aspirin or NSAIDs. Antidepressants are notorious for their anticholinergic effects. Theoretically, the antisecretory effects of well-known tricyclic antidepressants (TCADs) should palliate peptic disease. Prior to the arrival of the H_2-receptor antagonists, several studies demonstrated this helpful effect of TCADs on peptic ulcer patients. This line of investigation was discontinued after successful introduction of cimetidine and other more specific medications.

Could nortriptyline be a problem? Appetite stimulation, sedation, and weight gain may be TCAD side effects that promote GERD. Decreased gastric motility is a possible side effect. However, these are unlikely given the current subtherapeutic dose of nortriptyline.

6. *Cardiovascular problems.* Cardiac and pericardial conditions can present as atypical substernal pain with or without dyspepsia. Risk factors include male sex, family history, and overweight. The ECG demonstrates a PR interval of 200 ms and a QRS axis of −30 degrees. Thoracic aortic aneurysm can present as crushing pain that radiates to the back. However, there are no signs of ischemia, and these isolated findings are not sufficient to displace peptic disease syndrome as the working diagnosis.

7. *Hiatal hernia.* Mechanical possibilities include trauma, hernias, and anatomic variations (congenital, iatrogenic, and naturally occurring). There is no history of trauma, chest surgery, abdominal surgery, or caustic ingestion. Pectus excavatum has been associated with atypical chest pains, palpitations, and mitral valve prolapse. The presence of pectus in Mr. W. is an incidental finding that cannot explain his symptoms. An echocardiogram and/or CT of the chest is not indicated.

Hiatal hernia is prevalent in 20% to 50% of U.S. and Western European adults. Diaphragmatic hernias are rare. This patient has auscultable bowel sounds in the left lower chest. Should this finding be heavily weighted? These sounds can be heard at the edge of the left lower chest in 10% to 15% of normal adults. Therefore, the positive predictive value of this finding for diaphragmatic hernia is very low.

However, incarcerated diaphragmatic hernias can present acutely in adults. Continuous pain and dyspnea are characteristic. A normal chest x-ray and the history are not consistent with this possibility. Hiatal hernia is a strong possibility, particularly with the patient being 40 to 50 lb overweight. Hiatal hernia is an anatomic feature that promotes reflux and esophageal inflammation. Weight loss through diet and exercise should be recommended for Mr. W.

8. *Gastroesophageal reflux disease (GERD).* This can occur in the presence or absence of hiatal hernia. Esophageal inflammation can be painful or painless. The mucosal integrity is protected by the lower esophageal sphincter (LES). LES dysfunction can be associated with hiatal hernias, or it can be idiopathic. In infants, chalasia describes the condition in which LES relaxation permits reflux and pseudoregurgitation of meals.

In adults, this phenomenon bathes the esophageal mucosa with acidic gastric contents. Small amounts of reflux are well tolerated, but once an injury breaches the mucosal integrity, a vicious cycle begins. The wet environment, continued acid irritation, and the periodic passage of food make healing of esophageal lesions more difficult than healing of peptic lesions elsewhere. As peptic esophagitis advances, swallowing of food can become painful and difficult. Mr. W. does not exhibit overt dysphagia (mechanical difficulty with swallowing, such as food sticking), but his symptoms could be consistent with a mild dysphagia secondary to esophagitis. Chronic esophagitis can produce strictures. Usually these patients describe more difficulty swallowing solids than liquids, but this is also true with some cases of esophagitis. Pain avoidance can lead to severe or mild weight loss. Mr. W. has lost 5 lb.

Mr. W. has accurately self-diagnosed at least part of his problem as esophageal. The heartburn has been present for years, but this condition has dramatically worsened in the last few months. As adults age and their girth increases, reflux can become more severe. Discontinuation of evening meals should be expanded to an overall diet plan that includes an explicit weight-loss goal, an exercise plan, calorie restriction, and dietary awareness.

Fat, chocolate, and alcohol are notorious LES relaxants. Caffeine is probably not. Under normal conditions, small amounts (and even excesses) are tolerated. Once esophagitis begins, these foods and others should be monitored closely. Positional therapy for GERD has traditionally included placement of 4- to 6-in blocks under the legs supporting the head of the bed. This has not been proven in clinical trials, but seems prudent. Extra pillows should be discontinued because clinical studies have demonstrated that pillow-supported reclining postures can even increase the amount of reflux.

Antacids should be selected to achieve maximal effect. One tablespoon is not sufficient to neutralize normal stomach acid. However, standing upright and swallowing fluids can produce relief in patients who have been awakened or unable to sleep. A neutralizing equivalent of antacid is 140 mEq. This requires 30 ml Mylanta II, Maalox TC, Gelusil TC, and other high-potency antacids. Gaviscon may be an especially helpful option because the alginate component may create an additional barrier of protection for GERD patients. Patients need explicit, written instructions advising them to take 1 oz ("a shot glass" or "two tablespoons," but not "a swig") 1 and 3 hours after meals and at bedtime. Rx = 30 cc PO 1 and 3 hours after meals, also q.h.s. Mr. W. has not fully maximized the potential effect of antacids. This antacid regimen is a fundamental cornerstone of conservative therapy for all the peptic diseases (i.e., ulcers, gastritis, esophagitis, etc.). Lifestyle modification by diet, weight loss, and risk reduction are equally important cornerstones. A low cholesterol diet also will be indicated for the elevated cholesterol and cardiovascular risk profile of Mr. W.

9. *Duodenal ulcer.* The complaints of Mr. W. have gone beyond garden-variety heartburn and indigestion. Radiation of pain to the back and midcycle sleep awakening suggest more advanced disease that is less likely to respond to conservative measures. Additionally, upper abdominal pain occurring 1 to 2 hours after meals is characteristic of gastric and duodenal lesions rather than lesions limited to the esophagus.

Although pain can radiate to the back with esophageal lesions, this pain also can represent an ulcer on the posterior duodenal wall, gallbladder disease, pancreatitis, perforation, aneurysm, and others. The physical findings of epigastric tenderness and an ambiguous Murphy's sign can be found with inflammation of the liver, gallbladder, duodenum, stomach, and esophagus. These physical findings are consistent with but not pathognomonic of any one disease in particular.

Laboratory findings reveal elevations of amylase and alanine aminotransferase. These elevations are miniscule and insufficient to displace the working hypothesis of peptic disease syndrome with probable simultaneous involvement of the esophagus, stomach, and duodenum.

PLAN

Diagnostic. When the physician has considered and discounted those conditions requiring hospitalization, investigation and management commonly proceed in the office and by telephone. No further diagnostic tests are needed prior to the initiation of medical therapy.

Prior to 1985, there was controversy regarding the value of immediate radiologic contrast studies and/or esophagogastroduodenoscopy (EGD). An upper GI series with a small bowel follow-through (UGI/SBFT) was frequently ordered where EGD was not available. Similar to the controversy regarding air contrast barium enema (ACBE) versus colonoscopy in lower GI lesions, test selection depends on the patient's risk, the community's resources, and the physician's preference.

In contrast to ACBE versus colonoscopy, EGD has emerged as generally superior to UGI/SBFT (see Table 20–52). There are exceptions (i.e., motility disorders), and clinical judgment is necessary. Generally, the sensitivity of UGI/SBFT is 35% to 60% of EGD. On the

TABLE 20–52. COMPARISON OF DIAGNOSTIC METHODS FOR PEPTIC DISEASE SYNDROMES

VARIABLE	UPPER GI X-RAY	ESOPHAGOGASTRO-DUODENOSCOPY (EGD)
Operator dependent?	Yes	Yes
Average charge	$140–$240	$270–$670
Continuity of care possible?	No	By FP: Yes
		By consult: No
Biopsy possible on same visit?	No	Yes
IV sedation used?	No	Yes
Portable to the bedside?	No	Yes
Usable in the office?	No	Yes
Usable in the nursing home?	No	Yes
Hard copy of diagnostic images routinely retained?	Yes	By Video: Yes
		Fiberoptic: No
Sensitivity under ideal conditions:		
Cancer	30%–40%	60%–80%
Ulcer	40%–60%	90%–98%
Esophagitis	30%–50%	90%–95%
Motility disorder	60%–90%	10%–20%

Note: High specificity and a definite edge in sensitivity for peptic disease lesions favor EGD as the diagnostic test of choice except in suspected motility disorders of the esophagus. Complications are rare with both tests, but more frequent with EGD than with x-ray.

other hand, EGD detects histologically confirmed gastritis in 15% to 20% of healthy, asymptomatic controls. Other than this, EGD has a very good sensitivity (75%–98%) and high specificity (95%–99%) for peptic disease lesions. Specificity figures are confirmed by biopsy and brushing.

In 1985, the Health and Public Policy Committee of the American College of Physicians published a thoughtful and widely accepted consensus statement advocating empirical therapy for probable peptic disease syndrome. Further diagnostic tests are delayed pending the results of this therapy. This consensus concluded that "if all dyspeptic patients are treated empirically, considerable diagnostic resources will be saved."

Upper GI cancers are relatively uncommon, and the collective survival rate for upper GI cancers will not be improved significantly by universal detection 6 to 8 weeks earlier. Endoscopy should be reserved for two subsets of patients: (1) those who have no or minimal response to therapy after 7 to 10 days and (2) those (30%) whose illness improves but does not resolve after 6–8 weeks.

Therapeutic. Short-term therapeutic goals include prevention of complications, pain relief, and mucosal healing. Simultaneously, there is hypothesis testing with empirical therapy. Peptic disease is notoriously recurrent at an annual rate of 44% to 70%. A secondary therapeutic goal is the long-term prevention of recurrence.

Placebo-controlled studies of duodenal ulcers have demonstrated that a third of patients will resolve spontaneously over 8 weeks. Rigorous administration of 15 to 30 ml of antacids will significantly increase the healing rate to 85% to 87%. If the response is favorable, the 15-ml dose may decrease some of the side effects.

The inconvenience and bulk of liquids is a barrier to compliance. Dosage schedules requiring 7 daily doses are difficult to maintain. For these reasons, a variety of more convenient tablets have emerged as the drugs of choice (Table 20–53). These drugs are all effective and safe. The H_2-receptor antagonists can be prescribed in split doses, such as cimetidine 400 mg b.i.d. or 300 mg q.i.d., ranitidine 150 mg b.i.d., famotidine 20 mg b.i.d., and nizatidine 150 mg b.i.d.

For shift workers, a b.i.d. schedule may be better than a strict bedtime-only dosage. Most patients notice improvement in 24 to 72 hours with these medications. Based on the cumulative millions of patient-years of experience with cimetidine and ranitidine, long-term usage is probably safe. They cannot be used in pregnancy.

Sucralfate, a cytoprotective agent, can be given 2 gm b.i.d. It is an agent that preferentially binds to ulcerated mucosa. Since it does not act systemically, it probably is safe during pregnancy. Onset of effect may require 2 to 5 days.

A newer cytoprotective agent, misoprostol, is a prostaglandin analogue that promotes bicarbonate and mucus secretion by gastric mucosa. Omeprazole is a potent antisecretory agent that inhibits the H^+/K^+ ATPase proton pump. This pump is the final step in gastric acid secretion by the parietal cell. Bismuth agents may pro-

TABLE 20–53. COMPARISON OF HEALING RATES IN DUODENAL ULCER USING VARIOUS MEDICATIONS

DRUG	DOSAGE	PERCENT ULCERS HEALED	
		4 Weeks	*8 Weeks*
Cimetidine	800 mg q.h.s.	80–85	90–95
Ranitidine	300 mg q.h.s.	80–85	90–95
Famotidine	40 mg q.h.s.	80–85	90–95
Nizatidine	300 mg q.h.s.	80–85	90–95
Sucralfate	1 gm q.i.d.	75	86
Misoprostol	200 μg q.i.d.	70	80
Omeprazole	20 mg daily	90–95	95–100

mote duodenal and gastric ulcer healing by a bactericidal effect on *Helicobacter pylori*. These three agents are effective, but their properties and long-term benefits are not as well studied. In particular, the role of *H. pylori* as causal or secondary agent in peptic disease syndrome is poorly understood.

Esophageal lesions require a special treatment plan. Placebo trials confirm a 30% to 40% spontaneous improvement in erosive GERD. Sucralfate also will assist healing. Episodes that do not resolve may require larger doses and longer periods of traditional H_2-receptor antagonists (e.g., cimetidine 800 mg b.i.d. or ranitidine 300 mg b.i.d.). Despite 12 weeks of therapy, only 70% to 75% of patients may be healed.

Omeprazole has produced complete healing in 85% to 95% of esophagitis patients. However, once the omeprazole is stopped, there may be an 82% recurrence rate. Long-term maintenance with omeprazole has not been studied.

In summary, high-dose H_2-receptor antagonist therapy should be chosen for simultaneous treatment of probable gastric, duodenal, and esophageal disease. Additional prokinetic agents such as metoclopramide 5 mg b.i.d. or q.i.d. are recommended by some authorities.

Patient Education. Mr. W. is encouraged to consider a therapeutic contract for initiation and maintenance of lifestyle changes, including weight loss, exercise, avoidance of specific foods, and a calorie/fat diary. Alcohol should be avoided. The head of the bed can be elevated, but no more than one pillow should be used for sleeping.

Chewable or liquid antacids can be used as needed but should not be taken to interfere with absorption of the primary therapy—high-dose H_2-receptor antagonists b.i.d. Antacids within 2 hours prior to these pills may interfere with absorption.

Chewing gum may enhance esophageal clearance, thereby decreasing the amount of time that irritating substances are in contact with damaged mucosa.

Disposition. Reevaluate in 7 to 14 days. Mr. W. is requested to bring his calorie/fat content diary, which includes a daily weight. The diary will report exercise compliance also. He will anticipate a repeat cholesterol measurement.

Mr. W. is given a prescription for 2 weeks without refills. A phone call will be made by the office nurse at 7 to 10 days to determine if symptoms remain unchanged, have worsened, or have improved. Without improvement, Mr. W. will be prepared for EGD in the office by the family physician. Family physicians without EGD skills may request consultation.

FIRST FOLLOW-UP VISIT

SUBJECTIVE

Mr. W. reports only mild improvement in the dull epigastric pain that had been occurring 1 to 2 hours after meals. However, substernal pain has awakened him nightly for the past 3 nights. This pain does not radiate to the back, jaw, or shoulders. With upright posture and antacids, the pain gradually dissipates, allowing a return to sleep in 30 to 60 minutes.

Mr. W. has initiated the diet/exercise diary with a subsequent loss of an additional 2 lb. He admits difficulty following the diet and misses the camaraderie of "all-you-can-eat-night" at the hospital cafeteria. However, he is determined to succeed at weight and dietary control. He has come to the office NPO since midnight in anticipation of early morning EGD in the office. He has read and signed an informed consent.

OBJECTIVE

Mr. W.'s weight is 233 lb, and his vital signs are stable. Bowel sounds are present, and the epigastric pain to palpation is now gone. Otherwise the abdominal examination is unchanged. Twilight sedation is achieved with the gradual administration of diazepam 5 mg IV and meperidine 75 mg IV. The endoscopy report is attached (see Fig. 20–14).

Several biopsies are taken from the edge of the duodenal and esophageal ulcerations. Biopsies are taken from the gastric antrum and fundus. After an hour of observation, normal vital signs, and a return to clear sensorium, Mr. W. will be driven home.

ASSESSMENT

Based on signs and symptoms, healing of the probable gastritis and the probable duodenal ulcer is proceeding. However, the esophagitis is severe, and symptoms are worsening.

PLAN

The H_2-receptor antagonist will be discontinued, and omeprazole 20 mg daily will be started. Otherwise, Mr. W. is to continue with all other elements of the previously described management plan. If overt dysphagia develops, stricture formation will be suspected, and dilation could be necessary. A report on the biopsies will be available in 3 to 5 days, but Mr. W. is reassured that malignancy is unlikely. A minimum of an 8-week course of therapy is predicted, and maintenance therapy with an H_2-receptor antagonist will be necessary for at least an additional year.

SUGGESTED READING

Adelman AM. Management of Dyspepsia. Am Fam Physician 1987; 35(4):222–229.

DeGowin EL, DeGowin RL (eds.). Bedside Diagnostic Examination. New York, Macmillan, 1985.

Dooley CP, Larson AW, Stace NH, et al. Double contrast barium meal and upper gastrointestinal endoscopy: A comparative study. Ann Intern Med 1984; 101:538–545.

Goldsmith G, Patterson M. Irritible bowel syndrome: Treatment update. Am Fam Physician 1985; 31:191–195.

Rodney WM, Derezin M. Gastroenterology. In Rakel RE (ed.): Textbook of Family Practice, 4th ed. Philadelphia, W. B. Saunders, 1990.

Rodney WM, Hocutt JE, Coleman WH, et al. Esophagogastroduodenoscopy by family physicians: A national multisite study of 717 procedures. J Am Bd Fam Pract 1990; 3:73–79.

Silen W. Cope's Early Diagnosis of the Acute Abdomen. New York, Oxford University Press, 1979.

QUESTIONS

1. Which of the following statements is accurate regarding antacid prescriptions for peptic disease?
   a. Should be taken before meals.
   b. Different OTC brands are equally potent.
   c. Can interfere with absorption of H_2-receptor antagonists.
   d. Do not help esophageal lesions.
   e. An ounce per dose is too much.

2. Characteristic features of peptic disease syndrome include
   a. There is a continuum of illness ranging from subclinical to severe.
   b. Hospital-based investigations are required in a majority of cases.
   c. Prior to obtaining a specific tissue diagnosis, the physician is encouraged to prescribe empirically.
   d. Within 8 weeks, 60% to 70% of cases resolve spontaneously.
   e. Two to three daily cups of caffeinated coffee aggravate over 90% of cases.

3. Esophagogastroduodenoscopy is
   a. Not the diagnostic procedure of choice for all suspected esophageal disorders.
   b. A diagnostic and therapeutic skill that can be performed in the office by some family physicians.
   c. Generally more expensive than barium meal studies (i.e., UGI/SBFT x-rays).
   d. A procedure that usually requires intravenous sedation and close monitoring of the patient.
   e. All of the above.
   f. None of the above.

4. Nonulcerated gastritis is one histologic manifestation of the peptic disease syndrome. This entity
   a. Is painful in over 90% of cases.
   b. Can be detected with equal power by either EGD or UGI/SBFT x-rays.
   c. Is caused by *Helicobacter pylori*.
   d. Commonly presents with epigastric pain radiating to the back.
   e. Exists in up to 20% of asymptomatic healthy controls.
   f. All of the above.
   g. None of the above.

Answers appear on page 452.

Chronic Fatigue

JOSEPH HOBBS

INITIAL VISIT

SUBJECTIVE

Patient Identification and Presenting Problem. Jean, a 67-year-old white female, presents with a 6-month history of progressive generalized fatigue. The patient was well known to her physician, who had provided her comprehensive care for 15 years until 3 years ago, when church-related travel schedules began to conflict with her routine physician visits.

Present Illness. Jean was initially unable to associate her fatigue with any significant activity. However, her exercise tolerance had decreased significantly over the last 3 months, which made it difficult to negotiate inclines or stairs or walk long distances without becoming unusually fatigued and short of breath. The fatigue was not associated with chest pain, palpitations, or unexpected diaphoresis. Jean had no predisposing factors for coronary artery disease except her age and mild hypertension. She had never smoked or consumed alcohol, and previous cholesterol levels were within normal limits. Further, there was no history of melena, hematemesis, abdominal pain, epigastric pain, GI surgery, heat or cold intolerance, night sweats, or an increase in the frequency or severity of her arthralgias. Jean noted a 10-lb weight loss over this same 6-month period, which she attributed to poor appetite because food "no longer had its characteristic taste."

Although the fatigue had been a problem over the 6-month period, it was revealed by relatives that Jean's most frequent recent complaint had been coldness in the lower extremities that had persisted despite the warming weather of spring. Jean initially attributed her complaint to "poor circulation" but became concerned when she begin to note some mild periodic unsteadiness over the last 4 weeks. Jean also became aware of some mild dizziness when moving rapidly from a recumbent to a more erect position. There was no history of vomiting, diarrhea, polyuria, or fever.

Past Medical History. Jean has mild hypertension that is well controlled with hydrochlorothiazide 25 mg per day, and she receives prophylaxis against osteoporosis using 0.625 mg conjugated estrogens on days 1 through 21 of each month and 10 mg progestin on days 12 through 21 of each month. Jean has never consistently taken her prescribed potassium supplement, but over the last few years her monitored serum potassium levels have been within normal limits. She uses occasional acetaminophen 1000 mg PO q4h as needed for headaches and ibuprofen 200 mg PO q6h as needed for intermittent arthralgias. There is sonographic evidence of uterine fibroids, but these have been stable since their discovery 15 years ago.

Jean also has 2 days of light withdrawal bleeding when estrogens and progestins are withdrawn monthly, associated with mild dysmenorrhea controlled with ibuprofen. This pattern has not changed since she started estrogens and progestins 10 years ago. Jean's last mammogram was 36 months ago and was normal. Pap smears 39 months ago were class I for endocervical and ectocervical smears. Laboratory tests performed 42 months ago included a normal urinalysis, CBC, and glucose and electrolyte determinations.

Family History. Jean has lived alone since the death of her husband 10 years ago. Both Jean's parents are deceased, having died suddenly of unknown causes in their late seventies. Jean has three sisters and one brother, all younger, and they are in what she thinks is good physical health.

Social History. Jean owns her own home and appears active in community activities, including spearheading fund raising activities for her local church. She has been extremely active in other church activities and has been dating a friend from her church's "senior singles group" for 18 months.

Historical Problems

1. *Chronic fatigue.* Although no specific historical evidence exists, physical, laboratory, and other evaluations should focus on the possible presence of common problems such as anemia, hypothyroidism, hypokalemia, myocardial ischemia, non-insulin-dependent diabetes mellitus, occult malignancies, occult infections, psychosocial dysfunction, and anorexia of unknown cause (e.g., depression).

2. *Postural dizziness.* One must consider the possibility of diuretic-induced volume depletion; volume depletion secondary to decreased oral fluid intake, vomiting, and diarrhea; and occult diabetes mellitus. Decreased effective circulating volume secondary to left ventricular dysfunction, vasomotor dysfunction secondary to age, and medications also must be considered. Volume loss secondary to blood loss or other causes of anemia also should be considered.

3. *Cold feet.* We must evaluate the possible presence of peripheral vascular disease, venous stasis disease, and peripheral neuropathies.

4. *Hypertension.* This problem has been well controlled historically, but we must consider the possibility of excessive diuresis, which could lead to signs and symptoms of volume depletion and hypokalemia.

5. *Physiologic menopause.* This could be a cause of her chronic fatigue if symptoms are not well-controlled.

6. *Loss of spouse 10 years ago.* Continue to investigate the appropriateness of the patient's coping with the loss and the potential for occult depression even though on the surface she appears well adjusted.

7. *Family history of osteoporosis.*

8. *Anoxia.* Consider factors in 1 and 6 above.

9. Monthly estrogen/progestin *withdrawal uterine bleeding.* This could be a cause of iron-deficiency anemia.

10. *Uterine leiomyoma.*

11. *Mild dysmenorrhea.*

12. *Noncompliance* to scheduled appointments.

13. Frequent phone request for "medication refills."

14. Decreased or altered taste.

15. Weight loss possibly secondary to 1, 8, and 14 above. Consider other hypermetabolic states.

OBJECTIVE

Physical Examination. Jean is a pale-appearing white female in no acute distress, and she is oriented to time, place, and person. Her blood pressure is 130/92, with a pulse rate of 80 per minute lying down, and 110/68, with a pulse rate of 114 sitting, associated with complaints of mild dizziness. Her respiratory rate is 14 per minute and regular, and her temperature is 37°C. *Head:* Normocephalic without masses or evidence of trauma. *Ears:* Normal external ear canal with normal tympanic membranes bilaterally. *Eyes:* Pupils are equal and reactive to light and accommodation. Extraocular muscles are intact, and funduscopic examination is within normal limits, except for pale retinal backgrounds. The palpebral conjunctiva are also pale. *Nose:* Within normal limits, except pale nasal mucosa and evidence of old nasal mucosal bleeding. *Mouth:* Pale mucous membrane and a beefy red tongue that is KOH-negative. The remainder of the oropharynx is within normal limits. *Neck:* Supple without masses and no evidence of thyromegaly. There is no neck vein distension, and there is full range of motion of the neck. *Chest:* Clear to auscultation and percussion. *Breasts:* Symmetrical breasts with no evidence of masses, dimpling, nipple discharge, or tenderness. *Heart:* Regular rate and rhythm; S_1 and S_2 sounds are normal. There is a grade II/VI systolic ejection murmur heard best at the primary aortic area. Peripheral pulses are 2+ and palpable in all extremities. *Abdomen:* The contour of the abdomen is on plane and nontender. There is no organomegaly, and bowel sounds are normal. *Back:* Spine is midline and nontender to palpation. There is no paraspinal muscle tenderness, and Jean is able to bend and touch her toes without any difficulty, with the exception of some mild dizziness upon standing to a more erect position. *Pelvic:* Normal external genitalia. The vaginal mucosa is moist and pale. The cervix is parous and nonfriable. A Pap smear was obtained. A nodular, slightly enlarged uterus is present and is freely movable and nontender. No adnexal masses are noted. *Rectal:* Normal rectal sphincter tone. Stool is guaiac-positive. *Neurologic:* There is normal cerebral function. Jean demonstrates difficulty with tandem walking. There is good motor strength and function present. Sensory functions are intact, except decreased vibratory sensation distal to the midleg bilaterally and becoming more severe distally. *Skin:* No lesions, with the exception of skin pallor.

PHYSICAL EXAMINATION PROBLEM LIST

1. *Postural hypotension.* Consider decreased effective circulating volume caused by left ventricular dysfunction, absolute decrease in volume, decreased oncotic pressure, and/or decreased vascular tone.

2. *Skin pallor.* Consider decreased hemoglobin secondary to blood loss, decreased red blood cell production, or hemolysis at rates exceeding red blood cell production and the skin changes associated with hypothyroidism.

3. *Systolic ejection murmur* in primary aortic area. Consider valvular heart disease and high cardiac output state such as anemia and hyperthyroidism.

4. *Irregular uterine contour.* Consistent with history of uterine fibroids, but consider uterine malignancies.

5. *Decreased vibratory sensation* in distal lower extremities. Consider the possible presence of the peripheral neuropathy associated with diabetes mellitus and a deficiency of vitamin B_{12}.

6. *Heme-positive stools.* Consider the possibility of significant occult bleeding from the GI tract to include benign or malignant sources in both the lower and upper GI tract.

7. *Glossitis.* Consider chronic iron, B_{12}, and folate deficiencies as potential causes as well as candidiasis and other idiopathic causes.

Laboratory Tests. Diagnostic laboratory evaluation included measurement of the serum potassium level to determine whether or not Jean's fatigue was associated with hypokalemia in view of her use of a thiazide diuretic on a regular basis without potassium supplementation. The patient's pallor and fatigue prompted a CBC to evaluate for the presence of an anemia. A platelet count also was obtained to determine if the occult GI bleeding could be caused by a decrease in the quality and/or quantity of circulating platelets. A reticulocyte count was obtained to determine the body's response to what appeared physically to be an anemia. A serum glucose level was obtained to determine whether or not the fatigue was associated with the development of non-insulin-dependent diabetes mellitus, which also could account for the postural hypotension if polyuria and volume contraction associated with hyperglycemia had been present. Electrolytes studies were used to determine evidence of volume contraction associated with alterations in serum sodium concentration and the hypochloremic, hypokalemic metabolic alkalosis associated with excessive diuretic use. BUN and creatinine determinations would provide useful information about the presence of chronic renal disease or evidence of prerenal azotemia. Urinalysis would demonstrate the status of renal function, since urinary concentration after a water fast and the absence of protieunia would imply the lack of significant renal disease. Urinary sediment would provide information concerning the presence of urinary tract infection, renal calculi, and urinary tract malignancies. Because of Jean's age, an ECG would be beneficial to determine if she has subclinical organic heart disease. A chest x-ray would determine the presence or absence of atypical pneumonia and left ventricular dysfunction. A flexible sigmoidoscopic examination is essential to determine whether or not within the reach of the scope malignant or nonmalignant neoplasms or colitis are present that could account for the heme-positive stools. The presence of the hemoccult-positive stool in this setting also would dictate that not only should an endoscopic examination of the lower colon be performed but that the entire colon and upper GI tract should be studied to look for a bleeding source. Jean's fatigue prompted the evaluation of thyroid function to determine the presence of hypothyroidism or hyperthyroidism plus other endocrine disorders such as hypercalcemia.

RESULTS OF LABORATORY EVALUATION. WBC 2500, RBC 2.7, hemoglobin 7.0 mg/dl, hematocrit 21%, MCV 118 (normal 81–99 fL), MCH 33 (normal 27–31 pg/liter), MCHC 34 (normal 31.5–36 gm/dl), platelets 0.79 $\times$ 10⁵ (normal 1.50×10^5–4.0×10^5), corrected reticulocyte count 1.0. Peripheral blood smear revealed macrocytosis, hypersegmented neutrophils, and giant platelets.

CHEMISTRIES. Sodium 132 mEq/liter (normal 135–145), potassium 3.4 mEq/liter (normal 3.6–5.3), bicarbonate 27 mEq/liter (normal 24–32), chloride 105 mEq/liter (normal 100–110), BUN 13 mg/dl (normal 7–22), creatinine 1.9 mg/dl (normal 0.5–1.5), glucose 106 mg/dl (normal 60–110), calcium 8.1 mg/dl (normal 8.6–10.6), phosphorus 4.2 mg/dl (normal 2.6–4.8), CPK 75 μg/dl (normal 0–225), triglycerides 110 mg/dl (normal 30–150), cholesterol 211 mg/dl (normal 120–200), SGOT 72 U/liter (normal 0–40), LDH 4,722 U/liter (normal 100–200), serum iron 97 μg/dl, ferritin 120 ng/ml (normal 10–150), T_4 RIA 7 μg/dl (normal 5–9), and TSH 2.0 μU/ml (normal 0.015–6.2). *Urinalysis:* Urine specific gravity 1.30, urine pH 6.0, negative for glucose, nitrites, blood, and ketones. Urobilirubin was 1+, and urine sediment showed occasional RBCs and WBCs. Chest x-ray was within normal limits. Serum B_{12} and serum and RBC folate levels were drawn and sent to an outside laboratory.

LABORATORY PROBLEM LIST

1. *Macrocytic hypoproliferative anemia.* Consider folate deficiency secondary to decreased nutritional intake and all causes of vitamin B_{12} deficiency.

2. *Thrombocytopenia.* Consider causes of decreased platelet production and/or platelet destruction.

3. *Leukopenia.* Consider occult infection and other processes that can lead to WBC maturation arrest.

4. *Mild hyperbilirubinemia* and *2+ urobilinogen* on urinary dipstick. Consider intrinsic liver disease versus overproduction of heme degradation products secondary to increased RBC destruction.

5. *Heme-positive stools.* Consider bleeding from mucosal and benign, premalignant, and/or malignant GI tract neoplasms.

6. *Hyponatremia.* Consider appropriate ADH secretion in view of decreased effective circulating volume caused by chronic anemia.

7. *Hypokalemia* secondary to diuretic use without potassium supplementation.

8. *Elevated LDH.* Consider large cellular destruction secondary to hemolysis and hepatocellular disease.

9. *Elevated SGOT.* See number 8 above.

PLAN

A flexible sigmoidoscopy was scheduled, as well as an upper and lower GI tract fluoroscopy. Potassium elixir was started to replete body potassium stores. Jean is to return in 2 days for the results of pending laboratory studies and a flexible endoscopic examination with a 60-cm endoscope. Jean was asked to increase oral fluid intake. The diuretic was stopped temporarily to avoid exacerbation of postural hypotension.

SECOND VISIT (DAY 2)

SUBJECT

Jean returned to the office 48 hours later with persistent symptoms of fatigue but markedly decreased postural dizziness. Although Jean's physical assessment remained unchanged, she stated that she had been able to continue many of her routine activities at home.

OBJECTIVE

Physical assessment unchanged from initial evaluation of this problem. Flexible sigmoidoscopy performed after appropriate prep. The examination revealed inflamed internal hemorrhoids. B_{12} level returned to the office on the day of this visit, is 55 pg/liter (normal 180–900), serum folate is 9 ng/ml (normal >3), and RBC folate is 450 ng/ml (normal >300).

ASSESSMENT

1. *Hypoproliferative macrocytic anemia* secondary to B_{12} deficiency.
2. *Heme-positive stools* secondary to inflamed internal hemorrhoids, platelet dysfunction, or other GI tract lesions.
3. *Hypokalemia* caused by diuretic use without appropriate potassium repletion with KCl elixir.
4. *Cool extremities* potentially secondary to B_{12} deficiency–induced peripheral neuropathy.
5. *Unsteady gait* secondary to B_{12} deficiency–induced neuropathy, dorsal column signs, and/or volume contraction.

6. *Leukopenia* secondary to number 1 above.
7. *Thrombocytopenia* secondary to number 1 above.
8. *Elevated LDH* caused by ineffective erythropoiesis secondary to number 1 above.
9. *Elevated SGOT* caused by ineffective erythropoiesis secondary to number 1 above.
10. *Hyperbilirubinemia, mild hyperbilirubinea, and urobilinogen on urinalysis* caused by ineffective erythropoiesis secondary to number 1 above.
11. *Fatigue* potentially generated by number 1 above but must continue to consider multifactorial problems, especially the psychosocial ones.
12. *Hypertension* continuing to be well controlled.
13. *Inflamed internal hemorrhoids.*
14. *Glossitis* secondary to number 1 above.

PLAN

Therapeutic. Continue potassium repletion for Jean's hypokalemia until normokalemia ensues. Jean was instructed not to restart diuretic use until the results of the evaluation were complete. Jean received 1000 μg of B_{12} intramuscularly and was scheduled to receive another dose of B_{12} every 7 days for the next 2 weeks to replete B_{12} stores. Depending on the cause of the patient's B_{12} deficiency, a decision concerning long-term requirements of B_{12} repletion is to be made. If the B_{12} deficiency is secondary to pernicious anemia, B_{12} repletion will be required for life. If the B_{12} deficiency is secondary to a reversible problem with malabsorption, then B_{12} repletion may not be required continually. To determine the source of the B_{12} loss, Jean was scheduled to get a Shilling's test prior to the next appointment 1 week later. Jean also was instructed to increase dietary fiber and was started on stool softeners.

THIRD VISIT (DAY 10)

SUBJECTIVE

Jean returned with less exercise-induced fatigue after having received potassium repletion and the first loading dose of B_{12}. Jean also continued to drink increased amounts of fluids, and she did not restart her diuretic. She felt that her general sense of well-being had improved dramatically, and she was eating because she could taste her food.

OBJECTIVE

Physical examination is unchanged, except that postural blood pressure and pulse changes have resolved. Jean remains pale, and the decreased vibratory sensation in the lower extremities also remains. Jean is able to walk much better than during her last visit. Her tongue is not as red as it was initially.

Repeat CBC reveals a hemoglobin level of 8.1, with a corrected reticulocyte count of 16%, and WBC level of 4.0×10^3 and platelets of 1.72×10^5. Peripheral smear reveals hypersegment neutrophils, macrovalocytes, nucleated red blood cells, and shift cells.

Schilling's test was performed in the interim and revealed an abnormal Schilling's part I with a normal

Schilling's part II. Serum potassium determination performed during this office visit is 4.5.

ASSESSMENT

1. *Pernicious anemia*
2. *Peripheral neuropathy* secondary to pernicious anemia
3. *Hypokalemia,* resolved with potassium repletion
4. *Hypertension,* well controlled
5. *Fatigue,* more than likely secondary to number 1 above in large part but other causes of fatigue still sought, especially psychosocial ones
6. Effective circulating *volume depletion* secondary to overdiuresis, and anemia, symptomatologically improving

PLAN

Diagnostic. Jean was scheduled for an upper and lower GI series because of the presence of blood in her stool. Even though she has inflamed hemorrhoids, one must still evaluate the entire GI tract for signs of peptic ulcer disease, other mucosal lesions, and benign and malignant neoplasms. Jean's potassium repletion is continual, especially in view of the treatment of profound B_{12} deficiency anemia, which can make hypokalemia worse. Since her blood pressure is normal, it was elected to restart the diuretic on next office visit. Jean was scheduled for mammography in 1 month.

Disposition. In view of the historical, physical, and laboratory findings and the subsequent office visits of this 67-year-old white female, the following problems were noted:

1. Hyperproliferative macrocytic anemia secondary to B_{12} deficiency and lack of intrinsic factor (pernicious anemia)
2. Potassium deficiency secondary to kaluresis caused by hydrochlorothiazide without appropriate potassium supplementation
3. Hypertension under good control
4. Inflamed internal hemorrhoids
5. Heme-positive stool secondary to number 4 above, but must exclude other GI source of blood loss
6. Weight loss probably secondary to number 1 above
7. Fatigue secondary to numbers 1 and 2 above
8. Peripheral neuropathy secondary to number 1 above
9. Anorexia decreasing
10. Resolving glossitis
11. Decreased effective circulating volume secondary to anemia and overdiuresis improving

DISCUSSION

Fatigue is a frequent complaint of any primary care patient population, and although it can be the result of a multitude of factors, the most frequent cause is a psy-chogenic disorder such as depression or chronic anxiety.

Historical and physical findings suggestive of volume depletion raised the possibility that the utilization of a diuretic may have precipitated volume contraction associated with hypokalemia, accounting for both fatigue and postural hypotension. The finding of pallor and heme-positive stools increased the potential presence of an iron-deficiency anemia. The most common source of blood loss in patients this age is through the GI tract from mucosal and benign and malignant neoplasms. The fact that Jean had monthly withdrawal uterine bleeding was an additional source of blood loss.

However, the macrocytosis found on peripheral smears plus the hypersegmented neutrophils and the lack of reticulocytosis implies that Jean has an anemia that is probably caused by either B_{12} or folate deficiency. (See Table 20-54.) B_{12} deficiency appears to be the most likely cause of the presence of an unexplained distal peripheral neuropathy of recent onset. The presence of a megaloblastic anemia is confirmed by the presence of elevated levels of LDH, which signify ineffective erythropoiesis and intramedullary destruction of deformed blood cellular elements in the bone marrow. Further confirmation of a lack of iron deficiency is found by the presence of normal serum iron and ferritin levels, indicating appropriate body stores of iron. Although Jean had heme-positive stools, evidence suggests that GI

TABLE 20–54. CAUSES OF ANEMIA BASED ON BONE MARROW RESPONSE

I. Hypoproliferative bone marrow (decreased reticulocyte count)
   A. Microcytic hypochromic anemias
      1. Iron deficiency
      2. Thalassemias
      3. Sideroblastic anemia
      4. Chronic lead poisoning
   B. Macrocytic anemias
      1. Folate deficiency
      2. Vitamin B_{12} deficiency
      3. Chemotherapy with folate antagonist
   C. Normochromic normocytic anemias
      1. Anemia of chronic renal disease
      2. Anemia of chronic disease
      3. Anemia of chronic liver disease
      4. Anemia of myxedema
      5. Other causes of bone marrow failure

II. Hyperproliferative bone marrow (increased reticulocyte count)
   A. Acute hemorrhage
   B. Hemolytic anemias
      1. Enzymopathies (e.g., G-6-PD deficiency)
      2. Abnormal hemoglobin (e.g., sickle cell disease and hemoglobin C disease)
      3. Red blood cell membrane defect (e.g., hereditary sperocytosis)
      4. Increased nonimmune red blood cell environmental stress (e.g., traumatic hemolytic anemias such as March hemoglobinuria, anemia secondary to artificial heart valve and microangiopathic hemolytic anemia, malaria, clostridial infection)
      5. Increased immune environmental stress (e.g., immunohemolytic anemias with position Coombs' testing)

tract bleeding could not account for a significant part of this anemia. The definitive diagnosis was based on the low level of serum B_{12} and the normal level of serum folate, which implied that the megaloblastic process observed was secondary to B_{12} deficiency. (See Table 20-55.) Once the B_{12} deficiency was established as the cause of the megaloblastic anemia, it was then necessary to determine the cause of the lack of B_{12} stores by performing a Schilling's test. If the Schilling's test part I is abnormal and the replacement of intrinsic factor corrects the abnormality of B_{12} urinary excretion, then one must assume that the cause of the B_{12} deficiency is intrinsic factor deficiency or pernicious anemia. If intrinsic factor does not correct the abnormality, then the B_{12} deficiency is caused by intestinal absorption problems, such as blind loop syndrome, intestinal bacterial overgrowth, and other intestinal malabsorption syndromes. Part III of the Schilling's test requires the administration of antibiotics to remove bacteria as a source of competition for B_{12} absorption in the gut, and repeat of the Schilling's test then should be normal.

In this case, the most common cause of B_{12} deficiency is pernicious anemia. Because B_{12} is enterohepatically recirculated, it is unlikely that a patient will develop B_{12} deficiency merely because of dietary restriction of meat, milk, and milk products. Certain diseases of the terminal ileum caused either by surgical reconstruction or inflammatory bowel disease can remove or disrupt the

ileal reabsorptive sites of B_{12}–intrinsic factor complex. There also could be competition for intestinal B_{12} such as fish, tape worm infestation, and bacterial overgrowth that occurs in blind loop syndromes. There are certain drugs that interfere with absorption of B_{12}, such as alcohol, and some rare causes of B_{12} deficiency, such as transcolbalamine deficiency.

This patient also was reported to have persistently cold feet, which appeared not to be affected by changes in environmental temperature. Often patients will describe the sensation of neuropathy associated with diabetes and B_{12} deficiency as lower extremity coolness as opposed to numbness. This patient's neurologic problems helped differentiate the B_{12} deficiency from folate deficiency as a cause of the megaloblastic anemia.

The most common cause of folate deficiency is a lack of dietary intake, and this is usually seen in patients with extremely poor caloric intake of weeks' to months' duration. There is no way to distinguish the bone marrow pathology associated with B_{12} deficiency from that seen with folate deficiency. Megaloblastic disorders show anisocytosis and poikilocytosis with macrovalocytes. The neutrophils are usually hypersegmented, with an average neutrophil laboratory count of greater than 3.5. The presence of a neutrophil with 6 or more lobes would be indicative of megaloblastosis. In megaloblastic anemia secondary to folic acid deficiency, it would be necessary to measure RBC folic acid levels to ensure that there has been a chronic depression in the body's folate stores, since serum folate levels tend to fluctuate significantly with dietary lack or intake of folate sources. Also associated with ineffective erythropoiesis seen in megaloblastic anemias are elevated levels of bilirubin, increased serum iron, and elevated LDH levels. In pernicious anemia, patients usually have achlorhydria and a low reticulocyte index (a hyperproliferative anemia). There also may be antibodies directed against gastric mucosal cells and intrinsic factor as well as antithyroid antibodies.

Treatment required for B_{12} deficiency caused by pernicious anemia is 1000 μg of B_{12} intramuscularly every 7 days for 3 weeks and then 100 μg intramuscularly monthly for the rest of the patient's life. There are situations where there is a combination of B_{12} and folate deficiency. In these situations, folate deficiency should not be corrected until the B_{12} deficiency has been treated. Folic acid replacement with therapeutic dosages of folate prior to B_{12} deficiency treatment can exacerbate the neurologic manifestations of the B_{12}-induced neuropathies. Once B_{12} has been given, there is rapid reticulocytosis that peaks in about a week. The appearance of the bone marrow usually reverses in about 3 to 4 days from the characteristic megaloblastic picture to a hyperproliferative state. There is marked reticulocytosis in 3 to 7 days, with the appearance of nucleated RBCs and shift cells on peripheral smear. Platelet count also returns to normal during this time.

It also should be noted that B_{12} deficiency may be present without macrocytosis, hypersegmentation, and anemia, especially in elderly patients. The B_{12} deficiency is usually discovered as a part of routine evaluation of

TABLE 20–55. CAUSES OF MEGALOBLASTIC ANEMIA

I. B_{12} deficiency
  A. Inadequate B_{12} intake (e.g., strict vegetarians)
  B. B_{12} malabsorption
    1. Pernicious anemia (intrinsic factor deficiency)
    2. Total or partial gastrectomy
    3. Intestinal disorder
      a. Ileal resection
      b. Tropical and nontropical sprue
      c. Regional enteritis
  C. Competition for B_{12}
    1. Fish, tape worm infestation
    2. Bacterial overgrowth and blind loop syndrome
II. Folic deficiency
  A. Inadequate intake (e.g., inadequate diet secondary to old age, senility, chronic disease states, alcoholism, and fad diets)
  B. Malabsorption
    1. Tropical and nontropical sprue
    2. Drugs such as phenytoin, barbiturates, and ethanol
  C. Increased demand
    1. Pregnancy and lactation
    2. Infancy, especially prematurity
    3. Chronic hemolytic anemias
    4. Hemodialysis
  D. Drugs that interfere with folate utilization
    1. Folate antagonist (e.g., methyltrexate)
    2. Alcohol
III. Non–B_{12} or folate deficiency causes of megaloblastic anemia
  A. Hemopoietic malignancies
  B. Drugs that interfere with DNA synthesis (e.g., 5-fluorouracil)
  C. Megaloblastic anemias of unknown etiology

mental status change. This particular patient would not have required a transfusion to treat her anemia unless she had worsening angina, ischemic changes, or cardiac decompensation.

QUESTIONS

1. A 16-year-old previously healthy black male sustained an ankle injury while playing competitive high school basketball. After the injury, he received an ice pack and, as it was later discovered, an aspirin-containing compound provided by the basketball coach. Later that evening the student became unexplainably weak, and his parents noted that his eyes appeared "a little yellow." After 24 hours, the weakness persisted, and the parents became more alarmed because his eyes became progressively more yellow. On presentation to the family physician, the patient was found to have a Hgb of 8.5 gm/dl and a corrected reticulocyte count of 7.5%. Which of the following microscopic red blood cell findings would be most likely in this clinical case?

   a. Severe microcytosis
   b. Sickle cells
   c. Burr cells
   d. Heinz bodies
   e. All the above

2. If this young patient had an immediate screening test for the suspected red blood cell disorder described in question 1, which of the following findings would you anticipate to be present?

   a. Increased LDH levels
   b. Decreased folate levels
   c. Increased red blood cell fragility
   d. Positive G-6-PD screen
   e. Positive sickle-cell screen

3. A 72-year-old white female patient presents because of progressive difficulty with ambulation, leg pain, and forgetfulness over the last year and a half. Initial evaluation reveals decreased lower extremity vibratory sensation, an abnormal gait, and an ane-

mia characterized by an MCV of 120, hematocrit of 21%, LDH of 1637 units with hypersegmented neutrophils, WBC count of 1.7, and platelet count of 84,000. Which of the following best explains this presentation?

   a. Iron-deficiency anemia
   b. Folate deficiency
   c. Vitamin B_{12} deficiency
   d. Hereditary spherocytosis
   e. Bone marrow failure

4. A patient with an anemia, a low serum B_{12} level, and decreased urinary excretion of orally administered radioactive B_{12} did not have an increased urinary excretion of radioactive B_{12} when given intrinsic factor. These findings would be most likely secondary to which of the following?

   a. Intrinsic factor deficit
   b. B_{12} deficiency secondary to lack of dietary intake in a pure vegan
   c. Inflammatory bowel disease
   d. Status postgastrectomy without IM administration of monthly B_{12}

5. A 52-year-old white female reports with a 4-month history of progressive fatigue. Her physical evaluations during this time revealed no abnormalities. The patient's past medical history includes a hysterectomy for fibroids and dysfunctional bleeding 10 years prior to this presentation. The patient's laboratory results reveal a microcytic, hypochromic anemia with absence of significant reticulocytosis. Serum iron levels are depressed, and the ferritin level is also depressed. The patient has had a negative hemoccult test on three separate occasions. Which of the following should be included in the evaluation of this patient's anemia?

   a. A full workup for an occult GI source of blood loss
   b. Repeat hemoccult testing
   c. Therapeutic iron replacement for 3 to 4 months with mandatory follow-up
   d. Coombs' test

Answers appear on page 452.

Vomiting and Low Back Pain

DANIEL J. DERKSEN and HARRY E. MAYHEW

INITIAL VISIT

SUBJECTIVE

Patient Identification and Presenting Problem. Sally C. is a 60-year-old Hispanic female who presents to the Family Practice Center complaining that "I've been sick for 2 days." Her complaints include "a bad cold" associated with nausea, vomiting, low back pain, trouble breathing, chills, and fever.

Present Illness. Other than controlled hypertension, Sally had been well until 2 days prior to her office visit. Her illness started with severe bilateral low back pain associated with nausea, vomiting, and fever. The back pain improved but did not completely resolve. Sally became worried when she discovered that her temperature the morning of her office visit was 104.6°F. She also was concerned because she had shaking chills, was urinating less frequently than normal, and the urine had a foul odor.

Sally had not noticed any pain with urination or hematuria. She could not remember any back trauma or intense physical exertion prior to the present illness. Her bowel movements were normal. She was anorexic, and when she tried to eat, she vomited after intake of both solids and liquids.

Past Medical History. Sally has been a patient in the Family Practice Center for 1½ years. During this time, she has been treated for hypertension, which was diagnosed 5 years ago. Four months ago her treatment was changed from hydrochlorothiazide to verapamil, a calcium-channel blocker, to better control her hypertension and to correct hypokalemia. She has been on estrogen replacement since her hysterectomy and bilateral salpingo-oopherectomy 6 years ago for "heavy bleeding." Other surgeries include a cholecystectomy for cholelithiasis with incidental appendectomy 5 years ago. Eight years ago she had a stone in the left kidney that required surgical removal.

Family History. There is no family history of diabetes, myocardial infarction, kidney disease, hypertension, or breast cancer. Sally's mother is still living, at age 81, and is in good health. Her father died a few years ago at age 78 of "natural causes."

Social History. A few years ago Sally was divorced. Presently she lives with her 30-year-old mentally retarded daughter and relies on a small alimony payment and her daughter's disability income. She owns her house and her car. Since her divorce, Sally has not been sexually active.

Health Habits. Sally has never smoked, rarely drinks alcoholic beverages, and denies the use of any illicit drugs. She eats a diet high in saturated fat and cholesterol. During a typical week she eats six to eight eggs, beans cooked in lard, cheese, whole milk, pork, green chiles, tortillas fried in animal fat, and fried red meat. However, her last cholesterol test 3 months ago was normal. Sally rarely exercises. Her Pap smear and mammogram were normal less than 1 year ago. She could not remember when her last tetanus shot had been given.

Review of Systems. Sally has not lost any significant amount of weight over the last year. Since her present illness, she felt a little lightheaded when she stood up suddenly. She has not experienced any abdominal pain, nor has she noticed any blood or black, tarry stools. She has no known allergies and is not taking any over-the-counter medications or vitamin or mineral supplements.

OBJECTIVE

Physical Examination. Sally's vital signs are as follows: temperature is 101.5°F; respiratory rate is 22; pulse is 92; blood pressure is 110/80; there are no orthostatic changes in pulse and blood pressure; and her weight is 65 kg. *General:* Sally looks tired but is alert and seems to be a reliable historian. She is in mild to moderate distress with her back pain. *Mouth:* Dry mucous membranes. *Lungs:* Clear to auscultation and percussion. *CVS:* The heart PMI is not displaced; the rate and rhythm are normal; there is a grade II/VI early systolic murmur heard best in the supine position in the lower left sternal border, but the murmur does not radiate. *Abdomen:* A midline scar in the lower abdomen and a scar in the right upper quadrant are noted. Bowel sounds are present but diminished. The abdomen is soft and nontender. The liver and spleen are of normal size, and the kidneys are not palpable. *Back:* There is mild to moderate left CVA tenderness to fist percussion, normal range of motion. *Extremities:* Sally's two-point discrimination, vibratory sense, and deep tendon reflexes are normal. The peripheral pulses are also normal. *Breasts:* No masses palpated. *Pelvic:* No external lesions are noted. The vagina is atrophic, and no cervix is visible. The uterus and ovaries are not palpable. There are no adnexal masses, and the pelvic support is good without evidence of cystocele. *Rectal:* No masses. The stool is negative for occult blood.

ASSESSMENT

Working Diagnoses. Several possible diagnoses could explain Sally's symptoms:

1. *Urinary tract infection.* Sally's history of fever, malaise, back pain, nausea and vomiting, shaking chills, decreased urination, and foul-smelling urine is suggestive of an infection of the upper urinary tract. Sally's risk fac-

tors include her age (postmenopausal) and her history of surgery for a kidney stone.

2. *Nephrolithiasis.* Sally's history and physical examination are also suggestive of a stone in the upper urinary tract. The costovertebral angle tenderness to fist percussion on the left, fever, past history of nephrolithiasis, nausea and vomiting, shaking chills, and foul-smelling urine suggest that a stone and a secondary infection might be present.

The nausea and vomiting and the physical examination finding of diminished bowel sounds suggest that the stone(s) may be obstructing the upper urinary tract and causing gastric and small bowel ileus. Sally's history of a temperature to 104.6°F at home is of concern.

Differential Diagnoses

1. *Lower urinary tract infection.* This seems less likely because Sally does not complain of pain or burning during urination, frequency, or urgency. In addition, the patient reported a temperature to 104.6°F at home—a high fever is uncommon in lower urinary tract infections.

2. *Lower urinary tract stone (ureterolithiasis).* Sally's presentation makes this diagnosis unlikely. Her pain was vague, in the lower back with mild to moderate CVA tenderness. Ureterolithiasis more often presents as excruciating pain radiating from the flank down to the labia, scrotum, or inner thigh in association with diaphoresis and the patient having difficulty finding a comfortable position.

3. *Musculoskeletal injury.* Without a history of extreme exertion, heavy lifting, or trauma, this diagnosis seems unlikely. The associated findings of fever, shaking chills, and a foul-smelling urine do not support this diagnosis.

4. *Pancreatitis.* While Sally's history of nausea, vomiting, and back pain might suggest this diagnosis, foul-smelling urine, fever and chills, history of nephrolithiasis, and lack of epigastric tenderness point to the genitourinary tract rather than the pancreas. However, a common bile duct stone with pancreatic inflammation is a consideration in a patient with a history of cholelithiasis and this symptom complex.

5. *Gastrointestinal tract problem.* The diminished bowel sounds, nausea, vomiting, fever and chills, and back pain could be consistent with an acute abdominal process. However, Sally's past medical history reveals that she had an appendectomy and a cholecystectomy in the past. Diverticulitis or gastrointestinal tract cancer must be considered, but the stool is negative for blood and Sally has no weight loss, history of melena, change in caliber of stool, or bright red blood per rectum. No masses are palpated on rectal or abdominal examination. Also, Sally has no abdominal tenderness or guarding.

6. *Pelvic inflammatory disease.* This is very unlikely considering Sally's history of hysterectomy and salpingo-oophorectomy, age, and lack of sexual activity.

7. *Urinary tract tuberculosis.* This is a rare disease that is unlikely in this patient because of the acuity of the presentation and high-grade temperature.

8. *Mesenteric infarction.* Usually, infarction presents more suddenly, with rapid decline and death without surgical intervention. The time course (2 days), lack of peritoneal findings (rebound, guarding, or rigidity), and absence of blood in the stool make this diagnosis unlikely.

PLAN

Patient Education. Sally was told that she needed to be admitted to the hospital for treatment of her kidney infection and for further tests to determine if she had developed another kidney stone. While she realized that she was seriously ill, she was extremely concerned about who would pick up her retarded daughter from the day-care facility and care for her at home. Her anxiety was considerably decreased when Sally's sister was reached by telephone and agreed to care for her niece during the hospitalization. Sally demonstrated an understanding that the type of infection she had required treatment with parenteral antibiotics. She also realized the possibility of another kidney stone.

Diagnostic

1. Urinalysis with culture (catheterized specimen); CBC with differential; determination of electrolytes, amylase, lipase, BUN, and creatinine; and a plain film of the abdomen.

2. Renal ultrasound. A renal ultrasound could help determine if obstruction of the upper urinary tract had occurred by detecting the presence of hydronephrosis. In addition, a better localization of the stone in the urinary tract can be ascertained.

3. Intravenous pyelogram (IVP). An IVP is often used in the workup of a patient with a suspected stone, but the history of decreased urine output, evidence of dehydration, the possibility of pyelonephritis, and obstruction make renal ultrasound a reasonable alternative with fewer possible complications.

Therapeutic

1. Admission. Sally's problem required hospital admission because of the possibility of two emergency conditions: pyelonephritis and obstructive nephrolithiasis. In addition, Sally was not able to take oral fluids or medications.

2. Culture. Appropriate cultures were obtained prior to treatment and included cultures of the urine (catheterized specimen) and blood to check for sepsis.

3. Intravenous administration of antibiotics. Because of Sally's inability to take liquids or solids by mouth and the difficulty obtaining serum concentrations of antibiotic sufficient to treat pyelonephritis by oral antibiotics, IV administration of antibiotics was ordered. Ampicillin and an aminoglycoside were chosen to cover the most likely organisms in pyelonephritis. Ampicillin 1 gm every 6 hours IV and a loading dose of gentamicin equal to 2 mg/kg IV (65 kg $\times$ 2 mg/kg = 130 mg gentamicin) were given. Sally was put on a maintenance dose of 3 mg/kg IV gentamicin (65 kg $\times$ 3 mg/kg = 195 mg $\div$ 3 = 65 mg every 8 hours) to begin 8 hours after the loading dose. Peak (6–8) and trough

(<2) gentamicin levels were ordered to be drawn 30 minutes before and 30 minutes after administration of the third dose of gentamicin. In addition, Sally's creatinine would be followed closely while she received gentamicin.

4. Intravenous hydration. The nausea, vomiting, and evidence of mild dehydration on examination (dry mucous membranes) make IV fluid for maintenance necessary. Sally was designated NPO except sips of water or chips of ice and started on D_5NS with 30 mEq KCl per liter at 150 cc/h. Urine output, daily weight, and electrolyte determinations were ordered.

5. Renal ultrasound. Because of the severity of the illness and the possibility of obstruction of the upper urinary tract, an emergency renal ultrasound was ordered.

6. Treatment of chronic conditions. Sally's estrogen (0.625 mg daily) and verapamil sustained release (240 mg daily) were discontinued until she could take medication by mouth. Vital signs, including blood pressure, were ordered to be checked every 4 hours.

FIRST FOLLOW-UP VISIT (LATER IN THE DAY IN THE HOSPITAL)

SUBJECTIVE

Sally reports that she "feels about the same."

OBJECTIVE

Physical Examination. The physical examination is unchanged from the outpatient examination 4 hours previously. Sally is still febrile (102.5°F) and has moderate CVA tenderness and diminished bowel sounds.

Laboratory Tests. The results of the laboratory tests are as follows: sodium 128 (normal 135–145 mEq/liter), potassium 2.8 (normal 3.5–5.0 mEq/liter), chloride 93 (normal 100–110 mEq/liter), CO_2 25 (normal 25–30 mEq/liter), Cr 0.6 (normal 0.8–1.2 mg/dl), BUN 13 (normal 10–25 mg/dl), glucose 108 (normal 80–130 mg/dl), WBC 20.0 (normal 5–11 X10E3), Hct 38.4 (normal 37–47 gm/dl), neutrophils 85 (normal 31–71%), bands 1, lymphocytes 9.7 (normal 15–50%), amylase 37 (normal 23–115 IU/liter), lipase 54 (normal 46–208 IU/liter), urine sodium < 15, and urine osmolality 314. The chest x-ray (PA/LAT) is normal. The abdominal film shows calcified densities within the kidney outline on the left. The ECG shows evidence of left ventricular hypertrophy and nonspecific ST-T wave changes. *Urinalysis:* Specific gravity 1.020, +LCE, RBCs and WBCs too numerous to count. The renal ultrasound was reviewed with the radiologist. The left kidney was enlarged and showed evidence of three to four stones (0.5–2.2 cm) in the calyx with marked hydronephrosis of the left ureter. The right kidney was normal.

ASSESSMENT

The working diagnoses were correct—hydronephrosis due to ureteral obstruction secondary to nephrolithiasis. The patient's urinalysis, elevated WBC count, fever, and chills suggest a complicating pyelonephritis.

PLAN

Therapeutic

1. Evidence of obstruction on the renal ultrasound with associated pyelonephritis necessitated immediate urologic consultation and intervention.

2. Co-management with the urologist. The urologist recommended immediate placement of a nephrostomy tube to relieve the obstruction and continued treatment with IV antibiotics until Sally was medically stable. When the WBC count, fever, pain, and electrolyte abnormalities were corrected, the urologist would then perform percutaneous removal of the stones. Since one of the stones was greater than 2 cm in size and multiple stones were present, percutaneous removal was chosen over extracorporeal shock-wave lithotripsy (ESWL). Sally agreed with the recommendations.

Disposition. Sally underwent placement of a nephrostomy tube that evening. Once the tube was placed, pus was drained from the left renal calyx. Within 48 hours of nephrostomy tube placement and treatment with IV antibiotics, Sally defervesced and felt better. Her WBC count and electrolyte abnormalities returned to normal with IV hydration, replacement of sodium and potassium, and parenteral antibiotics. Sally was taken back to the operating room, and multiple, small stones were removed by percutaneous extraction through the nephrostomy site. The stones were sent for analysis. Two days later a nephrostogram was done, revealing no evidence of residual stones. The nephrostomy tube was clamped and then removed the next day. Urine culture done the day of admission grew out 10^5 *E. coli* sensitive to ampicillin. Sally was discharged on PO antibiotics (ampicillin) and did well postoperatively. She was seen frequently in the postoperative period, including visits 2 days and 2 weeks after discharge to have a follow-up urine cultures. Sally returned 4 weeks later to obtain a 24-hour urine collection. The specimen was sent for analysis, including calcium, citrate, oxalate, uric acid, and creatinine, to determine renal function, to decide whether further metabolic workup would be necessary, and to better advise Sally on how to prevent further stone formation.

DISCUSSION

Upper urinary tract stones are encountered commonly in Western countries. In the United States, calcium oxalate and calcium phosphate are the stones most frequently found, especially in the arid Southwest. While nephrolithiasis affects less than 1% of the population, the recurrence rate is quite high in patient's with a history of a previous stone (50%–80%). Since more than 80% of the stones contain calcium, most are visible on a plain film of the abdomen.

The pathogenesis of nephrolithiasis may be related to hypercalciuria. The cause of hypercalciuria may be excess absorption from the gut or excess leak of calcium from the renal tubules. Other causes of hypercalciuria include hypervitaminosis D, type I renal tubular acidosis, prolonged immobilization, drugs such as acetazolamide, sarcoidosis, or excess resorption of calcium from bone due to a parathyroid adenoma.

Patients suspected of a stone need a rapid assessment, including location of the stone, the degree of obstruction, determination of whether infection is present, and assessment of renal function. Stones greater than 6 mm in size are unlikely to be passed spontaneously. Evidence of obstruction or upper urinary tract infection (pyelonephritis) are emergency conditions that require immediate attention, including IV antibiotics and removal of the stone. Removal of the stone can be undertaken percutaneously with a grasping instrument or basket (percutaneous nephrolithostomy), by extracorporeal shock-wave lithotripsy (ESWL), or stone dissolution (alkalinizing the urine in patients with uric acid stones).

The most important issues to consider in the management of patients with urolithiasis include the following:

1. Stone analysis is important in all patients with urolithiasis.

2. Medical prevention of stones is important to reduce recurrence.

3. Spontaneous passage of ureteral stones is optimal (if possible).

4. Increased hydration is important in managing and preventing urolithiasis.

5. ESWL is effective for stones less than 2 cm in diameter.

    (a) Medical follow-up is necessary after ESWL treatment.

    (b) ESWL does not replace medical prevention.

    (c) ESWL can be used in combination with the percutaneous technique.

    (d) For asymptomatic stones less than 0.5 cm diameter, ESWL is controversial.

SUGGESTED READING

Frank SH, Resnick MI. Urolithiasis in primary care. Primary Care 1989; 16(4):967–979.

Jacobson EJ, Fuchs G. Nephrolithiasis. Am Fam Physician 1989; 39(3):233–245.

NIH Consensus Development Conference in the Prevention and Treatment of Kidney Stones. J Urol 1989; 141:705–808.

Selman SH, Mayhew HE. Urinary tract disorders. In Rakel RE (ed.): Textbook of Family Practice, 4th ed. Philadelphia, W.B. Saunders, 1990, pp. 1353, 1364–1367.

QUESTIONS

1. Management of a 32-year-old male with a symptomatic kidney stone 1.2 cm in size would include all the following *except*
   a. Extracorporeal shock-wave lithotripsy (ESWL).
   b. Oral hydration to obtain a urine output of more than 2 liters per day.
   c. Percutaneous removal of the stone.
   d. A 24-hour urine 4 weeks after the episode for calcium, oxatate, citrate, uric acid, and creatinine.
   e. IVP to assess for evidence of obstruction.

2. Which of the following are true concerning kidney stones?
   a. They are experienced by a majority of the population at some point during their life.
   b. Their assessment includes plain film of the abdomen because the stones can be seen on the x-ray most of the time.
   c. They are most often the result of an excess absorption of calcium from the gut.
   d. They can pass spontaneously if they are less than 5 mm in size.

3. Which symptom is not associated with uncomplicated passage of a kidney stone?
   a. Vomiting
   b. Hematuria
   c. Fever
   d. Back/flank pain
   e. Abdominal distension

4. Match the following.
   a. IVP
   b. Ultrasound
   c. Both
   d. Neither
       (1) Should be avoided in renal failure
       (2) Should be avoided in a dehydrated, elderly patient
       (3) Localizes kidney stones
       (4) Associated with allergic reactions

Answers appear on page 452.

Blurred Vision

ALEXANDER BERGER and EARL R. CROUCH, Jr.

INITIAL VISIT

SUBJECTIVE

Patient Identification.   Beatrice, a 43-year-old black woman, works as a cook at a local restaurant, a position she has held for the past 10 years. She is divorced and the mother of two grown children. She lives with her mother, who is a 64-year-old diabetic.

Presenting Problem.   Beatrice awoke this morning with pain behind her left eye and severe double vision with both eyes open. The diplopia is moderately disabling and is associated with dizziness and nausea. She wears a patch on her left eye in order to drive her car.

Past Medical History.   Beatrice is an insulin-dependent diabetic of 18 years' duration who manages to control her diabetes by repeated daily Accu-Check examinations and split doses of Humulin N and Humulin R insulin.

Beatrice had an episode of severe shortness of breath and orthopnea 6 months ago, at which time she was hospitalized for acute pulmonary edema. Her cardiovascular investigation demonstrated a normal-sized heart with ejection fraction of 55 but considerable thickening of her left ventricular wall, which was interpreted as diastolic congestive heart failure. She was started on Cardizem and Capoten for her cardiac disease, as well as Lasix 40 mg PO every other day.

Beatrice had hypertension of 12 years' duration that was well controlled prior to her congestive heart failure with Maxzide. The Maxzide was discontinued when Beatrice was started on Cardizem, Capoten, and Lasix. Her blood pressure remained in good control.

Because of the combination of diabetes, hypertension, truncal obesity, striae, and hirsutism, workup for adrenal hyperplasia (Cushing's syndrome) was undertaken. Evaluation was negative.

Beatrice's ophthalmic history included intermittent blurred vision until 5 years ago when she managed to bring her diabetes under better control. Over the last 12 months, Beatrice has noticed some blurred vision in her left eye.

Family History.   Beatrice's mother, age 64, is an obese, non-insulin-dependent diabetic with "heart trouble and kidney trouble." Beatrice never knew her father and has no siblings.

Health Habits.   Beatrice does not smoke and denies drinking alcohol. She adheres to a 1500-calorie ADA diet and maintains her weight at about 155 lb despite the fact that she does not exercise.

Review of Systems.   Prior to the onset of the present illness, Beatrice claims to have been doing quite well.

She denies chest pain but continues to have shortness of breath upon exertion. She denies orthopnea and paroxysmal nocturnal dyspnea since her treatment for diastolic congestive heart failure 6 months ago. Symptoms relating to her eyes, prior to the onset of her present illness, include blurred vision in her left eye for a period of approximately 1 year and "floaters" in both eyes that have worsened over the past couple of years. Pertinent negatives include no redness of either eye and no ocular pain. Beatrice has not had an ophthalmologic evaluation for the last 5 years although repeatedly advised to do so.

Beatrice complains of nocturnal pain in both legs and some paresthesias of her feet. She has lightheadedness that lasts for a few seconds when she gets up rapidly from a supine position.

OBJECTIVE

Physical Examination.   Beatrice appears noticeably upset and distraught, and her left eye is covered by a patch. Her vital signs are as follows: blood pressure 180/105, pulse 96 and regular, temperature 98.6°F, and respirations 22. Cardiac examination demonstrates an S_4 gallop, unchanged from previous examinations. Lungs are clear, and the abdomen is unremarkable. *Eyes:*   Approximately 3 mm of ptosis is noted in the left upper lid. Motility evaluation reveals that the left eye is deviated outward, or exotropic. It cannot be adducted, depressed, or elevated. The only major movement is in the abducted position outward. Extraocular movements of the right eye are normal. Pupils are equal and reactive to light and accommodation. Central vision in the right eye is 20/30; central vision in the left eye is 20/200. Gross examination of the peripheral vision using moving fingers seems to indicate normal visual fields in both eyes. There is no inflammation of either the conjunctival or ciliary vessels in either eye. The lens and vitreous are clear. Ophthalmoscopic examination using Mydriacyl 1% to dilate the pupils reveals bilateral microaneurysms and definite neovascularization around the right disc. The left eye shows macular hard exudates and scattered hard exudates of the fundus. Of note is the fact that during the examination of the eyes, one eye has to be covered in order to avoid attacks of vertigo and nausea.

ASSESSMENT

Working Diagnoses

1.   *Left exotropia and paresis of the extraocular muscles* secondary to diabetic 3rd nerve palsy
2.   *Diabetic retinopathy*

Differential Diagnoses

1.   A *posterior communicating artery aneurysm* most frequently arises at the artery's junction with the internal carotid. This is the most common cause of spontaneous acute 3rd nerve palsy with pupil involvement. Injury to

the oculomotor nerve is produced by the aneurysmal distension coupled with intraneural hemorrhage. Generally, the pupil is fixed and dilated. This is differentiated from patients with diabetic 3rd nerve palsies where the pupil is generally spared. Pain is common in almost 100% of cases and is the initial symptom in 90%. Aberrant regeneration of the 3rd nerve usually occurs. In diabetic 3rd nerve palsy, pain occurs in 50% of patients, and the pupil is spared in between 70% and 90% of patients. The diagnosis can be confirmed with CT scan and angiography.

2. *Traumatic basal skull fracture with 3rd nerve entrapment.* The 3rd nerve is less frequently injured in direct closed-head trauma than the 4th or 6th nerve. Traumatic basilar skull fractures may be associated with "blowout" fractures of the floor of the orbit. Entrapment of extraocular muscles (generally the inferior rectus) may be associated with this fracture. Other manifestations of basilar skull fractures may be rhinorrhea (drainage of CSF through the nose) or bleeding from the ear or behind the tympanic membrane. Generally, with basilar skull fractures, patients have had an episode of unconsciousness. Diagnosis can be made by history and confirmed by skull x-rays and CT scan.

3. *Cavernous sinus thrombosis* can occur with an inflammatory process, a granulomatous inflammation of the cavernous sinus, tumor, or aneurysm. If tumor is the etiology, the patient has a slowly progressive partial 3rd nerve palsy with diplopia and ptosis. Patients with aneurysms generally have periocular pain or vision loss. Skull films are abnormal in over 50% of patients. The CT scan is abnormal in virtually all patients with meningiomas and aneurysms.

4. *Intracavernous tumors.* Meningiomas are the most common intracavernous tumor. Generally, the patient has slowly progressive 3rd nerve palsy including diplopia, ptosis, and paresthesia of the scalp. Patients do not have periocular pain or vision loss. Diagnosis can be confirmed by skull films and CT scan.

5. *Demyelinating diseases such as multiple sclerosis.* Rarely, multiple sclerosis may present as a 3rd nerve palsy. More frequently, the 6th nerve is involved. Patients may present with transient attacks of diplopia as the initial symptom. More frequently, patients with multiple sclerosis will present with papillitis or retrobulbar neuritis. No single test establishes the diagnosis of multiple sclerosis. However, on CSF examination there is an elevation of IgG and an elevation of the IgG/albumin index. In addition, there is a presence of oligoclonal IgG bands. CT scan may be helpful in diagnosing acute multiple sclerosis, but this is generally more evident in more advanced cases.

PLAN

Beatrice has demonstrated several complications relating to her diabetes mellitus: Early on in her disease she described intermittent blurred vision that was most likely related to intermittent swelling of the lens resulting from fluctuations in blood sugar levels and changes in the lens's osmolarity related to deposition of sorbitol. At the time she presented to the office, she had a typical diabetic 3rd nerve paralysis, a very distressing symptom, but one with a generally favorable long-term prognosis.

Of much more concern were the eyeground findings, which suggested an advanced form of nonproliferative retinopathy with some evidence of proliferative changes. These changes, far more than the distressing 3rd nerve paralysis, require an urgent referral to an ophthalmologist. The need for laser intervention and the timing of such intervention and follow-up will be determined by the ophthalmologist.

DISCUSSION

Diabetic 3rd nerve palsy is a common occurrence in diabetics. A sudden onset of diplopia, caused by paresis of an extraocular muscle, may be the presenting sign and is due to infarction of the nerve. When the 3rd nerve is involved, pain may be a prominent symptom. Acquired 3rd nerve paralysis may be partial or complete. The pupil is not usually involved in 3rd nerve palsies that occur with diabetes mellitus. The pupil is involved generally with aneurysms of the posterior communicating artery. Acquired 3rd nerve palsy occurs rapidly with full involvement. Recovery is usually complete 6 months after onset. Many conditions can cause an acquired 3rd nerve palsy, including brainstem lesions, inflammatory conditions such as meningitis or polyneuritis, vascular lesions including aneurysm of the posterior communicating artery, intracranial tumors, demyelinating diseases such as multiple sclerosis, and trauma.

Treatment generally involves relief of the patient's diplopia. Occlusion therapy is the best initial solution to the patient's diplopia. Surgery is indicated only after 6 to 12 months for persistent strabismus if the patient's general condition permits.

Diabetic retinopathy is the most common cause of blindness in Americans between the ages of 20 and 74 years. Diabetics have 25 times greater incidence of becoming blind from diabetic retinopathy as compared with nondiabetics becoming blind from all other causes. Diabetic retinopathy is more common in women, but men appear to develop a more complicated and severe proliferative retinopathy. Ten years after diagnosis, 70% of diabetics have some form of retinopathy.

Diabetic retinopathy can affect both type I and type II diabetics. Type I diabetics (i.e. insulin-dependent diabetics, usually juvenile-onset) are generally free of retinopathy for the first 5 years after diagnosis of diabetes. Type II diabetics (adult-onset diabetics who may require insulin) are much more likely to develop retinopathy sooner after diagnosis. These patients should have an ophthalmologic evaluation at the time of their initial diagnosis.

Patients with diabetes for 4 years or less have a 15% incidence of retinopathy, whereas patients with diabetes for 15 years or greater have a 90% prevalence of retinopathy.

The pathogenesis of diabetic retinopathy appears to be related to the aldose reductase pathways and their inhibition. There is an increased retinal blood flow similar to the increased glomerular filtration in the kidneys. This leads to breakdown of the blood-related barrier that allows large molecules to enter the extracellular space of the retina, causing edema and deposition of lipids. Retinal ischemia induces the growth of new thin-walled vessels, which, because of their tendency to rupture, predisposes the patient to spontaneous vitreous hemorrhage and retinal detachment.

Diabetic retinopathy is divided into "background retinopathy," or "*non*proliferative retinopathy," and "proliferative retinopathy" (Table 20–56).

"Background (nonproliferative) retinopathy" accounts for 80% of all diabetic retinopathy. This condition rarely results in total blindness, but 5% to 20% of these patients will become legally blind within 5 years. Retinal findings in the early stages consist of microaneurysms, hemorrhages, and increased vascular permeability, resulting in edema and hard exudates in the central retina.

Microaneurysms are characteristic components of background retinopathy and are capillary aneurysms. On funduscopic examination, they appear as tiny red dots, separate from the arterioles and venules. Since these are capillary in origin, they are under low systemic pressure and do not have a great tendency to rupture and hemorrhage.

Basement-membrane changes common to capillaries throughout the body are also very prominent in the retina. The high glycosylation of glycoproteins in the basement membranes of capillaries result in leakier, thicker basement membranes. This leads to retinal edema. Because of the prominence of lipoproteins among proteins that leave the vessels, lipids are deposited in the retina and are seen as hard exudates. Plasma leakage is of particular clinical importance in the macula, the area of central, high-resolution vision. Macular edema can lead to moderate visual loss early in background nonproliferative diabetic retinopathy. Unfortunately, both symptoms and examination results, performed by the family physician, even when done correctly with dilated pupil and careful examination with the ophthalmoscope, often fail to detect early macular edema. The patient may not be aware of the loss of central vision because of maintained central vision in the contralateral eye and will often fail to report visual loss. Ophthalmologic examination may not reveal the edema to the same extent as careful examination with the biomicroscope by

an ophthalmologist. Fluorescein angiography is the most reliable method of detecting macular edema.

The preferred treatment for macular edema is focal treatment with laser, which results in an incidence of 14% of moderate visual loss at the end of 3 years as compared with 30% moderate visual loss without treatment. (These results were obtained from the ETDRS Study, a national cooperative study into the early treatment of diabetic retinopathy. The study demonstrates progressive disappearance of macular edema and regression or disappearance of hard exudates.)

The final, very significant component of nonproliferative retinopathy is retinal ischemia. This condition is associated with capillary nonperfusion and "capillary dropout." It signifies a high risk for subsequent proliferative retinopathy. It is often referred to as "preproliferative diabetic retinopathy." Retinal ischemia is manifest on funduscopic examination by "cotton wool" exudates, which are the result of closure of arterioles, damage to capillary endothelium, and leakage of plasma. Dilated capillaries are seen in this condition and are referred to as "intraretinal microvascular abnormalities" (IRMA). Another manifestation is "venous beading," which gives the venules an appearance of strings of beads. This occurs only in the presence of severe ischemia.

The results of the ETDRS Study show that in the presence of mild to moderate nonproliferative retinopathy, there is a 10% risk of progression to proliferative retinopathy in 1 year. However, in severe nonproliferative retinopathy, there is a 50% or higher risk of progression to proliferative retinopathy in 1 year. Therefore, it is clear that patients who have severe nonproliferative retinopathy need prompt ophthalmologic intervention and treatment.

"Proliferative retinopathy" is characterized by the new development of extraretinal fibrovascular tissue. Abnormal new blood vessels erupt to the surface of the retina and grow at the junction of the retina and the vitreous body. Neovascularization of the disc appears as a fine fishnet of blood vessels growing within and around the disc at the junction with the vitreous body. Neovascularization elsewhere in the retina (NVE) is the proliferation of new blood vessels on the surface of the retina or on the posterior vitreous body. Proliferative retinopathy causes far greater risks for loss of vision than nonproliferative retinopathy. The risk of visual loss in-

TABLE 20–56.   DIABETIC RETINOPATHY

NONPROLIFERATIVE RETINOPATHY	PROLIFERATIVE RETINOPATHY	TREATMENT	PREVALENCE
Most common (80%)	Least common (20%)	Reduces severe visual loss by 60%	15% within 4 years
5% to 20% legally blind in 5 years	50% blind in 5 years		90% within 15 years
Microaneurysms, hemorrhages	Vessel growth on disc and retina	Most effectively accomplished early, while patient is not symptomatic	
Macular edema and exudates	Retinal detachments, neovascular glaucoma		
Ischemia	Treatment: laser and vitrectomy		
Laser treatment of macular edema			

creases with the severity of proliferative retinopathy. The new vessels are particularly prone to tears and to vitreous hemorrhage because they have very thin walls and yet are under arterial pressure. They are also at the junction of the vitreous body and the retina. The causes of the loss of vision in proliferative retinopathy are largely vitreous hemorrhage and retinal detachment.

The Diabetic Retinopathy Study, another multicenter national study sponsored by the American Academy of Ophthalmology, showed that the treatment of high-risk eyes with panretinal photocoagulation slows the progression and reduces the visual loss in proliferative retinopathy. The study has demonstrated that severe visual loss occurred 50% less often in treated eyes than in nontreated eyes. Eyes with high grades of proliferative retinopathy should be considered for immediate laser surgery because the risk of visual loss is so great. Also, the risk of visual loss without treatment far outweighs the risk of visual loss after treatment. The treatment consists of scattered or panretinal photocoagulation. It consists of 1500 to 2000 individual applications of argon laser to the peripheral retina, sparing the macula. This treatment slows the increase in numbers of new vessels and the risk of complications. Macular edema, which is a possible complication of this method of treatment, tends to be transient and does not impair central vision permanently.

In cases of vitreous hemorrhage, retinal traction, or retinal detachment, vitrectomy can be performed. The effectiveness of treatment depends on the timing the treatment is applied; therefore, it is crucial that all diabetic patients undergo systematic ophthalmologic examinations on the following schedule: Diabetics whose age at onset of the disease was 0 to 30 years should have their first examination 5 years after the onset, with yearly follow-ups. If the age of onset is greater than 31 years, the first ophthalmologic examination should be at onset and then yearly. After retinopathy has been diagnosed, follow-up is dependent on the findings and may need to be as frequent as every 4 to 6 weeks.

It is clear that blood sugar levels over 200, when encountered over significant periods of time, increase the risk of retinopathy. It also has been shown that optimal control of the diabetes and the associated control of hypertension and renal disease do indeed reduce the risk of diabetic retinopathy.

SUGGESTED READING

Benson WE, Tasman W, Duane TD. Diabetic retinopathy. In Duane TD (ed.): Clinical Ophthalmology. Hagerstown, Maryland, Harper & Row, 1990, vol. 3. chap. 30, pp. 1–20.

Bresnick GH. Diabetic maculopathy: A critical review highlighting diffuse macular edema. Ophthalmology 1983; 90:1301–1317.

Diabetic Retinopathy Study Research Group. Photocoagulation treatment of proliferative diabetic retinopathy: Clinical applications of Diabetic Retinopathy Study (DRS) findings (DRS report number 8). Ophthalmology 1981; 88:583–600.

Diabetic Retinopathy Study Research Group. Photocoagulation treatment of proliferative diabetic retinopathy: The second report from the Diabetic Retinopathy Study. Ophthalmology 1978; 85:82–106.

Diabetic Retinopathy Study Research Group. Four risk factors for severe visual loss in diabetic retinopathy: The third report from the Diabetic Retinopathy Study. Arch Ophthalmol 1979; 97:654–655.

Early Treatment Diabetic Retinopathy Study Research Group. Photocoagulation for diabetic macular edema (Early Treatment Diabetic Retinopathy Study report number 1). Arch Ophthalmol 1985; 103:1796–1806.

Lauritzen T, Larsen H-W, Frost-Larsen K. Effect of 1 year of normal blood glucose levels on retinopathy in insulin-dependent diabetics. Lancet 1983; 1:200–203.

Parks MM. Cranial nerve palsies. In Duane TD (ed.): Clinical Ophthalmology. Hagerstown, Maryland, Harper & Row, 1986, vol. 1. chap. 19, pp. 153–164.

QUESTIONS

1. Findings that occur with a diabetic 3rd nerve palsy include all the following *except*

   a. Ipsilateral ptosis and contralateral exotropia.

   b. Contralateral ptosis and ipsilateral exotropia.

   c. Ipsilateral ptosis, pupillary dilation, and ipsilateral exotropia.

   d. Ipsilateral ptosis, ipsilateral exotropia, and pupillary sparing.

2. Primary characteristics of diabetes type I include all the following *except*

   a. Insulin-dependent.

   b. Generally free of nonproliferative retinopathy for the first 5 years after diagnosis.

   c. Generally juvenile-onset.

   d. Patients develop proliferative retinopathy within the first 5 years after initial medical diagnosis.

3. Background retinopathy (nonproliferative retinopathy) includes all the following *except*

   a. Retinal detachments and neovascular glaucoma.

   b. Macular edema and exudates.

   c. Microaneurysms and hemorrhages.

   d. Retinal ischemia.

4. The primary treatment for diabetic retinopathy includes all the following *except*

   a. Laser or photocoagulation for macular edema.

   b. Vitrectomy for proliferative diabetic retinopathy.

   c. Krypton photocoagulation to the trabecular meshwork.

5. The primary treatment of diabetic 3rd nerve palsy includes all the following *except*

   a. Patching for diplopia.

   b. Therapeutic cycloplegics.

   c. Surgery between 6 and 12 months after stabilization of the patient's general diabetic condition.

Answers appear on page 452.

Headache

ROBERT SMITH

INITIAL VISIT

SUBJECTIVE

Patient Identification. Joyce L. is a 35-year-old school teacher who came to the office complaining of severe headache and nausea. She had recently moved into the area with her husband and two small children and this was her first visit.

Presenting Problem. Joyce states that she is healthy except for her headaches. She is happily married, and she has just started teaching sixth grade in a local school. She believes she manages her busy life well. She had normal pregnancies, and her husband had been promoted when transferred and has been sympathetic and supportive when she has one of her bad headaches.

Present Illness. This headache began at work 24 hours previously. It was preceded by Joyce's seeing "bright sparkling lights" in her field of vision, followed 1 hour later by an aching pain that began over her right eye and gradually spread to the right temple and then posteriorly to the right side of the neck. The pain was deep-seated and throbbing and made worse on head movement. It now involved the whole head. As the headache worsened, Joyce felt nauseated and began vomiting. She took two Fiorinal tablets prescribed by her previous physician, and although she retained them, they did not relieve the headache. She left work and went to bed. She took two more tablets and also used a rectal ergotamine suppository. Finally, she obtained some relief, but some pain and nausea persisted that prevented her from sleeping. She took sips of water as had been prescribed by her previous physician, but this morning the headache was still severe. She had taken a total of six Fiorinal tablets as well as the suppository. She felt very weak and cold. In the past, the medication usually controlled her headaches, but recently she noticed that pain tablets were losing their effect and she had increased the number she took for an attack. Her headaches were lasting longer and becoming more frequent. This was the worst attack she could remember.

Past Medical History. Joyce has had no previous serious illnesses. Apart from her two pregnancies, she has never been hospitalized. She has never had head or other trauma. She has no allergies. Her headaches began as a teenager and always involved the right side, occurred about once a month related to her periods, and lasted 4 to 8 hours, usually responding to aspirin or acetaminophen. Now the headaches occur two to three times per month and last 2 to 3 days. Joyce is now rarely without some sort of headache. This makes her worried and depressed because her headaches are beginning to interfere with her work and family life.

She remembers that during her pregnancies she was free of headache, but afterwards they recurred, and when she began taking birth control pills, the headaches became severe. When she stopped taking the pill, the headaches improved, but they never returned to the milder headaches before her pregnancy.

Joyce has noticed that oversleeping on weekends causes headache. She does not think stress is a factor; on the contrary, her headaches are more likely to occur when she is relaxed. She is a nonsmoker and has avoided cigarette smoke because this triggers attacks, as do noise and bright lights. She has noticed that a strong perfume used by a colleague at work makes her headaches worse. Smells in general become stronger and nauseating when she has a severe attack. Chocolate and red wine give her headaches. Before attacks she feels depressed, but afterwards she feels very happy and energetic. She thinks she passes more urine during attacks. She has a strange sensation that the side of her head feels enlarged during an attack, and it hurts to comb her hair. She obtains some relief by applying cold compresses to her right eye and temple. She has marked bad breath during an attack and feels drowsy and irritable and does not want her husband or children near her. She feels clumsy and has knocked into furniture. Her vision becomes blurred, and she cannot focus to read or concentrate. Sleep often relieves the headache, but recently she has been awakening in the early hours with severe headache, and now she is beginning to fear sleeping. On several occasions she has noticed that the right side of her face and right forearm get numb for 1 to 2 minutes before an attack, and she cannot speak properly and her arm feels limp. She is frightened because the last time this happened she was driving a car.

Family History. Joyce's mother suffered from migraine, as did an older sister. Her mother is now in her sixties and is almost free of headache. Her maternal grandmother died suddenly of stroke in her fifties, as did her mother's sister. Joyce is worried that she might also have a stroke. Her father is well, and there is no history of headache on his side of the family.

Health Habits. Joyce does not smoke or drink, and she states that she has never used illicit drugs. She feels guilty because her attacks interfere with family functioning. She also feels bad about the increasing number of analgesic drugs she takes and is embarrassed to ask for refills. On several occasions in the past year she was made to feel like a "drug addict" when she went to the hospital emergency room seeking headache relief. She plays tennis and jogs, but recently she has given up both because she believes they aggravate her headache. She watches her weight and avoids foods containing too much fat because her last physician told her she must reduce her cholesterol. She drinks two cups of coffee at breakfast and a total of six or seven cups daily. She has tried without success to switch to decaffeinated drinks because she has been told caffeine is bad for her headaches. She avoids dairy products, especially strong cheese, and Chinese food for the same reason.

Social History. Joyce married her high-school sweetheart at age 21. She describes her marriage as "perfect." She majored in psychology and continued by taking a diploma in teaching. She interrupted her training to have a child and took time off from teaching for the second child, now age 3. No further children are being planned, although she knows that pregnancy would provide her with headache relief. Her husband is an "outdoor type," but increasingly Joyce is unable to take part in outings and picnics because of her headaches. She now had cut back on other activities such as church socials and teaching Sunday school.

Review of Systems. Joyce has increased weight recently by several pounds. Her pain medication gives her indigestion. She has no chest, abdominal, or limb pain, nor has she any breathing difficulty on exercise. When she has no headache, she feels fit and is able to cope fully with her work and family activities. Her periods are regular and normal, and her sexual life is normal, although recently she has increasingly been avoiding intercourse because of her headaches.

OBJECTIVE

Physical Examination. Joyce is a normal-appearing Caucasian female; her weight is 129 lb; her height is 65 in; her blood pressure is 130/80; and her pulse rate is 80 and regular. Joyce looks pale and anxious and clasps her hands tightly on her lap, leaning forward as she speaks. Neurologic examination is normal. There is no sensory loss; tendon and abdominal reflexes are normal. Pupils are equal and respond normally to light; both fundi are normal, as are the ocular muscles and accommodation reflex. *Head and Neck:* Joyce's lower jaw moves normally, with normal bite and without tenderness or cracking sensation over the temporomandibular joints. She is tender over the right temporal area, and there is neck tenderness, most marked in the right suboccipital area. There is pain in this area on lateral movement of the neck in both directions. There is no neck rigidity. There are no carotid bruits. *Chest:* Breath sounds are normal, and the apex beat is not displaced. A midsystolic click is heard at the apex. There are no murmurs. *Abdomen:* No tenderness or masses are felt. Joyce is menstruating.

Laboratory Tests. The urine was not examined. An executive multiphasic fasting blood screen was drawn.

ASSESSMENT

The history and presentation confirm the previous diagnosis of migraine. Changes in the headache pattern have occurred, and new neurologic symptoms and increasing headache severity have developed. The follow-

TABLE 20–57. HEADACHE CLASSIFICATION

1. Migraine
2. Tension-type headache
3. Cluster headache and chronic paroxysmal hemicrania
4. Miscellaneous headache with no structural lesion
5. Headache and head trauma
6. Headache and vascular disorders
7. Headache and nonvascular intracranial disorders
8. Headache and substances or their withdrawals
9. Headache and noncephalic infection
10. Headache and metabolic disorders
11. Headache or facial pain and disorders of cranial neck or cranial structures
12. Cranial neuralgias
13. Headache not classifiable

ing headache diagnoses should be considered (see Tables 20–57 and 20–58):

1. *Migraine with typical aura* (classification: migraine 1.2.1). Previously used terms: classic migraine, classical migraine, ophthalmic, hemiparesthetic, hemiparetic, hemiplegic, or aphasic migraine, migraine accompagnee. *Description:* Idiopathic recurring headache manifesting with attacks of neurologic symptoms unequivocally localizable to cerebral cortex or brainstem, usually gradually developed over 5 to 20 minutes and usually lasting less than 60 minutes.

2. *Tension-type headache* (classification: tension-type headache 2). Previously used terms: tension headache, muscle-contraction headache, stress headache, psychologic headache. *Description:* Recurrent episodes of headache lasting minutes to days. Pain is pressing/tightening in quality, mild or moderate in severity, and bilateral. Nausea is absent, but photophobia or phonophobia may be present. May become chronic (classification: 2.2).

3. *Mixed migraine and tension-type headache.* Sometimes migraine develops a chronic tension headache component. More frequently, episodic tension-type headache becomes chronic. In both instances, overuse

TABLE 20–58. MIGRAINE CLASSIFICATION

1. Migraine
 1.1 Migraine without aura
 1.2 Migraine with aura
  1.2.1 Migraine with typical aura
  1.2.2 Migraine with prolonged aura
  1.2.3 Familial hemiplegic migraine
  1.2.4 Basilar migraine
  1.2.5 Migraine aura without headache
  1.2.6 Migraine with acute-onset aura
 1.3 Ophthalmoplegic migraine
 1.4 Retinal migraine
 1.5 Childhood periodic syndromes that may be precursors to or associated with migraine
  1.5.1 Benign paroxysmal vertigo of childhood
  1.5.2 Alternating hemiplegia of childhood
 1.6 Complications of migraine
  1.6.1 Status migrainus
  1.6.2 Migrainus infarction
 1.7 Migrainus disorder not fulfilling above criteria

of drugs frequently plays a role in aggravating the disorder.

4. *Headache associated with substances or their withdrawal* (classification: 8.2). Headache can be induced by chronic use of ergotamine and analgesics when these have been taken for a headache disorder, not when they have been taken for other disorders. The headache is diffuse, pulsating, and distinguished from migraine by absent attack pattern and/or associated symptoms. The diagnosis can only be made after withdrawal of ergotamine and/or analgesics relieving the induced but not the primary headache.

The clinical picture includes features of all the above. Tension headache as the primary headache probably is least likely. Although the history and examination indicate the presence of stress, temporal and neck tenderness is unilateral, as is often found in migraine. The onset of new neurologic symptoms is a cause of some concern. The aura, which had been a scintillating scotoma common in migraine, now is associated with short periods of paresthesia and discoordination of the right face and arm, as well as a bizarre body image effect (head felt enlarged in the area of the headache).

PLAN

Immediate CT scan and EEG are deferred because of the absence of objective neurologic findings. An ECG is performed because of the midsystolic click. Mitral valve prolapse has been reported as occurring more frequently in migraine patients. Chest x-ray and cardiac sonogram are deferred.

Diagnostic. Fasting executive multiphasic screen was ordered because of chronic medication overuse and history of hyperlipidemia. The urine was not tested because Joyce is menstruating.

Therapeutic

1. *Some pain relief was immediately obtained* by subcutaneous infiltration of the tender areas in the temporal and occipital regions with 0.5 to 1 cc of a mixture of equal parts of short- and long-acting local anesthetic without epinephrine (2% lidocaine and 0.25% bupivicaine). This avoids the use of narcotic analgesics and ergotamine, which are probably contributing to the problem, and provides immediate temporary relief and often completely aborts the attack.

2. A *drug withdrawal* regimen was begun, replacing the narcotic analgesics and ergotamine in a phased manner with nonsteroidal analgesics. To suppress any withdrawal symptoms, clonidine 0.12 mg was prescribed twice daily.

3. A *preventive program* was started using a small daily amount of the beta-blocker nadolol (10 mg each morning). Joyce was instructed to call the office if she noticed any symptoms of hypotension. This was unlikely because of the small amounts of clonidine and nadolol used.

4. *Dietary control.* Joyce's history indicated dietary trigger factors. At this stage, an exclusion diet was strongly recommended. This excludes *alcohol* (especially beer and red wine), *tyramine* (aged or processed cheese, chocolate, cola drinks, pickled herring), *nitrates* (preservative found in ham, bacon, sausage, lunch meats, wieners), *monosodium glutamate* (MSG) (flavor enhancer in many Chinese foods and commercially prepared foods), and *excessive salt* in foods. *Note:* Large amounts of the above eaten on an empty stomach are more likely to act as a trigger. Missing meals may induce "hunger headache," which in a migraine sufferer may develop into an acute attack.

5. *Relaxation therapy.* Relaxation tapes and biofeedback are worth considering to educate Joyce about the role of stress in headache and the part played in chronic pain syndromes by mind–body interaction. The value of this depends greatly on the individual's willingness to "buy in" to this approach. Centrally acting agents with anxiolytic action should be avoided because of danger of habituation and dependence.

6. *Psychometric evaluation.* The Minnesota Multiphasic Personality Inventory (MMPI) is not warranted at this stage. Depression is commonly caused by chronic recurring headache. Depression per se is an uncommon primary cause of headache. Stress is commonly associated with headache, although with migraine to a lesser degree than with tension headache. The whole question of emotional factors in migraine should be handled carefully, since they usually are overemphasized, creating feelings of frustration and anger in many patients because of the implied inadequacy in their ability to cope.

7. *Record keeping.* A daily headache record was started. This provides the physician with the headache pattern and helps identify any association with trigger factors (menstruation, "letdown" weekend headache, seasonal problems, shift work). Joyce is gratified by the physician's interest, and confidence in the overall therapeutic approach is heightened.

Patient Education. Several books on migraine for the lay public are available. These explain the pathogenesis of migraine in simple terms and help to diminish guilt feelings. They emphasize that the patient is not at fault, that the condition is probably genetic, and that, although incurable, the condition can be controlled when the patient and physician can work on the problem together. A strong therapeutic relationship must be developed and sustained, especially in the early months when the response may be slow.

Disposition. Joyce was given medication for 4 weeks (nadolol, clonidine, ergotamine suppositories, and nonsteroidal analgesics) and asked to return in 4 weeks. She was instructed to have her blood pressure checked by the office nurse in 1 week, to report progress, and, if necessary, have her medication adjusted. If her blood pressure remains within the normal range, the beta-blocker should be increased from 10 to 20 mg daily. The clonidine should be maintained until transfer to a nonnarcotic nonergotamine therapeutic regimen has been stabilized. Joyce also was instructed to call if very severe headache attacks occurred.

FIRST FOLLOW-UP

Within 48 hours, Joyce's husband phoned to report that after 1 day completely free of headache, a very severe attack had recurred and Joyce was very ill. Joyce was directed to the emergency room, and when she was seen, her headache appeared to be even more severe than when she was previously seen in the office. She had numbness on the right side, now present for 2 to 3 hours. Previously, numbness lasted only about 1 minute. She had increased tendon reflexes present in her right upper and lower limbs and loss of sensation to light touch on the right side of her face and right forearm. There was some loss of sensation to pinprick in some areas. She was slightly dehydrated.

ASSESSMENT

The lack of response to treatment and the symptom crescendo and persistence of neurologic deficits suggested (1) headache associated with a transient ischemic attack (TIA) (headache classification 6.1.2.1) or (2) headache with thromboembolic stroke (headache classification 6.1.2).

PLAN

Therapeutic. Joyce was treated with IV saline and given prochlorperazine (Compazine) 5 mg IV over 1 minute. A CT scan was ordered, and when it was performed 3 hours later, Joyce was free of all symptoms. The CT scan revealed a large arteriovenous malformation in the right occipital area of the brain. Joyce was admitted to neurosurgery for further investigation and treatment.

A carotid arteriogram confirmed the diagnosis. An MRI indicated no recent or previous hemorrhage from the malformation. Because of the size of the mass, bleeding was considered a decided risk. There was surgical risk to adjoining visual cortex. Radiotherapy to the area would reduce the mass considerably and could be repeated in 2 years to deal with any residual malformation. The risk of homonymous hemianopia is less with this procedure than with surgery.

The persistence of the symptoms and their clearing within 24 hours ruled out a thromboembolic stroke. The prolongation of the aura over several hours indicated the presence of a true transient ischemic attach (TIA) in this case. The relationships between migraine TIA and vascular malformations are poorly understood. The worsening of the migraine, the lack of response to treatment, and the development of newly associated symptoms indicated a possible intracranial abnormality and the need for admission and further neurological workup.

Disposition. Joyce is likely to continue to have migraine attacks in the future even after surgery, but the condition should then respond better to routine migraine treatment. Joyce should be informed of this and firmly assured on this point. The outcome effect on aura and on future TIAs remains to be seen. It is important for Joyce to continue with the beta-blocker treatment and to add a daily aspirin. These medications will be required long term, but if the migraine symptoms improve, the use of the beta-blocker may be gradually withdrawn.

Final Diagnosis. Migraine with aura associated with TIA and with an unruptured occipital arteriovenous malformation (headache classifications 6.1. and 6.4.1).

SUGGESTED READING

Chung MK, Kraybell DE. Headache: A marker of depression. J Fam Pract 1990; 31:360–364.

Classification and diagnostic criteria for headache disorders, cranial neuralgias and facial pain. Report of Committee of International Headache Society, Jes Olesen, Chairman. Cephalalgia 8 (suppl. 7) 1–96; 1988.

Smith R. Scalp tenderness, pain threshold and headache relief. Cephalalgia 1989; 9(suppl. 10):206–207.

Smith R. Headache and depression (editorial). J Fam Pract 1990; 31(4):357–358.

Rakel RE (ed.). *Textbook of Family Practice,* 3rd ed. Philadelphia, W. B. Saunders, 1984, pp. 1160–1165.

QUESTIONS

1. All the following drugs are useful in preventing migraine *except*
   a. Cardioselective beta-blockers.
   b. Noncardioselective beta-blockers.
   c. Methysergide.
   d. Calcium-channel blockers.
   e. Valproic acid.

2. All the following are known trigger factors in migraine attacks *except*
   a. Too much sleep.
   b. Too little sleep.
   c. Hyperlipidemia.
   d. Tyramine-rich food.
   e. Weather change.

3. All the following statements are correct *except*
   a. Auras preceding migraine are of short duration.
   b. Aspirin prevents migraine aura.
   c. Migraine aura is not a stroke precursor.
   d. New-onset migraine prodromes merit a CT scan.
   e. Transient ischemic attacks (TIAs) do not last longer than 24 hours.

Answers appear on page 452.

H. JAMES BROWNLEE

INITIAL VISIT

SUBJECTIVE

Patient Identification. Anne B. is a 69-year-old married Caucasian female who presents for her first visit.

Presenting Problems. Anne presents with a complaint of chronic progressive fatigue accompanied by stiff joints and muscles. There has been some pain with the stiff joints, for which the patient consulted a rheumatologist on her own. The rheumatologist diagnosed the patient as having moderate osteoarthritis of her hips and knees but felt she needed further evaluation for a probable neurodegenerative disorder, since her disability did not appear to be limited strictly to her joints.

Present Illness. Anne indicates she led a very active life until the past 3 years, when her "arthritis" started to slow her down. She indicates that she feels weak most of the time, with an increasing need recently to take a nap each afternoon. She does indicate problems with sleep at night because "my legs shake." On further questioning, Anne indicates that her right leg started to shake first, but after about a year, both legs began to shake. She now indicates that her hands also have begun to tremble. When questioned further, Anne denies reduction of the tremors after ingesting alcohol. Getting out of a soft chair, in and out of the car, and climbing stairs have recently become significant problems for her. Although she has not fallen yet, she feels a bit unsteady. Her husband has had to help her lately with getting dressed and undressed. Her only medications include a nonsteroidal anti-inflammatory drug, naproxen (Naprosyn), 500 mg twice daily, for her arthritis.

Past Medical History. Anne has had multiple hospitalizations in the past for kidney stones with related urosepsis; however, no further hospitalizations have been necessary after undergoing a right heminephrectomy at age 59 for removal of a large staghorn calculus. Anne is $G_6P_5Ab_1$, with menopause occurring at age 53. She is allergic only to sulfa drugs.

Family History. Family history reveals that Anne's father died at age 73 of a myocardial infarction and her mother died at age 83 of congestive heart failure. There were four siblings; three are living, and one died of a brain tumor. There is a history of "degenerative" arthritis in Anne's mother. There is no family history of "neurodegenerative illnesses or tremors." Anne's husband has coronary artery disease that is well controlled on oral medication. They have five children, ages 42, 41, 39, 38, and 31, all in good health.

Health Habits. Anne never smoked on any regular basis and rarely ingests alcoholic beverages. She always wears a seatbelt, but she requires the assistance of her husband to insert and release the buckle for her.

Social History. Anne has been married for 44 years to a recently retired general practitioner. Anne worked episodically as a registered nurse in doctors' offices and in a local emergency room. She quit her emergency room job and began working as a phlebotomy nurse for the blood bank when the emergency room nursing became too demanding for her physically.

Review of Systems. Anne has noted progressive hearing loss, for which she has been fitted for a hearing aid, but she prefers not to wear it because of the excessive extraneous noise it produces. She has worn glasses since nursing school, and her vision has not changed recently. She notes some difficulty swallowing chewy foods. She has seen her dentist, who indicates that her dentures are fine. Her children often complain that she does not talk loudly enough when speaking with them on the telephone; however, she has to use the phone to communicate with them because "my writing has become so difficult to read." Anne has noted increased constipation the past year and has been relying on over-the-counter laxatives on a fairly regular basis. She denies urinary incontinence, although she has to be careful not to wait too long to empty her bladder, since it takes longer to ambulate to the bathroom. Her weight has decreased by approximately 5 lb this past year, which she attributes to lack of appetite.

OBJECTIVE

Physical Examination. Anne's height is 62 in; her weight is 139 lb; her pulse is 84; and her blood pressure is 136/86. *HEENT:* Thinned/fine hair; no localized alopecia. *Eyes:* Full range of motion in all quadrants with no gaze abnormality. *Nose and Ears:* Clear. Decreased hearing bilaterally, with no hearing aid in place. *Mouth:* Upper dentures complete, partial lower; otherwise normal. *Neck:* Thyroid normal; no bruits. *Lungs:* Clear to auscultation. *Heart:* Normal sinus rhythm without murmur. *Abdomen:* Mildly obese, right nephrectomy scar, no hernias, no organomegaly. *Pelvic/rectal:* Deferred to be completed at future visit. *Extremities:* Bilateral mildly hypertrophic knee joints; no overt inflammation and minimal swelling. No other joint deformity. Peripheral pulses 2+ and equal bilaterally. Trace bilateral edema of both ankles. *Skin:* Mild facial seborrheic dermatitis of chin and forehead. *Neurologic:* Oriented to place, time, and person. Anne shows difficulty in arising from the examining room chair when asked to sit on the examining table. After several attempts to stand, by using her hands on the arms of the chair, Anne is able to arise, although her balance seems a bit unstable initially. She requires the assistance of the physician to step up and sit on the end of the table. A slow-frequency bilateral hand tremor, right greater than left, is noted when Anne has her hands on her lap. The tremor disappears when she is asked to grab the physician's fingers. There is some resistance without cogwheeling to extension of the elbow and rotation of wrist joints. The cranial nerves all appear intact; however, Anne appears to have little facial expression, appearing somewhat sad. There is no focal motor or sensory deficit. Testing of the patient's gait shows her to be slow to initiate gait, and she shuffles her feet somewhat. There is a lack of arm flexion at the elbow and very limited arm swing while walking.

Laboratory Tests. Office laboratory analyses ordered with the first visit included a CBC, which was normal except for a slight decreased hemoglobin of 11.9 with normal indices, a normal urinalysis, a normal chemistry profile, except for a cholesterol of 238.

ASSESSMENT

Working Diagnoses

1. *Idiopathic Parkinson's disease.* This is a chronic progressive neurodegenerative disorder. The classic tetrad of symptoms and signs, including resting tremor, rigidity, bradykinesia, and postural reflex impairment, is manifested to some degree in this patient.
2. *Osteoarthritis.* This was already diagnosed by a rheumatologist clinically prior to this visit.
3. *Mild anemia* with normal indices. This is an anemia of chronic disease, although a mixed nutritional disorder is possible.
4. *Mild hypercholesterolemia*
6. *Seborrheic dermatitis* of the face

Differential Diagnoses. The purpose of Anne's presentation is to discuss Parkinson's disease. There are no laboratory or radiologic tests at this time that can be used to make a diagnosis. Instead, these tests help rule out other neurodegenerative disorders. The diagnosis of Parkinson's disease is purely a clinical diagnosis. Other conditions to consider include

1. *Essential tremor.* This usually occurs during sustained posture and during motion rather than at rest, as noted in Anne. An essential tremor can affect the hands, usually bilaterally, but it also commonly causes head tremor, which is rare in Parkinson's disease patients. Alcohol did not reduce this patient's tremor, whereas small amounts of alcohol often markedly reduce an essential tremor. A family history of essential tremor exists in over 50% of patients with this disorder.
2. *"Parkinson's plus" syndrome.*
   a. *Progressive supranuclearpalsy.* This is very similar to Parkinson's disease clinically but is differentiated by a patient's loss of voluntary downward and lateral gaze.
   b. *Shy–Drager syndrome.* This "syndrome" consists of classic Parkinson's but with much more severe autonomic nervous system impairment, including profound orthostatic hypotension.
   c. *Olivopontocerebellar atrophies.* Patients with these disorders likewise manifest parkinsonian symptoms but are differentiated by marked cerebellar dysfunction, most commonly ataxia.
   d. *Striatonigral degeneration* is a disorder very similar to Parkinson's disease, but it is differentiated by more limited tremor, and dementia is uncommon. The diagnosis can be supported by lack of response to levodopa.
3. *Secondary parkinsonism.*
   a. *Postinfectious.* This is seen especially during the convalescent phase of encephalitis.
   b. *Drug induced.* Those drugs which block dopamine receptors, especially the neuroleptic agents, as well as metoclopramide and reserpine, an antihypertensive agent not prescribed much today.
   c. *Toxin-induced.* This includes exposure to carbon monoxide, carbon disulfide, manganese, cyanide, methanol, and the synthetic heroin analogue MPTP (1-methyl-4-phenyl-1,2,3,6-tetrahydropyridine).
   d. *Hereditary diseases,* especially Wilson's disease, involving a defect in copper metabolism that first appears in the second or third decade and is treatable with chelating agents and diet.
   e. *Elderly.* Often the elderly will manifest some parkinsonian features, such as kyphosis, stooped posture, balance impairment, and a shuffling gait, and yet have no neurodegenerative process and not respond to anti-Parkinson's medications.
4. *Hypothyroidism.* The fatigue and lack of energy require one to consider this hypometabolic state. Weight gain and slow pulse are both features classically seen in hypothyroidism, but they are not manifested in this patient.

PLAN

Diagnostic

1. Rediscuss key symptoms and signs in Anne's history and examination to help rule in or rule out a diagnosis of Parkinson's disease.
2. Serum chemistry laboratory work to include liver function tests to evaluate for Wilson's disease, creatine phosphokinase to evaluate for muscle disease, a thyroid-stimulating hormone (TSH) level to evaluate for hypothyroidism. A serum copper level to evaluate for Wilson's disease should not be necessary, since Anne's symptoms and signs developed in her sixth decade.
3. Magnetic resonance imaging (MRI) of the brain to evaluate for other neurodegenerative processes, since MRI is not of benefit for making the diagnosis Parkinson's disease.
4. An anemia profile is ordered to attempt to iden-

tify a treatable nutritional deficiency as a cause of the anemia.

5. Cerebrospinal spinal fluid analysis to evaluate for other neurologic disorder presenting with parkinsonism (optional).

Therapeutic. A full explanation of the diagnosis and treatment of Parkinson's disease is given to Anne and her husband. Anne is begun on Sinemet (carbidopa–levodopa) 25 mg/100 mg to be taken once a day for 3 days with food, then increased to twice a day for 3 days, and then increased again to three times a day. After 2 weeks, Anne is to take the medication at least 1 hour before meals.

A prescription for 1% hydrocortisone cream twice a day was given to Anne to use on the facial seborrheic dermatitis until improved and then as needed. Anne also was placed on a cholesterol-lowering diet and was advised to continue taking her present arthritis medication.

Patient Education

1. Anne is told to take the carbidopa–levodopa with meals initially to limit the most common side effect of the medication—nausea. However, after 2 weeks of gently increasing the dosage, the medication ingestion time is advanced to 60 minutes prior to eating to eliminate competitive inhibition between the medication and food (especially protein) in the intestine as well as at the blood–brain barrier.

2. Anne is asked to maintain a symptom diary as the medication dosing increases. She is advised to bring the symptom diary with her to all future visits.

3. Anne is encouraged to maintain a program of exercise and social activity to keep physically and mentally healthy, yet to balance these activities with the necessary rest and precautions required of patients with this disease.

Disposition. Anne is asked to complete the diagnostic testing, initiate the medication previously discussed, and return in 4 weeks.

FIRST FOLLOW-UP VISIT

SUBJECTIVE

Anne noted some nausea when the carbidopa–levodopa was first begun, especially on a day when the pill was taken without food. There is no nausea now. She indicates that she seems to have developed "some more strength." She still needs a nap, but she finds getting out of chairs and climbing stairs is easier. Her unsteadiness is still the same, however. She also notes that her legs still shake in bed at night, but her hands "don't tremble as much." Her only concern is that when she gets up quick, she gets lightheaded, but this resolves quickly.

OBJECTIVE

Physical Examination. No change from the previous physical findings, except the following: The seborrheic dermatitis on her forehead and chin are much improved. Anne is able to move from the examining room chair to the table with less hesitancy. She still requires assistance to step up to and sit on the examining table. Anne's resting tremor is still present, but it is less visible. The elbow and wrist joint rigidity has almost disappeared. Anne's facial movements and gait are both more animated, although her gait is still shuffled, especially when she turns a sharp corner.

Laboratory Tests. The serum chemistries, including liver function tests, creatine phosphokinase, and thyroid-stimulation hormone, were all normal except for mildly decreased serum albumin and serum calcium levels that correct to normal in relation to the decreased albumin. The anemia profile reveals normal folate, serum iron, and ferriten levels and a mildly elevated vitamin B_{12} level. The MRI of the brain shows mild cerebral atrophy, not unusual for age; otherwise normal. CSF studies were not obtained.

ASSESSMENT

1. Idiopathic Parkinson's disease—improved by symptomatic treatment with carbidopa/levodopa. Anne's history, essentially normal laboratory results, and positive response to carbidopa/levodopa help support this diagnosis.
2. Osteoarthritis
3. Anemia profile supports the initial presumptive diagnosis of anemia of chronic disease.
4. Mild hypercholesterolemia. Not retested at this time; to be checked at the next visit.
5. Seborrheic dermatitis—improved with the use of a mild topical steroid cream.

PLAN

The carbidopa–levodopa dose will not be altered at this time, allowing Anne further adjustment time to the medication. Anne is given a Parkinson's symptom documentation flowsheet to indicate times of most strength and mobility related to the timing of doses.

Patient Education. Anne and her husband were given the phone number and address of the local Parkinson's support group to contact for further education and social support.

Disposition. Anne is scheduled to return for office follow-up in 1 month (sooner if there is any deterioration in her condition). A repeat lipid profile will be completed at the next office visit.

DISCUSSION

Parkinson's disease is the second most common neurodegenerative disorder (Alzheimer's disease is more common), affecting over 500,000 Americans. Parkinson's disease usually manifests itself clinically in patients aged 55 to 70 years, after 75% of the dopaminergic neurons in the substantia nigra are destroyed by mechanisms not fully understood at this time. It is a difficult disease to diagnose because many of its signs and symptoms are characteristic of several other disease entities. The classic symptoms and signs of Parkinson's disease include a resting tremor (most commonly of the hands, but not limited to or necessary for the diagnosis); rigidity, especially of the upper extremities, which is called "cogwheel rigidity" if there are superimposed tremors; bradykinesia or akinesia (lack of or reduced muscle movement); and postural reflex impairment causing patients to be unstable and fall. Very important, the diagnosis of Parkinson's disease does not require all four of these symptoms and signs to be present. In fact, early Parkinson's disease is often without balance problems. The diagnosis, however, is purely a clinical diagnosis, since there are no specific, reliable laboratory or radiologic studies that confirm the diagnosis of Parkinson's disease. Laboratory and radiologic studies are performed, however, to help rule out other disease entities that can cause similar symptoms and signs. Other, more subtle signs and symptoms of Parkinson's disease include drooling due to impairment of swallowing and increased salivation; hypophonia (a soft, monotonous voice due to the loss of the ability to vary speech intensity); micrographia (very small handwriting, probably a component of bradykinesia); depression (either endogenous or reactive); and autonomic nervous system dysfunction, which can include excessive perspiration, seborrhea, and orthostatic hypotension.

The treatment of Parkinson's disease includes not only medications but also patient and family education, as well as physical therapy to help keep the patient mobile. There are various national Parkinson's disease organizations available to assist patients and their families in dealing with the social and physical implications of this illness.

Most experts agree that medication for the treatment of Parkinson's disease should be started whenever any disability from the disease interferes with the activities of daily life.

Carbidopa–levodopa combinations continue to be the foundation of present-day drug treatment of Parkinson's disease. Although dopamine deficiency is the primary abnormality in Parkinson's disease, dopamine itself cannot be given to patients because it is not able to cross the blood–brain barrier. Levodopa, however, is converted in the brain to dopamine, although it also can be converted to dopamine outside the blood–brain barrier. If significant conversion of levodopa to dopamine occurs outside the blood–brain barrier, side effects, especially nausea, can be quite a problem. Carbidopa was therefore combined with levodopa, since it is able to effectively block much of the conversion of levodopa to dopamine outside the brain. A minimum of 75 mg carbidopa per day is usually necessary to block the peripheral conversion of levodopa. Another way to limit the nausea with carbidopa–levodopa combinations is to start with low doses and build up to therapeutic doses gently. It also may benefit the patient to initially take the medication with food to blunt rapid intestinal absorption, allowing the vomiting center (area postrema) to

modulate itself to become less sensitive to levodopa and dopamine. After several weeks, the medication should be given approximately 1 hour prior to meals to increase intestinal absorption. The most commonly accepted starting dose of carbidopa–levodopa combination is 25 mg/100 mg three times a day. The dose is then slowly increased until symptoms improve or until side effects limit further dosing increases. Overdosage side effects of carbidopa–levodopa combinations include dystonia, confusion, dizziness, and hallucinations. Increasing the frequency of doses from three to four times a day is often more beneficial initially than increasing the dosage amount when more medication is needed. A new controlled-release formulation will likely assist in better side-effect control.

Anticholinergic drugs play a very limited treatment role in the illness. These drugs work by reducing the cholinergic overdrive seen in Parkinson's disease. These drugs are most helpful in reducing tremor and rigidity, but they do little to reduce the bradykinesia and gait/balance abnormalities that are more disabling to Parkinson's patients. The side effects of these drugs (confusion, urinary retention, constipation) can be quite bothersome, especially in the elderly, so treatment is begun with very low doses and is increased very slowly.

Amantadine, which was used for years as drug prophylaxis against influenza A, has some therapeutic benefits for patients with early Parkinson's disease. Amantadine's therapeutic benefits appear to be derived from its ability to enhance the release of stored dopamine from neurons. The normal starting dose is 100 mg twice a day, but it must be adjusted to lower doses if renal function is impaired. Side effects seen with other Parkinson's disease medications, including dystonias, nausea, and confusion, are also seen with this medication.

Dopamine agonists are ergotamine compounds that are most effective when given in combination with carbidopa–levodopa, but they may be administered alone. Bromocriptine mesylate has been used for years, starting with an initial dosage of 1.25 mg/day for 1 week and then increasing the dose by 1.25 mg every week until symptoms are controlled or side effects occur. The newer of the dopamine agonists, pergolide mesylate, is longer acting and more potent, since it stimulates a greater number of dopamine receptors than bromocriptine. The initial dosing of pergolide is too complex to discuss here; however, low doses and slow dosage increases are as essential as the previously discussed Parkinson's disease drug regimens. Side effects of these dopamine agents include GI distress, dyskinesias, and orthostatic hypotension.

Selegiline is one of the newest drugs for the symptomatic treatment of Parkinson's disease. Recent investigations with this medication also have suggested a probable neuroprotective effect; however, not all Parkinson's disease experts endorse this suggestion. Selegiline, a monamine oxidase B inhibitor, slows down the oxidative metabolism of dopamine.

Selegiline is presently approved by the Food and Drug Administration only for use as an adjunct with carbidopa–levodopa therapy needing further symptomatic control. The approved dose is 5 mg twice a day; however, lower doses, such as 2.5 to 5.0 mg/day, are often initially utilized to avoid side effects. A reduced dosage of simultaneous carbidopa–levodopa therapy by 10% to 30% is often recommended, since inhibition of dopamine metabolism occurs, potentially inducing clinical manifestations of dopamine toxicity. Selegiline is an amphetamine, so dosing should occur in the morning and at noon to reduce nausea and limit evening "amphetamine" overstimulation.

Surgical procedures for the treatment of Parkinson's disease include stereotactic thalamotomy and tissue transplantation. Computer-assisted stereotactic thalamotomy is helpful only for selected patients who have notable disability secondary to tremor not controlled by medications. Autologous adrenal medulla tissue transplantation is no longer performed or recommended at most centers in this country. This approach still holds promise for the future.

SUGGESTED READING

Ahlskog JJE, Wilkinson JM. New concepts in the treatment of Parkinson's disease. Am Fam Physician 1990; 41(2):574–584.

Hallett M. Classification and treatment of tremor. JAMA 1991; 266(8):1115–1117.

Hopfensperger K, Koller WC. Recognizing early Parkinson's disease. Postgrad Med 1991; 90(1):49–59.

Lieberman AN. Treatment of Parkinson's disease (editorial). Mayo Clin Proc 1988; 63:1046–1049.

Marsden CD. Parkinson's disease. Lancet 1990; 334:948–952.

Parkinson study group. Effect of deprenyl on the progression of disability in early Parkinson's disease. N Engl J Med 1989; 321(20):1364–1371.

Pergolide and selegiline for Parkinson's disease (editorial). Med Lett 1989; 31:81–83.

QUESTIONS

1. Which of the following is a common characteristic of tremor of Parkinson's disease?
   a. A family history of tremor
   b. A head tremor
   c. Alcohol reduces the tremor
   d. A resting tremor

2. The most important laboratory test to order to confirm a diagnosis of Parkinson's disease is
   a. Indirect bilirubin.
   b. MPTP (1-methyl-4-phenyl-1,2,3,6-tetrahydro-pyridine).
   c. Serum calcium.
   d. Thyroid-stimulating hormone (TSH).
   e. None of the above.

3. The four classic symptoms and signs of Parkinson's disease include all the following *except*
   a. Dystonias.
   b. Tremor.
   c. Rigidity.
   d. Bradykinesia.
   e. Postural reflex impairment.

4. Which of the following class of drugs is *not* helpful in the treatment of Parkinson's disease?
   a. Anticholinergic agents
   b. Dopamine agonists
   c. Levodopa preparations
   d. Monamine oxidase B inhibitors
   e. Phenathiazines

Answers appear on page 452.

Sexual Dysfunction

CHARLES E. DRISCOLL

INITIAL VISIT

SUBJECTIVE

Patient Identification.   James L. is a 58-year-old married Caucasian male who presents for his first visit to have a "general checkup."

Presenting Problem. James is in for a general checkup, but he quickly relates that he has had type II diabetes for the past 2½ years, hypertension since his early thirties, and occasional difficulties with a sliding hiatal hernia with reflux. He had recently been informed by his usual physician that he should find a new doctor because the physician was entering retirement within 3 months. The agenda established by the patient for this visit was to "become acquainted and refill some prescriptions."

Present Illness. James has recently encountered symptoms of urinary frequency and dysuria that went untreated because he was traveling for his job. Those symptoms have resolved, but he noted during that episode blood sugar levels in the range of 400 by home glucose monitoring. Now his sugar levels are in the 200 range, and because he has been gaining weight over the last 6 months, he feels it is "time to become more serious about this blood sugar problem and lose 20 pounds." His medication program includes glyburide (Micronase) 2.5 mg daily. He also takes diltiazem (Cardizem) 60 mg three times daily for hypertension. Other symptoms related to his diabetes include a secondary complication of some left leg neuropathy with numbness and tingling and waxing and waning difficulties with blurry vision that he attributes to fluctuations in his sugar level. James relates that he once saw an endocrinologist who personally offended him with comments about his weight, and he refused to see that person again.

James has a good energy level and states that he is "in good health except that I have to travel a lot and find it difficult to regulate the diet." He currently denies polyuria, polydipsia, polyphagia, or problems with appetite. Two years ago he experienced several episodes of hypoglycemia when he was started on medication (glyburide) at a dose of 5 mg/day. He voluntarily reduced the dose without consulting his physician. He denies pruritus, dry mouth, chest pain, or problems with his nerves.

Past Medical History. James had type A hepatitis at age 16, mononucleosis at age 25, and a pneumonia secondary to influenza sometime in his late twenties. Two hospitalizations were reported, surgery 14 years ago for a right inguinal hernia repair and a 3-day in-hospital workup 4 years ago for chest pain that was attributed to symptoms from a hiatal hernia. Blood pressure medication was changed from a diuretic to a calcium-channel blocking drug at that time. There are no known drug allergies or sensitivities.

Family History. Family history reveals type II diabetes in James's paternal grandfather, father, mother, and brother. James's father died at age 87 of cancer of the gallbladder, and his mother died at age 89 of a coronary. There were three male siblings, two now alive and one dead of oral cancer. One living brother has a history of substance abuse. James's mother and a brother suffered heart attacks and have high blood pressure. James's wife is alive and in good health, and there is one son, age 27, in good health.

Health Habits. For 10 years during his thirties James smoked approximately 1½ packs of cigarettes daily; he has not smoked for 19 years. He has three to seven alcoholic beverages per week, reports always using seat belts, and rides an exercise bicycle three times weekly when not traveling.

Social History. James is married with one child and is a health professional with 11 years of education after high school.

Review of Systems. Positive findings include a 15- to 20-decibel hearing loss which James states is familial. James has worn glasses since high school. Immunizations are not current, with the last tetanus booster over 15 years ago. He reports seasonal hay fever and an allergy to sunflower seeds. He has noticed over the past couple of years some pain in the calves of his legs when he walks distances more than two blocks. The pain disappears after a short rest. His energy level has been good, and he denies a history of depression, hot flashes, or genital trauma or infection.

During review of the genitourinary (GU) system, James hesitantly admits to some "sexual difficulties." With prompting, he volunteers that he has experienced erectile difficulties since his hospitalization for chest pain 4 years ago. He and his wife have discussed this at length, and he admits that they both would like "something done about it." He denies any extramarital relationships. His erections are partial erections, occasionally firm enough for intercourse, but he has failed as many times as he has succeeded. His wife does not place a lot of demand on him, although he feels that there is some psychologic component to his problem. He strongly believes that most of his trouble may relate to his blood pressure medication. He has a normal sexual desire. He also has noted a decrease in the firmness of his erection upon awakening or with masturbation. His relationship with his wife is described as "very good, very open."

OBJECTIVE

Physical Examination. James's vital signs are as follows: His height is 186 cm; his weight is 94.5 kg; his pulse is 72; and his blood pressure is 140/80. HEENT examination is negative, no retinal changes noted. His thyroid is normal. His neck is without bruits, and his lungs are clear to auscultation. His heart is in normal sinus rhythm without murmur. Some actinic keratoses are present on both forearms, and there is a wart on the left parietal area of the scalp. Abdominal examination shows a healed right inguinal herniorrhaphy, no bruits, and no hernias. The testicles descended, the penis is uncircumcised, and the foreskin will not retract all the way past the corona of the glans. No anatomic abnormalities of the genitalia can be detected. Rectal examination reveals no masses. Stool for occult blood is negative. The prostate gland is of normal size. Bones, joints, and extremities are unremarkable, except for a fungal infection under the right great toenail and trace edema bilaterally. Peripheral pulses seem only slightly diminished and are equal.

Laboratory Tests. Laboratory analyses ordered with the first visit include a urinanalysis, which shows 0 to 1 white cells, otherwise completely negative; hemoglobin A_1C 10.8, serum potassium 5.0, glucose 165, liver functions and electrolytes normal, cholesterol 217, HDL 48, and LDL 150. The CBC is normal. BUN is 14; serum creatinine is 1.3.

ASSESSMENT

Working Diagnoses

1. *Type II diabetes mellitus with poor control.* This is a chronic problem and the one for which James sought

treatment. There is some suggestion of a secondary complication of neuropathy with numbness and tingling sensation in the left leg and visual difficulties. Diabetes is also the systemic disorder most frequently associated with erectile dysfunction, probably mediated through vascular and neurologic complications associated with the disease.

2. *Essential hypertension.* Because he is male, has an elevated cholesterol level, and has a positive family history for heart disease, diabetes, and hypertension, James has multiple risk factors for coronary artery disease. James has a strong suspicion that his antihypertensive medication is somehow related to his erectile dysfunction. Antihypertensives are one of the three most common drug categories (antihypertensives, antihistamines, psychopharmacologics) that cause erectile dysfunction.

3. *Hiatal hernia with reflux.* This has been proven by x-ray and is a documented cause for James's chest pain.

4. *Seasonal hay fever.* With the use of unsupervised medication to control his symptoms of hay fever, James may increase his blood pressure or adversely affect his erectile function. All these problems are interrelated.

5. *Erectile dysfunction.* There are many risk factors present for an organic impotence, yet James admits to some degree of psychologic interference with his ability to have a satisfactory erection. Erectile dysfunction may be caused by neurogenic factors, endocrinologic factors, psychogenic factors, drugs, or vasculogenic factors. More than one factor is usually involved.

Differential Diagnoses. James's symptoms and physical findings suggest that the following conditions could be occurring either alone or in combination:

1. *Pure psychogenic impotence.* The gradual onset and apparent openness to discussing the problem with his wife suggest that other factors are operational. This is a secondary erectile dysfunction and seems to be present in sexual stimulation with and without his partner present. Some emotional concern may play a contributing role.

2. *Male "menopause."* Failure of testosterone secretion can occur, but it is usually accompanied by depression, fatigue, and sometimes "hot flashes." Erectile dysfunction without these other symptoms present makes testosterone failure less likely.

3. *Neurogenic impotence.* Disorders affecting the parasympathetic sacral spinal cord can cause partial or complete erectile dysfunction. More common neurologic disorders associated with impotence are spinal cord injury, multiple sclerosis, and peripheral neuropathy due to diabetes or alcoholism. The presence of some peripheral neuropathy in the left leg makes this possibility more important in the differential diagnosis.

4. *Vasculogenic impotence.* Alterations in blood flow into and out of the penis are perhaps the most frequent cause of organic impotence. Peripheral pulses are slightly diminished, and a history of claudication was given. Common risk factors are present for atherosclerotic occlusive disease, although renal function appears normal.

5. *Drug-induced impotence.* This possibility should be explored first, since the patient attributes his erectile dysfunction to his medication. It is temporally associated, and if some degree of vasculogenic impotence is present, drug administration may potentiate the problem. This diagnosis also should deserve strong consideration because it may be the easiest to treat by altering the patient's medication program.

6. The most likely cause of this man's problem is a *combination* of several of these factors.

PLAN

Diagnostic

1. Rediscuss the problem with both husband and wife present. Initial impressions should be corroborated by a complete sexual and psychologic history of both partners. Look for situational factors. Assessment of the sexual satisfaction and relationship factors of the partners should further rule out a principally psychogenic cause and be helpful in the later treatment of this condition.

2. Perform a sexologic examination, and include the cremaster and bulbocavernosus reflexes. Check breasts for gynecomastia and nipple discharge. Palpate the penile shaft for plaquelike fibrosities. Assess the size of the testicles.

3. Serum testosterone determination. An elevated testosterone level may suggest hypothyroidism, whereas a low testosterone level may be associated with hyperprolactinemia. Low testicular output could be verified by a serum testosterone level less than 300 ng/dl.

4. Nocturnal penile tumescence testing. Normally, three to five spontaneous erections lasting 25 to 35 minutes occur each night in association with rapid eye movement (REM) sleep. In this patient, a quantitative assessment would be helpful, and this can be done by monitoring the changes in the circumference of the penis at the base and at the tip with strain gauges and a special recording device in a sleep lab facility. This also may be an important pre- and postassessment where removal of medication therapy is planned. If the patient is unwilling to do this test, he may be willing to use the snap-gauge (Dacomed) in the privacy of his home.

5. Vascular testing. Penile artery flow can be assessed in the flaccid state using a Doppler ultrasound probe to determine systolic blood pressure. Systolic pressure may be compared with that in the brachial artery, and a penile–brachial artery flow ratio of less than 0.7 can be considered evidence for significant vascular flow reduction.

Therapeutic. The calcium-channel blocker diltiazem can be gradually withdrawn over a week's period. After 3 days of no blood pressure therapy, James is to start enalapril (Vasotec) at 5 mg/day. Although enalapril also has been occasionally associated with sexual side effects, so have most other antihypertensives. This change in class (i.e., from a calcium-channel blocker to an ACE inhibitor) may work satisfactorily for this individual. Changes should be made until sexual side effects abate.

A record of home blood pressure readings is to be returned to the office at the next visit.

Patient Education

1. James and his spouse are encouraged to enjoy noncoital sexual activity. James can be instructed to keep a diary of successful and unsuccessful attempts at erection. Although James is to keep a diary, the couple is cautioned against "spectatoring" in an attempt to make adjustments to the erectile function.

2. The couple are given a videotape describing treatment options of intracavernosal injection therapy and vacuum constriction devices (Erecaid system). They are encouraged to have a discussion after watching the videotape about their preferences.

3. James and his wife are instructed by the nurse in taking home blood pressures with their own equipment. James chose assessment with the snap-gauge and was instructed in its use on three consecutive nights at home. He also was instructed to increase his glyburide to 5 mg twice daily.

Disposition. Return in 4 weeks.

FIRST FOLLOW-UP VISIT

SUBJECTIVE

James had no difficulty in tapering the diltiazem, and the highest blood pressure off medication was 155/90. Since starting the Vasotec, his pressures have averaged 138/85. Home glucose monitoring has shown sugar levels ranging from 125 fasting to 180 at 4:00 p.m. James and his wife watched the videotape and prefer to try the vacuum constriction device, having an aversion to injection therapy. He reports erections seem to be improved, as confirmed by his diary. He feels that the enalapril is without side effects.

OBJECTIVE

Physical Examination. Weight 97 kg, pulse 72, and blood pressure 138/88. No new physical findings.

Laboratory Tests. Blood sugar 133, hemoglobin A_1C 9.4. Examination of the snap-gauge device shows that two of three plastic bands have broken, indicating partial erections occurring. Vascular testing revealed a penile–brachial artery flow ratio of 0.75, indicating borderline vascular flow. Serum testosterone measurement was within the normal range.

ASSESSMENT

1. *Type II diabetes.* Control has improved, and the hemoglobin A_1C level, although still elevated, is declining toward normal. Random blood sugar has nearly normalized.

2. *Essential hypertension.* Blood pressure is now under good control, and medication therapy is without apparent side effects. James feels that his erections are improving following discontinuation of the previous antihypertensive. Multiple risk factors for coronary artery disease are still present, but improvement is noted. Mild hyperlipidemia should have dietary counseling provided.

3. *Erectile dysfunction.* This patient's problem is a combined vascular, neurogenic, and psychologic impotence. The effects secondary to drug administration have been minimized, and with compliance, further improvement is expected. Endocrine factors have been ruled out.

PLAN

Diagnostic

1. Continued monitoring of diabetes is necessary to ensure compliance with treatment plan. Obtain hemoglobin A_1C and blood sugar determinations in 4 months.

2. A repeat lipid profile is planned in the next 4 to 6 months.

3. Home blood pressure monitoring and home glucose monitoring are to be done. Reassessment of renal function with BUN and creatinine determinations, a CBC, and a serum potassium determination will be done to ensure that no adverse effects of drug therapy occur.

Therapeutic. In addition to the diagnostic plans, James was given a prescription for a vacuum constriction device to assist erections. He was asked to use a demonstration Erecaid system at home for 1 week and then purchase his own if it was satisfactory. Patients who are motivated to use this device find a high degree of acceptance and improved performance.

Patient Education. James was given preliminary instruction in dietary control of cholesterol and was advised to purchase and utilize the *American Heart Association Cookbook*.

Disposition. James was asked to return in 4 months for follow-up of these problems. He was to call or write with his impression of the use of the vacuum system and to allow him an opportunity to clarify any questions about its use.

DISCUSSION

Erectile dysfunction is estimated to occur in 1 in 10 American men. Until medical technology was capable of making accurate assessments, 90% of erectile dysfunctions were believed to be psychogenic in origin. Now, however, with more sophisticated evaluation equipment, researchers have estimated that erectile dysfunction has a physical cause in approximately 80% of patients. Both psychogenic and organic factors usually interplay to cause erectile impotence. Treatment must be based on a careful evaluation, and both psychologic and biomedical therapies must be offered.

When patients have a documented organic erectile impotence (e.g., diabetes or medication-induced), therapy is directed toward removing offending medications and modifying the erectile response either pharmacologically or with vacuum-assist devices. In extreme cases, vascular surgery or penile implants may be indicated.

In the last 5 years, investigators have focused on injection therapy, with intracorporeal injections of papaverine or another vasoactive medication. The drug causes a marked relaxation of the cavernous smooth muscle as well as dilation of the arterial vessels. Patients with neurogenically based erectile dysfunction are most suited for these drugs; however, some patients with vascular impotence also will benefit. The major problem with intracorporeal injection therapy is the development of fibrosis in the penis which may later impede the placement of prosthetic devices. Injection therapy should be initiated only with the consultation of a urologist. Other potential complications include pain, hematoma, hypertension, tachycardia, and prolonged erection.

This patient may well be a candidate for later diagnostic vascular imaging followed by revascularization surgery. The claudication in the lower extremities suggests compromised penile blood flow, as does the low-normal penile–brachial artery flow ratio. This ratio can be monitored, and when further decline is detected, referral for vascular study would be indicated.

The vacuum-constriction device has the advantage of assisting the partially erect penis to become more rigid without significant side effects. A vacuum-generated negative pressure creates accumulation of blood in the penile shaft, and a constriction band placed at the base of the penis impedes drainage of the blood and maintains the erection. In this patient, the foreskin may impede full erection mechanically produced by this device. One must be cautious in use of this device in an uncircumcised penis with an inability to completely retract the foreskin, because a painful erection may result.

The use of penile prostheses is reserved for those patients who have failed other forms of therapy. The last 10 years have seen an improvement in the technology, with a wide variety of penile prostheses now available. There is a strong likelihood that the patient may require later additional surgery. One worrisome complication is erosion of the penile prosthesis through the skin. Additionally, the morbidity of surgery, the cost, and availability are matters for consideration. The inflatable type of prosthesis is generally thought to provide more natural function. If infection does not occur (incidence of about 3%) and the prosthesis functions normally, the patient with complete erectile failure can have about a 90% success rate after the implant.

The wives of impotent men may be depressed and impatient with this problem. A continued working relationship with the couple (not just the patient) is an important key to successful resolution of this problem. Refocusing the couple on noncoital sexual activity and lowering the demand for performance will alleviate most of the psychogenic component. The spouse must be reassured that she is attractive to her mate and that the failure of erection does not imply feelings of rejection or avoidance. The couple should attempt to meet the wife's sexual needs by kissing, caressing, and manual or oral stimulation. Continued open communication is important to avoid the self-blame, resentment, and rejection feelings that often accompany this problem.

SUGGESTED READING

Allen J, Ellis DJ, Carroll JL, et al. Snap-gauge band vs. multidisciplinary evaluation in impotence assessment. Urology 1989; 34(4):197–199.

Driscoll CE, Hoffmann GS. Sexual health care: A life cycle approach. In Rakel RE (ed.): Textbook of Family Practice, 4th ed. Philadelphia, W. B. Saunders, 1990, pp. 1517–1546.

Fein RL. Classification of sexual dysfunction for management of intracavernous medication-induced erections. J Urol 1990; 143:298–301.

Fishman IJ. Treating erectile dysfunction: New approaches. Drug Ther 1989; 19:102–111.

Korenman SG, Viosca SP, Kaiser FE, et al. Use of a vacuum tumescence device in the management of impotence. J Am Geriatr Soc 1990; 38:217–220.

Krane RJ, Goldstein I, de Tejada IS. Impotence. N Engl J Med 1989; 321(24):1648–1659.

Segraves RT. Effects of psychotropic drugs on human erection and ejaculation. Arch Gen Psychiatry 1989; 46:275–284.

Susset JG, Tessier CD, Wincze J, et al. Effect of yohimbine hydrochloride on erectile impotence: A double-blind study. J Urol 1989; 141:1360–1363.

Swartz CM. Low serum testosterone: A cardiovascular risk in elderly men. Geriatr Med Today 1988; 7(12):39–49.

QUESTIONS

1. Intracorporeal vasodilator drug injection is most successful in the treatment of
   a. Drug-induced impotence.
   b. Male menopause.
   c. Neurogenic impotence.
   d. Vasculogenic impotence.

2. The problem of erectile dysfunction is
   a. Best treated by a combination of counseling and medical therapy.
   b. Easily treated by self-help books given to the patient.
   c. Usually a psychogenic problem requiring little investigation.
   d. Generally responsive to hormone therapy with testosterone and with vitamin E.

3. The penile–brachial artery flow ratio is used as an indication of
   a. Endocrine cause.
   b. Neurogenic cause.
   c. Psychogenic cause.
   d. Vasculogenic cause.

Answers appear on page 452.

Genetic Counseling

ANDREW M. BARCLAY and RICHARD E. LUTZ

INITIAL VISIT

SUBJECTIVE

Patient Identification. Lennea G. is a 28-year-old married white female who presents with concerns regarding future pregnancies.

Presenting Problem. Two years ago, Lennea's first pregnancy ended with the delivery of a baby boy with Down syndrome (DS) who died 3 days after birth from congenital heart disease. Lennea was surprised to learn that 80% of infants with Down syndrome are born to women under the age of 35. She asked, "What is my risk of having another baby with Down syndrome?" Lennea is frightened that a second baby also may have Down syndrome and is concerned about raising a child, if it lives, who is mentally retarded.

Family History. Lennea states that there had been no other cases of Down syndrome in her family or that of her spouse, Earl, who is also age 28. A family genogram offers no additional information regarding genetic conditions or multiple miscarriages. Of note, Lennea's grandmother recently developed senile dementia of Alzheimer's type at age 85. Lennea mentions that chromosomal analysis of the baby confirmed Down syndrome, but she does not know what type. A chromosome study has not been performed on Lennea or Earl.

Past Medical History. No surgery, accidents, or major illness. Lennea is currently taking an oral contraceptive.

Social History/Habits. Lennea does not smoke, but her husband smokes one pack of cigarettes a day. They both drink about a six pack of beer per week. Since the loss of the baby, their relationship has been rocky at times. Lennea works as clerk in a department store, and Earl is an auto mechanic.

Review of Systems. Lennea does not feel pregnant now and has not missed any oral contraceptive pills. Her periods are regular both on and off the oral contraceptive pill. Menarche was at age 13. Lennea denies breast, gastrointestinal, or cardiovascular symptoms. She states that she was rubella-immune during her last pregnancy and that she was rhesus-positive.

OBJECTIVE

Physical Examination. Physical examination in the office was unremarkable, with the exception of signs of anxiety.

ASSESSMENT

1. *Genetic concern: need for information and counseling.* Ninety-three percent of cases of Down syndrome are of the nondisjunction type. "Nondisjunction" occurs during meiosis and develops two populations of cells, one with trisomy 21 and one with monosomy 21 (the latter gamete is usually not viable). Of younger siblings of persons with Down syndrome, 0.5% to 2% will have Down syndrome or another chromosomal abnormality. Two percent of Down syndrome infants are mosaics. Following nondisjunction in a fertilized zygote, some cases of DS have two cell lines, one normal and one with 47 chromosomes. The relative proportion of each cell line is highly variable. These individuals with two cell lines are "mosaics" and demonstrate a different number of features of Down syndrome. Five percent of Down syndrome individuals have a "translocation" type of chromosomal abnormality, and the risk of Down syndrome in future siblings is higher. In about 25% of children with a translocation type of Down syndrome, a balanced translocation will exist in one of the parents. Accordingly, these parents should be genetically tested if they plan future pregnancies. Seventy-five percent of the parents will both be chromosomally normal, and these parents have a 1% to 2% risk of having another baby with the translocation type of Down syndrome (gonadal mosaicism). If the balanced translocation exists in the mother, the risk of having another Down syndrome baby is approximately 10%; if it exists in the father, the risk is 2.5%.

2. *Unresolved grief and marital dysfunction.* The couple may have guilt associated with having a chromosomally abnormal child, the death of that child, and the fact that the child was mentally retarded. Guilt, anger, and blame are common features in couples who sustain a loss of this type, and they should be counseled about these feelings. They need to share their feelings with each other in a nondestructive manner.

PLAN

Therapeutic

GENETIC CONCERNS. To be sure that Lennea and Earl have no increased risk in the future (above 0.5% to 2% of all parents who have a child with DS), the physician should obtain the results of the chromosomal analysis of the baby with Down syndrome. Genetic testing of the parents (the cost is approximately $400 each) is not indicated unless the baby had the translocation type of Down syndrome or there had been a family history of miscarriages or trisomies. If the couple decides on another pregnancy, tests such as the maternal serum alpha-fetoprotein (MSAFP) test and sonography may be done during the pregnancy at 12 to 16 weeks. The MSAFP test is only 30% sensitive for Down syndrome, but when combined with human chorionic gonadotrophin (HCG) and serum estriol determinations, this is more sensitive for detecting DS. Chorionic villus sampling and amniocentesis are available and are sensitive but more expensive. Lennea said that she did not believe in abortion and was not sure what she would do if the fetus had Down syndrome. Many couples who discover a pregnancy with Down syndrome chose to continue the pregnancy. Professional counseling is essential regarding the decision.

UNRESOLVED GRIEF. Lennea and Earl should come in together to discuss the possibility of another pregnancy. During this visit, the possibility of unresolved grief should be addressed, since 50% of all couples who sustain a loss of a baby divorce within a year. The genetic service at the University Medical Center 200 miles away was mentioned as a resource, but Lennea did not wish to go there, since that was the site of her son's death. Because of her cesarean section in a hospital 200 miles away, she was unable to get to the University Medical Center before her son's death and feels additional grief and guilt because of this. More information is needed so that this couple can make reasonable plans for the future and deal with their feelings in a straightforward fashion.

FIRST FOLLOW-UP VISIT

PLAN

Therapeutic

GENETIC CONCERNS. The hospital records from the University Medical Center confirm that the infant died from congenital heart disease, and a diagnosis of Down syndrome had been made and confirmed by karyotype. There was evidence of nondisjunction, which puts the couple at a risk of 0.5% to 2% for Down syndrome in future pregnancies. The normal risk of any chromosomal abnormality is 0.1%. The infant showed classical features of Down syndrome, including marked hypotonia, flat occiput, epicanthal folds, and a wide interdigital space between the first and second toes. Expensive karyotyping of Lennea and Earl was therefore not necessary. The couple should be advised that their risk of a chromosomal abnormality in each subsequent pregnancy is 0.5% to 2%, but that this risk will increase in accordance with age-specific risks. Other major congenital problems could occur at normal rates. It should be emphasized that nothing they did during the course of the first pregnancy was responsible for the baby having Down syndrome and that they were not responsible for the baby's death. Because of their concerns, an MSAFP test and sonography could be performed if they choose to attempt another pregnancy. Amniocentesis (or chronic villus sampling) would provide more specific information about the risk of Down syndrome.

Lennea decides that she would like to try to become pregnant again, and she is advised to avoid oral contraceptives for a least 2 months before trying to become pregnant so that the lining of the uterus will be better able to sustain a pregnancy. A daily prenatal vitamin with 1 mg folic acid is recommended prior to conception to reduce the risk of neural tube defects.

GRIEF. The birth and death of their son and the very difficult situation in which they were placed is reviewed:

1. They had no warning that the infant would not be perfect, and Lennea had unfortunately not had a routine MSAFP test during her first pregnancy.

2. The infant was taken to another hospital rapidly, without much time for Lennea or Earl to bond with the infant or to process this deviation from their expectations.

3. The couple had no idea how they were going to cope with a child who had both heart defects and mental retardation.

4. Many couples experience a feeling of relief that a baby with these severe problems has died. This feeling of relief promotes feelings of great guilt, and both Lennea and Earl should be advised that the feelings of relief and the feelings of guilt are normal and very human responses.

5. All these factors contributed to a detached view of the loss of their baby with the development of unresolved grief.

Like many couples in this situation, both Lennea and Earl felt that they were being blamed by the other for the genetic problem and "would not have had this deficient child if they had married a different partner." Following the death of their son, they had been advised by relatives that it was "God's will" and "just as well," which did not relate to their feelings at the time, with the result that they felt isolated and alone after their initial grieving period. Well-meaning friends and relatives are often not very helpful in these situations because they are desperately trying to think of something useful to say. A feeling of tremendous isolation is common, and Lennea and Earl should be congratulated for their marriage surviving one of the toughest life events (Holmes and Rahe scale). They are encouraged to work on communication skills with each other, and they will need to be open with each other during an anxious second pregnancy.

DISCUSSION

Genetic counseling is, of necessity, a task for many family physicians, especially those practicing in a rural area. The principles of genetic counseling include accurate diagnosis, informative counseling, supportive counseling, and follow-up. Specific directions or recommendations as to whether a couple should attempt further pregnancies are not a role of the genetic counselor. Such a decision remains one for the family.

SUGGESTED READING

Rakel RE (ed.). Textbook of Family Practice, 4th ed. Philadelphia, W. B. Saunders, 1990, pp. 19–40, 1552–1565.

Stray-Gundersen K (ed.). Babies with Down Syndrome: A New Parent's Guide. Kenington, Md., Woodbine House, 1986.

QUESTIONS

1. Which of the following are features of a newborn who has Down syndrome?

   a. Hypotonia
   b. Long ears
   c. Wide space between the first and second toes
   d. High risk (50%) for congenital heart disease

2. Which of the following options are components of genetic counseling?

   a. Diagnosis
   b. Informative counseling
   c. Specific advise as to a couple's future reproductive efforts
   d. Supportive counseling
   e. Follow-up

3. Following the delivery of a baby with Down syndrome in a karyotypically normal couple under the age of 30, what is their risk of delivering another chromosomally abnormal baby?

   a. 0.5% to 2%
   b. 10%
   c. 25%
   d. 50%

4. What percentage of Down syndrome babies are born to women under the age of 35?

   a. 1%
   b. 10%
   c. 50%
   d. 80%

Answers appear on page 452.

Palpitations and Sweating

JOHN P. GEYMAN, WAYNE J. KATON, and NANCY GRAY STEVENS

INITIAL VISIT

SUBJECTIVE

Patient Identification. Molly P. is a 35-year-old Caucasian woman who was first seen in the Family Medical Center 2 years ago for advice about contraception/infertility, dysmenorrhea, irregular periods, and malar rash.

Present Illness. After more than 2 years without a visit, Molly presented, at the urging of a friend, with numerous somatic complaints, including frequent urination, irregular periods, premenstrual breast pain, headaches, night sweats, and intermittent sore throat. She also complains of several episodes over the last 2 months while driving and at other times of the feeling of some unnamed impending problem. At these times she feels that "the world is closing in around me and I have trouble breathing." These episodes are usually accompanied by palpitations, sweating, and trembling. Sometimes she also has a headache with these episodes, sometimes not. Questions about current life events reveal that her husband is considering quitting his job of many years and starting a new business and her 14-year-old son to whom she has been very close for years has begun to rebel and separate from her. Because of the complexity of her numerous complaints and the physician's suspicion that her life stresses may be a significant contributor to her symptoms, some diagnostic studies were obtained and another office visit was scheduled to get a more complete assessment. A CBC, erythrocyte sedimentation rate, ANA, M-12, and thyroid studies were ordered at this visit. The possibility that her physical symptoms may be related in part to her current stresses was suggested to her, but Molly did not want to further explore that area at that time.

Molly returns as scheduled 2 weeks later and describes two additional episodes of palpitations, shortness of breath, sweating, and a sense of impending doom. These also were associated with headache (starting in the neck and spreading up over the occiput). There was no associated chest pain, nausea, vomiting, abdominal pain, dizziness, or other complaints. The episodes again occurred while Molly was driving, despite her attempts to prevent them. Molly initially attributed these symptoms to low blood sugar. She attempted to alleviate these episodes by taking along candy and a carbonated drink while driving, but since these approaches were not successful, she then began to avoid driving and other situations, such as attending basketball games, which she has enjoyed in the past. She has recently restricted her activities, avoiding public gatherings and situations where she feared she would lose control of herself. She even canceled a referral appointment to a dermatologist for her malar rash because it would mean driving in an unfamiliar area. Molly is quite disabled by her symptoms and her self-imposed limitations to avoid them and is now requesting treatment.

Past Medical History. Molly has had no surgery, serious illnesses, or accidents and has never been hospitalized, except for delivery of her son 14 years ago. There is no history of child or sexual abuse. She takes no medication on a regular basis and denies allergy to any drugs. She has been followed for a malar rash and a presumptive diagnosis of acne rosacea, including past consultation with a dermatologist. She has not used any contraceptive method since the birth of her son. More recently, she has begun to worry about the possibility of pregnancy and has avoided intercourse for the last 2 years because of her fear of pregnancy.

Family History. Both Molly's parents are alive and live only several miles away in Seattle. Her father, age 70, has recently undergone surgery for carcinoma of the colon. Her mother, age 67, is described as a passive, dependent person who has restricted her normal activities over the years. She has not had serious illnesses or hospitalizations other than for childbirth. She has had "nervous" episodes through the years, has been heavily dependent on her husband for care, and has never learned to drive. As a result of Molly's father recent illness, he is less able to care for her mother, and the burden of her care has shifted to Molly. Molly's only sibling, a sister age 32, works full time and is not expected by Molly's parents to be available to help. However, they expect Molly to be available to help at any time, especially since she is "not working."

Health Habits. Molly does not smoke, drinks only occasionally in small amounts, and denies use of any illicit drugs. Until recently, Molly has exercised regularly as part of a group exercise program (without significant limitation of physical activity by shortness of breath). Her dietary preferences are for carbohydrates and sweet foods.

Social History. Molly married in 1969 at age 18 upon graduation from high school. She describes her marriage in neutral terms, and she and her husband have one son, now 14. Molly has not worked outside the home since her marriage. Her husband previously wanted her not to work, but recently he has been considering starting his own business and has been urging Molly to do the bookkeeping for the business. Molly is ambivalent about having more children and does not want to undertake work outside the home. This has caused her considerable stress, both to avoid the perceived criticism of many of her peers and to confront her husband concerning her role in his business venture. Molly also felt under increased stress within the family because of the growing demands of her parents for assistance and her perception that her husband and son are often allied as a pair. She and her son were very close until quite recently, and the separation is very difficult for her.

Review of Systems. Molly has retained a good appetite, and her present weight of 140 lb is average within her usual range of 130 to 150 lb. Her height is 68 in. She denies sleep problems but has nocturia three to four times each night with a history of copious water intake but without dysuria or history of urinary tract infections. She has had occasional night sweats without known fever or chills. She denies a history of heart disease, peptic ulcer, joint complaints, visual changes, or other symptoms.

OBJECTIVE

Physical Examination. Molly's vital signs are within normal limits, including a blood pressure of 110/80, heart rate of 80 and regular, an oral temperature of 36.5°C, and a weight of 140 lb. She is very pleasant and cooperative, speaks at a rather fast rate, and seems tense and apologetic in describing her symptoms. Her physical examination is notable for a malar rash with areas of inflammatory and pustular changes, and her palms are moist. The thyroid gland is normal to inspection and palpation. Cardiac examination is normal without murmur or opening click. Neurologic and mental status examinations are likewise within normal limits. No lymphadenopathy is noted, and the liver and spleen are not enlarged.

Laboratory Tests. The CBC is normal, with a hematocrit of 38%, at lower range of normal. Routine urinalysis is also normal, as are sedimentation rate (8 mm/h) M-12 panel, thyroid function studies, and ANA. All these studies were ordered at the previous office visit 2 weeks ago and were completed during the interval before this office visit.

ASSESSMENT

One must consider a number of organic and psychiatric diagnoses to explain Molly's symptoms and findings, including the possibility of multiple diagnoses:

1. *Lupus erythematosus.* The malar rash and fatigue raise initial suspicion of lupus erythematosus, but this remote possibility can be discounted in view of the skin rash more typical of acne rosacea; the absence of fever, joint effusions, hepatosplenomegaly, or adenopathy; and the normal sedimentation rate and ANA.

2. *Hyperthyroidism.* This is unlikely because of the absence of weight loss, hypertension, resting tachycardia, tremor, or other physical findings of hyperthyroidism, and it is ruled out by normal thyroid function studies.

3. *Diabetes mellitus.* This is suggested by a possibility that increased water intake could represent polydipsea with secondary nocturia, but it is easily ruled out by the lack of further clinical manifestations of diabetes, the normal urinalysis, and the normal serum glucose level.

4. *Pulmonary disease.* Intermittent episodes of shortness of breath without chest pain raise the possibility of pulmonary disease. This diagnosis was discounted early in view of the absence of a history of asthma, dyspnea on exertion, or pulmonary disease and the normal physical findings. A chest x-ray was considered, but it was not felt to be indicated at this time.

5. *Tension headaches.* This is a distinct possibility,

particularly in view of the nature of headaches, with origin in neck muscles and spread up over the occiput. Auras, gastrointestinal symptoms, and other features of migraine and other types headaches are absent. The presence, however, of associated "panic" symptoms suggests that the symptoms are probably not directly due to tension headaches per se, although Molly may well have coexisting tension headaches.

6. *Generalized anxiety disorder.* This is unlikely owing to the absence of chronic and pervasive anxiety and worry over an extended period (i.e., more than 6 months). In this instance, the clearly episodic nature of the symptoms provides further evidence that the underlying problem is not generalized anxiety.

7. *Adjustment disorder with anxious mood.* This disorder typically follows a known psychosocial stressor(s) as a result of dysfunctional occupational, social, or interpersonal relationships. Continued, nonepisodic nervousness, worry, and trouble falling asleep are usually present. Although some dysfunctional family dynamics probably contribute to Molly's stress level, the episodic nature of her symptoms, together with the extent of associated somatic symptoms (e.g., shortness of breath and tachycardia) argue against this diagnosis as the primary problem.

8. *Depression.* It has been demonstrated by numerous studies that patients with anxiety disorders have a high frequency of depression, either as a coexisting disorder or as part of a previous history of depression. The reverse is also true, with about 60% of patients with major depression also having a concurrent anxiety disorder. In Molly's case, therefore, one must have a very high index of suspicion for depression and screen for it as needed. In Molly's case, the episodic nature of her symptoms, together with absence of sleep disorder, depressed mood, weight change, and cognitive symptoms such as decreased self-esteem, guilt, helplessness, hopelessness, or suicidal ideation, suggests that depression is not the major problem.

9. *Panic disorder with agoraphobia.* Tables 20–59 and 20–60 present diagnostic criteria for panic disorder with agoraphobia. Molly fully meets these criteria in terms of the nature and recurrence of typical panic attacks. Her anticipatory anxiety of future panic attacks and avoidance behavior of public settings (e.g., basketball games) where she fears an uncontrollable episode represent classic features of agoraphobia.

PLAN

Diagnostic. Initial laboratory studies were obtained at a previous visit. In past visits Molly's physician raised the possibility of panic disorder, and Molly exhibited reluctance to consider therapy. During this visit, Molly requested therapy. In view of a strong patient–physician relationship ensuring future follow-up and continuity of care, further diagnostic studies were not considered necessary at this point. The contemplated use of a tri-

TABLE 20–59. DIAGNOSTIC CRITERIA FOR PANIC DISORDER

I. At some time during the disturbance, one or more panic attacks (discrete periods of intense fear or discomfort) have occurred that were unexpected* (i.e., did not occur immediately before or on exposure to a situation that almost always caused anxiety) and were not triggered by situations in which the person was the focus of others' attention.†

II. Either four attacks, as defined in criterion I, have occurred within a 4-week period or one or more attacks have been followed by a period of at least 1 month of persistent fear of having another attack.

III. At least four* of the following symptoms developed during at least one of the attacks:

    A. Shortness of breath (dyspnea) or smothering sensations
    B. Dizziness, unsteady feelings, or faintness
    C. Palpitations or accelerated heart rate (tachycardia)
    D. Trembling or shaking
    E. Sweating
    F. Choking
    G. Nausea or abdominal distress
    H. Depersonalization or derealization†
    I. Numbness or tingling sensations (paresthesias)
    J. Flushes (hot flashes) or chills
    K. Chest pain or discomfort
    L. Fear of dying
    M. Fear of going crazy or of doing something uncontrolled

IV. During at least some of the attacks, at least four of the symptoms in III developed suddenly and increased in intensity within 10 minutes of the beginning of the first symptom noticed in the attack.

V. It cannot be established that an organic factor initiated and maintained the disturbance (e.g., amphetamine or caffeine intoxication or hyperthyroidism).‡

Source: Reprinted with permission from the Diagnostic and Statistical Manual of Mental Disorders, 3rd ed, revised. Copyright 1987 by the American Psychiatric Association, pp. 237–238, with permission.

*Attacks involving four or more symptoms are panic attacks; attacks involving fewer than four symptoms are limited symptom attacks.

†"Depersonalization" is manifest by a feeling of detachment from and being an outside observer of one's body or mental processes or of feeling like an automaton or as if in a dream. "Derealization" is evidenced by a strange alteration in the perception of one's surroundings so that a sense of the reality of the external world is lost. Alteration in the size or shape of objects in the external world is commonly perceived.

‡Mitral value prolapse may be an associated condition, but it does not preclude a diagnosis of panic disorder.

TABLE 20–60. DIAGNOSTIC CRITERIA FOR PANIC DISORDER WITH AGORAPHOBIA

I. Meets the criteria for panic disorder.

II. Agoraphobia: Fear of being in places or situations from which escape might be difficult (or embarrassing) or in which help might not be available in the event of a panic attack. (Include cases in which persistent avoidance behavior originated during an active phase of panic disorder, even if the person does not attribute the avoidance behavior to fear of having a panic attack.) As a result of this fear, the person either restricts travel or needs a companion when away from home or else endures agoraphobic situations despite intense anxiety. Common agoraphobic situations include being outside the home alone, being in a crowd or standing in a line, being on a bridge, and traveling in a bus, train, or car.

Specify current severity of agoraphobic avoidance:

Mild: Some avoidance (or endurance with distress), but relatively normal lifestyle (e.g., travels unaccompanied when necessary, such as to work or to shop; otherwise avoids traveling alone)

Moderate: Avoidance results in constricted lifestyle (e.g., the person is able to leave the house alone but not to go more than a few miles unaccompanied)

Severe: Avoidance results in being nearly or completely housebound or unable to leave the house unaccompanied

In partial remission: No current agoraphobic avoidance, but some agoraphobic avoidance during the past 6 months

In full remission: No current agoraphobic avoidance and none during the past 6 months

Specify current severity of panic attacks:

Mild: During the past month, either all attacks have been limited symptom attacks (i.e., fewer than four symptoms) or there has been no more than one panic attack.

Moderate: During the past month, attacks have been intermediate between "mild" and "severe."

Severe: During the past month, there have been at least eight panic attacks.

In partial remission: The condition has been intermediate between "in full remission" and "mild."

In full remission: During the past 6 months, there have been no panic attacks or limited symptom attacks.

Source: Reprinted with permission from the Diagnostic and Statistical Manual of Disorders, 3rd ed, revised. Copyright 1987 by the American Psychiatric Association, pp. 238–239.

cyclic antidepressant would provide appropriate treatment for both panic disorder and underlying depression, if present.

Therapeutic. A tricyclic antidepressant, desipramine, was selected and started at a low dose of 25 mg at bedtime. In addition, Molly was asked to keep a diary of the frequency, setting, and nature of any future panic episodes. Reassurance was given concerning the therapeutic effectiveness of the medication for this condition. Psychiatric consultation was considered but was not felt to be indicated at this time.

Patient Education

1. Molly was advised that she may have some side effects from desipramine but that these should be mild and self-limited. A low starting dose is being used, and this may cause dry mouth and possible dizziness. The possibility of a stimulant effect was discussed, in which case the daily dose should be taken in the morning instead of at bedtime. The stimulant side effect also might be an indication to decrease the initial dosage to as low as 10 mg, followed by gradual 10-mg increases.

2. The high prevalence of panic disorder in the general population was explained. Further reinforcement was given that Molly could look forward to full alleviation of symptoms with appropriate adjustment of medication dosage and that she could expect to again un-

dertake activities in previously feared situations without recurrence of panic attacks.

3. Molly was informed about the similarity between a panic attack and the autonomic nervous system's "fight or flight" response to danger. Panic attacks are believed to be "fight or flight" responses occurring at inappropriate times when there is no real danger. The symptoms produced by this autonomic response are often quite frightening to the patient.

4. In addition, Molly's separation from her son and need to set limits with her parents were discussed, and she was encouraged to work on these issues to reduce the stress in her life.

Disposition. The physician plans to call Molly in 2 or 3 days to see how she is doing, and Molly is to return in 2 weeks for follow-up.

FIRST FOLLOW-UP VISIT

SUBJECTIVE

Molly returns as scheduled, reporting mild symptoms of dry mouth on desipramine as well as dramatic improvement in her panic symptoms. She describes several examples of progress, including being able to drive again, even in traffic, without any recurrence of panic symptoms. She is starting to get more involved with many of her previous activities. Despite this increased level of activity, she reports no recurrence of panic symptoms and expresses confidence in further expanding her future activities.

OBJECTIVE

Molly appears much less anxious than on her previous visit. She looks visibly relieved of worry, and her mood seems optimistic. Her diary shows no panic symptoms but still some lingering anticipatory anxiety of certain situations.

ASSESSMENT

1. Panic disorder with agoraphobia—responding to desipramine at a low dose.
2. Molly's dramatic response to a small bedtime dose of desipramine, together with her positive outlook and general improvement, adds further evidence that major depression is not a concurrent problem.

PLAN

Diagnostic. No additional tests are indicated at this time.

Therapeutic. Since Molly has tolerated the initial low starting dose of desipramine well, and since the goal is complete control of her symptoms, her bedtime desipramine dosage is increased to 50 mg.

Patient Education. Molly was counseled again regarding side effects of desipramine. Further reinforcement also was given that previous activities and settings that she had avoided due to panic symptoms could confidently be approached without concern.

Disposition. A return visit is scheduled in 3 weeks.

FOLLOW-UP NOTE

By the next visit, Molly's panic symptoms have completely resolved, despite full involvement in previously threatening situations. She is able to drive her car anywhere alone, including in rush-hour traffic. She has successfully tried out to join a follies program and has purchased dancing shoes. In addition, she is starting to set some limits for the first time on the demands of her mother, and she is able to be more assertive in stating her own needs within the family. She is a most grateful patient and is continued on desipramine 50 mg h.s.

DISCUSSION

The successful diagnosis and management of Molly's panic disorder was facilitated by a strong and trusting physician–patient relationship. The diagnosis is easily missed in primary care by the unwary physician who might ascribe the patient's symptoms to hypochondriasis, somatization disorder, or other anxiety disorders or even to consider the patient as a "difficult patient." In this instance, a high level of personal continuity of care was maintained, and Molly's physician was able to raise the possibility of panic disorder over sequential visits and to overcome the patient's initial reluctance to recognize and treat the problem. Thus the value of regular office visits with the same physician is demonstrated, together with a partnership effort between patient and physician in diagnosis and management.

The physician's workup for panic disorder effectively ruled out other differential diagnoses in a cost-effective way without resorting to a full battery of possible studies. For example, an echocardiogram was not ordered despite the common association of mitral valve prolapse in patients with panic disorder (this is usually a mild, asymptomatic type requiring no treatment). A graded workup is the norm in primary care, however, and further studies can be ordered later based on continuing reassessment of the patient's course, changing physical findings, and/or response to treatment.

This case also illustrates the value of further history on follow-up visits by the physician regularly reassessing the patient for possible additional underlying or new problems. In this instance, the patient had been followed for several years for various problems, including dysmenorrhea, irregular menses, and ambivalence to contraception/conception, with a high level of background stressful life events. Further history, particularly the clearcut episodic nature of new panic symptoms and the possible maternal history of panic disorder, tipped off the alert physician to this new problem.

Panic disorder is common in everyday practice. In one study, Katon et al. found that 20% of primary care patients had panic disorder at some time in their lives, while an additional 18% had infrequent attacks not meeting all the diagnostic criteria for panic disorder. The highest 6-month prevalence has been found to be in the 25- to 44-year age group, but panic disorder has been observed from the midteens to the 60-year age group. Most studies show about a twofold increased prevalence in females over males with panic disorder. Panic disorder occurs in approximately 30% of first-degree relatives of patients with anxiety attacks. Also, the concordance rate in monozygotic twins is up to five times higher than the concordance rate in dizygotic twins.

Molly's presenting symptoms were representative of many patients with panic disorder. In one study of primary care patients, Katon found the three most common presenting symptom complexes to be cardiologic (chest pain, tachycardia, and/or irregular heart beat), gastrointestinal (particularly epigastric distress), and neurologic (headache, dizziness, syncope or paresthesias). Other recent studies have associated panic disorder with migraine headache and irritable bowel syndrome. Within the common presenting symptom groups, however, there is wide variation from patient to patient. Thus, in Molly's case, she experienced no chest pain or epigastric pain, which commonly occur in other patients with panic disorder and usually lead to negative cardiac and GI workups. Across the entire spectrum of patients presenting with possible panic disorder, Katon and colleagues have found that the single most sensitive question in the history targeting the diagnosis is, "Do you ever have sudden episodes of rapid heartbeat, shortness of breath, shakiness, and sweatiness, and feeling that something frightening is happening to you."

With respect to treatment, Molly had a typical dramatic response to tricyclic antidepressant drug therapy. Although imipramine has received most attention in studies of panic disorder, it appears that any of the tricyclic antidepressants are equally effective in treating this problem. Desipramine was a good choice in view of its relatively low frequency of side effects, whether anticholinergic, sedation, or orthostatic hypotension. This patient had a full therapeutic response to a comparatively low dose of desipramine, both in terminating the panic attacks and in allowing successful reentry into previously avoided situations without recurrence of symptoms. The usual daily dosage range for most tricyclic antidepressants for treatment of panic disorder is 100 to 300 mg, with some patients responding to 25 to 50 mg, as in this case, and others requiring up to 300 mg. High-potency benzodiazepines (clonazepam, alprazolam, and lorazepam) and monoamine oxidase inhibitors (phenelzine) also have been shown to be effective in treating panic disorder in double-blind placebo-controlled trials. Since this patient had no complicating problems of alcohol or other substance abuse, was not depressed, and had no prior history of obsessive–compulsive disorder or posttraumatic stress syndrome, a favorable prognosis can be anticipated with the use of a low-dose tricyclic antidepressant. This medication should be continued for 6 months after successful treatment and then tapered gradually over 1 to 2 months. Crucial to this successful outcome, however, was a precise diagnosis of panic disorder, enabling specific effective therapy.

SUGGESTED READING

Friedman I, Jaffe A. Anxiety disorders. J Fam Pract 1983; 16:145–152.

Grant B, Katon W, Beitman B. Panic disorder. J Fam Pract 1983; 17:907–914.

Katon W. Panic disorder and somatization: A review of 55 cases. Am J Med 1984; 77:101–106.

Katon W. Panic Disorder in the Medical Setting. Rockville, Md., U.S. Department of Health and Human Services, Public Health Services, National Institute of Mental Health, 1989, p. 11.

Katon W, Vitaliano PP, Russo J, et al. Panic disorder: Epidemiology in primary care. J Fam Pract 1986; 23:233–239.

Katon W, Vitaliano PR, Russo J, et al. Panic disorder: Spectrum of severity and somatization. J Nerv Ment Dis 1987; 175(1):12–19.

Rakel RE (ed.). Textbook of Family Practice. 4th ed. Philadelphia, W. B. Saunders, 1990, pp. 1566–1581.

Reid WH, Wise MG. DSM-III-R Training Guide. New York, Brunner/Mazel, 1989.

QUESTIONS

1. The most common serious anxiety disorder in primary care is
   a. Generalized anxiety.
   b. Posttraumatic stress syndrome.
   c. Panic disorder with agoraphobia.
   d. Adjustment disorder with anxious mood.
   e. Obsessive–compulsive disorder.

2. Panic disorder is most frequently seen in
   a. Young-adult and early-middle-aged females.
   b. Young-adult and early-middle-aged males.
   c. Adult females aged 45 to 65.
   d. Adult males aged 45 to 65.
   e. Adolescent years equally in both sexes.

3. The element in the history most useful in differentiating panic disorder from other anxiety disorders is
   a. Family history.
   b. History of depression.
   c. History of mitral valve prolapse.
   d. Duration of symptoms.
   e. Episodic nature of symptoms.

4. The best initial therapy for panic disorder is
   a. Reassurance without drug therapy.
   b. A benzodiazepine.
   c. A hypnotic-sedative.
   d. A tricyclic antidepressant.
   e. A monoamine oxidase inhibitor.

Answers appear on page 452.

Excessive Sleepiness and Fatigue

THOMAS L. SCHWENK and JAMES C. COYNE

INITIAL VISIT

SUBJECTIVE

Patient Identification. Karen E. is a 35-year-old female nurse who presents at a routine office visit with concerns about fatigue.

Presenting Problem. Karen describes general good health until 3 months ago, when she experienced increasing fatigue. She does not initially express concern about other symptoms or mood alterations. She says that she has a long history of iron-deficiency anemia and wants a CBC done.

Present Illness. Karen describes her fatigue as a problem with hypersomnolence, sleeping 10 to 12 hours per day. Despite this excessive sleeping, Karen reports morning fatigue and difficulty getting through her work day. She is concerned about anemia and is somewhat obsessed with this potential diagnosis and doing appropriate laboratory tests to investigate it. She also wonders about testing for hypothyroidism. She initially denies mood disturbance or other neurovegetative complaints such as change in appetite or weight or decreased sexual interest. She also denies anxiety or suicidal intent. Upon further questioning, Karen describes the fatigue as a decreased enthusiasm for her usual activities and an inability to maintain her usual family and personal responsibilities. She describes her usual day as feeling tired upon awakening, going to work and performing satisfactorily, and coming home without any interest or energy to exercise or pursue other pleasurable activities. She is accustomed to pursuing a fairly vigorous exercise program, running 3 to 4 miles three times per week. She is not involved in an active sexual relationship, but when questioned more closely, she suggests that she has minimal sexual interest. She also reports some emotional lability with occasional episodes of crying for unexplained reasons.

Karen denies other problems, except for a mild intermittent tension-type headache. She denies other pain or cardiac, metabolic, skin, or gastrointestinal symptoms. She also denies cognitive dysfunction at work.

Past Medical History. Karen reports a long history of anemia, for which she was told in the past to take iron supplements, but she cannot provide details or specific blood values. She denies other chronic illness or hospitalizations, except one uncomplicated obstetrical delivery. Karen reports an episode of severe "breakdown" in her late teens or early twenties but cannot be more specific and does not seem to relate her current illness to this episode.

Family History. Karen is divorced and does not have custody of her teenage daughter, who lives with her father in a city several hours' drive away. Karen sees her daughter occasionally, but the relationship is strained and a source of considerable stress. Karen was raised as one of four children in a family she describes as strict in its discipline but without sexual or physical abuse. She reports that one brother and one sister are currently being treated with antidepressants, but she does not know specific details about their diagnoses. She knows of no psychiatric diagnoses in her parents or other relatives. There is no hereditary disease in the family otherwise.

Health Habits. Karen used to exercise regularly but has lost interest in exercise in the last few months. She does not smoke, and she drinks alcohol only very occasionally. She takes no illicit or prescription drugs and is very wary of taking any medication, especially psychotropic medication, because of fears about possible addiction.

Social History. Karen works on an inpatient surgical unit at University Hospital as a registered nurse. She lives alone and does not have a current sexual relationship. She has few close personal friends and has lost contact with friends in the last few months.

Review of Systems. Negative for other symptoms.

OBJECTIVE

Physical Examination. Karen's vital signs are within normal limits. Her weight has increased 10 lb, from 140 to 150 lb, over the past 6 months, according to chart records. A brief physical examination with an emphasis on neurologic, cardiac, and metabolic systems is negative, including an absence of focal neurologic findings and no vascular or skin abnormalities.

Laboratory Tests. No tests were done at the time of the visit, but a CBC and thyroid function studies were ordered.

ASSESSMENT

Working Diagnosis. The most likely diagnosis for Karen is *major depressive disorder*. She does not fully fit the DSM-III-R criteria (see Table 20–61) based on the information available at this visit. She reports anhedonia plus three additional criteria-based symptoms (fatigue, weight change, and sleep disturbance), but further investigation at the next visit has a high likelihood of providing additional information that will bring her into a full fit with these criteria (such as psychomotor retardation or feelings of worthlessness or guilt). Karen's report of fatigue includes an element of moderately severe anhedonia or loss of pleasure and involvement in usual daily activities such as exercise. Patients frequently do

TABLE 20–61. DSM-III-R CRITERIA FOR MAJOR DEPRESSIVE DISORDER

At least five of nine of the following symptoms, at least one of which is depressed mood or loss of interest or pleasure
1. Depressed mood
2. Loss of interest or pleasure
3. Significant weight change (>5% of body weight in 1 month) or appetite change
4. Sleep disturbance
5. Psychomotor agitation or retardation
6. Fatigue or loss of energy
7. Feelings of worthlessness or excessive guilt
8. Cognitive dysfunction
9. Recurrent suicidal ideation

No organic cause or relationship to normal bereavement
No delusions or hallucinations
No associated psychiatric morbidity, such as schizophrenia

Source: Adapted from American Psychiatric Association. Diagnostic and Statistical Manual of Mental Disorders, 3rd ed.—revised. Washington, D.C., American Psychiatric Association, 1987, with permission.

not comprehend more abstract phrasing of questions about loss of interest or pleasure, but Karen was able to identify this loss specifically in relation to her interest in running and exercise. The excessive sleep is usually of poor quality, resulting in morning fatigue. Karen exhibits a weight gain of 6% to 7% but is not aware of an associated appetite disturbance, so the weight change may be due to decreased exercise. Her mood and psychomotor and cognitive functions are apparently not disturbed, and the length of the routine office visit does not allow much exploration of feelings of worthlessness or guilt. The presence of these feelings would bear closer questioning and scrutiny, particularly with regard to her relationship with her daughter. She does describe significant emotional lability with occasional crying for no apparent reason. She has experienced these symptoms for several months, during which she had several periods of consistent symptoms exceeding 2 weeks.

Karen's positive past history and family history increase the likelihood of the diagnosis of major depressive disorder (MDD). The details of the "breakdown" episode in her past are unclear, but it likely was a first episode of MDD, which is common in the third or fourth decade of life. The fact that Karen did not relate the current illness to this earlier episode is not uncommon, since depressed patients often have distorted recall about past illnesses. The fact that two siblings are currently taking antidepressants strongly suggests that they have a diagnosis of MDD, but this would require further elaboration. Karen's family and social history are otherwise not particularly remarkable, especially for the lack of physical or sexual abuse, but a divorced, single mother (even without child custody) has an increased risk for MDD. A history of physical or sexual abuse is increasingly identified as a risk factor for the development of MDD, possibly due to the resultant poor self-esteem involved.

A lack of other physical complaints or chronic illness tends to draw attention away from other biomedical illness, particularly metabolic or hematologic diseases, which are usually multisymptom in presentation. In summary, Karen shows evidence of anhedonia and three

additional criteria of MDD present for more than 2 weeks.

Differential Diagnoses. Karen's symptoms suggest several other diagnostic possibilities, although none is nearly as likely as MDD:

1. *Dysthymia.* Karen's emotional disturbance could be characterized as a less severe depression, such as dysthymia (see Table 20–62), except that the symptoms have been present for only a few months. Her symptoms of tearfulness and possible social withdrawal are criteria for dysthymia, but the intensity of the vegetative symptoms and their presence for a shorter length of time argue against dysthymia.

2. *Adjustment disorder.* The constellation of symptoms could fit an adjustment disorder diagnosis, except that no obvious precipitating event can be identified.

3. *Hypothyroidism.* Karen shows no additional stigmata of hypothyroidism and has neurovegetative symptoms beyond simple fatigue.

4. *Anemia.* The past history of anemia is pertinent, but Karen shows no pallor or weakness in support of this diagnosis. This diagnosis is easily confirmed or refuted with a hematocrit/hemoglobin determination.

5. *Chronic fatigue syndrome.* Fatigue was the presenting complaint for Karen, but upon further questioning, her complaint is really a lack of motivation to pursue usual activities. She is functional in her work and home roles but has no pleasure in usual recreational activities. She also reports no initiating illness or acute onset.

6. *Generalized anxiety disorder.* Many patients with depression present with anxiety, and vice versa. Karen shows none of the psychologic, physical, or autonomic hyperreactivity symptoms or findings required for a diagnosis of anxiety.

PLAN

Diagnostic. As noted earlier, CBC and thyroid-stimulating hormone level were ordered.

TABLE 20–62. DSM III-R CRITERIA FOR DYSTHYMIA

Depressed mood for most of the day, more days than not, for at least two years

Presence, while depressed, of at least two of the following:
1. Poor appetite or overeating
2. Insomnia or hypersomnia
3. Low energy or fatigue
4. Low self-esteem
5. Poor concentration or difficulty making decisions
6. Feelings of hopelessness

No evidence of Major Depresssion Episode, Manic Episode, or Hypomanic Episode

Not superimposed on a chronic psychotic disorder, such as Schizophrenia or Delusional Disorder

No evidence of an organic cause, e.g., prolonged administration fo an antihypertensive medication

Source: Adapted from American Psychiatric Association. Diagnostic and Statistical Manual of Mental Disorders, 3rd ed.—revised. Washington, D.C., American Psychiatric Association, 1987.

TABLE 20–63. CHARACTERISTICS OF COMMONLY USED ANTIDEPRESSANTS

GENERIC NAME	TRADE NAME(S)	EFFECT ON SEROTONIN UPTAKE	EFFECT ON NOREPINEPHRINE UPTAKE	SEDATING EFFECT	ANTICHOLINERGIC EFFECT	ORTHOSTATIC EFFECT	USUAL DOSE AND DOSAGE RANGE (MG/DAY)
Tricyclic Tertiary Amines							
Amitriptyline	Elavil, Endep	++++	++	++++	++++	++++	150(75–300)
Imipramine	Tofranil, SK-Pramine	++++	++	++	+++	++++	150(75–300)
Doxepin	Sinequan, Adapin	+++	++	+++	++	++	150(75–300)
Tricyclic Secondary Amines							
Desipramine	Norpramin, Pertofrane	+++	++++	+	+	+	150(75–300)
Protriptyline	Vivactil	+++	++++	+	+++	+	30(15–60)
Nortriptyline	Pamelor	+++	+++	++	++	+	75(50–150)
Others							
Amoxapine	Ascendin	++	+++	++	++	++	150(75–300)
Maprotaline	Ludiomil	+	++	++	+	++	150(75–200)
Trazodone	Desyrel	+++	+/−	+++	−	++	300(200–600)
Fluoxetine	Prozac	++++	+/−	+	+	+	20(20–60)
Monamine Oxidase Inhibitors							
Isocarboxazid		−	−	−	−	−	20(10–50)
Phenelzine		−	−	−	−	−	60(45–90)
Tranylcypromine		−	−	−	−	−	20(10–50)

Note: −, absent; +, slight; ++, moderate; +++, strong; ++++, very strong.
Source: From Rakel RE. Textbook of Family Practice, 4th ed. Philadelphia, W. B. Saunders, 1990, with permission.

Therapeutic. Because of the significant hypersomnolence and early morning fatigue, a prescription for desipramine 25 mg 2 hours before bedtime was offered. Desipramine was chosen because of a slight energizing effect and minimum anticholinergic effects in most patients (see Table 20–63). It can cause appetite suppression due to nausea, although not nearly to the degree that fluoxetine can. Fluoxetine might ultimately be a better choice because of its anorectic effect with resultant weight loss, a characteristic of all seritonergic antidepressants, but a trial of low-dose antidepressant in a patient for whom a diagnosis of MDD is not yet made is less convenient because of its fixed dosage availability and its slower onset of action. Karen was told that the low dose of desipramine did not mean a firm diagnosis of MDD had been made, but that it would be helpful for the sleep and energy disturbance irrespective of future diagnoses and treatments. Increasing the desipramine dosage to a therapeutic antidepressant level would be negotiated at future visits.

Psychotherapy and Patient Education

1. The interview helped to clarify for Karen the full constellation of symptoms that suggest the diagnosis of MDD and helped to deemphasize the possibility of anemia or hypothyroidism as an explanation for her symptoms. Significant discussion ensued regarding the consequences of this possible diagnosis, the pertinence of her past and family history, the ways in which MDD can cause her symptoms, and the potential treatments.

2. Karen was given a detailed pamphlet from the National Institute of Mental Health to read and was encouraged to purchase additional reading material, such as the book *Feeling Good*, by David Burns, M.D.

3. Karen was encouraged to resume at least a portion of her previous exercise program at a reduced intensity and length, perhaps doing up to 30 minutes of aerobic activity three times per week.

4. Karen was asked to consider what relatives or friends were potential sources of support not yet tapped. She suggested a friend who lived in another city, with whom she had not had contact recently, due primarily to her own lack of initiative. She agreed to consider calling her friend in the next week to tell her how she was feeling and discuss the possibility of depression as an explanation for her illness. She also was asked if she had any significant decisions to make in the coming week, and she reported that she had been avoiding writing or calling her daughter but wished to do so. She was encouraged to follow through with this plan.

5. Above all, Karen was told that several possible diagnoses would be explored and that a resolution of her fatigue was likely. She was also told that if depression was the eventual diagnosis, her prognosis was reasonably good, given that she had experienced relatively few recurrences and had been symptomatic a relatively short time for this episode. Karen also was encouraged to consider pursuing specific psychotherapy related to her family stress, irrespective of subsequent diagnoses.

Disposition. Karen was asked to return in 1 week after completing the various reading, exercise, and personal assignments. She was asked to consider the possibility of additional counseling in the future and to contact the physician should any significant suicidal ideation develop.

FIRST FOLLOW-UP VISIT

SUBJECTIVE

Karen returns in one week reporting moderate improvement in sleep, having slept a lesser time each night and feeling more energetic in the morning. She is somewhat more receptive to the diagnosis of MDD after reading the assigned material. She has also called her sister with questions about her illness and has found that she is taking an antidepressant at therapeutic doses for MDD, as is her brother. This information appears to make Karen more receptive to the diagnosis of MDD, especially after she admits to looking up her laboratory values on the hospital computer system and finding them to be normal. She continues to report no actual mood disturbance, but she elaborates more fully on significant stress and interpersonal conflict with her daughter and ex-husband. She was unable to reach her friend for other support but is relatively satisfied with how she has felt during the past week. She has exercised twice in the past week, to her considerable satisfaction.

OBJECTIVE

Karen's vital signs are normal, and she has lost 1 lb. Her mood appears stable, without evidence of lability, and she has manifested no suicidal ideation. Her hematocrit is 40.2%, and her TSH level is 3.5 mU/liter.

ASSESSMENT

Karen has responded well to a low dose of antidepressant, with the primary benefit being an improved quality of sleep that had probably been quite disturbed unbeknownst to her. She also has responded to the hope and support offered at the previous visit and was compliant with most assignments. She is more receptive to an increased antidepressant dosage as a result of discussions with her sister. No other biomedical cause for her

TABLE 20–64. ORGANIC ILLNESSES ASSOCIATED WITH DEPRESSION

Rheumatologic—systemic lupus erythematosus, rheumatoid arthritis
Cardiac—mitral valve prolapse, myocardial infarction, hypertension
Endocrine—hyperthyroidism and hypothyroidism, diabetes mellitus, hypercalcemia, Cushing's syndrome, postpartum state
Gastrointestinal—cirrhosis, inflammatory bowel disease, pancreatitis, intestinal bypass
Hematologic—sickle-cell anemia
Nutritional deficiencies—B12, folate, iron, thiamin, niacin
Infectious—encephalitis, hepatitis, influenza, infectious mononucleosis, pneumonia, tuberculosis
Renal—renal transplant, uremia
Neoplastic—intracranial, leukemia, pancreatic, lymphoma
Neurologic—subdural hematoma, multiple sclerosis, CVA, Parkinson's uncontrolled epilepsy
Miscellaneous—psoriasis, sarcoidosis, drugs

Source: From Rakel RE. Textbook of Family Practice, 4th ed. Philadelphia, W. B. Saunders, 1990, with permission.

symptoms has been found, nor are there other symptoms to suggest that further testing should be done. No other causes for a secondary MDD have been found (see Table 20–64).

PLAN

1. The dose of desipramine is increased to 75 mg, again 1 to 2 hours before bedtime, and Karen is told that the dose will be increased again in 1 to 2 weeks.

2. Karen is encouraged again to contact her friend and is also asked to contact her daughter as a way to clarify the impact of the current estrangement and conflict on her illness.

3. Karen is encouraged to increase her exercise consistent with her energy level.

4. Karen is asked again to consider pursuing outside psychotherapy, particularly concerning her family relationships.

SUBSEQUENT FOLLOW-UP VISITS

Karen is seen weekly for two more visits, during which the dose of desipramine is increased to 125 mg q.h.s. and held there. She reports sleep normalization and markedly increased energy levels. Her exercise program is continuing to develop. As her knowledge about depression increases, from reading and talking to friends, she becomes very accepting of the diagnosis of MDD and adds additional buttressing evidence to support the criteria for MDD, particularly more pronounced feelings of guilt related to her daughter. She is accepting of a referral for counseling in this regard, particularly focused on her feelings of poor self-worth due to a perception of having failed in her relationship with her daughter. During several visits Karen denies suicidal ideation.

Karen improved in function, mood, and energy level over the course of several months. She continued at the desipramine dosage of 125 mg at bedtime and did not require an increase to more typical therapeutic levels of 150 to 200 mg. She also continued on a reduced dose of desipramine (75 mg at bedtime) when the antidepressant dosage was tapered after 6 months of treatment. She continued in therapy and was seen every 3 months by the physician to monitor the low-dose desipramine treatment.

DISCUSSION

This patient demonstrates several characteristic features of patients with MDD seen by family physicians, including (1) presentation with a somatic emphasis on the chief complaint and related symptoms, including an actual denial of mood disturbance and an interpretation of anhedonia as fatigue for which a biomedical explanation was sought, (2) a past history of probable MDD in the late teens or early twenties, (3) being a divorced women with significant family and child relationship disturbances, and (4) a rapid and productive response to moderate doses of a standard antidepressant. Overall, 70% to 80% of patients with MDD respond to antide-

pressant therapy, but a higher percentage of primary care MDD patients probably respond, often to only a modest dosage.

Karen is somewhat atypical but not rare in her presentation with hypersomnia. The most common sleep problem in depression is insomnia, which is usually mild. About 15% to 30% of depressed patients report hypersomnia, and it is usually part of a picture that includes increased appetite and weight gain rather than the more common decreased appetite and weight loss. More than other depressed patients, those with hypersomnia report depression in a first-degree relative, agitation, earlier age of onset, and headaches.

There are several indications for referral of MDD patients to a psychiatrist (Table 20–65) for more specialized psychopharmacology, electroconvulsive therapy, or associated psychotherapy. However, patients with these indications for referral constitute only 10% to 20% of the MDD patients in a typical family practice. A majority of patients have relatively uncomplicated presentations and respond well to usual treatments. The biggest challenge for the family physician is to uncover the MDD diagnosis in the face of a strong bias (on the part of both the patient and the physician) toward a biomedical explanation of somatic symptoms, particularly chronic pain and neurovegetative problems.

With severe depression, some combination of medication and psychotherapy is usually indicated. With mild to moderate depression, the choice of one or the other treatment or a combination depends somewhat on the presentation of the patient and the preferences of the patient and clinician. When vegetative symptoms predominate and patients do not give evidence of significant stresses in their lives, treatment with antidepressant medication may prove sufficient. However, depression tends to occur in a stressful interpersonal context, and there are several reasons for considering psychotherapy or counseling. Many patients want the opportunity to discuss their psychosocial problems, and an opportunity to participate in psychotherapy increases their adherence to medication and allows them to focus more specifically on the effectiveness and side effects of their medication in physician office visits. Also, medication has limited effect on the psychosocial problems that precipitate or accompany depression, and its effect on veg-

TABLE 20–65. INDICATIONS FOR REFERRAL TO A PSYCHIATRIST

Moderate or high suicidal risk
Severe cognitive dysfunction with difficulty in daily living or nutritional deficiencies
Psychotic or delusional symptoms
Lack of family support for observation or care
Significant physical illness complicating antidepressant treatment
Uncertain diagnosis or complicating psychiatric diagnosis such as alcoholism
Bipolar disease
Lack of response to antidepressants (combined with severe neurovegetative symptoms, suggesting need for electroconvulsive treatment)

Source: From Rakel RE. Textbook of Family Practice, 4th ed. Philadelphia, W. B. Saunders, 1990, with permission.

etative symptoms and mood may be diminished when these problems persist. Psychotherapy may thus be indicated to resolve problems not affected by the medication, to increase the effectiveness of the medication, and to reduce the probability of a relapse or recurrence.

Karen proved to be an excellent candidate for brief, problem-focused therapy targeting her relationship with her daughter and her need to get on with her own life, irrespective of the divorce and the lack of custody of her daughter. In six sessions of therapy, Karen gained an appreciation of how she had encouraged her daughter in her manipulative and exploitative behavior by being overly solicitous and too willing to accept full responsibility for the divorce and the daughter's problems. She composed a letter in which she expressed disappointment over her daughter's treatment of her, including her decision not to spend Christmas with her. Instead of mailing the letter, Karen telephoned her daughter. In the conversation, Karen rejected her daughter's attempts to dwell on Karen's shortcomings. After a brief period without contact, the daughter asked to visit and apologized for past behavior. Although contact remains limited, it is markedly improved in quality and free of the turmoil that previously characterized the relationship.

Psychotherapists are increasingly recognizing the efficacy of relatively brief, structured, problem-focused therapy for depression. That a patient presents with depression and serious psychosocial problems does not necessarily indicate the need for long-term, insight-oriented therapy. Myths about the incompatibility of psychotherapy and medication are also being discarded. Family physicians would do well to identify psychotherapists who are prepared to work in a brief, collaborative, goal-oriented manner.

The indication for antidepressant therapy is primarily the presence of neurovegetative symptoms suggesting an underlying neurotransmitter abnormality. The selection of a specific antidepressant is somewhat dependent on matching the side-effect profile of a specific medication with the patient's symptoms (see Table 20–63), although some evidence suggests that patients with psychomotor retardation and fatigue will respond to a sedating antidepressant, and vice versa, owing to the correction of the underlying neurotransmitter deficiencies. However, patient acceptance and compliance are very low in these situations. Therefore, selection of an antidepressant that complements the patient's symptoms is helpful. Specific guidance includes avoiding medications with strong orthostatic effects in elderly patients, being careful about the anticholinergic effects of some medications (leading to prolonged QT intervals in patients with cardiac disease), choosing medications with an anorectic effect (such as desipramine and fluoxetine) in patients who are trying to lose weight, and avoiding the use of trazodone in male patients due to the risk, albeit small, of priapism. Antidepressants should be started at a low level to minimize side effects, but they should be increased rapidly to a therapeutic level over a few weeks. Most tricyclics begin to show an effect in 1 or 2 weeks, and the dosage can be adjusted according to response.

QUESTIONS

1. All the following symptoms are accepted criteria for the diagnosis of major depressive disorder *except*
   a. Feelings of worthlessness or excessive guilt.
   b. Chronic pain without biomedical explanation.
   c. Loss of pleasure in usual activities (anhedonia).
   d. Significant mood disturbance.
   e. Psychomotor agitation or retardation.

2. Which of the following statements about the diagnosis of major depressive disorder is *not* true?
   a. A patient who complains of a physical symptom such as fatigue should have all possible biomedical explanations explored before the diagnosis of depression is considered.
   b. Several different types or categories of depression can be difficult to distinguish in an initial office visit.
   c. Patients who present with significant symptoms of anxiety or agitation have a significant likelihood of being depressed.
   d. Divorced or single women, particularly with single-parent responsibilities, have a markedly increased risk of major depression.
   e. A past history of depression is helpful in making an accurate diagnosis of a current illness episode.

3. Which of the following statements about the treatment of major depressive disorder is true?
   a. Joint psychotherapy and antidepressant treatment is contraindicated due to mutually exclusive objectives and occasional confounding interactions between these two approaches to depressed patients.
   b. Starting antidepressant therapy at an initial high dose increases the likelihood of an early favorable response.
   c. Matching the side-effect profile of a specific antidepressant with the somatic complaints of a patient may improve the patient's compliance with therapy.
   d. Antidepressant therapy should be withdrawn as soon as the patient improves so as to decrease the risk of medication tolerance.
   e. Since depressed patients often suffer from feelings of worthlessness and low self-esteem, they should not be asked to complete specific assignments, such as contacting supportive friends, exercising, or reading about depression.

4. Which of the following statements about psychotherapy in depressed patients is true?
   a. Referral for psychotherapy is always indicated in depression because of the inability of most primary care physicians to provide this type of complicated psychosocial care.
   b. Psychotherapy is clearly more effective than an-

tidepressants in patients who are severely or moderately depressed.

c. Treatment of depressed patients with both antidepressants and psychotherapy is often indicated and can work in a complementary or synergistic fashion.

d. Brief, focused psychotherapy is rarely indicated in depressed patients owing to the complex psychosocial problems and history of most such patients.

e. The primary care physician should rarely give specific assignments, such as personal contacts, exercise, or reading, to depressed patients because of their inability to make decisions and follow through effectively.

Answers appear on page 453.

Upset Stomach and Headache

ERICH E. BRUESCHKE and SUSAN VANDERBERG-DENT

INITIAL VISIT

SUBJECTIVE

Patient Identification. Bill G. is a 37-year-old Hispanic salesman who is being seen for somatic complaints that include vague physical complaints, digestive upset, headaches, and "feeling shaky."

Presenting Problem. Bill describes himself as a nervous individual who has been experiencing loose bowels, nausea, gas pain and bloating, a "knot in his stomach," increased perspiration, and poor concentration for several months. He has also recently found a lump on his testicle, and he is concerned about cancer. In addition, he has poor sleep, weight loss of approximately 5 lb over the last 4 months, and frequent headaches. He has a number of concerns about poorly defined aches and pains.

Present Illness. Bill has described himself as having a lifelong history of somatic complaints, nervousness, worrying, and anxiety. Over the past 3 months, he has had a variety of gastrointestinal symptoms, which he attributes to a bout of flu he had about 3 months ago. Of note is that Bill was diagnosed with an ulcer about 2½ years ago, which was treated with ranitidine and apparently resolved.

He reports that he experiences cramping and a "full" sensation in his abdomen that occurs several times daily but is unrelated to position, activity, or meals. He frequently belches, but this only temporarily relieves the discomfort. His symptoms are not relieved by taking antacids. His bowel movements are of normal color, unformed, but not watery, occurring three to four times daily. He denies any blood per rectum, fecal incontinence, or awakening to defecate.

In discussing Bill's background, he recalls that he has always been a nervous person who always feared the worst, always was worried about catastrophes, and always took the negative view. Although he reports performing well on his job, he constantly questions whether or not he will be able to complete his projects and whether he is doing as well as he should. A variety of physical symptoms have ebbed and flowed throughout his life, almost always associated with stress. Over the years, he has seen physicians for tiredness and fatigue, muscle weakness, and generalized pain in the extremities. None of these has been a significant problem recently.

Bill has occasionally experienced bilateral chest discomfort and palpitations that are sometimes related to abdominal pain. His symptoms tend to be relieved somewhat when he drinks alcohol.

Past Medical History. Bill has had no surgery or accidents, although he was hospitalized for peptic ulcer about 2½ years ago. He has no known allergies and does not take any medications on a regular basis. He has never had psychologic treatment for stress, although he was once prescribed alprazolam (Xanax) 0.5 mg t.i.d. by his family physician for "stress" about 4 years ago.

Family History. Bill's mother, age 58, is in good health but is described as a chronic worrier. She was once hospitalized for depression. She drinks several beers and some hard spirits each day. He is the eldest of seven children: three brothers and three sisters. One of his sisters has been treated for depression; one sister was treated for anxiety; two brothers are alcoholics; and one brother is described as "very nervous." Bill has two maternal uncles who are alcoholics, and his maternal grandfather is also an alcoholic. His father, age 59, has no particular health problems, has apparently no problems with stress or nervousness, but is rarely home because he works long hours during the day and frequently at night. Emotional problems, especially stress, tend to be expressed in his family as somatic complaints.

Bill is worried about the possibility of inheriting a predisposition for alcoholism, about cancer because of the lump on his testicle, and about what he describes as a lack of satisfaction with life. There is some suggestion that Bill's mother may have trained the children to be nervous by constantly warning them of the danger of even the most minute actions, such as crossing the street, eating chicken (a bone may get stuck in your throat and you will suffocate), and falling asleep while driving. As a child, Bill remembers that his mother was always threatening to leave the children if they misbehaved.

Health Habits. Bill does not smoke, but he does drink one to two cocktails two or three times weekly and occasionally several drinks when he is particularly nervous. He is more preoccupied with his physical complaints of stomach problems, the lump on his testicle, racing heart, and weight loss than about anything else. He wears a seatbelt when he drives his car, and he exercises sporadically. He has no particularly strong interest in a balanced diet, since no one in his family has died from a heart attack.

Social History. Bill is single and lives with his parents. He has been seeing one girlfriend irregularly for the last 2 years and is sexually active but exclusively with her. They have no plans for marriage, but he describes the relationship with her as close and supportive. He has several additional friends but is preoccupied with his physical problems. He is worried about his relationship with his peers and his girlfriend, even though he reports they are loyal and seem to enjoy his presence.

Review of Systems. Bill has had no change in appetite, but he has had an approximate 5-lb weight loss over the last 4 months. He is increasingly worried about his stomach problems, the lump on his testicle, weight loss and headaches, how he is doing at work, and the relationship he has with his girlfriend. He denies early morning awakening and says that despite all his difficulties, he is somewhat optimistic about the future. He denies suicidal thoughts. Review of systems is otherwise noncontributory.

OBJECTIVE

Physical Examination. Bill's vital signs are all within normal limits, except for his blood pressure, which is 146/92, right arm, seated, and a regular heart rate of 94. His height is 72 in, and his weight is 178 lb. Bill is a young Hispanic male who is alert, cooperative, and in no acute distress. He appears somewhat nervous, and he periodically sighs. *Skin/Hair:* Cool and moist. There is no pallor or cyanosis. There are a few acne lesions on face and chest. He has normal hair distribution, but there is some male-pattern balding. *HEENT:* Pupils equal and reactive; intact extraocular motion. There is no exophthalmos or lid lag. The fundi are normal. Tympanic membranes are clear. The nose is clear. There are no oral lesions or tonsillar erythema or exudate. His

teeth are in good repair. The thyroid gland is not enlarged, and no nodules are palpated. There is no cervical adenopathy. Brisk carotid pulses are palpated. *Chest:* Lungs clear to auscultation and percussion. There is no axillary adenopathy. The heart rate is regular, 94/minute; PMI palpable in 5th intercostal space at midclavicular line. Normal S_1 and S_2 sounds are heard, and no S_3 or S_4 sounds, clicks, or murmurs are auscultated. *Abdomen:* The abdomen is flat, without scars. Bowel sounds are diffusely hyperactive with normal pitch. The abdomen is soft and nontender to palpation, and there are no masses or hepatosplenomegaly. *Genitourinary:* Circumcised penis without lesions. No testicular masses or swelling is palpated. There is a small left-sided varicocele. *Rectal:* No mass, normal prostate, negative fecal occult blood. There was some pain on tapping the posterior rectal mucosa. *Extremities:* No edema or joint swelling, full range of motion. There is no muscle atrophy or weakness. Radial, dorsalis pedis, and posterior tibialis pulses are all full and symmetrical. *Neurologic:* Cranial nerves II to XII are intact. Deep tendon reflexes are 2+ and symmetrical. Bill has intact balance, proprioception, and sensory examination. No tremor is seen.

Laboratory Tests. This was an initial visit, and no laboratory tests were ordered in advance.

ASSESSMENT

Working Diagnoses

1. *Generalized anxiety disorder.* Patients with generalized anxiety disorder (GAD) have unrealistic or excessive worry about one or more life circumstances for 6 months or more during which they are bothered more days than not by these concerns. From a list of 18 symptoms, patients must have at least 6 from these three categories: motor tension, autonomic hyperactivity, and vigilance and scanning (Table 20–66). Bill has unrealistic and excessive worry (apprehensive expectation) about his job, even though he is doing well at work, and he is worried about his interactions with peers, including his girlfriend, even though there seems to be no underlying problem. Bill exhibits 8 of the listed symptoms, including 3 symptoms of motor tension (feeling shaky, muscle aches, and easy fatigability), 3 symptoms of autonomic hyperactivity (palpitations, sweating, and abdominal distress), and 2 symptoms of vigilance and scanning (feeling keyed up and on edge and sleep difficulties). Thus he exceeds the 6 symptoms required, all of which are somatic symptoms, as well as the other elements listed in Table 20–66.

2. *Irritable bowel syndrome.* Bill's symptoms of gaseous distension, cramping, and loose stools are consistent with irritable bowel syndrome (IBS). In patients with IBS, disagreeable abdominal sensations are commonly associated with nonspecific somatic symptoms (e.g., bloating, nausea, headache, fatigue, anxiety, and difficulty with mental concentration). The pain on tapping the posterior rectal mucosa is commonly seen in IBS. Stress exacerbates the symptoms of IBS; a chroni-

TABLE 20–66. DIAGNOSTIC CRITERIA FOR GENERALIZED ANXIETY DISORDER

I.   Unrealistic or excessive anxiety and worry (apprehensive expectation) about two or more life circumstances, e.g., worry about possible misfortune to one's child (who is in no danger) and worry about finances (for no good reason), for a period of 6 months or longer, during which the person has been bothered more days than not by these concerns. In children and adolescents, this may take the form of anxiety and worry about academic, athletic, and social performance.

II. If another axis I disorder is present, the focus of the anxiety and worry in I is unrelated to it; e.g., the anxiety or worry is not about having a panic attack (as in panic disorder), being embarrassed in public (as in social phobia), being contaminated (as in obsessive–compulsive disorder), or gaining weight (as in anorexia nervosa).

III. The disturbance does not occur only during the course of a mood disorder or a psychotic disorder.

IV. At least 6 of the following 18 symptoms are often present when anxious (do not include symptoms present only during panic attacks):
   A. Motor tension:
   1. Trembling, twitching, or feeling shaky
   2. Muscle tension, aches, or soreness
   3. Restlessness
   4. Easy fatigability
   B. Autonomic hyperactivity
   1. Shortness of breath or smothering sensations
   2. Palpitations or accelerated heart rate (tachycardia)
   3. Sweating or cold clammy hands
   4. Dry mouth
   5. Dizziness or lightheadedness
   6. Nausea, diarrhea, or other abdominal distress
   7. Flushes (hot flashes) or chills
   8. Frequent urination
   9. Trouble swallowing or "lump in throat"
   C. Vigilance and scanning:
   1. Feeling keyed up or on edge
   2. Exaggerated startle response
   3. Difficulty concentrating or "mind going blank" because of anxiety
   4. Trouble falling or staying asleep
   5. Irritability

V.   It cannot be established that an organic factor initiated and maintained the disturbance, e.g., hyperthyroidism, caffeine intoxication.

Source: Reprinted with permission from American Psychiatric Association. Diagnostic and Statistical Manual of Mental Disorders, 3rd ed., revised. Washington, D.C., American Psychiatric Association, 1987, pp. 252–253 with permission.

cally anxious individual like Bill is almost constantly stressed by worries.

3. *Strong family history of alcoholism.* Bill has several alcoholic male relatives; his mother is likely also alcoholic. This puts him at risk for alcoholism or other substance abuse, as well as the psychological sequelae of an alcoholic family of origin.

Differential Diagnoses

1. *Somatization disorder.* Somatic symptoms are frequently a patient's way of handling persistent anxiety or depression (see Table 20–67). When specific criteria are met, the diagnosis of somatization disorder may be made. This condition is characterized by recurrent and multiple somatic complaints over many years, usually starting during young adulthood and involving many organ systems. While Bill has a number of somatic symptoms, he does not have the breadth of symptoms involving many organ systems and starting before the age of 30 that must be seen to diagnose somatization disorder. The DSM-III-R diagnostic criteria also require a lifetime history of at least 13 unexplained somatic symptoms from a list of 37. At most, Bill meets only 7 of these criteria, namely, abdominal pain, nausea, bloating, pain in extremities, palpitations, chest pain, and muscle weakness. He does not have the history of numerous surgeries and/or hospitalizations common to the disorder.

2. *Hyperthyroidism.* This entity can cause many of Bill's symptoms, but it can be readily ruled out by nor-

mal thyroid studies. He also has no specific signs of hyperthyroidism (enlarged or tender thyroid gland, tremor, exophthalmos), but nonspecific signs such as tachycardia and borderline blood pressure elevation are present.

3. *Panic disorder.* Bill does not report discrete panic episodes (intense fear or discomfort), nor are his symptoms reliably produced by situations that precipitate panic, such as crowds, churches, and stores. His anxiety is more chronic and pervasive. Panic disorder is also more common in women.

4. *Posttraumatic stress disorder.* Bill demonstrates no catastrophically stressful life event, so this diagnosis is not pertinent.

5. *Obsessive–compulsive disorder.* Obsessive ideation and/or compulsive–ritualistic behaviors are not part of Bill's behavior.

6. *Depression.* Bill complains of poor sleep but does not demonstrate early morning awakening characteristic of depression. He also has not experienced a depressed mood or suicidal ideation, and his degree of weight loss is not as rapid as that seen in major depression. Bill has some suggestive symptoms such as loss of concentration, but he does not fulfill criteria for the diagnosis of major depression.

7. *Essential hypertension.* One borderline blood pressure reading does not confirm a diagnosis of hypertension. At least two elevated readings must be documented. Bill's blood pressure should be rechecked within 2 months. This can be done at his follow-up visits for other problems.

TABLE 20-67. POSSIBLE SOMATIC MANIFESTATIONS OF ANXIETY BY ORGAN SYSTEM

ORGAN SYSTEM	SYMPTOMS	SIGNS
Cardiovascular	Angina Palpitations Substernal pressure Precordial pain Facial flushing	Arrhythmias Tachycardia Elevated systolic blood pressure Functional systolic ejection murmur
Pulmonary	Difficulty breathing Smothering sensations	Hyperventilation Increased frequency of sighing respiration
Gastrointestinal	Epigastric distress, belching, heartburn, dyspepsia "Lump in throat" Diarrhea, constipation Anorexia, compulsive eating Dry mouth Difficulty swallowing Abdominal pain	
Genitourinary	Frequent urination Amenorrhea, excessive menstrual flow and cramps Impotence, premature ejaculation	
Nervous	Muscle tension Aches or soreness Difficulty concentrating Lightheadedness, irritability Exaggerated startle response Feeling shaky Sleep disturbances Ill-defined fear Easy fatigability Headaches, poor coordination Trembling, numbness, and tingling	Strained facial expression Stereotypical behavior Cold, clammy handshake Pacing, restlessness Fine tremors or twitches

8. *Hypochondriasis with cancer neurosis.* Although Bill has fear that he has cancer because of the lump he feels in his testicle, this is probably a realistic concern. Patients with hypochondriasis appear to have abnormal responses to normal sensations or amplified responses to minor abnormal sensations. Hypochondriacs have an unrealistic, persistent fear of having or getting a serious disease with which they are preoccupied for at least 6 months that is not supported by appropriate physical evaluation. Bill's concerns are neither unrealistic nor have they been present for a sufficient time.

9. *Peptic ulcer disease.* Bill has a prior history of ulcer disease and recurrence is possible. His stomach symptoms are not relieved by eating, nor do they occur 1 or 2 hours postprandially. Bill's pain is more diffuse, as opposed to the usual epigastric location of peptic ulcer disease. The lack of response to antacids also points away from ulcer disease.

10. *Inflammatory bowel disease.* Bill does not have frank diarrhea; he has not passed bloody stools; and he does not awaken at night with diarrhea. Also, he has not suffered significant weight loss.

PLAN

Diagnostic

1. Urinalysis. This is a good initial test in a new patient with abdominal complaints and a one-time elevation of blood pressure.

2. Complete blood count. This is useful to rule out anemia as a cause of fatigue and an important test in a person with weight loss.

3. Blood chemistry, SMA-12.

4. Serum T_4 assay and T_3 resin uptake to help exclude hyperthyroidism.

5. Electrocardiogram (ECG). Bill complained of palpitations, and although unlikely to show abnormalities, a normal ECG may provide useful reassurance.

Therapeutic

1. *Relaxation techniques.* Concepts were introduced to deal with acute and chronic anxiety, which included deep breathing and progressive muscle relaxation as a first step in helping Bill control his anxiety and his somatic symptoms. Treatment is supportive and palliative. The physician's sympathetic understanding and guidance are of overriding importance. Counseling with a clinical psychologist should be considered to allow the patient to gain insight into the etiology of his negative thinking patterns and develop more successful coping methods, as well as to deal with the impact of his dysfunctional family of origin.

2. *Instruction in stress-management techniques* will be essential to successfully manage the gastrointestinal symptoms. Additionally, a bulk agent such as psyllium mucilloid (e.g., Metamucil) should help to normalize his stool pattern. Psyllium hydrophilic mucilloid can be

taken with two glasses of water to stabilize the water content of the bowel and provide bulk. A high-fiber diet and avoidance of spicy, fried, and fatty foods were recommended as a treatment for his somatic symptoms.

3. *Nonsedating anxiolytic.* Since Bill fits the criteria for generalized anxiety disorder, and since he is experiencing considerable problems necessitating pharmacologic treatment, an anxiolytic is indicated. Since Bill is at increased risk because of his family history of alcoholism and his use of alcohol to control anxiety, a nonsedating anxiolytic would be the drug of first choice. An azapirone, buspirone, was therefore chosen. This was started at 5 mg t.i.d.

Patient Education

1. The role of bulk in a diet for irritable bowel syndrome as well as the contribution of stress to the disorder was outlined.

2. The benign nature of the varicocele was stressed, and Bill was reassured that the testicular examination was entirely normal. He was instructed in testicular self-examination.

3. Bill was asked to keep a 7-day food diary and an ongoing diary of his somatic experiences.

4. The likelihood of improvement in his anxiety, and consequently his somatic symptoms, was discussed. Physical complaints were presented as his body's way of controlling stress.

5. Bill was cautioned that since the anxiolytic prescribed did not cause sedation or euphoria, he should not expect to experience any immediate "drug effects."

6. Bill was cautioned about the use of alcohol to control anxiety and/or stress.

Disposition. Bill is asked to return in 1 week for follow-up of his laboratory studies, somatic symptoms, blood pressure, and anxiety.

FIRST FOLLOW-UP VISIT

SUBJECTIVE

Bill returns 1 week after his initial visit. He is feeling somewhat better due mainly to his relief from the fear of cancer and some improvement in his abdominal complaints. He is working at the relaxation techniques. He is still having some chest discomfort and palpitations. He wonders if the drug he was prescribed is doing any good. He reports that his concentration is improving.

OBJECTIVE

Bill is less nervous. His heart rate is 80, and his blood pressure is 138/88, right arm, sitting. His food diary shows good progress on a high-fiber diet, and his symptoms diary shows a small decline in somatic complaints.

The following laboratory results were received: *CBC:* Hemoglobin 14.8, hematocrit 43.9%, WBC count 7800, platelets 210,000. *Chemistries:* Fasting glucose 89 mg/dl, total cholesterol 170 mg/dl. All other chemistries are normal. *Thyroid function:* Serum T_4 7.2

$\mu g/dl$, T_3 resin uptake 30%. *ECG:* Sinus rhythm, rate 90, axis +30 degrees, no ectopic beats, conduction disturbances, or ischemic changes. All these studies are within normal limits.

ASSESSMENT

1. Normal blood pressure.

2. Normal laboratory findings. Bill is informed that he is not anemic and that his blood sugar and cholesterol are not elevated. He is also informed that his thyroid gland is functioning normally. Bill is reassured that there is no evidence of heart disease detected on his ECG.

3. Generalized anxiety disorder—mild, responding well to reassurance, behavioral modification, and the nonsedating anxiolytic, as evidenced by reduction in somatic complaints. Bill also noted an improvement in concentrating ability, which is an early sign of azapirone effectiveness.

4. Irritable bowel syndrome—responding to stress-reduction strategies, high-fiber diet, and Metamucil.

PLAN

Diagnostic. None needed.

Therapeutic

1. Continue to counsel the patient on relaxation techniques and strategies for handling stress.

2. Diet. Continue dietary restrictions of spicy and fried foods. Continue Metamucil.

3. Generalized anxiety disorder. Continue with buspirone t.i.d. It was decided to increase the dose to 7.5 mg t.i.d. to be in the normal therapeutic range.

Patient Education

1. The process of psychologic support by the family physician was explained, with an emphasis on a brief series of planned, not "as needed" office visits to deal with the problems and to address any new somatic complaints. The possibility of family counseling was broached. These follow-up visits and their linkage to the symptomatic treatment of the irritable bowel syndrome were covered.

2. A general discussion on a healthy lifestyle and a balanced diet was held, along with a discussion of the role of exercise in reduction of risk factors for cardiovascular disease.

3. Questions were answered concerning the relatively benign nature of Bill's irritable bowel syndrome, with a focus on the role of stress and diet.

4. Bill was cautioned again to refrain from using alcohol as a method to control stress. This was done to reinforce the concept.

5. Bill was asked to continue his symptom diary as a mechanism to report his progress to the physician.

Disposition. Bill is asked to return in 2 weeks for a further assessment of his stress, somatic symptoms, and medication response.

TABLE 20–68. FOLLOW-UP TREATMENT PRINCIPLES

1. Educate the patient about the problems, and use this as an opportunity to gain the confidence of the patient.
2. Modify current factors that are maintaining the physical symptoms.
3. Directed physical examination at each encounter, concentrating on area of somatic complaint.
4. Address the more long-standing, deeper issues, which may include referral to appropriate mental health professionals.
5. Avoid hospitalization, diagnostic procedures, surgery, and laboratory tests unless clearly indicated.
6. Therapy should follow from the assessment. Patients with chronic somatic complaints have become adjusted to the sick role and need treatment of anxiety as well as counseling.
7. Medications, especially the antidepressants and the anxiolytics, can be beneficial in the management of the somatic patient.
   a. *Antidepressants:* best for depression-related somatization and panic attacks. Sedating antidepressants are good for patients with marked sleep disturbances and are the treatment of choice for panic attacks.
   b. *Anxiolytics:* Not for panic attacks, except possibly alprazolam. Thus question about panic attacks to avoid inappropriate prescribing. Patient with acute environmental stressors associated with physical symptoms may benefit from a short-term trial of an anxiolytic. For the patient with persistent underlying anxiety with associated physical or autonomic symptoms or both, a nonsedating anxiolytic may offer significant relief.
8. Recommend scheduled, regular visits at 2- to 4-week intervals, not "as needed." Later extend visit interval to 4 to 6 weeks.
9. Specifically inquire about symptoms at the end of 2 weeks and at the end of 4 weeks of therapy.

DISCUSSION

The treatment of the somatic patient with significant anxiety involves the series of treatment principles shown in Table 20–68. Treatment for generalized anxiety disorder involves psychologic and pharmacologic approaches. Drug treatment may be either a heterocyclic antidepressant, a benzodiazepine, or an azapirone. Bill had few depressive symptoms or signs, and thus an antidepressant would not be the pharmacologic agent of first choice. One would ordinarily have an array of anxiolytics from which to choose. However, since Bill has a family history of alcoholism and has used alcohol to control anxiety and stress, he is at greater risk for substance abuse. Because of the euphoria and sedation associated with their use, benzodiazepines would present some risk for abuse for this patient. A nonsedating anxiolytic is available that has a negligible risk of abuse. This class of anxiolytics, the azapirones, of which buspirone is the first available agent, would therefore be a good choice as an initial trial of therapy.

Buspirone is not a p.r.n. drug. It should be taken three times a day in divided doses. The typical initial dose is 5 mg three times a day, with dose increases only every 1 or 2 weeks, since there is a lag period of about 1 week before anxiolytic effects are manifest. Since buspirone produces little, if any, euphoria or sedation, there are no immediate drug side effects to indicate to the patient that the drug is "working." This lack of euphoria and sedation must be understood by the physician as well as the patient, especially if the patient has used benzodiazepines (such as diazepam, chlordiazepoxide, alprazolam, or others) in the past, since such effects, which can be a signal of drug effect, do not occur. The actual anxiolytic effects of both the benzodiazepines and the azapirones take about 1 week to be manifest, and in some cases, it may take several weeks. Full therapeutic effects generally become evident during the second week of treatment. During the first 4 weeks of treatment, buspirone can be increased to 10 mg three times a day in small increments if necessary.

It is important to consider several factors in monitoring the patient on buspirone. Most important, the onset of anxiolytic effects can be quite subtle, which in some ways mirrors a natural improvement of symptoms. Symptoms such as worry, poor concentration, and irritability tend to improve first, followed by improvement in somatic symptoms. This focus on symptom improvement rather than drug effects is an important concept that must be appreciated by both the patient and the physician. Some groups of patients, such as the elderly, tend to focus on somatic complaints. Effective monitoring involves regular patient interaction, wherein specific questions are asked concerning both emotional and physical symptoms.

Both generalized anxiety disorder and panic disorder, when not adequately diagnosed or treated, have been shown to result in multiple physician consultations, frequent and often unnecessary diagnostic tests, and an annual medical expenditure of 5 to 10 times that of the nonanxious patient. Chronic anxiety may be constant or may wax and wane over many years. In some of these patients, panic disorder or a depressive disorder may develop. The role of psychotherapy in the management of mildly ill chronic GAD patients appears promising, but well-designed, prospective studies are still needed. Recent research on anxiolytic treatment of GAD seems to indicate that long-term buspirone therapy, on which some patients were followed up to 40 months, produces a more permanent level of improvement than did the benzodiazepines. This suggests that pharmacologic therapy for such patients should be continued for a number of months, along with scheduled office visits every 2 or 4 weeks for monitoring of symptoms and counseling.

SUGGESTED READING

Katon W, Geyman J. Anxiety. In Rakel RE (ed.): Textbook of Family Practice, 4th ed. Philadelphia, W. B. Saunders, 1990, p. 1571.
Rickels K, Schweizer E. The clinical course and long-term management of generalized anxiety disorder. J Clin Psychopharmacol 1990; 10(3):1015–1105.

QUESTIONS

1. For patients with a lifelong history of somatic complaints, there are a number of principles that should be followed. These include
   a. New symptoms in such patients are very likely to have an organic basis.
   b. Multiple physician visits for a variety of somatic complaints suggest anxiety.
   c. Problems with anxiety or stress in other members of the family are of little diagnostic value.
   d. Such patients frequently "doctor shop."

2. When monitoring a patient on anxiolytic therapy,
   a. Worry and irritability will improve more rapidly than will somatic symptoms.
   b. Full therapeutic effect of anxiolytic therapy should be present within 1 week of starting treatment.
   c. Dosages should be increased if necessary no more frequently than every 1 to 2 weeks.
   d. Office visits should be scheduled regularly for the first few visits (every 2 to 4 weeks even if the patient is improving).

3. Irritable bowel syndrome is helped by
   a. Stress-management training.
   b. Fiber restriction.
   c. Avoidance of greasy foods.
   d. An alcoholic beverage at bedtime.

4. Match the drug with the appropriate statement.
   a. Tricyclic antidepressant
   b. Benzodiazepine
   c. Azapirone
   d. Psyllium
   b (1) Habituation is a potential side effect
   a (2) Best choice for panic disorder
   c (3) Anxiolytic effects without sedation or euphoria
   d (4) Specific therapy for irritable bowel syndrome

Answers appear on page 453.

Approaches to Patients Who Smoke

ALAN BLUM

Robert W., a 31-year-old firefighter and father of four, visits the family practice center because of abdominal pain 1 week ago that lasted 20 minutes. Apart from three previous episodes in the past 2 months, he states that he has been in good health. He drinks four cups of coffee and three cans of Lite beer daily. He admits to financial worries and fears of being laid off from work, and he has recently increased his consumption of cigarettes from one and a half to two packs per day of Marlboro Mediums. "But my chest x-ray was normal in the preemployment physical exam last year," he adds.

At the same time, Andy B., a 50-year-old executive at a major corporation, has come to the center at the insistence of his wife. She is extremely concerned about her husband's increasing shortness of breath over the past 3 months. In addition to being in a sedentary occupation, he is 40 lb overweight and has smoked a pack of Kent cigarettes each day for 32 years.

Jane L., a 28-year-old psychologist, is also waiting to see her family physician for her annual well-woman examination. In addition, she is concerned about an article in the *Woman's Home Magazine* that she has just read in the waiting room. The author warned of dangers associated with the use of oral contraceptives by women who smoke. Accordingly, she is interested in stopping the pill and in being fitted for a diaphragm.

Another young lady, 15-year-old Paula D., has just arrived at the center, having been referred by the high school nurse because of constant coughs and colds that have led to frequent absences. She has a hoarse voice and stained teeth and notes on the health questionnaire that she has smoked a pack a day of Virginia Superslims for 2 years.

Paula had received a ride from a fellow patient, Jeannie W., a 48-year-old food service supervisor at the high school, who has recently been diagnosed as having essential hypertension and has come for a check of her blood pressure. She is on her feet all day long, gets no exercise, and is 50 lb overweight. Her mother died at age 50 from a stroke. Since being told she has high blood pressure, she has switched from Salem Longs cigarettes to Carlton Menthol Lights 100s and continues to smoke at least a pack a day.

Sitting next to her is Bess T., age 24, who is in the 16th week of her first pregnancy. She has an unremitting, nonproductive cough; moreover, she has gained only 1 lb in the past 2 months. She has assured her physician that she would never buy a brand of cigarettes with the label that warns of injury to the fetus; rather, she seeks out the brands with the label that says only that cigarette smoke contains carbon monoxide.

Ted K., a 62-year-old disabled Korean War veteran suffering from Buerger's disease, has just been added to the schedule because of a worsening of his condition and the possibility of gangrene in his right foot. Since basic training in the army more than 40 years ago, he has smoked two packs a day of Camel regular cigarettes.

Regardless of the additional history and physical findings that the family physician would glean in the examining room, the cessation of smoking is the most crucial action that can be taken to improve the health of each of these seven patients. Cigarette smoking is the major preventable cause of numerous fatal diseases, including cancer of the lung, larynx, nasopharynx, and esophagus; emphysema; coronary heart disease; Buerger's disease; and cerebrovascular disease. It is also associated with cancers of the pancreas, bladder, kidney, stomach, and uterine cervix; indeed, 40% of all deaths from cancer are caused by smoking. Smoking is almost synonymous with chronic bronchitis and is frequently found in association with peptic ulcer disease. The common factor in the three leading causes of death—coronary heart disease, cancer, and cerebrovascular disease—is cigarette smoking. In short, cigarette smoking is the chief avoidable cause of death in our society.

Although it may come as a shock to the firefighter, Robert W., detection of a lung cancer on an x-ray does not improve the survival rate. Many benefits from stopping smoking can be demonstrated at all ages, even in the case of Ted K., the older man with Buerger's disease. And while several factors may be contributing to Robert W.'s abdominal pain, removing cigarettes from the picture is the most elemental, economical, and sensible measure that may afford relief. Granted, it may not be easy to stop smoking, much less to motivate a patient to do so, but therein lies a creative intellectual challenge far exceeding that of refilling a prescription for an antibiotic for chronic bronchitis or an H_2 antagonist for peptic ulcer disease. Most gratifyingly, in retrospective studies, patients report that the physician's active involvement in motivating them to stop smoking was a significant impetus. Such informative dialogue may well be what patients are seeking when they criticize physicians for not listening to them. A variety of factors may inhibit the physician from addressing this issue, such as the perceived lack of time or lack of reimbursement by insurance carriers for such counseling. Nonetheless, the physician may well find that an enhanced role in promoting smoking cessation, regardless of the minimal extra income, helps build a practice as word spreads about the doctor who cares.

None of these patients presents with a primary concern about smoking, and none of them expects a lecture on smoking at this time. However, in each case, the family physician has an opportunity to lead the patient to make the connection between the improvement of the predominant health problem and the cessation of smoking. The physician's active role in encouraging patients to stop smoking—akin to his or her role in the prevention of smoking among teenagers—can be the determining factor in the patient's success. In only a few minutes, there is much the physician can do to motivate patients to stop using cigarettes, in lieu of relegating this task to ancillary personnel, a smoking cessation clinic, or a pamphlet off the shelf.

LOOKS, SEX, AND MONEY

The key to successfully enhancing the motivation of patients to stop smoking is a positive approach. Although admonitions about the diseases caused by smoking and the harmful constituents of tobacco smoke are important, the benefits of not *buying* cigarettes must be emphasized at least as strongly.

As with any patient encounter, the overall approach must be individualized, taking into account social, cultural, and ethnic factors. Different methods will be needed for a blue-collar worker beginning to show symptoms of a cigarette-related illness, a seriously ill executive, a health professional who acknowledges the hazards of smoking but continues her habit, and a high school girl who is relatively new to smoking.

Solely educating patients about the facts of smoking in a single office visit is unlikely to result in behavioral change. On the other hand, the family physician can, through the use of creative analogies related to the patient's hobbies, romantic interest, or occupation, succeed in changing the patient's entire attitude toward smoking. For example, listing the toxic gases in tobacco smoke, such as cyanide, formaldehyde, carbon monoxide, and ammonia, may mean little at first, but by noting that ammonia causes the odor in urine and cat litter, the physician is likely to cause the patient to think about smoking a bit differently.

The use of an everyday, nonmedical vocabulary is essential for patient education in general and smoking cessation efforts in particular. Instead of the medical term "pack-year history," which merely refers to the approximate number of packs per day multiplied by the number of years the patient has smoked, a more relevant term for the patient is the "inhalation count." A 20-cigarette (pack-a-day) smoking patient will breathe in upwards of 1 million doses of poisonous fumes in less than 15 years, not including the inhalation of the smoke of co-workers and family members. Another nonthreatening way to emphasize the enormous waste of smoking is to restate the amount smoked in financial terms: A pack-a-day cigarette buyer will spend in excess of $800 a year or in excess of $10,000 in a decade.

INDIVIDUALIZE AND DEMYTHOLOGIZE

Thus, whereas smoking cessation rests on the knowledge of the deleterious aspects to health, the cognitive component alone is insufficient. Both the physician and the patient must be motivated to succeed. The three keys to motivating the patient are to individualize, personalize, and demythologize. Individualizing the message to the patient is the cornerstone of success. The same words cannot be used for a high school girl, a firefighter, or an executive already showing signs of emphysema. The teenager, perhaps more anxious about her self-image than any of the other patients (and therefore more susceptible to the glamorous images in cigarette advertisements and promotions), may or may not respond to a discussion about lung cancer and heart disease; it is usually more helpful to focus on the cosmetic unattractiveness of yellow teeth and bad breath, as well as the diminution of athletic ability and the drain on the pocketbook. Rather than acknowledging that smoking is an adult custom, the physician should refer to it as a childish and silly-looking habit like picking one's nose. The most important comment the physician can make to an adolescent is, "You still smoke? Come on, that's for little kids."

The psychologist who diligently reports for an annual Pap smear may seem well-motivated about maintaining her health, yet she chooses to give up the pill rather than stop smoking. She has been misinformed about the relative risks involved. A straightforward presentation of the facts should occur before any cervical smear is taken, to clarify the proper health priorities.

For the firefighter, the best approach might be to talk about the chances of increased fitness for work, athletic ability, and even an improved sex life were he to stop smoking. Money saved and the reduced risk of fire at home are worth mentioning.

In talking with Andy B., the executive, it is especially important to explode various myths about smoking, such as that the low-tar cigarettes he is smoking are safer. To the contrary, use of so-called low-tar brands, which should be referred to as "low-poison" by the physician, results in compensatory deeper inhalation of greater concentrations of poisonous gases and chemical additives that increase the risk of heart attack and emphysema. One way to highlight the absurdity of the belief that low-tar cigarettes are safer is to ask rhetorically, "Safer than what? Fresh air?" or to wonder aloud if it is safer to jump from the 50th floor of a skyscraper instead of the roof. Another analogy is to point out that one would never buy a loaf of bread that was advertised as containing only "2 mg of cancer causers." Similarly, Jeannie W., the food service worker, might be intrigued, if not astonished, to learn that menthol is an anesthetic agent that deadens the throat and creates the impression that the cigarette is not as irritative. An additional analogy is that paying $2.50 for a pack of cigarettes (which costs less than a nickel to manufacture) is like spending $100 for a pound of baloney.

The physician must learn to personalize approaches to smoking cessation by reviewing existing pamphlets and other audiovisual aids, as one would with a new drug or medical device. Personally handing a brochure to a patient while underlining certain points or illustrations provides an important reinforcing message.

EXPLODING CONSUMER MYTHS

The most important myth surrounding smoking is that it relieves stress. This can be debunked by pointing out that the stress that is relieved is that which resulted from being dependent on cigarettes; this is the essence of addiction. At the same time, it is important to point out that deep breathing in and of itself has a relaxing effect. An equally sad myth, reinforced in advertisements for Virginia Superslims and other brands of long, thin cigarettes aimed at young women, is that smoking keeps weight off. Upon hearing this rationalization from a patient, the famous chest surgeon Dr. Alton Ochsner would reply, "So who wants to be a svelte corpse?" Aside from pointing to all the overweight women who smoke, one must emphasize that smoking is a far greater health risk. Smoking inhibits appetite by damaging taste buds and other digestive tract cells, and one may well start to gain weight on stopping smoking as the body feels better. Weight gain does not follow, however, if one will learn to enjoy walking or other exercise.

Once the physician has succeeded in enhancing the patient's motivation to stop smoking, it must be pointed out that accomplishing this may not be as difficult as the patient believes. Too much sympathy and coddling of the patient concerning the challenge of breaking the power of nicotine addiction serves only to reinforce the obstacles to change. The patient should be encouraged to transfer the guilt and anger over smoking away from oneself and onto those who are pushing the cigarettes, namely, the manufacturers. In this way, the physician is no longer a finger-wagging lecturer on the dangers of smoking but rather a consumer advocate who points out the cheap and defective nature of the product that has been purchased in good faith by the consumer/patient. Unfortunately, the medical profession has been slow to put aside its authoritarian image on this issue, and virtually all other published or promoted methods for smoking cessation focus on "the smoker" and "nicotine addiction" without even mentioning the product itself or its promoters. There is scant science in the field of smoking cessation, the result of which has been to witness 95% of persons who smoke today switching to low-tar filter brands in the misguided belief that these are safer. (The tobacco advertisers could be called our leading health educators.)

Unfortunately, too, despite little evidence to back up their claims, expensive commercial aids for smoking cessation abound. These include acupuncture, hypnotherapy, aversive conditioning with electric shock, special filters, pocket calculators for tracking cigarette consumption, and a host of pharmacologic agents, including antihypertensive medications, minor tranquilizers, nicotine substitutes, and nicotine itself in the form of chewing gum or skin patches. The most widely promoted of these are Nicorette and Nicoderm. Even the manufacturer of these medications acknowledges that they can be of help only in concert with a comprehensive behavior modification effort such as can be facilitated by the physician. Prior to recommending this adjunct for smoking cessation, therefore, a simpler and less expensive method should be tried, such as the use of very sour lemon candies as an oral substitute for cigarettes along with various situational modifications that postpone or otherwise inhibit the situations in which one is most likely to light up a cigarette.

Promotions for various pharmacologic agents, mail-order gadgets, and smoking cessation clinics reinforce the notion that smoking is primarily a medical problem (a nicotine addiction) with a simple, prescribable, non-individualized solution. Yet time and commitment on the part of the family physician will result in greater success and a tremendous feeling of satisfaction on the part of physician and patient alike.

QUESTIONS

1. The most effective approach to assist in smoking cessation that affects the largest number of people is
   a. Hypnotherapy.
   b. Prohibition of smoking in the workplace.
   c. Nicorette.
   d. Biofeedback.
   e. Prohibition of smoking in schools.

2. Which of the following are essential components of effective patient education?
   a. Demythologize
   b. Individualize
   c. Personalize
   d. Proselytize

3. Which of the following features of cigarettes *do not* help reduce the risk of lung cancer, emphysema, or heart disease?
   a. Low tar
   b. Low nicotine
   c. Filter
   d. Menthol

4. Which of the following myths are widely believed by persons who smoke?
   a. Smoking relieves stress.
   b. Smoking reduces ulcers.
   c. Low-tar cigarettes are safer.
   d. Switching to pipes or cigars lessens the risk of oral cancer.

Answers appear on page 453.

Memory Loss

RICHARD E. FINLAYSON

INITIAL VISIT

SUBJECTIVE

Patient Identification. Martha T. is a 66-year-old single retired public school teacher accompanied by a concerned friend.

Presenting Problem. Memory problems have been developing since the death of Martha's mother 6 months ago. In addition, Martha has continued to grieve and feel "very depressed" about her loss.

Present Illness. Martha's mother had come to live with her 16 years ago after Martha's father died. The mother died at age 86 as a result of a myocardial infarction. In the days following the funeral, Martha had much difficulty with sleep, and her brother, a physician, wrote a prescription for flurazepam (a long-acting benzodiazepine), 15 mg at bedtime as needed. One capsule nightly was enough initially, but now Martha sometimes needs two capsules. At this time she is taking the flurazepam five nights out of seven. Her sleep is still interrupted by waking periods, and it is difficult for her to get back to sleep. Martha has anorexia without weight loss, lacks energy, and is withdrawn, but she says that she has some interest in doing things if she could "just get going." She denies having anger about her mother's death, guilt feelings, or suicidal thoughts.

A few days ago the telephone company shut off her service because she forgot to pay the bill. Martha's friend volunteered that she had noted these memory problems for about a year before the death of Martha's mother, but they are "much worse now."

Martha has fallen at home twice within recent weeks, but she says that she did not strike her head or seem to have a serious injury.

Past Medical History. Martha has enjoyed generally good health. She has essential hypertension, diagnosed at age 42 years, for which she takes a thiazide diuretic daily and follows a no-salt-added diet.

Family History. Martha's mother had maturity-onset diabetes mellitus, hypertension, and memory problems. Her grandmother died in a public mental institution because of "senility" caused by "hardening of

*Portions of this section were previously published in Finlayson RE. Dementia. In Rakel RE (ed.): *Textbook of Family Practice,* 4th ed. Philadelphia, W. B. Saunders, 1990, pp. 1642–1647, by permission of Mayo Foundation. Copyright 1991 by the Mayo Foundation.

the arteries.'' Her father died at age 72 as a result of prostate cancer. Martha's brother, age 64 years, is well, but he was treated for depression after his first wife died.

Health Habits. Martha has been moderate in her approach to activity, diet, and recreation. She likes to go for daily walks, but she has done little of this since her mother died. Alcohol use is minimal. She does not use tobacco.

Social History. Martha likes to care for her small yard and work in her vegetable garden. Her neighbors are friendly, but she has not been particularly close to any of them. She belongs to a church and attends services, but she is not active in any of its organizations or special activities. Her nearest relative, her brother, lives about 200 miles away.

Review of Systems. Martha has a dull discomfort in her head and says that thinking is difficult. The discomfort is not relieved by analgesics such as aspirin. She is also constipated because, as she explains, ''I just do not eat right these days.''

OBJECTIVE

Physical Examination. Martha's height is 66 in; her weight is 132 lb; her blood pressure (sitting) is 154/92; and her pulse rate is 84 with regular rhythm. The positive findings on the physical examination include a grade 1 hypertensive retinopathy, and there are resolving ecchymoses over the right elbow and forearm and the left hip area. The lung fields are clear, and the heart sounds and rhythm are within normal limits. Results of the neurologic examination are normal.

Laboratory Tests. Results of a hematology group study and urinalysis are normal. The chest radiograph shows mild cardiomegaly.

Mental Status Examination. Martha's posture is somewhat slumped, and eye contact is fair. Her speech is slurred (dysarthria). She seems to have difficulty finding words to express her thoughts (anomia). Her affect is moderately flat. The underlying mood is depressed. Psychomotor activity is moderately slowed. Depressive themes are noted in her thinking, but she is not psychotic or suicidal.

The ''mini-mental status examination'' (Folstein et al.) score is 24/30; deficiencies are noted in orientation to time, arithmetic, short-term memory, and in reproducing a geometric design.

ASSESSMENT

Differential Diagnoses. Martha presents with symptoms common to several disorders that frequently occur alone or in combination in her age group:

1. *Dementia.* Of persons this age who have dementia, dementia of the Alzheimer's type (DAT) occurs in 50%

TABLE 20–69. CATEGORIES OF DEMENTIA BASED ON REVERSIBILITY: EXAMPLES OF SOME CAUSES AND DISORDERS

CAUSES THAT CAN BE REMOVED OR REVERSED	PROGRESSIVE DEGENERATIVE DISEASES
Intoxications	Without important neurologic findings other than dementia
Prescription drugs	Alzheimer's disease
Illicit drugs	Pick's disease
Carbon monoxide	With important neurologic findings with or without dementia
Heavy metals	
Drug combinations	Parkinson's disease
Infections	Huntington's disease
Any agent capable of affecting brain	Progressive supranuclear palsy
Metabolic disorders	Many others
Endocrinopathies	
Encephalopathy of renal/ hepatic failure	
Wilson's disease	
Nutritional disorders	
Thiamin deficiency	
Folate deficiency	
Niacin deficiency	
Vascular	
Hypertension	
Atherosclerosis	
Vasculitis	
Embolic disease	
Cardiac disease	
Space-occupying lesions	
Chronic subdural hematoma	
Brain tumor	
Affective disorders	

Source: Data from the Office of Medical Applications of Research, National Institutes of Health (1987), with permission.

to 60%, multi-infarct dementia (MID) occurs in about 15% (estimates vary greatly), and various less common conditions occur in the remainder (Table 20–69). In Martha's case, MID must be considered because of the history of hypertension, although it is unusual for the syndrome to occur without evidence of past or current cerebrovascular accidents. Table 20–70 describes the standard diagnostic studies for a basic workup for someone suspected of having dementia; these should be supplemented with specialty consultation and additional tests as recommended. Table 20–71 presents the diagnostic criteria for dementia.

TABLE 20–70. STANDARD DIAGNOSTIC STUDIES FOR NEW-ONSET DEMENTIA

Complete blood cell count
Electrolyte panel
Screening metabolic panel
Thyroid function tests
Determination of vitamin B_{12} and folate concentrations
Tests for syphillis and, depending on history, for HIV*
Urinalysis
Electrocardiogram
Chest radiograph

*HIV, human immunodeficiency virus.
Source: Data from the Office of Medical Applications of Research, National Institutes of Health (1987).

TABLE 20–71. DIAGNOSTIC CRITERIA FOR DEMENTIA

I. Demonstrable evidence of impairment in short- and long-term memory. Impairment in short-term memory (inability to learn new information) may be indicated by inability to remember three objects after 5 minutes. Long-term memory impairment (inability to remember information that was known in the past) may be indicated by inability to remember past personal information (e.g., what happened yesterday, birthplace, occupation) or facts of common knowledge (e.g., past presidents, well-known dates).

II. At least one of the following:
   A. Impairment in abstract thinking, as indicated by inability to find similarities and differences between related words, difficulty in defining words and concepts, and other similar tasks
   B. Impaired judgment, as indicated by inability to make reasonable plans to deal with interpersonal, family, and job-related problems and issues
   C. Other disturbances of higher cortical function, such as aphasia (disorder of language), apraxia (inability to carry out motor activities despite intact comprehension and motor function), agnosia (failure to recognize or identify objects despite intact sensory function), and "constructional difficulty" (e.g., inability to copy three-dimensional figures, assemble blocks, or arrange sticks in specific designs)
   D. Personality change (i.e., alteration or accentuation of premorbid traits)

III. The disturbances in I and II significantly interfere with work or usual social activities or relationships with others.

IV. Not occurring exclusively during the course of delirium.

V. Either A or B:
   A. There is evidence from the history, physical examination, or laboratory tests of a specific organic factor (or factors) judged to be etiologically related to the disturbance.
   B. In the absence of such evidence, an etiologic organic factor can be presumed if the disturbance cannot be accounted for by any nonorganic mental disorder (e.g., major depression accounting for cognitive impairment).

Criteria for Severity of Dementia:

Mild: Although work or social activities are significantly impaired, the capacity for independent living remains, with adequate personal hygiene and relatively intact judgment.

Moderate: Independent living is hazardous, and some degree of supervision is necessary.

Severe: Activities of daily living are so impaired that continual supervision is required (e.g., unable to maintain minimal personal hygiene; largely incoherent or mute).

Source: From American Psychiatric Association. Diagnostic and Statistical Manual of Mental Disease, 3rd ed, revised. Washington, D.C., American Psychiatric Association, 1987, p. 107, with permission.

2. *Depression.* Martha's symptoms are suggestive of a major depression. In persons who are bereaved, such as Martha, development of a depressive illness is common. Her brother's history of a depressive illness in response to a similar loss suggests a possible familial vulnerability for affective illness. The diagnosis of depression does not exclude dementia—depression also develops in about 30% of persons with DAT. In most situations, the diagnosis of depression is based on the history and results of the mental status examination.

3. *Abnormal or unresolved grief.* Although this disorder should be considered in any case in which psychopathology accompanies bereavement, Martha's history does not suggest this diagnosis (see Discussion).

4. *Drug intoxication.* This disorder is suggested by Martha's history of taking a long-acting benzodiazepine during much of the course of her recent illness. Even though Martha may not have abused this drug, it could have accumulated in her fatty tissues to the extent that she is now impaired due to central nervous system depression. A toxicology screen would not be particularly helpful in her case unless other drug or alcohol use is not acknowledged but is suspected.

PLAN

Diagnostic

1. Chemistry group study, Pap smear, thyroid function tests, determination of vitamin B_{12} and folate concentrations, tests for syphilis, and ECG.

2. Minnesota Multiphasic Personality Inventory (MMPI).

3. Neurologic and psychiatric consultation.

Therapeutic

1. Martha's friend, a widow, offered to stay with her to provide domestic help and psychologic support.

2. Use of flurazepam will be stopped; an equivalent dose of chlordiazepoxide will be given and tapered over 2 weeks.

Patient Education

1. The symptoms are probably due to the influence of various factors (bereavement, depression, medication, and possibly an undiagnosed medical disorder).

2. It will be necessary to taper the dose of flurazepam slowly over at least 2 weeks. This process will be under direct medical supervision. Possible complications of the taper include tremors, fast pulse or palpitations, excessive sweating, and a feeling of anxiety.

Disposition. Martha is to return every 3 to 4 days for assessment of the progress of the drug taper, monitoring of her mental status, supportive counseling, and blood pressure checks. The next full visit for summarization of diagnostic studies and additional treatment recommendations will be in 4 weeks.

FOLLOW-UP VISIT AT 4 WEEKS

SUBJECTIVE

Martha has tolerated the drug withdrawal generally well. She has, however, experienced a worsening of her insomnia, and her mood is more depressed. She continues to process her grief well.

OBJECTIVE

Martha's blood pressure is 162/96. The only laboratory abnormality is a creatinine value of 1.2 mg/dl. The ECG shows "left-axis deviation." The neurologic and psychiatric consultations, supported by MRI of the head, electroencephalography, and psychologic testing, suggest the presence of generalized organic cerebral impairment (as evidenced by deficits in memory, language, abstract reasoning, and constructional ability). No evidence of focal neurologic disease is found. The depressive disorder does not adequately explain Martha's cognitive problems. The psychiatric consultant recommended a trial of an antidepressant and ongoing psychosocial support.

ASSESSMENT

Martha's affective state has worsened. This progression is not explained by normal grief. A drug-abstinence syndrome seems unlikely. Her blood pressure has increased, and better control is needed. The workup to date has not revealed a general medical disorder to explain her symptoms. MID seems unlikely because of the clinical course and laboratory findings. DAT is the most likely explanation for Martha's cognitive problems.

PLAN

Diagnostic. No additional tests are planned at this time.

Therapeutic

1. Start use of trazodone (an antidepressant), 50 mg twice a day. A tricyclic antidepressant is best avoided because of the risk of postural hypotension complicating her cardiovascular status.
2. Replace thiazide as antihypertensive treatment with a calcium-channel blocker.
3. Have Martha report initial response to trazodone by telephone in 2 days.

Disposition. A conference with Martha, her brother, and a social worker from county social services is arranged. The goal of the meeting will be to discuss the implications of Martha's diagnoses and the community resources that are available to Martha for coping with illness and aging issues. The next visit to the clinic is in 2 weeks.

DISCUSSION

The elderly, compared with younger persons, are more likely to present to a physician with diverse symptoms that do not lead to a specific diagnosis or define a "case." This is particularly so with the syndrome of dementia, as Martha's history illustrates. Her very earliest symptom, as reported by her friend, was memory loss. It may be difficult to differentiate the early stages of dementia from "age-associated memory impairment" (Crook et al.). This latter phenomenon is experienced by most people as they age and is accepted as "normal" because the frequency and intensity of memory lapses do not seriously interfere with a person's life. Treatment of a psychologic disturbance or pain in an older person with benzodiazepines, barbiturates, narcotics, or other central nervous system depressants will occasionally unmask an underlying previously unrecognized dementia.

Affective symptoms may be the first observed evidence of a dementing illness, particularly with so-called subcortical dementia (Albert et al.). This syndrome has been linked to various diseases, including progressive supranuclear palsy, Huntington's disease, Jakob–Creutzfeldt disease, Parkinson's disease, lacunar state, dementia associated with human immunodeficiency virus (HIV), and others. The earliest symptoms may include apathy, slowed thinking, depressive moods, restlessness, insomnia, and somatic complaints that may reflect a disturbed affective state. DAT has been identified as a "cortical dementia," but this distinction based on cortical versus subcortical is controversial. The important point is that affective symptoms arising from various causes may contribute in a significant way at any stage to the manifestations of dementia. Because of their diverse characteristics, affective symptoms alone do not easily lead to or provide a basis for a diagnosis of dementia. Affective symptoms may, of course, represent a psychologic response to stress, a primary affective disorder, or an affective disorder secondary to a general medical illness. In the case presented, the affective symptoms seemed to arise in association with the death of a parent late in the patient's life, and depression then evolved.

One of the diagnostic issues confronted in this case was whether the patient was experiencing abnormal or unresolved grief. Symptoms to look for are hostility toward the deceased or another person closely related to the death, overidentification with the deceased, symptoms like those of the deceased during his or her final illness, failure to mourn or process feelings (seeming to be too happy or euphoric), and giving away possessions in a reckless or foolish fashion. Complicated grief usually requires active intervention with grief counseling and sometimes psychotherapy.

The scope of personality changes in dementia is broad. Personality traits that seemed adaptive, or at least were well tolerated by others, may become exaggerated and cause considerable social tension. Sometimes one observes what seems to be a complete reversal of personality. In Martha's case, she had been a rather private person who had had a close relationship with her mother, but she had little interaction with the community. This isolation became exaggerated during her illness.

The clinical history is the single most important source of information in the diagnosis of dementia. An awareness of the wide range of psychobehavioral disturbances and diverse causes is essential to accurate diagnosis. There were clues in this case study for both affective illness and dementia. Both disorders may be present. Major depression, when accompanied by overt cognitive problems, may mimic dementia. The brother's history of treatment for depression under a similar circumstance should raise that diagnostic possibility. There is evidence of genetic vulnerability for some types of affective illnesses and dementia. The history that Martha's grandmother had died as a result of "senility" due to "hardening of the arteries" should be questioned, unless this was confirmed by a tissue diagnosis. Many such persons so diagnosed years ago probably had DAT.

Once a physician suspects the dementia syndrome from the history, it is important to document (or rule out) the presence of cognitive impairment. A structured mental status examination such as the "mini-mental state," as was used in Martha's case, is very useful and much to be preferred over a hit-or-miss attempt at bedside assessment of mental status. This examination will help to identify cognitive impairment, but it is not sufficient to make a diagnosis of dementia. The historical search for clues leading to an explanation for cognitive impairment must cover a wide variety of conditions (see Table 20–69). Some of these are reversible causes of dementia.

The physical examination of an older patient should be performed with a knowledge of findings that are related to aging per se. In this case study, the findings related to hypertension suggested a possible cerebrovascular source for cognitive loss. Other physical findings were unremarkable, except for the bruising related to her falls. Some examples of physical findings that might reflect an illness causing dementia are hypoactive deep tendon reflexes in hypothyroidism, a gait disturbance in subdural hematoma, and hepatomegaly in alcoholism.

Table 20–70 presents standard diagnostic laboratory studies for new-onset dementia. Beyond this basic workup, one might consider neurologic and psychiatric consultation, especially when the question of depression versus dementia arises. Neuropsychologic assessment is most useful when the history and examination results are equivocal, and it also provides a baseline estimation of cognitive performance. The diagnosis of dementia is based on all available evidence, but not infrequently it remains tentative. In the special settings in which advanced brain imaging is available (such as positron-emission tomography), very early evidence of brain dysfunction may be obtained, but even then a specific diagnosis is unlikely. Table 20–71 provides the diagnostic criteria for dementia according to the *Diagnostic and Statistical Manual of Mental Diseases* (DSM III-R). Observation over a period of months may be necessary in order to make a reasonably firm diagnosis. Martha's case presentation ends with a strong suspicion of DAT. The completion of detoxification and successful treatment of the depression are helpful for defining her baseline mental status (e.g., level of cognitive impairment).

Once a dementia is moderately advanced, it is readily discernible to persons living and working in close association with the person that cognition is impaired. The person may get lost on the way home. Because self-care diminishes (to various degrees), poor hygiene and inappropriate dress result. A steady progression is characteristic of DAT. Patients eventually require assistance in being clothed, fed, and bathed and in handling secre-

tions. Language is lost. The person can no longer sit up and finally becomes comatose.

The typical course of MID is one of abrupt onset (usually in conjunction with a stroke), and the deterioration is stepwise. Personality is relatively spared, but emotional lability can be intense. Focal neurologic findings are common. There may be prolonged stable periods.

The primary focus of this case study is the early manifestations of dementia and the conditions that may overlap and interact with its symptoms. The wise physician will keep in mind the possibility of multiple causes of dementia in a given patient. A program that addresses the obvious medical disorders that are treatable and provides psychosocial management from the outset is most desirable. The involvement of Martha's brother and the social agency serving her early in the course of her illness provided a good starting point for long-term management.

SUGGESTED READING

Albert ML, Feldman RG, Willis AL. The "subcortical dementia" of progressive supranuclear palsy. J Neurol Neurosurg Psychiatry 1974; 37:121–130.

Crook T, Bartus RT, Ferris SH, et al. Age-associated memory impairment: Proposed diagnostic criteria and measures of clinical change—Report of a National Institute of Mental Health work group. Dev Neuropsychol 1986; 2:261–276.

Finlayson RE. Dementia. In Rakel RE (ed.): Textbook of Family Practice, 4th ed. Philadelphia, W. B. Saunders, 1990, pp. 1642–1647.

Folstein MF, Folstein SE, McHugh PR. "Mini-mental state": A practical method for grading the cognitive state of patients for the clinician. J Psychiatr Res 1975; 12:189–198.

QUESTIONS

1. Which one of the following is not a cause of dementia that can be removed or reversed?
   a. Chronic subdural hematoma
   b. Pick's disease
   c. Endocrinopathies
   d. Folate deficiency
   e. Wilson's disease

2. Which of the following clusters best describes dementia of the Alzheimer's type?
   a. Stepwise course, labile emotions, senile plaques
   b. Progressive course, senile plaques, neurofundibular angles
   c. Stepwise course, personality spared, labile emotions
   d. Progressive course, senile plaques, neurofibrillary tangles

3. Which statement is most correct with reference to the relationship of affective symptoms and dementia?
   a. Affective symptoms usually develop late in the course of dementia.
   b. Depression develops in about a third of patients with Alzheimer's disease.

c. Huntington's disease is generally considered a type of cortical dementia.
d. Depression and dementia are likely to present as clearcut syndromes in older people.

4. Which of the following is *not* a DSM III-R criterion for the diagnosis of dementia?

a. Impairment of short-term memory
b. Delirium
c. Impairment in abstract thinking
d. Aphasia
e. Agnosia

Answers appear on page 453.

ANSWERS

Chapter 1 The Family Physician

1. a, c, d

Comment: Continuing comprehensive care is the most concise and crisp definition of family medicine. The wide variety of problems encountered provide the stimulation that makes this specialty exciting. Family Physicians are personal physicians whose familiarity with the patient provides significant advantages in diagnosis and therapy.

2. c, d

Comment: This commission was chaired by John S. Millis, president of Case Western Reserve University in Cleveland, Ohio. Published in 1966, it was a timely and powerful influence toward the establishment of the American Board of Family Practice as the twentieth medical specialty board in the United States.

3. a (5), b (1), c (4), d (1), e (4), f (5), g (4)

4. a, b, c, d

Comment: The American Board of Family Practice was the first specialty board to require periodic recertification to remain a diplomat of the Board. In order to maintain certification a diplomat must pass a written examination every 6 years but cannot sit for that examination unless first qualifying by maintaining 50 hours of approved continuing medical education annually and by completing an audit of medical records from his or her practice.

5. a, c, d, e

Comment: Although assisting at surgery is a skill of family physicians and experience at the operating table during residency enhances the family physician's ability to diagnose and manage surgical cases, major surgery is not a necessary skill of today's family physician. Experience managing common problems as seen in the model office and the ability to treat emotional problems are essential components of residency training.

Chapter 2 Scope of Family Practice

1. a, c, e

Comment: The classic and frequently quoted study published in 1961 by White and others, showed that during an average month 750 of every 1000 adults will experience an injury or illness, 250 will consult a physician, 9 will be hospitalized, 5 will be referred to another physician, and only one will be admitted to a university medical center where the great majority of medical education takes place. This study emphasizes the need for more teaching in the outpatient setting so physicians learn to manage those problems that never reach the teaching hospital.

2. a, c, d

Comment: The NAMCS study defines primary care in the United States by documenting the kind and the frequency of problems seen in the outpatient setting. It includes physicians in all specialities who see patients in an office or clinic. Hypertension is consistently the most frequently encountered diagnosis.

3. a, b, c, d

Comment: These data from the National Ambulatory Medical Care Survey in 1991 emphasize the importance of primary care to our health care system. The magnitude to primary care can be recognized when only 1% of all office visits result in hospitalization and less than 3% of patients are referred to another physician for consultation or treatment.

4. b

Comment: It is estimated that in Great Britain and Canada 70% and 50% respectively of practicing physicians are in primary care whereas in the United States this figure is only 30%. The percent of the gross national product in each country that is devoted to health care is inversely proportional to the number of primary care physicians. It is 5% in Great Britain, 9% in Canada, and 12% in the United States. An efficient health care system requires a broad base of primary care physicians rather than the specialty maldistribution that currently exists in the United States.

Chapter 3 Ethics in Family Medicine

See text and references for discussions of these questions.

Chapter 4 Family Dynamics

1. e   2. b   3. b   4. e   5. c   6. b

Chapter 5 The Family's Influence on Health

1. b	2. e	3. c	4. e	5. b	6. d	7. a
8. b	9. a	10. c	11. d	12. b	13. c	
14. d	15. e	16. b	17. d	18. c		

Chapter 6   The Family Impact of Illness and Disability

Multiple Choice Questions

1. a, c, d   2. a, b   3. c   4. d   5. b, c, e
6. d   7. a   8. b   9. False   10. a, c, e

Short Essay
See text and references for discussions of these questions.

Chapter 7   Care of the Dying Patient

1. c   2. a, b, c, d   3. a, b, c, d

Chapter 8   Home Care

1. a, b, c, d, e

Comment: Total parenteral nutrition (TPN) provides all the essential nutrients to patients who are unable to take in sufficient nutrition orally. These include those unable to eat adequate amounts of food, those with inadequate absorption of food, and those with excessive metabolic needs due to burns or draining wounds. All of the above are included in TPN.

2. a, b, d

Comment: The physician must not only assess the adequacy of family members to provide care but also monitor them frequently for signs of burnout. Although a variety of health professionals will be involved in the care, the physician is expected to be the leader who designs the nature and extent of care. Knowledge of community resources is essential, but hospital privileges, although desirable, are not required.

3. a, d

Comment: Burnout can be a significant problem since family members provide 80% of home care and one third of them also hold jobs outside the home. The primary caregiver is usually an adult child, and most of them will provide care for 1 to 4 years.

4. a, b, c, d

Comments: All of the above are important benefits of the home visit. Each of these concerns can be touched on during routine office visits, but they can be explored with greater ease and depth by means of the home visit.

5. c, d.

Comments: Although the folk remedies, alternative healers, and compliance issues should be addressed during home visits, they are not associated principally with elder abuse. The caregiver most likely to abuse a patient is the one whose family has a history of violence and who suffers fatigue, anxiety, depression, or low morale.

Chapter 9   Developing Communication Skills

1. c

Comment: Although specific questions and those requiring a yes or no answer are useful under certain circumstances, open-ended questions will obtain the most information and often elicit useful, hidden information. Silence is also a useful facilitating technique and would be the next best answer.

2. (c) 1,   (a) 2,   (d) 3,   (b) 4

Comment: Mirroring is a useful technique for facilitating rapport and indicates that two people are in agreement. In our culture feelings such as sadness are often disguised by the more socially acceptable smile. The nose rub is a form of the respiratory avoidance response. It can be a non-verbal indication of discomfort with what the speaker is saying or hearing. "Micro-expressions" may last only $\frac{1}{25}$th of a second, but they reflect a person's true feelings before the expression is suppressed or neutralized.

3. d

Comment: The eyes are the principal organs of expression and are the best indication that the speaker is sincere. A smile and a handshake are good rapport building gestures but they are not as convincing as the eyes.

4. a, b, c, d

Comment: All of the above are components of Neurolinguistic Programming. Although the eye-accessing cues are not universally accepted because of their inconsistency, these are useful signs to be aware of since they can be clues to a person's inner thoughts. Rapport can be enhanced by mirroring another person's body position and by using their preferred forms of verbs and adjectives. Patients thus feel comfortable and understood.

Chapter 10   Interviewing Techniques

Single-Answer Multiple Choice

1. d   2. c   3. e   4. b   5. c   6. c

Match:

7. c   8. a   9. a   10. b   11. b   12. b
13. c   14. a   15. c   16. b

True or False

17. (a) F,   (b) F,   (c) T,   (d) F,   (e) T   18. (a) T,
(b) T,   (c) T,   (d) T   19. (a) F,   (b) T,   (c) F,
(d) T   20. (a) T,   (b) T   (c) T,   (d) T,   (e) T

Chapter 11   Patient Compliance

1. d   2. c   3. a   4. d   5. e

Chapter 12   Disease Prevention

1. b   2. b, d   3. a, c, d, e   4. c   5. d   6. a
7. a, b, c   8. b, c   9. c   10. c, e   11. a, c
12. a, c, d   13, c, d, e   14, a, c   15, c   16. d
17. a   18. b   19. e   20. c, f

Chapter 13   Using Consultants

1. e

Comment: The American Board of Ophthalmology was the first specialty board and was established in 1917. The American Board of Family Practice, established in 1969, was the twentieth primary specialty Board. There are now twenty-three primary specialty boards and fifty-one subspecialty boards in the United States.

2. c

Comment: Although the referring physician may not provide adequate information to the consultant, the most frequent breakdown is the lack of a report from the consultant back to the referring physician. Most studies show that a report is not sent 40% of the time and university medical centers are the poorest responders.

3. d

Comment: When selecting a consultant, the family physician must consider knowledge, technical skill, and the personality of the consultant to ensure that his or her patient will be well served. Patient dislike of a consultant is a less common reason to avoid further referrals than failure to receive a report.

4. a

Comment: Well-trained family physicians can competently manage 97% of the problems presented to them in practice. As can be seen in Table 13–1 or 13–2, a large number of studies show a referral rate of between 1 and 3.8% with an average of 3%.

5. b

Comment: As seen in Table 13–1 or 13–2, the majority of referrals in the studies published are to orthopedic and general surgeons with otorhinolaryngologists and obstrician/gynecologists next in line.

Chapter 14   Problem Oriented Medical Record

1. b

Comment: The problem list is the most important single component of the POMR and is a useful addition to a medical record system even if the other components are not implemented. The problem list provides a unique picture of each individual's health, including potential risks as well as current and past medical problems.

2. a, b, c, d, e

Comment: The data base contains all of the basic information including history, physical examination and laboratory data. Thus all of the above are correct.

3. c

Comment: Although the acronym SOAP stands for Subjective, Objective, Assessment, and Plan an almost correct answer would be the more traditional terms that these words stand for, i.e, history, physical findings, diagnosis, and treatment. The terms are not synonymous, however, since Assessment includes an honest description of the problem even though there may not be a diagnosis. Similarly, Plan includes diagnostic studies and patient education in addition to treatment.

4. a, b, c

Comment: Items that can be monitored using a flow sheet are laboratory results, physiologic data and medications. Diet, non-drug therapy, and patient education can also be included. Although the problem list and consultant reports are important components of the problem oriented medical record they are not included in the flow sheet.

5. a, b, c, d, e

Comment: Although all of the above are standard components of a genogram some are more important than others. The purpose of the genogram is to document the occurrence of significant disease in at least three generations in order to recognize the potential risk to subsequent generations.

6. c, d, e

Comment: The usefulness of a standard genogram can be expanded by adding functional symbols, but they should be used sparingly to preserve clarity and ease of interpretation. Functional charting includes symbols showing the strength of interpersonal relationships and friction or discord when it exists.

Chapter 15   The Economics of Medical Practice

Matching Questions

1. e   2. c   3. a   4. d   5. h   6. k   7. g
8. i   9. j   10. b   11. f   12. b   13. a
14. g   15. c   16. d   17. e

True or false questions

18. (a)F,   (b)T,   (c)F,   (d)T,   (e)F,   (f)F   19. c
20. (a)T,   (b)T,   (c)T,   (d)T

Chapter 16   Research In Family Medicine

1. c   2. b   3. a   4. c   5. d   6. c   7. d
8. a   9. c   10. b

Chapter 17   How To Read Medical Journals

1. (a) F,   (b) F,   (c) T,   (d) T,   (e) T   2. (a) F,
(b) T,   (c) T,   (d) F   3. d   4. a   5. c   6. d
7. a   8. (a) T,   (b) F,   (c) T,   (d) F   9. c
10. (a) T,   (b) T,   (c) T,   (d) T

Chapter 18   Problem Solving in Family Medicine

1. b   2. c   3. b   4. e   5. b   6. d   7. c
8. d   9. b   10. c   11. c.   12. d

Chapter 19   Interpreting Laboratory Tests

1. b   2. c   3. c   4. b   5. d   6. a   7. c
8. e   9. a   10. a   11. e   12. d   13. e
14. a   15. e   16. d   17. b   18. c   19. a
20. e

Chapter 20   Clinical Case Studies

WEIGHT LOSS AND DIARRHEA

1. c   2. b   3. c   4. c

COUGH

1. A lobar distribution of infiltrates, particularly in association with a pleural effusion, is the most important radiographic sign suggesting that a pneumonia is not due to *Chlamydia*, *Mycoplasma*, or a virus.

2. A cough that is of psychogenic origin may be strongly suggested by its character and its timing. Where a cough is becoming a habit tic, the cough will frequently occur in a series or have a fixed number and may only occur following completion of a sentence or series of phrases. It may occur only in the immediate presence of others or may disappear on weekends, during the evening hours, and almost invariably during sleep. In persistent cough due to organic factors, sleep is commonly disrupted by the cough. Cough due to asthma is commonly worse during the evening hours and nighttime. Cough of psychogenic origin is usually nonproductive and unaccompanied by other systemic symptoms.

3. The most common causes of persistent cough include asthma, inflammation of the nasal mucosa, postinfectious bronchitis sustained either by environmental factors including smoking, and a combination of the aforementioned. Less common causes of persistent cough include endobronchial tumors, both benign and malignant; congestive heart failure; interstitial lung disease; and esophageal abnormalities. Bronchoscopy may, on rare occasions, be necessary to exclude endobronchial lesions.

FEVER AND CHEST PAIN

1. The clinical signs most suggestive of an underlying bacterial pneumonia include a marked degree of illness or toxicity, the presence of focal chest pain, the sudden onset or worsening illness following on a relatively mild prodrome, and the presence of vigors. The presence of a pleural friction rub or signs suggesting pleural effusion increase the likelihood that one is dealing with a bacterial process.

2. The principal causes of atypical pneumonia syndromes include viruses, *M. pneumoniae*, and *C. pneumoniae*. The latter organism principally causes pneumonia in young people. Its frequency varies tremendously; it seems more common in Scandinavia than in the United States.

3. Diabetes mellitus is probably the most common underlying disease associated with complicated pneumonia, although the precise immune defect is not understood. There is an increased frequency of *S. pneumoniae* and gram-negative pneumonia in patients with diabetes mellitus, and the course tends to be prolonged. Patients with alcoholism or chronic obstructive pulmonary disease tend to have complicated episodes, and the course is usually prolonged. Other disease states predisposing to severe pneumonia include granulocytopenia from any cause, immunosuppressive medication, chronic lymphocytic leukemia, or multiple myeloma. It is now recognized that patients infected with human immunodeficiency virus (HIV) may have recurrent bouts of bacterial pneumonia that are frequently bacteremic.

FEVER AND RUNNY NOSE

1. d   2. e   3. d   4. a

SINUS CONGESTION

1. a   2. a (4),   b (3),   c (2),   d (1)

RECURRENT EAR INFECTIONS

1. d   Serum IgE levels can be normal in atopic allergic disease depending on the time of the year and amount of exposure the allergic person experiences. Although occasionally helpful, serum total IgE determination is only supportive in making a diagnosis.

2. e   Purulent nasal discharge is most often associated with infection. Although allergic individuals can, and frequently do, develop secondary infections, this is not seen with acute allergen exposure.

3. a. True.   Prior to instituting any other forms of therapy, these drugs should be used. The newer, nonsedating antihistamines are preferred, but are not cleared for use in children under age 10.

b. False.   Skin testing should be reserved for those patients in whom "conservative" measures fail to control symptoms.

c. False. Environmental control of dust, dander, smoke exposure, and other home irritants should always be done prior to considering immunotherapy in *all* allergic patients.

4. a, b, c

MULTIPLE ALLERGIES

1. c Asthma is a reversible, obstructive pulmonary disease having periods of time without symptoms and occurring at any age.

2. d Hemoptysis is not associated with a primary diagnosis of asthma. Although "asthmatics" can develop mild hemoptysis with infection, pulmonary infarctions and neoplastic processes should be considered first.

3. (a) T, (b) T, (c) T, (d) T 4. (a) T, (b) T, (c) T, (d) F, (e) F

DIARRHEA

1. d The literature clearly shows that diarrhea is the major presenting symptom in almost 100% of cases. This is followed by fatigue (72%–97%), abdominal pain (61%–83%), foul stool (75%–79%), bloating (63%–79%) and weight loss (59%–73%).

2. b Chronic giardiasis is characterized by flatulence (94%), upper abdominal pain (84%), epigastric gnawing (75%), nervousness (72%), and weight loss (53%). It is important to recognize that diarrhea represents only 41% of the cases.

3. c The "string test" (Enterotest, HDC Corporation, Mountain View, Calif.) is the office procedure of choice. It can be performed in the office setting in about 5 hours. Trophozoites are rarely found in the stools.

4. d This broad-spectrum antibiotic is poorly absorbed after oral administration, and nearly all the drug is recoverable in the stool. The drug should be used with caution in persons with ulcerative lesions of the bowel. A decision to treat during pregnancy should be based on the severity of the illness. Metronidazole has been used in the 2nd and 3rd trimester of pregnancy.

NORMAL PREGNANCY

1. b   2. b   3. b   4. True

NEWBORN CARE

1. b   2. d   3. d

SHORT CHILD

1. b Although the average height of both parents is 66 in, the midparental height averages the parents' heights after adding 13 cm to the mother's height for boys or subtracting 13 cm from the father's height for girls. This corrective vactor allows for the later and greater growth of boys when they enter puberty.

2. c For a normal individual, chronologic age = bone age = height age.

3. (1) a, (2) b, (3) a, (4) a Short stature due to endocrine deficiencies often result in delayed bone age, enabling catch-up growth once these deficiencies are restored. Growth retardation and delayed puberty are common manifestations of hypothyroidism. Children with constitutional growth delay have a retarded bone age, which allows them a longer growth interval to achieve their true adult height. Children with familial short stature are genetically programmed to be short and have a normal bone age.

ABDOMINAL PAIN

1. c   2. d   3. e   4. e

BREAST DISCOMFORT

1. d   2. d   3. a (4), b (3), c (2), d (5)   4. b, c, e

LACERATION

1. b   2. b, c   3. a (3), b (1), c (2)

VAGINITIS

1. b   2. c   3. a (4), b (1), c (2), d (3)   4. a, b, d

AMENORRHEA

1. d Failure to withdraw to either progestin or estrogen and progestin implies end-organ failure such as due to Asherman's syndrome (intrauterine synechiae) or uterine or vaginal agenesis. In all other conditions, a normal uterus will respond to either progestin or estrogen plus progestin.

2. a A positive progestin challenge test implies enough function of the hypothalamic–pituitary–ovarian axis to produce circulating estrogen sufficient to cause withdrawal bleeding. When the patient fails to ovulate, no progestin is produced because no corpus luteum is produced. Therapy is exogenous progestin on a monthly basis to provide orderly withdrawal periods and to counteract the unopposed estrogen stimulation that can lead to endometrial cancer. If the patient is sexually active and no pregnancy is desired, birth control pills can accomplish the same purpose.

3. c A negative withdrawal to progestin rules out anovulation. The positive withdrawal to estrogen plus progestin rules out end-organ failure. The normal prolactin level and normal sella turcica rule out pituitary disor-

ders. The normal LH and FSH levels rule out ovarian failure. The diagnosis of exclusion is hypothalamic amenorrhea.

4. e   If the LH and FSH are both greater than 40, this is consistent with ovarian failure. The same values will be found in a menopausal patient.

5. a (3)   If the anovulatory patient is not sexually active, she needs no contraception but does need monthly progestin withdrawal to protect her from the unopposed estrogen stimulation that can lead to endometrial hyperplasia or cancer. If she were sexually active, birth control pills would be satisfactory.

b (2)   The patient with premature ovarian failure needs estrogen replacement therapy because she is hypoestrogenic and at risk for osteoporosis. This patient does not require birth control pills because she had a tubal ligation, so estrogen replacement therapy is the best choice.

c (1)   The patient with hypothalamic amenorrhea also needs contraception as well as estrogen replacement therapy, so birth control pills are her best choice. If she were not sexually active, estrogen replacement therapy would be acceptable.

VAGINAL BLEEDING

1. c   In a viable pregnancy, the β-HCG doubles every 48 to 72 hours. In general, the minimal rise consistent with a viable pregnancy in 48 hours in 67%.

2. d   The concept of the "discriminatory zone" of β-HCG states that above this zone almost all intrauterine pregnancies will be seen on ultrasound. An unusual exception is a miscarriage that has just passed most or all of the products of conception, giving an empty appearance on ultrasound and a β-HCG that began above 1000 and is falling because of the spontaneous abortion but at the time the ultrasound and β-HCG are performed the level is still above 1000. A repeat β-HCG will, of course, document the falling trend. Many ectopics cannot be seen on ultrasound at all at any β-HCG level. Likewise, ectopics can occur at any β-HCG level depending on the gestational age and size of the ectopic at the time of diagnosis. Similarly, an ectopic is never ruled out in any specific β-HCG level. Only when an IUP is documented on ultrasound is an ectopic effectively ruled out. Lastly, there are some occasions to do further β-HCG determinations above the "discriminatory zone." Once an ectopic is ruled out by seeing the fetal pole in ultrasound, serial β-HCG determinations may be helpful to document fetal viability if no cardiac motion is seen yet.

3. c   Once an intrauterine pregnancy is clearly demonstrated, the chance of a combined pregnancy is remote. A closed os on pelvic examination is consistent with a threatened spontaneous abortion, normal intrauterine pregnancy, or an ectopic. Examination consistent with 6 weeks is likewise consistent with ectopic or an early intrauterine pregnancy, since the uterus will swell slightly with the hormone effect of the pregnancy even in an ectopic. If the uterus is much larger than 6 to 8 weeks, however, it makes intrauterine pregnancy more likely and ectopic less likely. An intrauterine pregnancy seen on ultrasound, of course, is the most reliable way to rule in (not rule out) an ectopic. Rising β-HCG levels are consistent with a viable early pregnancy, whether intrauterine or ectopic, although the rise in ectopics is frequently not as rapid as in intrauterine pregnancy.

4. d   A normal early intrauterine pregnancy with a β-HCG level greater than 1000 mIU should be visualized easily on ultrasound. This is the basis for the concept of the "discriminatory zone." If the uterus is empty, it most likely represents an ectopic pregnancy (tubal or abdominal), but an empty uterus also can be seen in the case of the just completed or nearly completed spontaneous abortion, in which all or most of the products of conception have just been passed, resulting in an empty uterus. The β-HCG in this instance may have begun at a level greater than 1000 but is now falling and the level happened to be greater than 1000 at the moment the β-HCG was drawn. Subsequent levels will show the downward trend in these cases.

CONTRACEPTION

1. a   Of the options listed, combination estrogen–progestin oral contraceptives are the most effective, with typical failure rates of 3% in the first year and a lowest expected rate of 0.1%. Condoms with spermicide and vaginal sponges are barrier methods, which have higher failure rates. The calendar method is the least effective of the periodic abstinence techniques.

2. a, c   Breast cancer is one of the potentially estrogen-dependent malignancies and is thus a reason to avoid OCs completely. A history of deep-vein thrombosis (thrombophlebitis) or pulmonary embolism at any time in a woman's life means she should never take estrogen-containing oral contraceptives. Obese women may take OCs, as many women with fibrocystic breasts. In fact, some studies suggest that OC use protects against fibrocystic disease. However, if there is a discrete breast lump that might be malignant, cancer should be excluded by biopsy before hormones are considered. A history of preeclampsia (pregnancy-induced hypertension) does not contraindicate OC use, as long as the hypertension resolves after delivery. Women with a history of preeclampsia are at no greater risk of hypertension or other complications of OCs than women who had normal pregnancies.

3. a, c, e   Trichomonal vaginitis is a sexually transmitted disease and therefore contraindicates use of an IUD. Likewise, PID is a sexually transmitted disease. A woman who has had PID once is at high risk of recurrence; therefore, IUD use would be inappropriate. Irregular vaginal bleeding should be worked up before an IUD is inserted to exclude cancer and other contraindicating conditions. "Multiparity" means having lots of children and is not a reason to avoid the IUD. Hyper-

tension is a reason to avoid OCs, but it does not contra-indicate IUD use.

4. d The family physician's task is to apprise women or couples of their contraceptive options, including the advantages and disadvantages of each, and to assist patients in making an informed choice. Low health risks, high effectiveness, and reversibility are all desirable characteristics, but they must be weighted in the context of the individual's situation and preferences. Explaining which method is the best choice implies that it is the physician's prerogative to state which is best, and this leaves the patient out of the decision-making process.

SHORTNESS OF BREATH

1. c 2. e 3. a, b, c, d 4. a, b, c, d

NOSEBLEED

1. a (3), b (3), c (4), d (2) 2. d 3. a, b, e
4. a, b, d, e

CHEST PAIN

1. a, b, c, e 2. a (4), b (2), c (3), d (1) 3. d

PRESCHOOL PHYSICAL EXAMINATION

1. b 2. c 3. c

SEVERE LETHARGY

1. b 2. c 3. e 4. c

CONFUSION WITH LETHARGY

1. c 2. c 3. d 4. d

LEG PAIN

1. b, c, d 2. a, c, d 3. a 4. None are true.

KNEE INJURY

1. c 2. b, c, e 3. a (3), b (1), c (5), d (2)
4. d 5. a, c, d

LOW BACK PAIN

1. d 2. d 3. a, b, d 4. d 5. e

STIFFNESS IN FINGERS

1. b, e 2. a, b, d, e 3. c

SKIN IRRITATION

1. a, b, c, d 2. c 3. d 4. a, b

RECURRING RASH

1. d 2. a, b, e 3. b

DIABETES MELLITUS

1. a (2), b (2), c (2), d (2), e (1) 2. c, d 3. a, b, d 4. c, d

INTERMITTENT TACHYCARDIA

1. a 2. a, c 3. a 4. a (3), b (2), c (2), d (3), e (1) 5. c

NUTRITIONAL PROBLEMS IN THE ELDERLY

1. c A no-salt-added diet (about 4-gm sodium). The 6-gm sodium diet would likely be too liberal, and the 1-gm sodium diet would not be palatable.

2. c For females, 100 lb plus 5 lb for each inch over 5 ft. (For males, it is 106 lb plus 6 lb for each inch over 5 ft.) These values should be considered to be within a range; the range may be quite higher for a large-frame person.

3. a, b, c A recent significant weight loss in the elderly is often the result of causes that are reversible if assessed and treated early. A highly restrictive diet can contribute to poor intake and further weight loss. Unless the elderly patient is highly physically active, quick weight loss will primarily be lean muscle mass. Because the turnover rate for albumin is slow, serum albumin will decrease slowly with weight loss secondary to poor intake.

4. c, d Soluble and insoluble dietary fibers exert different effects on GI function. Soluble fibers bind water and can reduce watery diarrhea. Insoluble fibers can decrease constipation if adequate fluid is consumed.

FATIGUE

1. b 2. e 3. c 4. c

HEARTBURN

1. c 2. c 3. e 4. e

CHRONIC FATIGUE

1. d   This case is consistent with hemolytic anemia because of the presence of a decreased hematocrit and a reticulocytosis. This case suggests that the young patient had undiagnosed G-6-PD deficiency and was innocently given an oxidant drug for his ankle injury. Agents that can produce a red cell membrane oxidation and homolysis in patients with G-6-PD deficiency include aspirin, phenacetin, and other aspirin-containing compounds. Sickle cells would be found in sickle-cell disease and would be unlikely in this case, since this 16 year-old male's previous medical history is essentially unremarkable and not punctuated by crisis and the other complications associated with sickle-cell disease. Burr cells, which have a scalloped perimeter, are more likely found in uremia, and microcytosis would be more likely found in iron-deficiency anemia. Heinz bodies, which are dark purple, irregularly shaped inclusions seen by crystal violet stains, represent denatured hemoglobin that occurs after oxidant drug consumption in G-6-PD deficiency. Macro-ovalocytes, which are large, oval-shaped cells, are more likely seen in megaloblastic anemias.

2. a   When large quantities of red cells are lysed, intracellular enzymes such as LDH are released in abundance. Sickle-cell screening identifies patients with both sickle-cell disease and sickle-cell trait. Although 12% of the black American population may carry the sickle-cell trait, this case does not support this diagnosis. A red blood fragility test would be helpful only in the setting of suspected membranous red blood cell defect, such as hereditary spherocytosis. There is no information to suggest that this young student has a folate deficiency. In G-6-PD deficiency associated with black persons, young red cells have an appropriate amount of functioning G-6-PD and therefore are resistant to oxidant stress. As these cells age, G-6-PD activity decrease significantly, making them susceptible to oxidant stress and premature hemolysis. After an acute hemolytic crisis, all the older cells deficient in G-6-PD are hemolyzed by the oxidant, leaving mostly younger cells that still possess an appropriate amount of functional G-6-PD. Therefore, the screening immediately after a hemolytic crisis in G-6-PD deficiency could be negative and would require rescreening for the suspected enzyme deficiency 2 to 4 weeks after the acute event.

3. c   Neurologic manifestations of B_{12} deficiency include a peripheral neuropathy characterized by pain, decreased peripheral vibratory sensation, and at times an abnormal gait. The neurologic manifestations of B_{12} deficiency also can manifest themselves as CNS alterations, and in fact, patients can develop psychosis. In this case, the patient has hemologic findings characteristic of a megoblastic anemia. To include an elevated LDH level, elevated RBC indices, and hypersegmented neutrophils, since folate deficiency does not cause neurologic manifestations, vitamin B_{12} deficiency is the most likely cause of this presentation.

4. c   The absorption of B_{12} and its urinary excretion were not altered by the addition of intrinsic factor in the Schilling's test, which is inconsistent with pernicious anemia or B_{12} deficiency associated with gastrectomy. Although pure vegans can, although rarely, have a dietary lack of B_{12}, intrinsic factor production should be intact, and therefore, urinary excretion of orally administered radioactive B_{12} would be normal. Failure of orally administered intrinsic factor to correct the urinary excretion of B_{12} is consistent with many forms of inflammatory bowel disease, which inhibit the absorption of the B_{12}–intrinsic factor complex.

5. a   In this 52-year-old woman with no gynecologic source of blood loss, the most likely source of iron loss would be bleeding through the GI tract. The microcytic hyperchromic anemia with low serum iron and ferritin levels would indicate iron-deficiency anemia. The presence of a negative hemoccult test does not of itself exclude the GI tract as the source of the blood loss. There is no evidence of hemolysis in this case presentation, since the patient does not have an anemia associated with a reticulocytosis. Therapeutic replacement of iron in a patient of this age with iron-deficiency anemia only delays what will eventually will be required: a full investigation of the GI tract for occult benign, premalignant, and malignant sources of blood loss.

VOMITING AND LOW BACK PAIN

1. c   2. b, c, d   3. c   4. (1) a,   (2) a,   (3) c,   (4) d

BLURRED VISION

1. d   2. d   3. a   4. c   5. b

HEADACHE

1. a   2. c   3. b

STIFF JOINTS

1. d   2. e   3. a   4. e

SEXUAL DYSFUNCTION

1. c   2. a   3. d

GENETIC COUNSELING

1. a, c, d   2. a, b, d, e   3. a   4. d

PALPITATIONS AND SWEATING

1. c   2. a   3. e   4. d

EXCESSIVE SLEEPINESS AND FATIGUE

1. b   2. a   3. c   4. c

UPSET STOMACH AND HEADACHE

1. b, d   2. a, c, d   3. a, c   4. a (2),   b (1),
c (3),   d (4)

APPROACHES TO PATIENTS WHO SMOKE

1. b   2. a, b, c   3. a, b, c, d   4. a, c

MEMORY LOSS

1. b   2. d   3. b

Note: Page numbers in *italics* refer to illustrations; page numbers followed by the letter *t* refer to tables.